Medication Administration

Lena L. Deter, MPH, RN

First Edition

**Educational Translator
DELHEC, LLC
Educational Services and Consulting**

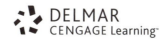

DELMAR
CENGAGE Learning™

Australia • Brazil • Japan • Korea • Mexico • Singapore • Spain • United Kingdom • United States

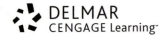
DELMAR
CENGAGE Learning™

Medication Administration, 1st Edition
Lena L. Deter, MPH, RN

Vice President, Career and
  Professional Editorial: Dave Garza

Director of Learning Solutions: Matthew Kane

Acquisitions Editor: Matt Seeley

Managing Editor: Marah Bellegarde

Product Manager: Laura J. Wood

Editorial Assistant: Samantha Zullo

Vice President, Career and
  Professional Marketing: Jennifer Baker

Marketing Director: Wendy E. Mapstone

Senior Marketing Manager: Kristin McNary

Marketing Coordinator: Scott A. Chrysler

Production Director: Carolyn Miller

Senior Art Director: Jack Pendleton

Technology Project Manager: Chris Catalina

For product information and technology assistance, contact us at
Cengage Learning Customer & Sales Support, 1-800-354-9706

For permission to use material from this text or product,
submit all requests online at **www.cengage.com/permissions**.
Further permissions questions can be e-mailed to
permissionrequest@cengage.com

Library of Congress Control Number: 2010930030

ISBN-13: 978-1-4354-8172-5

ISBN-10: 1-4354-8172-0

Delmar
5 Maxwell Drive
Clifton Park, NY 12065-2919
USA

Cengage Learning is a leading provider of customized learning solutions with office locations around the globe, including Singapore, the United Kingdom, Australia, Mexico, Brazil, and Japan. Locate your local office at: **international.cengage.com/region**

Cengage Learning products are represented in Canada by Nelson Education, Ltd.

To learn more about Delmar, visit **www.cengage.com/delmar**
Purchase any of our products at your local college store or at our preferred online store **www.cengagebrain.com**

Notice to the Reader
Publisher does not warrant or guarantee any of the products described herein or perform any independent analysis in connection with any of the product information contained herein. Publisher does not assume, and expressly disclaims, any obligation to obtain and include information other than that provided to it by the manufacturer. The reader is expressly warned to consider and adopt all safety precautions that might be indicated by the activities described herein and to avoid all potential hazards. By following the instructions contained herein, the reader willingly assumes all risks in connection with such instructions. The publisher makes no representations or warranties of any kind, including but not limited to, the warranties of fitness for particular purpose or merchantability, nor are any such representations implied with respect to the material set forth herein, and the publisher takes no responsibility with respect to such material. The publisher shall not be liable for any special, consequential, or exemplary damages resulting, in whole or part, from the readers' use of, or reliance upon, this material.

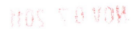

Printed in the United States of America
1 2 3 4 5 6 7 15 14 13 12 11 10

*To the frontline caregivers who
spend their days
and nights caring for our ill,
disabled, and elderly.*

Contents

MODULE I | ETHICAL AND LEGAL ASPECTS

Chapter 1

Chapter 2

Chapter 3

Alfred A. Gray, Esq

MODULE II MEDICATION FUNDAMENTALS

Chapter 4

Introduction to Medications 51

Chapter 5

Medication Orders 71

MODULE III   MEDICATION ADMINISTRATION

Chapter 8

Administration of Oxygen   176

Chapter 9

Administration of Enemas   204

MODULE V — COMMUNICATION AND DOCUMENTATION

MODULE VII ADDITIONAL KNOWLEDGE AND SKILLS

Chapter 32
Mathematics: Weights and Measures 713

Chapter 33
Vital Signs 725

Chapter 34
Care of Individuals
with Epilepsy 749

Chapter 35

Substance Abuse   781

Preface

Medication Administration prepares Unlicensed Assistive Personnel for the task of medication administration. This text provides the learner with the basic knowledge and skills to perform medication administration safely and effectively.

Medication administration by Unlicensed Assistive Personnel, although a controversial concept, is not a new concept. It was born out of need as our health care system shifted from a primary focus of institutional care to one of community-based care. As the baby boomers age and our disabled population lives longer, the increasing need to shift basic task-oriented care to our frontline caregivers, Unlicensed Assistive Personnel, will increase. Medication administration is just one of these basic tasks. The challenge put before us is to find the safest, most effective way to transfer these tasks to our frontline caregivers.

The challenge arises as we try to separate the task from the advanced skill of clinical assessment. In the past, these actions have been enmeshed. Our fear is that as we separate the two, the business world will presume that unskilled Unlicensed Assistive Personnel, who lack the necessary advanced education, are able to perform the assessment skills, leaving the individuals under our care in unsafe situations. On the other hand, training Unlicensed Assistive Personnel to perform basic tasks, providing the required clinical oversight under which these tasks are performed, and providing the ongoing clinical assessment of the individuals under our care will all ensure that these tasks, such as medication administration, are performed safely and effectively.

This textbook sets out to address each one of these areas. First, the textbook provides a thorough training for all staff who will be administering medications. Throughout this manual, the role of the Unlicensed Assistive Personnel is clearly defined. At no time does the Unlicensed

Assistive Personnel function as an independent practitioner. The Unlicensed Assistive Personnel is taught to observe, report, and record. Assessment skills are not taught. It is not the intention of the textbook to create nurses; rather, it is to provide the basic knowledge and skills for Unlicensed Assistive Personnel to administer medications safely and effectively under the clinical direction of the licensed health care provider and supportive clinicians.

Second, this textbook is written with the expectation that adequate clinical oversight will be provided to the Unlicensed Assistive Personnel. Throughout the textbook, Unlicensed Assistive Personnel are instructed to consult licensed health care providers, pharmacists, supervisors, and other licensed clinicians at any time for any change in the individuals for whom they are caring. At no time are the Unlicensed Assistive Personnel taught to make an independent decision, with the exception of calling for emergency medical services.

Last, all individuals receiving medications require ongoing clinical assessment both by the licensed health care provider ordering the medications and by licensed clinicians in the field. In the past, these assessments were performed each time a task was completed or a medication was administered by a licensed nurse. When shifting medication administration to the Unlicensed Assistive Personnel, this ongoing assessment is changed. The Unlicensed Assistive Personnel becomes the eyes and ears of the licensed nurse.

Unlicensed Assistive Personnel are taught to observe, report, and record. Unlicensed Assistive Personnel are taught to immediately report any change in an individual to his or her designated supervisor or clinical consultant. However, the need for ongoing assessment is not replaced by the observations of the Unlicensed Assistive Personnel. Although altered, the role of the licensed nurse remains as strong as ever.

Medication administration by Unlicensed Assistive Personnel varies considerably across the United States. Some states do not permit this practice at all in any setting. Other states permit Unlicensed Assistive Personnel to administer medications in limited settings, such as residential settings, for individuals with developmental disabilities. Still others permit Unlicensed Assistive Personnel to administer medications in long-term care facilities and assisted living facilities.

To date, there are no federal guidelines or regulations regarding the training and certification of Unlicensed Assistive Personnel for medication administration as there are for certified nursing assistants. Although medication administration is occurring in various states, to the knowledge of this author, only Massachusetts has standardized testing provided by an independent contractor for medication certification *and* recertification for Unlicensed Assistive Personnel, which went into effect in 1999.

As with testing, to date, federal regulations defining the minimum guidelines for curriculum development for Unlicensed Assistive Personnel regarding medication administration are nonexistent in the United States. State departments have created their own guidelines to meet state regulations and/or program needs.

On August 9, 2007, the National Council of State Boards of Nursing, Inc. (NCSBN), approved a 100-hour *Medication Assistant Certified (MA-C) Model Curriculum*. The curriculum provides a course outline, both didactic and clinical, that prepares Unlicensed Assistive Personnel to administer medications in those states where regulation permits them to do so.

This textbook was written inclusive of the requirements of the NCSBN's model curriculum. The textbook presents training materials in such a manner that an instructor is able to go to one complete source, choose the materials desired, and move forward with course presentation. The textbook, learner workbook, and Instructor Resources CD-ROM include the materials needed to present a comprehensive course on medication administration for Unlicensed Assistive Personnel. The only two additional pieces of information required to teach this course are individual state regulations and individual workplace policy and procedure manuals.

ORGANIZATION OF CONTENT

The content is presented in a clear, easy-to-understand format. The text consists of thirty-five chapters that are divided into seven modules.

Module I discusses the ethical and legal aspects of medication administration. Chapter 1 provides a brief history of health care in the United States and the development of the role of the Unlicensed Assistive Personnel in medication administration. The role of Unlicensed Assistive Personnel is described. Regulations are discussed as they pertain to the scope of function of Unlicensed Assistive Personnel. Chapter 2 discusses state and federal regulatory issues surrounding medication administration. Chapter 3 delves into the medical and legal issues or challenges Unlicensed Assistive Personnel may experience.

Module II provides the learner with the fundamentals of medication administration. Chapter 4 begins the learner's introduction into pharmacology and medications. Chapter 5 introduces the learner to medication orders, prescriptions, medication records, and labeling. Chapter 6 instructs the learner on the principles of medication administration: the Six Rights, the Three Checks, the basic guidelines, handwashing, and the use of gloves.

Module III teaches the learner the procedures of medication administration. Chapter 7 discusses the nonparenteral routes of medication administration. Chapter 8 teaches the administration of oxygen, pulse oximetry, incentive spirometer, CPAP, and other relevant information related to respiratory care of an individual. Chapter 9 provides instruction on the administration of various types of enemas. Chapter 10 delves into the care and use of gastrostomy and jejunostomy tubes, including checking for residual feeding, flushing of the tubes, the administration of tube feedings, and medication administration via gastrostomy and jejunostomy tubes. Chapter 11 teaches the administration of epinephrine via the EpiPen Auto-Injector.

Module IV presents information on medications and their effects on the body. Chapter 12 briefly reviews the systems of the body. Chapters 13 to 27 present medications and their effects on the systems of the body, including cardiovascular, respiratory, gastrointestinal, urinary, endocrine, musculoskeletal, nervous, reproductive, and sensory systems. Features of the chapters highlight the following:

- Each major medication classification includes:
  - Description
  - Action
  - Uses
  - Contraindications
  - Adverse reactions/side effects
  - Special considerations
  - Tables that summarize currently used medications

Module V deals with effective communication and documentation. Chapter 28 introduces the learner to the importance of trust, the need to build relationships and teamwork, and effective communication. The chapter provides specific detail regarding the duties of Unlicensed Assistive Personnel in medication administration. Observation, reporting, and recording are discussed in detail along with the guidelines for documenting. Chapter 29 teaches principles of basic and advanced transcription, verification of orders, and monthly quality reviews.

Module VI covers the topic of safety in medication administration. In Chapter 30, the administration of over-the-counter medications is presented. Medication interactions, medication use in the elderly, medication errors, medication losses, and medication refusals are also presented. Chapter 31 discusses poison control.

Module VII provides the learner with additional knowledge and skills useful in medication administration. Mathematics: weights and measurements are taught in Chapter 32 along with oral dose calculations for adults. Since Unlicensed Assistive Personnel may be required to take vital signs as part of the process of administering medications, Chapter 33 includes a section on vital signs. Chapter 34 presents information on the care of individuals with epilepsy. Substance abuse, both by the individuals being cared for by Unlicensed Assistive Personnel and by their coworkers, is discussed in Chapter 35.

REFERENCES

The references of all materials used throughout the text are listed.

APPENDICES

Appendix A provides a Table of Authorities used in Chapter 4.

Appendix B consists of a list entitled *"Use Caution—Avoid Confusion."* The list includes the names of those medications that are commonly confused due to similarities in their names.

Appendix C provides a list of medications that should not be crushed.

Appendix D provides a list of suggested readings and resources.

INDEX

A comprehensive index includes a general listing of the topics and a list of the medications described in the text.

SPECIAL FEATURES

- This text was written specifically for Unlicensed Assistive Personnel. Care was taken throughout the text to present the material in an easy-to-read, user-friendly format. Wherever possible, materials are presented in outline form.

- A comprehensive glossary is provided at the rear of the text.

- In addition, a rolling glossary is included. Learners have a quick reference to spelling and definitions of terms throughout the text.

- Figures and tables are utilized to provide explanation of complex materials and to provide examples.

- Review questions are at the end of each chapter. Clinical scenarios are also at the end of those chapters where appropriate.

- Web site addresses are provided for pharmacology-related information.

ADDITIONAL RESOURCES
Instructor Resources CD-ROM

ISBN-13: 978-1-4354-8174-9

The Instructor Resources CD-ROM is a robust, computerized tool for your instructional needs—a must-have for all instructors. This comprehensive and convenient CD-ROM contains:

- The Instructor's Manual, with suggestions for implementing the curricula. It eases the burden of planning classes and permits the instructor to concentrate more time on the learners. The Instructor's Manual contains the following information:

  - Recommendations for using *Medication Administration* in the classroom.

  - Answers to the review questions, practice exercises, and clinical scenarios found at the end of each chapter.

  - Performance record and skill checklists.

  - Resources for the instructor that include reference information such as Internet and educational resources, health-related organizations, and continuing education programs.

- Instructor slides enhance class presentation for both the learner and the instructor. Instructor slides are created using Microsoft PowerPoint®. Slides are available for each of the thirty-five chapters.

- The ExamView® Computerized Test Bank is organized by chapter and includes over 1500 questions. This test bank assists the instructor in creating personalized chapter tests, midterm, and final exams. Features include:

- An interview or "wizard" to guide the instructor through the steps to create a test in less than 5 minutes.*

- The capability to edit questions or to add an unlimited number of questions in order to adapt tests to fit your teaching style or to meet unique state standards.

- Online and computer-based testing capabilities. Tests students in a distance learning, hybrid course, or traditional classroom environment using a paperless test.

- A sophisticated word processor. Incorporates artwork and symbols and performs spell checks using similar capabilities as found in any word processor.

- Numerous test layout and printing options.

Medication Administration Workbook

ISBN-13: 978-1-4354-8173-2

The workbook provides the learner with hands-on learning. Here the learner may practice transcribing health care providers' orders, calculate doses, read labels, complete telephone order forms, and much more. For those of us who have taught adult learners, we know from experience that the more one practices, the more one retains.

The workbook includes:

- Multiple-choice questions

- Fill-in-the-blank questions

- Short essay questions

- Matching questions

- Diagrams and forms to complete

- Performance record and skills checklists

Medication Administration: Math Module

ISBN-13: 978-1-4354-8175-6

The Math Module includes a Math Pretest followed by a general review of fractions, decimals, percentages, ratio and proportions, and basic conversion along with additional information on the apothecary, household, and metric systems. The Math Module complements the basic review offered in Chapter 32 of *Medication Administration*.

---

*With ExamView® you can customize tests by using the QuickTest Wizard to pull from various chapters in order to create midterm or final examinations. ExamView® lets you select the chapters used and the length of each exam. The software automatically randomizes the order and questions that appear on each exam based on the pool of questions you select. This provides you with a unique exam every time you build a test.

Medication Administration: Caring for Individuals with Diabetes Module

ISBN-13: 978-1-4354-8176-3

The Module "Caring for Individuals with Diabetes" discusses types, treatments, and complications of diabetes. Included is a discussion of oral antidiabetic medications and the administration of insulin. The responsibilities of the Unlicensed Assistive Personnel are described. Blood glucose monitoring, acetone, and the importance of record keeping are detailed. Sick day guidelines are reviewed.

Medication Administration: Medicating Children Module

The Module "Medicating Children" provides a general discussion of administering medications to children from birth through the age of eighteen (18). In addition, this module briefly discusses children with diabetes and children with epilepsy and reviews the procedures for taking vital signs for children.

Instructor Online Companion

ISBN-13: 978-1-4354-8172-5

For instructor's only, this online companion includes an Instructor's Manual, slides, and test banks to accompany each of the three modules available with this product. Contact your sales representative or log on to login.cengage.com to access the instructor companion.

ABOUT THE AUTHOR

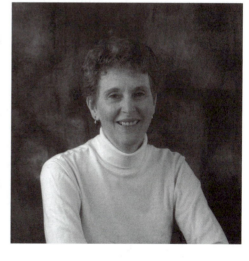

Lena Deter is the founder and clinical consultant for DELHEC, LLC.

As an educational translator, Lena merges research and clinical practice, creating culture change in the health care environment. Her expertise lies in her ability to provide knowledge, guidance, and support to staff, facilities, and providers so that they may (1) create a vision for change, (2) develop a pathway for transformation, and (3) sustain the cultural change they achieve. Her extensive clinical background and achievements include the development of innovative training programs and curricula, proven cross-cultural communication skills, change management skills, and interagency networking qualifications. Lena is talented at creating an empowering and participative learning environment that instills clinical concepts while promoting interdisciplinary team building. Having served in a wide range of clinical, training, and advisory capacities, Lena possesses a wealth of experience and a history of leading health care improvement initiatives.

After graduating from St. Vincent Hospital School of Nursing, Lena progressed through staff nurse, charge nurse, IV therapy, and assistant director of nursing positions with several of Massachusetts's regional hospitals and long-term care facilities. She successfully transitioned into health care administration, working for the American Red Cross, Trivalley Elder Services, and the Committee to End Elder Homelessness. It was also during this time that Lena graduated summa cum laude from Worcester State College with a BS in health education. She went on to earn a master's degree in public health from Boston University, where she concentrated in both health services and social behavioral studies.

In 1996, Lena began as a clinical reviewer for the Massachusetts Department of Public Health (DPH), where she oversaw the implementation of the Medication Administration Program (MAP) within more than 2,200 Department of Developmental Services (DDS) and Department of Mental Health (DMH) programs. She played an instrumental role in defining and instituting clinical and training benchmarks to establish uniformity among sites throughout the state. She also led the successful development and launch of the program's clinical review process as well as the revision of the Medication Occurrence Reporting System.

Because of Lena's achievements with DPH, she was hired as the director of health services for the DDS. In this newly created position, she built on her clinical and training innovations with the continued development of the MAP in more than 1,800 residential programs while simultaneously contributing to several other DDS health service systems. Among her key contributions and achievements was the creation of a formal training curriculum and certification process for the MAP. It was also during this time that Lena pioneered the new Professional Oversight Model for Nursing, which received support from the Massachusetts Board of Registration in Nursing and was presented to the Joint Health Care Committee.

In 2000, Lena accepted a corporate trainer position with Oriol Health Care to lead the development, implementation, and assessment of training programs for licensed and unlicensed staff at three nursing facilities. She recognized the need for an expanded CNA certification course to meet the training requirements of a multinational staff. The result was the creation of a 180-hour course that realized a 100% certification rate and delivered significant improvements in patient care and interdisciplinary collaboration. Lena also designed seminars to develop the leadership, communication, and team-building skills of nurses.

As a clinical consultant for Diligent Services, Lena traveled throughout the northeastern portion of the United States assisting hospitals and long-term care facilities implement Safe Patient Handling Programs. Lena's work with Diligent exemplified her ability to effectively provide relevant and needed consultation and training in a variety of health care fields.

Currently, Lena is a clinical nurse specialist in education at Hebrew Rehabilitation Center (HRC). Here she develops, coordinates, and/or teaches educational sessions for nursing and rehabilitation staff in collaboration with members of HRC's Department of Professional Development. In addition, Lena is involved with creating the culture change needed to implement a social model of care for HRC's new Continuing Care Retirement Community.

Lena continues to expand on the training programs and curricula she developed throughout her career and has created customized programs to meet the specific needs of facilities. It is her consistent ability to inspire and challenge people to learn that makes Lena a respected and successful trainer. It is her forward-thinking attitude and commitment to excellence that makes her a valuable asset and adviser to administrators and others in the health care industry.

ACKNOWLEDGMENTS

To Darlene S. Barnes, LPN, BS, in health administration for her expertise in the adult learning model, curriculum development, and mentoring in the acute care and long-term care settings.

To Stephanie Deter, MS in information technology, for her expertise in computer information technology, employee training and development, management, and client relations.

And last, but not least, to my husband, John, for his understanding and patience as I devote time to my passion of writing.

CONTRIBUTORS

Alfred A. Gray Jr. is a partner in the Boston office of Bowditch & Dewey, LLP. Prior to entering private practice in 2000, he served as the deputy general counsel for the Massachusetts Department of Developmental Services. Among many other duties and responsibilities, Mr. Gray served as the legal adviser for all facets of the Massachusetts Medication Administration Program (MAP), including its creation and implementation. Mr. Gray's current practice focuses on providing advice, counsel, and representation in the health care services field, including long-term care facilities, assisted living centers, special education schools and programs, providers for disabled persons, and various individuals. Mr. Gray also practices in the area of labor and employment within and outside the health care industry.

REVIEWERS

Deborah S. Hartman, RN, MSN, CHPN
Assistant Professor of Nursing
Blue Ridge Community College
Weyers Cave, Virginia

Linda Londre, RN,C, CEN, MSN
Program Director Nursing
Chippewa Valley Technical College
Eau Claire and River Falls, Wisconsin

Barbara McGraw MSN, RN, CNE
Nursing Faculty
Central Community College
Grand Island, Nebraska

Drew Strong, RN, MSN
Assistant Professor of Nursing
Blue Ridge Community College
Weyers Cave, Virginia

Valerie Taylor RN,C, MSN, MEd
Assistant Professor
Lorain County Community College
Elyria, Ohio 44035

FEEDBACK

Comments may be sent to the author by contacting Delmar, Cengage Learning at 800-998-7498.

MODULE I
Ethical and Legal Aspects

Chapter 1
Introduction to Medication Administration

Learning Objectives

After reading this chapter and completing the review questions, you should be able to:

1. Spell and define terms.
2. Briefly describe the development of institutional care in the United States.
3. Describe three changes in health care in the United States over the past forty (40) years.
4. List three goals of deinstitutionalization.
5. List five settings in which Unlicensed Assistive Personnel (UAPs) might work.
6. Explain three purposes of the Nurse Practice Act.
7. Describe four models of nursing care.
8. List the five rights of delegation.
9. Explain the two choices a UAP has when a task is assigned to her.

Key Terms

Adult Foster Care

almshouses

assisted living facilities

cognitive disorders

deinstitutionalization

delegation

Five Rights of Delegation

habilitation model

hospice

"least restrictive setting"

long-term care facilities

Medicaid

Medicare

mental retardation

multidisciplinary team

normalization

prevocational programs

regulations

sanatoriums

scope of function

scope of practice

supportive housing

tuberculosis (TB)

Unlicensed Assistive Personnel

INTRODUCTION

In the United States, the practice and tradition of caring for individuals in institutions and facilities began in the late 18th and early 19th centuries. At the beginning, care was given to the ill and disabled in places called **almshouses**. Other individuals living in the almshouses provided the care (Williams & Torrens, 1993).

Later, community and voluntary hospitals were built. These hospitals cared for individuals with acute illnesses and injuries. Individuals with infectious diseases and mental illness were not allowed in. By 1850, large hospitals, such as Massachusetts General Hospital in Boston and Bellevue Hospital in New York, were being built. These hospitals offered organized health care by staff with specialized training (Williams & Torrens, 1993).

With the entrance of the 20th century, medical schools as we know them today began to grow. Soon city and county hospitals were built to care for the poor. **Sanatoriums** were built to care for individuals with infectious diseases like **tuberculosis (TB)**. State mental hospitals were built by state governments to care for individuals with mental illness and **mental retardation**. Changes in funding and legislation in the 1960s encouraged the building of **long-term care facilities** (nursing homes).

By the mid-1900s, individuals were looking for ways to pay for health care. Health care insurance plans were created and expanded. In the 1960s, the government began to pay for medical care through **Medicare** and **Medicaid**. The government also started to provide money for medical research and for the building of hospitals.

As our health system grew and technology improved, our costs increased greatly. By the latter part of the 20th century, the government was looking for ways to limit the system's growth. By limiting resources (including money), by passing laws to slow the system's growth, and by changing the way payment and care were given, the government has been able to change our health care system (Williams & Torrens, 1993).

CHANGES IN HEALTH CARE IN THE UNITED STATES

Because of the controls put into place by our government over the past years, our health care system has changed the way care is provided. In the past, individuals were cared for in hospitals for long periods of time. Individuals today experience short hospital stays. Healing occurs more often at home. Death may occur at home.

For this to happen, care must be provided by visiting nurses and home health assistants in individual's homes. Home health care is one of the oldest parts of our health care system. Today, it is one of the fastest-growing areas of health care. **Hospice** provides an alternative way to care for the dying. It came into existence in this country in the 1970s. It also is becoming more popular as individuals are being cared for more at home.

Long-term care facilities now provide care for individuals who no longer need to be cared for in a hospital but who are not able to return home.

almshouses
Privately financed homes for the poor.

sanatoriums
Facilities for the care of the chronically ill.

Tuberculosis (TB)
A chronic infectious disease, mainly of the lungs; may be contagious.

long-term care facilities
Nursing homes and other facilities that provide care to individuals who are chronically ill or severely injured.

Medicare
A government program that partially pays for health care for individuals over the age of sixty-five (65) or who are permanently disabled.

Medicaid
A government reimbursement system through which the federal government issues money to the states. The states use the monies to pay for the care of individuals who have no money of their own.

hospice
A facility or program that provides care to individuals who are dying and to their families.

assisted living facilities
Facilities that provide daily supervision and/or assistance with daily activities as needed to individuals who are able to live on their own. Medical care and nursing care are not provided.

Adult Foster Care
A state-funded program that offers elderly and/or disabled individuals (adults) the opportunity to live in private homes in the community.

supportive housing
Offers disabled individuals ongoing levels of support so that they may live in their own apartments in the community.

"least restrictive setting"
Caring for an individual in a setting that permits him to have as much freedom as possible while at the same time providing care that meets all of her needs.

deinstitutionalization
The process of moving or shifting individuals from living in large facilities, hospitals, state schools, and other large settings to living in homes, apartments, and other community settings.

prevocational programs
Programs that prepare individuals to enter work programs.

Some individuals stay at the facilities until they die. Others stay for only short periods of time until they heal. Once healed, they return home. **Assisted living facilities** allow individuals to live on their own. Assistance may be provided if and when needed.

There are many nontraditional ways to provide care for individuals today. New ways are being created every day. These include programs such as **Adult Foster Care** and **supportive housing** for the homeless and for individuals who have chronic illnesses and disabilities. With every new program comes an increasing role for unlicensed assistive personnel in the community.

HISTORY OF DEINSTITUTIONALIZATION

In the 1950s, new medications were discovered that allowed individuals with mental illness to be treated effectively in the community. Institutionalization was no longer the only alternative for safe and effective care. New innovative approaches needed to be developed (Williams & Torrens, 1993).

In 1955, Congress passed the National Mental Health Study Act. The act paid for a three (3)-year study of the care of individuals with mental illness in the United States. As a result of the study's findings, legislation was passed. Federal funding was made available for outpatient services. The new federal funding helped build community mental health centers. The centers provided care to individuals in the community who were being discharged from the state mental hospitals. The centers also offered care to individuals who did not have access to mental health services before (Williams & Torrens, 1993).

Beginning in the 1960s, patients who had been institutionalized, many for long periods of time, began to legally challenge the state mental health systems. Because their constitutional rights had been violated, they won their cases. As a result, care being provided today to individuals with mental health problems must be provided in the **"least restrictive setting"**. Several landmark cases included *O'Connor v. Donaldson*, *Addington v. Texas*, *Foucha v. Louisiana*, and *Alberta Lessard v. Schmidt* (see Table of Authorities, Appendix A).

This process of **deinstitutionalization** that began in the 1950s has resulted in a large decrease in the number of individuals being treated in state and county mental hospitals. In their book *Introduction to Health Services* (4th ed.), Williams and Torrens (1993) state that the number of individuals in state and county mental hospitals decreased from 559,000 to 138,000 between 1955 and 1980.

According to statistics from the Massachusetts Department of Public Health, the Massachusetts Department of Mental Health experienced a decrease of 14,500 patients in 1967 to 2,150 in 1982 in its state hospitals. The Massachusetts Department of Mental Retardation saw a decrease of 9,646 individuals in 1967 to 3,850 in 1982 in its state schools.

Discharges from the state facilities were to full-time residential programs and short-term vocational training programs, including community residential programs, apartment programs, social and **prevocational programs**, work day treatment programs, adult day programs, crisis intervention programs, and community support programs. Most often these programs were primarily for adults (Frechette & Massachusetts Department of Public Health, 1982). For the most part, the staff working in these programs were unlicensed direct care staff.

In summary, the goals of deinstitutionalization were:

- To encourage individuals to live and behave as nondisabled, healthy individuals as much as possible

- To control the costs of health care

- To provide settings that were like "normal" family living—a philosophy called **normalization**

WORK SETTINGS OF UNLICENSED ASSISTIVE INDIVIDUAL

Unlicensed Assistive Personnel (UAPs) work in a variety of settings. Each setting has its own set of **regulations**. Each set of regulations serves to define the role and responsibilities of the UAP.

The settings one might work in include:

- Full-time residential programs

- Short-term vocational training programs

- Community residential programs or apartment programs

- Social programs

- Prevocational programs

- Work day treatment programs

- Adult day programs

- Crisis intervention programs

- Community support programs

- Rest homes/room-and-board facilities

- Long-term care facilities/nursing homes

- Assisted living facilities

- Schools (public and private)

- Day camps

- Hospices

- Detox centers or clinics

- Physicians' offices or practices

- Homeless shelters

- Home care

- Other community settings

Different work settings permit different practices (Table 1-1).

normalization
A principle or concept that helps us create an environment for individuals with developmental disabilities that is as close to normal as possible. It allows us to offer the individuals the same types of treatment and care as others of their own age. Focus is on the positive qualities and strengths of the individual rather than the negative qualities or weaknesses.

Unlicensed Assistive Personnel
Unlicensed direct care staff working in health care or in the human service field.

regulations
A set of laws.

Table 1-1 Work Settings

	DEPARTMENT OF MENTAL HEALTH RESIDENTIAL PROGRAM*	DEPARTMENT OF MENTAL RETARDATION RESIDENTIAL PROGRAM*	REST HOME*	NURSING HOME/ LONG-TERM CARE FACILITY*
Medication	Administration by UAPs to adults: may administer oral medications; ear, eye, and nose drops; use of an EpiPen	Administration by UAPs to adults: may administer oral medications; ear, eye, and nose drops; rectal and vaginal medications; use of an EpiPen	Administration by UAPs to adults: may administer oral medications; ear, eye, and nose drops	No administration by UAPs
Tube feedings	Not permitted	Permitted by UAPs with specialized training	Not permitted	Not permitted
Change a simple sterile dressing	Not permitted	Permitted by UAP with additional training	Permitted by UAP with additional training	Not permitted
Perform clean catheterization	Not permitted	Permitted by UAP with additional training	Not permitted	Not permitted

* In the state of Massachusetts
Source: Clifton Park, NY: Delmar, Cengage Learning.

It is the UAP's responsibility to:

* Know the regulations for each setting she works in
* Do only those tasks that the regulations permit her to do

OVERSIGHT/SUPERVISION/DELEGATION

The type of supervision the UAP has at work will depend on her work setting. In a community residential program, her immediate supervisor may be a licensed nurse or may be a nonmedical, unlicensed staff, depending on the state regulations. In a health care facility like a nursing home or a home health care agency, the UAP's immediate supervisor will be a licensed nurse.

When caring for individuals with mental illness, developmental disabilities, Alzheimer's disease, or other **cognitive disorders,** the setting the UAP works in may follow the philosophy of the **habilitation model**. This philosophy allows an individual to participate as fully as possible in all aspects of her life, including her family, community, and social life. The UAP provides a wide range of support, from personal care (activities of daily living), health care, transportation, and advocacy to social and recreational assistance and employment support depending on the setting in which she works. The UAP's role is to help the individual direct her own life.

cognitive disorders
Affect intellect, memory, and/or attention.

Working in a setting that believes in the habilitation model, the UAP will learn to follow a concept or principle known as normalization. Normalization helps us create a home and place of work that are as close to "normal" as possible. These settings allow us to offer individuals the same types of treatment and care as others of their own age. Focus is on the individual's positive qualities and strengths rather than the negative qualities or weaknesses.

In this setting, supervision of UAPs may be done by their immediate supervisor (unlicensed staff) or by nursing. If supervision is provided by nonmedical, unlicensed staff, states will most often require clinical consultants. State regulation will determine the level and type of supervision that will take place. It is the UAP's responsibility to know and follow her state regulations.

In a setting where nursing oversees, monitors, or supervises the UAP's work, there are many different models or ways in which this may be done. A few of the models currently used today are:

- Functional Nursing: Assignments are made by a charge nurse according to the type of task and the work to be done. For instance, one staff member is assigned to take vital signs, another staff member passes medications, another staff member gives showers, and so on.

- Team Nursing: The registered nurse(RN)/licensed practical nurse (LPN) (known as the team leader) organizes the activities/duties of the licensed staff and UAPs to provide care for a group of patients.

- Total Patient Care: A staff of only RNs is assigned to provide all the care needed by a group of patients.

- Primary Care Nursing: One nurse (RN) has the total responsibility of managing nursing care for a specific group of patients for the entire 24 (twenty-four)-hour period of hospitalization. The RN writes and supervises the plan of care. Associate RNs/LPNs on other shifts carry out the plan of care.

- Case Management: The RN organizes the services of a **multidisciplinary team** and may or may not provide direct care.

- Professional Oversight: This model was developed specifically to provide oversight for UAPs in community settings for administration of medications. The RN provides monitoring of the medication administration program and practices of the medication certified UAPs.

multidisciplinary team
A team of professionals and paraprofessionals who work together to provide care to an individual and her family.

NURSE PRACTICE ACTS AND STATE REGULATION

Each individual entering the health care field to work must know and understand the federal and state laws that affect her day-to-day work. Throughout the United States, each state has passed its own Nurse Practice Act. The act regulates nursing practice within a state. It is important to note that although Nurse Practice Acts are alike in many ways, they also are different in each state. Therefore, nurses and UAPs must know about the act in the state where they are working.

Nurse Practice Acts:

- Protect the health, welfare, and safety of the citizens living in the state
- Define the scope of practice for licensed nurses as well as other health care workers
- Allow the revocation or suspension of a nursing license (or, in some states, a UAP's certification) for such reasons as:
  - Practicing outside one's scope of practice
  - Performing one's duties in an incompetent manner
  - Being negligent or abusive
  - Other reasons
- Are used to determine the nursing tasks the UAP may perform
- Are used to formulate legal and advisory opinions about UAPs

If a UAP performs a task or skill beyond her scope of practice, the UAP could be practicing nursing without a license, creating problems for both the UAP and the nurse supervising the UAP (Sorrentino, 2008).

A **scope of practice** is the legal limits of one's role in health care. It is:

- What a health care worker can do
- What a health care worker cannot do

Note: **In many work settings, a UAP must work under the direction of an RN and/or an LPN at all times.**

The UAP's scope of practice is determined by:

- The Nurse Practice Act
- Federal regulations under the Omnibus Budget Reconciliation Act
- State regulations for the setting in which she is working
- Legal and advisory opinions
- The UAP's training and experience
- The employer's *written* policies and procedures

Note: **In the health care field, many words and phrases change over time as duties, responsibilities, and understandings change. Recently, the term "scope of practice," when used in reference to Unlicensed Assistive Personnel (such as CNAs in long-term care), has been replaced with the term scope of function. Throughout the rest of this textbook, the phrase "scope of function" will be used, but the learner should be aware that in some long-term care settings and other settings or in some reading materials, the phrase "scope of practice" may still be used.**

scope of practice
The legal limits within which one may work.

scope of function
The legal limits within which the UAP may work.

As with all things, there are basic rules to follow. The UAP:

- *Immediately* reports any changes in an individual's physical and/or mental status. When reporting, the UAP follows the chain of command.

- *Never* makes medical decisions about what should or should not be done for an individual. Medical decisions are to be made only by licensed health care providers such as nurses and physicians.

- *Never* makes a diagnosis or prescribes treatments or medications for an individual.

- Does only those tasks that she has been trained to do. If a UAP does not understand instructions or directions, she must ask for an explanation *before* doing the task.

- *Never* does a task or skill that she has not been trained to do or that she does not feel comfortable doing *without* additional training and proper supervision.

- *Never* provides confidential information. The UAP refers the individual requesting information to her supervisor or charge nurse.

- *Never* just ignores an order or request to do something that she cannot do or that is beyond her scope of function. The UAP notifies her supervisor of her inability to fulfill a request (Sorrentino, 2008).

According to the Nurse Practice Acts, nurses assign tasks or duties to UAPs through a legal process called **delegation**. Delegation is defined in a state's Nurse Practice Act as:

> The legal responsibility under which an RN, through supervision, assigns a task or skill to another RN, LPN, or UAP. Some Nurse Practice Acts allow an LPN, under the supervision of an RN, to assign a task or skill to a UAP. Although the task or skill is delegated and performed by another, the RN or LPN remains legally responsible and accountable for the outcomes of that delegation (Sorrentino, 2008).

delegation
The legal act of assigning tasks or duties.

Note: Nurse Practice Acts in some states define LPNs as independent practitioners. In these states, LPNs may independently delegate tasks and skills to UAPs.

The legal responsibility of delegation includes:

- RN/LPN is responsible for the actions and/or inactions of the UAP to whom she delegates.

- RN/LPN must make sure that the task or skill is done safely and correctly.

- RN/LPN is responsible for *all* care given by the UAP (Sorrentino, 2008).

- UAPs *cannot* delegate. For example, Sally is instructed by the nurse to give Joe his medication at 3 p.m. Sally cannot ask another staff member to give Joe his medication at 3 p.m. If Sally is unable to give Joe his medication, Sally needs to contact the nurse (National Council of State Boards of Nursing Delegate Assembly, 2007).

- Delegation of medication administration to the UAP is *always* individual specific and situation specific. In other words, administering medication to one individual does not mean that the UAP may administer medication to all individuals. Also, administering medication to an individual in one situation does not mean the UAP may administer medication to the individual in all situations (National Council of State Boards of Nursing Delegate Assembly, 2007).

- Delegation should always result in the best care for the individual (Sorrentino, 2008).

Note: **Delegation is used mainly in a medical model of care. Not all work settings follow a medical model of care. It is the UAP's responsibility to know her state regulations and workplace policies regarding the model of care used in her work setting.**

For a nurse to delegate a task to a UAP, the nurse must follow the **Five Rights of Delegation:**

1. Right task—Can the task be safely delegated?

    - Does the state permit the task to be delegated?

    - Was the UAP trained to do the task?

    - Does the UAP have the experience to do the task?

    - Is the task in the UAP's job description?

2. Right circumstance—What are the individual's physical, mental, emotional, and spiritual needs at this time?

    - Is the UAP trained, experienced, and able to meet the individual's needs at this time?

    - Does the UAP understand the purpose of the task?

    - Can the task be performed safely by the UAP under the circumstances?

    - Does the UAP have the necessary equipment and supplies to safely do the task?

    - Does the UAP know how to properly and safely use the equipment and supplies?

3. Right individual—Does the UAP have the training and experience to safely do the task for this individual?

    - Is the UAP comfortable doing the task?

    - Are all the UAP's questions and concerns about the task addressed?

4. Right direction and communication—The nurse must give clear directions. The nurse tells the UAP what to do, when to

do it, what observations to make, and when to report back. The nurse allows time for questions and helps the UAP set priorities.

- Are the nurse's instructions clear?
- Were the directions understood by the UAP?
- Did the nurse review the task with the UAP?
- Does the UAP understand what the nurse expects?

5. Right supervision—The nurse guides, directs, and evaluates the care the UAP gives. The nurse demonstrates tasks as necessary and is available to answer questions. To help the UAP learn, the nurse tells the UAP what she did well and what she can do to improve her work.

- Is the nurse nearby to answer the UAP's questions?
- Is the nurse available if there is a change in the individual's condition or if the UAP has a problem? (Sorrentino, 2008).

Note: According to the National Council of State Boards of Nursing, when delegating medication administration to a UAP, the licensed nurse must (1) determine the level of supervision, monitoring, and accessibility she must provide the UAP; (2) have effective communication, interpersonal, and organizational skills; (3) be available to monitor the progress of the individual being medicated, to note the effect of the medication being administered to the individual, and to assess the need for prn medication; and (4) must periodically review licensed health care provider orders and individual medication records (National Council on State Boards of Nursing Delegate Assembly, 2007).

When a nurse delegates or assigns a task to the UAP, the UAP has two choices. The UAP may (1) agree to do the task or (2) refuse to do the task (Sorrentino, 2008).

WHEN ACCEPTING A TASK:	TO REFUSE A TASK:
The UAP is responsible for her action(s). The UAP must complete the task safely and properly.	The UAP must have a valid reason. • The task is beyond the UAP's scope of function. • The task is not in the UAP's job description. • The UAP is not trained to do the job safely. • The individual's condition is unstable. • The UAP does not know how to use the equipment or supplies. • The nurse's request is unethical, illegal, or against policy. • The nurse's directions are unclear or incomplete. • The nurse is unavailable for supervision.

A UAP may *not* refuse to do a task simply because the UAP does not:

- like to do the task

- want to do the task

- agree with the nurse's decision (Sorrentino, 2008)

A UAP must never ignore an order or an assignment to do a task. If the UAP is unable to complete a task, she needs to explain to the nurse her concerns and inability to do it (Sorrentino, 2008).

All the nursing models discussed use the process of delegation except for the Professional Oversight Model. In the Professional Oversight Model:

- UAPs train, test, and become medication certified by taking a state certification examination similar to the CNA state certification examination.

- Nurses provide the initial and ongoing training of the UAPs.

- Nurses provide monitoring of the medication administration program and practices of the medication certified UAPs but are not legally accountable for the UAP's practice.

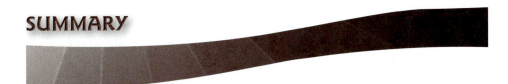

SUMMARY

Health care in the United States today looks very different from fifty (50) or even twenty-five (25) years ago. Through the process of deinstitutionalization, which began in the 1950s, individuals were moved from large institutions into the community. Because of this movement, the majority of individuals are now cared for in the community. To meet the needs of these individuals, the role of the UAP has undergone changes. The responsibility for skilled tasks, such as medication administration and feeding by gastrostomy tube, that were once performed by licensed health care workers is shifting to the UAP. States have passed laws and established regulations to address these changes. Formal training and testing have been developed. Some states now have certification requirements and programs to demonstrate that the UAP has knowledge and skills in different areas.

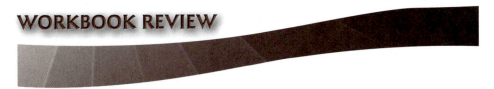

WORKBOOK REVIEW

Go to the workbook and complete the exercises for Chapter 1.

REVIEW QUESTIONS

1. In the 1960s, the federal government began to pay for medical care through:
   a. Medicine and Medical
   b. Medicare and Medicaid
   c. Money and Medicine
   d. Magazine and Manicure

2. Providing care to individuals with mental health problems in the least restrictive setting is a result of a process called:
   a. hospice
   b. assisted living
   c. deinstitutionalization
   d. hospitalization

3. An alternative to hospitalization in the United States *today* may be:
   a. almshouse
   b. assisted living
   c. sanatorium
   d. all of the above

4. In the 1960s, individuals being discharged from state and county mental hospitals went to programs such as:
   a. community individual programs
   b. social prevocational programs
   c. community support programs
   d. all of the above

5. "Normalization" is a philosophy that promotes:
   a. making individuals act "normal" in their daily life
   b. providing a setting that is like "normal" family living
   c. giving individuals medications to help them act "normal"
   d. teaching individuals to be "normal" during work

6. An individual's scope of practice is:
   a. what one can and cannot do in one's job
   b. how long one can practice a task before getting it right
   c. what one feels like doing at one's job
   d. what one sees when looking through a telescope

7. The rule(s) that helps to define the UAP's scope of practice is/are:
   a. the UAP reports any changes in the individual's physical and/or mental status within twenty-four (24) hours of noticing the change
   b. the UAP makes medical decisions as long as they are not important ones
   c. the UAP may change an individual's medication but only once
   d. the UAP does only those tasks she has been trained to do

8. The philosophy of the habilitation model of care is:
   a. the individual is totally dependent on staff for all aspects of her life
   b. the individual lives in a habitat
   c. the individual goes to rehabilitation
   d. the individual participates as fully as possible in all aspects of her life

9. The legal process of delegation is defined as:
   a. the responsibility under which an RN assigns a task to another RN, LPN, or UAP
   b. the responsibility under which an RN trains another RN, LPN, or UAP to do a task
   c. the responsibility under which an RN performs her daily tasks
   d. the responsibility under which an RN documents at the end of her shift

10. The Five Rights of Delegation, followed by an RN when delegating a task to a UAP, include:
   a. Right task
   b. Right date
   c. Right place
   d. Right documentation

11. When a nurse delegates or assigns a task to a UAP, the UAP may:
   a. do it when she feels like it
   b. agree to do the task or refuse it
   c. call her supervisor to complain
   d. write a note in the communication book about it

12. A valid reason for refusing a delegated task would be:
   a. the task is beyond one's scope of practice
   b. the UAP is trained to do the job safely
   c. the individual's condition is stable
   d. the nurse's directions are clear or complete

Chapter 2
Regulatory Issues

Learning Objectives

After reading this chapter and completing the review questions, you should be able to:

1. Spell and define terms.
2. Explain the three purposes of the Pure Food and Drug Act of 1906.
3. Name two oversight agencies that deal with medications and drugs.
4. List five of the rules from the Federal Food, Drug and Cosmetic Act of 1938 with their amendments of 1951 and 1965.
5. List four of the rules of the Controlled Substance Act, which was written to set tighter controls on a specific group of drugs and medications.
6. Give two examples of each of the five schedules of drugs/ medications.
7. Explain how state laws may differ from federal laws.
8. List the three legal terms used for medications and explain how they differ from each other.

Key Terms

administer	drug standards	pharmaceutical company	schedules
controlled substances			

INTRODUCTION

The main purpose of laws in the United States is to protect people. This is no different when it comes to medications. Changes due to scientific advances, progress, and changes in our society throughout the 1900s required our government to pass laws that created drug standards and oversight agencies.

FEDERAL LAWS

drug standards
Rules made so that we, the people, get what we pay for when we fill our prescription medications.

Drug standards are rules that were made so that we, the people, get what we pay for. The laws say that all medications called by the same name must have the same strength, quality, and purity. Because of these standards, when an individual takes a prescription to a pharmacy to be filled, he can be sure that he is getting the same basic medication in the same amount and quality. It does not matter which pharmacy he takes it to. It does not matter what part of the country he is in. It does not matter if he orders medications through a mail-order company. A prescription is filled the same way with the same basic medication everywhere he goes.

pharmaceutical company
A company that makes and sells medications.

According to the drug standards, a **pharmaceutical company** must not add other active ingredients or other chemicals to a medication. Companies must meet the federally approved drug standards for the specific strength, quality, and purity of the medication. Unlike in years past, we no longer have to be concerned about the ingredients in our medications.

The Pure Food and Drug Act passed in 1906 established the drug standards. The law was the government's first act in protecting our supply of food and drugs (medications). In addition, the law addressed two other issues:

1. It demanded that medications containing morphine be in a labeled container stating that one of the ingredients was morphine.

2. It created two references of *officially* approved medications. Before 1906, information about medications was handed down from generation to generation. There were no official written resources. After the passage of the Pure Food and Drug Act in 1906, there were references that stated the *official* U.S. standards for the making of each medication. These were the *United States Pharmacopoeia (USP)* and *National Formulary (NF)*. These two references have since been combined into one reference.

Two oversight agencies were created by law during the mid-1900s. The Food and Drug Administration (FDA), under the United States Department of Health and Welfare, was created in 1938. The Drug Enforcement Administration (DEA) was created in 1970 as a bureau of the Department of Justice. Each department enforces the requirements of a specific law.

In addition to creating the FDA, the Federal Food, Drug and Cosmetic Act of 1938 with amendments of 1951 and 1965 set up more specific rules to prevent tampering with medications, food, and cosmetics. These rules included the following:

1. All labels must be accurate.

2. All labels must include generic names.

3. All new products must be approved by the FDA before being released to the public.

4. Warning labels must be on certain products. For example, labels must say "may cause drowsiness," "may cause nervousness," or "may be habit forming."

5. Certain medications must be labeled with the legend (message) "Caution—federal law prohibits dispensing without a prescription." The term *legend drugs* refers to prescription medications.

6. This law states which medications can be sold without a prescription.

7. Prescription and nonprescription medications must be shown to be effective as well as safe.

The Controlled Substance Act of 1970 not only created the DEA but also set much tighter controls on a specific group of drugs/medications (controlled substances). This group of drugs/medications was being abused by society and therefore needed to be controlled. They include depressants, stimulants, psychedelics, narcotics, and anabolic steroids. Rules set up by this act are as follows:

1. The abused and addicting drugs/medications are grouped into five levels, or **schedules**, according to how dangerous they are:

    C-I, C-II, C-III, C-IV, and C-V (Table 2-1).

    These drugs/medications were named **controlled substances**.

2. The Controlled Substance Act demanded security of the controlled substances. Anyone who dispenses, receives, sells, or destroys these substances must keep on hand special DEA forms. These DEA forms tell the exact current inventory and a two (2)-year inventory of every controlled substance transaction.

3. The act set limitations on the use of prescriptions. It set guidelines for each of the five schedules of controlled substances, stating the number of times a medication may be prescribed in a six (6)-month period. It also stated which schedule prescriptions may be phoned in to the pharmacy and so on.

4. The act demanded that each individual (physician, dentist, pharmacist, or veterinarian) who writes a prescription register with the DEA. This individual then receives a DEA registration number. When the prescription for the controlled substance is written, the DEA registration number must be included on it.

5. Pharmaceutical companies must also register with the DEA. They also receive a DEA registration number.

schedules
The groups or levels of certain prescription medications that have the danger of addiction and abuse.

controlled substances
Prescription medications that because of their danger for addiction and abuse have additional federal regulations.

Table 2-1 Five Schedules of Controlled Substances

SCHEDULE NUMBER	ABUSE POTENTIAL AND LEGAL LIMITATIONS	EXAMPLES OF SUBSTANCES
C-I	High abuse potential Limited medical use	Heroin LSD Marijuana Mescaline
C-II	High abuse potential May cause serious dependence Written prescription only No phoning in of prescription by office health care worker No refills May be faxed, but original prescription must be handed in to pick up prescription In an emergency, physician may phone in prescription, but handwritten prescription must go to pharmacy within seventy-two (72) hours	Morphine Codeine Methadone Percocet Tylox Dilaudid Ritalin Cocaine Concerta
C-III	May cause limited dependence Written, faxed, or verbal (phoned in) prescription by physician only May be filled up to five times in six (6) months	Paregoric Empirin with codeine Tylenol with codeine Fiorinol Anabolic steroids
C-IV	Lower abuse potential than the above schedules Prescription may be written out by the health care worker but must be signed by the physician Prescription may be phoned in by the health care worker or faxed May be filled up to five (5) times in six (6) months	Valium Ativan Chloral hydrate Phenobarbital Librium Darvon Restoril Ambian
C-V	Low abuse potential compared to the above schedules Consists mainly of medications for cough suppressants containing codeine and medications for diarrhea (e.g., opium tincture)	Cheracol syrup Robitussin-A-C Expectorant DAC Donnagel-PG Lomotil

Source: Based on Woodrow (2007), Table 1-1.

Drugs/medications are grouped into the five schedules based on how likely they are to be abused and how dangerous they may be. Drugs in Schedule C-I, such as heroin, have the potential to be the most dangerous and are most likely to be abused. Medications in Schedule C-5, such as Robitussin AC Cough Syrup, pose the least danger and are less likely to be abused. Therefore, Schedule C-I has the strictest controls and rules.

Medications/drugs are often added, removed, or moved from one schedule to another. For example, if the DEA decides that a drug or medication is becoming more of a problem in society (e.g., causing an increase in overdoses), that drug or medication may be moved from one schedule to another; for example, a Schedule C-IV medication may be changed to Schedule C-III.

Because controlled substances are stored and handled differently than other medications, it is important for the UAP to know whether a medication is a controlled substance. He can get this information from a drug reference book, a pharmacist, the label on the medication bottle, drug packages, and drug inserts. These are discussed later in the training manual.

The UAP will learn to recognize the schedule of the controlled substance by noting a capital "C" with or without a Roman numeral on the different items mentioned previously. The symbols may be as simple as a red "C" on a medication label, the capital "C" followed by the Roman numeral (C-I), or a capital "C" with the Roman numeral inside the curve of the "C," as shown in Figure 2-1. Each state may even use a different method or code to show that a medication is a controlled substance. It is the UAP's responsibility to know the method or code used in his state.

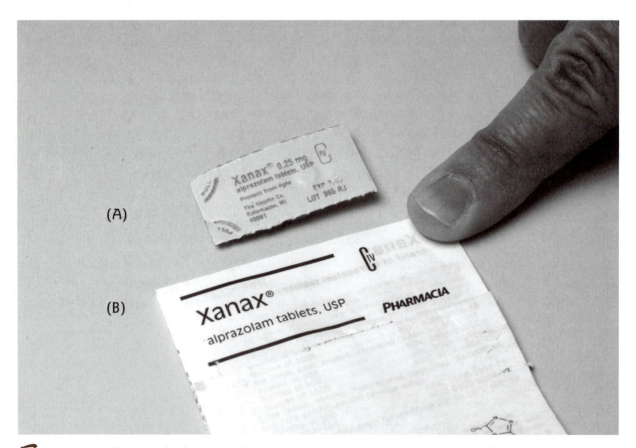

Figure 2-1 Controlled substance schedule numbers appear in a variety of drug information resources, including A) drug packages and B) drug inserts. Schedule numbers are also found in drug reference books.

(Delmar/Cengage Learning)

STATE LAWS

administer
To dispense or to give; for example, to give medication.

States may decide to follow the federal laws as written, or they may decide to set stricter guidelines. It is the responsibility of every individual who **administers** medications within a state to know both the federal laws and his own state laws regarding the handling, storage, and administration of medications in the setting in which he works.

For example, in some states there are six schedules of controlled substances, not five as discussed previously. Schedule C-VI includes all prescription medications not included in Schedules C-I through C-V, such as ampicillin, Ditropan, oxygen, and erythromycin. Schedule C-VI medications, for the most part, usually do not need to be double-locked or counted every twenty-four (24) hours as is federally required for Schedules C-II through C-V.

Other differences the UAP might see among the states are as follows:

- Health care workers may not be permitted to write out prescriptions for the physician to sign even though this is permitted for Schedules C-IV and C-V under federal law.

- Health care workers may not be permitted to phone in or fax prescriptions to a pharmacy even though again this is permitted for Schedules C-IV and C-V under federal law.

- UAPs may not be permitted to administer medications OR may be permitted to administer medications in only certain settings in a state.

- Controlled substances (Schedules C-II through C-V) may need to be counted and reconciled every eight (8) hours instead of every twenty-four (24) hours.

- Schedule C-VI medications may need to be double-locked along with Schedules C-II through C-V medications.

- Medications may need to be packaged in a special way, such as in "blister" packaging or "bubble" packs. (Packaging of medications is discussed later in the training manual.)

- The amount of medication kept on-site (e.g., at the nursing home or group home) may be limited to a certain amount.

- Medications may need to be stored in a special or specific way.

- UAPs may not be permitted to split, cut, or break a tablet, pill, or capsule or other unit of a medication.

- There may be certain medication(s) that UAPs are not permitted to administer.

Remember that the UAP must follow his state regulations for the setting in which he works. Regulations will differ from state to state. They will differ from setting to setting. They will also be different for a nurse or other licensed clinician than for a UAP. The UAP must be sure to follow the regulations for his scope of function.

Table 2-2 Legal Description of Medication

OTC (OVER-THE-COUNTER)	LEGEND (PRESCRIPTION) MEDICATION	CONTROLLED SUBSTANCE
• Purchased over-the-counter • No restrictions by the FDA	• Determined by the FDA as unsafe for over-the-counter purchasing because of possible harmful effects if taken indiscriminately • Includes birth control pills, antibiotics, cardiac medications, hormones, and so on • Indicated in drug references by the symbol to the far right of the trade name	• Controlled by prescription requirement because of the danger of addiction and/or abuse • Indicated in references by schedule numbers C-I to C-V

Source: Delmar/Cengage Learning

COMMON LEGAL TERMS

As one can easily see, medication administration involves the law. Because of this, there are common legal terms used in any program where medication is administered. Table 2-2 provides a brief description of the legal terms used to describe the different types of medications that one may administer to an individual. Note that medications can be described in other ways, such as classification, generic name, trade name, chemical name, or official name. These other ways are discussed further in Chapter 4. For now, refer to the legal description.

SUMMARY

Wherever the UAP works, if he administers medications, he will be responsible for their safe handling, storage, and administration. This will include complete and proper documentation of the administration of the medication to an individual or individuals as well as a record of the inventory of the medication itself. The UAP will need to track medications:

- As they enter the workplace
- When they are administered
- When they are destroyed
- When there is a medication error
- When medications are missing

Topics such as the storage of medications, the procedure for administering medications, the procedure for counting and tracking the inventory, the procedure for medication disposal, and the procedure for reporting medication errors and losses are discussed in future chapters.

WORKBOOK REVIEW

Go to the workbook and complete the exercises for Chapter 2.

REVIEW QUESTIONS

1. Drug standards ensure that an individual gets:
   a. the same basic medication in the same amount and quantity from any pharmacy
   b. a different medication, depending on which pharmacy one goes to
   c. a different medication when one orders through a mail-order company
   d. a different medication, depending on where one is in the United States
2. According to the drug standards, pharmaceutical companies must:
   a. mix in additives and other chemicals when manufacturing medications
   b. color all of their pills blue, white, or green
   c. not add other active ingredients or other chemicals to a medication
   d. provide lunch whenever they give an in-service in a health care provider's office
3. The Pure Food and Drug Act, passed in 1906, addressed the following issues:
   a. it was demanded that all over-the-counter medications were labeled
   b. it required that all medications have a prescription
   c. it created one primary reference of official approved medications—the *United States Pharmacopoeia*
   d. it demanded that medications containing morphine be in a labeled container stating that one of the ingredients was morphine
4. Two food and drug oversight agencies created during the mid-1900s were the:
   a. Federal Deal Administration and the Drug Enactment Agency
   b. Food and Drug Administration and the Drug Enforcement Administration
   c. United States Department of Health and Human Services
   d. United States Department of Justice

5. Some of the specific rules set by the Federal Food, Drug and Cosmetic Act include:
   a. all cosmetics must have a warning label
   b. all new products must be approved by the Department of Justice before they are offered to the public
   c. warning labels, such as "may cause drowsiness" or "may cause nervousness," must be on all products that contain morphine
   d. all labels must be accurate and must include generic names

6. "Legend drugs" are drugs that:
   a. must be labeled with the message "Caution—federal law prohibits dispensing without a prescription"
   b. are legendary for their potency
   c. are mentioned when telling fables or legends
   d. are dispensed with a set of descriptive symbols similar to a map legend

7. The Controlled Substance Act of 1970 has set a very tight control on a specific group of drugs abused by society, including:
   a. depressants, narcotics, and stimulants
   b. aspirin, Motrin, and Tylenol
   c. Colace, Mylanta, and Maalox
   d. none of the above

8. The five schedules or levels of danger of controlled substances are:
   a. A, B, C, D, and E
   b. a, b, c, d, and e
   c. C-I, C-II, C-III, C-IV, and C-V
   d. 1, 2, 3, 4, and 5

9. The DEA forms for tracking controlled substances tell:
   a. who has taken the controlled substance in the facility
   b. who has dispensed the controlled substance in the facility
   c. the exact current inventory and a two-year inventory of every controlled substance transaction
   d. which pharmacy has supplied the controlled substance to the facility

10. When talking about the five schedules of controlled substances:
    a. drugs in Schedule C-I have the potential to be the most dangerous and are most likely to be abused
    b. drugs in Schedule C-V have the potential to be the most dangerous and are most likely to be abused
    c. drugs in Schedule C-IV are more dangerous than those in Schedule C-II
    d. drugs in Schedule C-III are more dangerous than those in Schedule C-I

11. When looking at the label of a controlled substance medication, you will notice:
    a. a blue "C" on the label
    b. a capital "C" followed by a the numbers 1, 2, 3, 4, or 5
    c. the abbreviation "CS"
    d. a capital "C" with the Roman numeral inside the curve of the "C"

12. When handling medications including controlled substances, one must:

    a. follow the regulations for your scope of function

    b. follow the instructions of the RN on duty, even if they are beyond your scope of function

    c. count the controlled substances every twelve (12) hours

    d. split, cut, or break a tablet, pill, capsule, or other unit of a medication before giving it to a resident

Chapter 3
Ethical and Legal Issues
Alfred A. Gray, Esq.

Learning Objectives

After reading this chapter and completing the review exercises, you should be able to:

1. Spell and define terms.
2. List the three health care documents regarding an individual's rights and describe six items these documents have in common.
3. Describe the difference between ethical standards and legal standards.
4. List three ethical principles that are important to the UAP.
5. Describe the role of an ethics committee.
6. List the basic rules for sharing information.
7. Describe various legal theories.
8. Describe the four elements of negligence.
9. Explain three legal situations that UAPs should avoid.

Key Terms

abuse	comparative negligence	financial abuse	liable
advance directives	criminal liability	grievance	licensed health care provider
aiding and abetting	discrimination	harm	
breach	diversion	HIPAA	malpractice
causation	duty	informed consent	misappropriation of funds
civil liability	ethical standards	involuntary seclusion	
Client's Bill of Rights	ethics committee	legal standards	mistreatment

national origin

neglect

negligence

Omnibus Budget
    Reconciliation Act
    of 1987

Patient Care
    Partnership:
    Understanding
    Expectations, Rights
    and Responsibilities

physical abuse

psychological abuse

Resident's Bill of Rights

Respondeat Superior

sexual abuse

sexual orientation

statute of limitations

theft

verbal abuse

INTRODUCTION

**Omnibus Budget
Reconciliation Act
of 1987**
The law that regu-
lates the education
and certification of
nursing assistants
in long-term care
facilities.

In the United States, people receiving health care have the right to make
sure that they receive quality care. The **Omnibus Budget Reconciliation
Act of 1987** (OBRA), passed by the federal government, legislates the
rights of residents in long-term care facilities such as nursing homes.
The American Hospital Association adopted the Patient's Bill of Rights
in 1973. Their document is now called the Patient Care Partnership: Understanding Expectations, Rights and Responsibilities. The Client's Bill
of Rights is used in home care.

HEALTH CARE DOCUMENTS

Resident's Bill of Rights
A document that
states the rights
of residents living
in long term care
facilities.

**Patient Care Partnership:
Understanding
Expectations, Rights
and Responsibilities**
A document
developed by the
American Hospital
Association that
describes the basic
rights that a patient
is entitled to while in
the hospital or outpa-
tient clinic.

Client's Bill of Rights
A document that
states the rights of
individuals receiving
home health care.

In the health care setting, these are three different documents used to
inform people of their right to receive quality health care. The type of
document used depends on where the care is being given. A copy of the
Resident's Bill of Rights is given to each individual (resident) or her
representative on admission to a skilled nursing facility such as a nursing home (Figure 3-1). The **Patient Care Partnership: Understanding
Expectations, Rights and Responsibilities** is given to each individual
(patient) on admission to a hospital, day surgery, outpatient clinic, or
other similar setting (Figure 3-2). An individual receiving care in her
home from staff of a home health care agency will receive a copy of the
Client's Bill of Rights (Figure 3-3).

On receiving a copy of the Bill of Rights, the individual is asked to sign
a statement stating that she has received the document. However, if the individual is unable to read or understand the Bill of Rights provided to her,
the document is given to a family member or the individual's legal representative. If the family member or representative receives the document,
then the family member or representative signs that she has received it.

All staff working in health care need to be familiar with the different types of Bills of Rights. Supporting the rights of the people the UAP
cares for helps the UAP to give more effective care. All the documents
mentioned earlier are similar. All three stress the right of the patient,
resident, or client to:

- Be treated respectfully and in a dignified manner. Each individual has the right to privacy and confidentiality.

- Have open and honest communication with her caregivers.

- Have an active role in decision making for treatment choices
  and the planning of her care. To do this, the individual must have

Resident's Rights

This is an abbreviated version of the Resident's Rights as set forth in the Omnibus Budget Reconciliation Act. This document must be given to all residents and/or their families prior to admission to a long term care facility.

1. The resident has the right to free choice, including the right to:
   — choose an attending physician
   — full advance information about changes in care or treatment
   — participate in the assessment and care planning process
   — self-administer medications if the resident is assessed as being able to do so
   — consent to participate in experimental research

2. The resident has the right to freedom from abuse and restraints, including freedom from:
   — physical, sexual, mental abuse
   — **corporal punishment** (the use of physical force) and **involuntary seclusion** (isolating a resident without a medical reason)
   — physical and chemical restraints

3. The resident has the right to privacy, including privacy for:
   — treatment and nursing care
   — receiving/sending mail
   — telephone calls
   — visitors

4. The resident has the right to confidentiality of personal and clinical records.

5. The resident has the right to accommodation of needs, including:
   — choices about life
   — receiving assistance in maintaining independence

6. The resident has the right to voice grievances.

7. The resident has the right to organize and participate in family and resident groups.

8. The resident has the right to participate in social, religious, and community activities, including the right to:
   — vote
   — keep religious items in the room
   — attend religious services

9. The resident has the right to examine survey results and correction plans.

10. The resident has the right to manage personal funds.

11. The resident has the right to information about eligibility for Medicare/Medicaid funds.

12. The resident has the right to file complaints about abuse, neglect, or misappropriation of property.

13. The resident has the right to information about advocacy groups.

14. The resident has the right to immediate and unlimited access to family or relatives.

15. The resident has the right to share a room with the spouse if they are both residents in the same facility.

16. The resident has the right to perform or not perform work for the facility if it is medically appropriate for the resident to work.

17. The resident has the right to remain in the facility except in certain circumstances.

18. The resident has the right to use personal possessions.

19. The resident has the right to notification of change in condition.

Figure 3-1 Resident's Bill of Rights *(Delmar/Cengage Learning)*

informed consent. **Informed consent** means that the individual gives permission for care or procedures *after* knowing all information about their purpose, their benefits, and any risks involved.

- Be advised about **advance directives**. These are documents, such as a will, a power of attorney, or a health care proxy, that tell

informed consent
Permission given for care or treatment after knowing all information.

The Patient Care Partnership:
Understanding Expectations, Rights and Responsibilities

When you need hospital care, your doctor and the nurses and other professionals at our hospital are committed to working with you and your family to meet your health care needs. Our dedicated doctors and staff serve the community in all its ethnic, religious and economic diversity. Our goal is for you and your family to have the same care and attention we would want for our families and ourselves.

The sections explain some of the basics about how you can expect to be treated during your hospital stay. They also cover what we will need from you to care for you better. If you have questions at any time, please ask them. Unasked or unanswered questions can add to the stress of being in the hospital. Your comfort and confidence in your care are very important to us.

What to Expect During Your Hospital Stay

- **High quality hospital care.** Our first priority is to provide you the care you need, when you need it, with skill, compassion, and respect. Tell your caregivers if you have concerns about your care or if you have pain. You have the right to know the identity of doctors, nurses and others involved in your care, and you have the right to know when they are students, residents or other trainees.

- **A clean and safe environment.** Our hospital works hard to keep you safe. We use special policies and procedures to avoid mistakes in your care and keep you free from abuse or neglect. If anything unexpected and significant happens during your hospital stay, you will be told what happened, and any resulting changes in your care will be discussed with you.

- **Involvement in your care.** You and your doctor often make decisions about your care before you go to the hospital. Other times, especially in emergencies, those decisions are made during your hospital stay. When decision-making takes place, it should include:

  - *Discussing your medical condition and information about medically appropriate treatment choices.* To make informed decisions with your doctor, you need to understand:
    — The benefits and risks of each treatment.
    — Whether your treatment is experimental or part of a research study.
    — What you can reasonably expect from your treatment and any long-term effects it might have on your quality of life.
    — What you and your family will need to do after you leave the hospital.
    — The financial consequences of using uncovered services or out-of-network providers.

    Please tell your caregivers if you need more information about treatment choices.

  - *Discussing your treatment plan.* When you enter the hospital, you sign a general consent to treatment. In some cases, such as surgery or experimental treatment, you may be asked to confirm in writing that you understand what is planned and agree to it. This process protects your right to consent to or refuse a treatment. Your doctor will explain the medical consequences of refusing recommended treatment. It also protects your right to decide if you want to participate in a research study.

  - *Getting information from you.* Your caregivers need complete and correct information about your health and coverage so that they can make good decisions about your care.
    That includes:
    — Past illnesses, surgeries or hospital stays.
    — Past allergic reactions.
    — Any medicines or dietary supplements (such as vitamins and herbs) that you are taking.
    — Any network or admission requirements under your health plan.

(continues)

Figure 3-2 The Patient Care Partnership: Understanding Expectations, Rights and Responsibilities
(*Source: Reprinted with permission of the American Hospital Association, copyright 2003*)

- *Understanding your health care goals and values.* You may have health care goals and values or spiritual beliefs that are important to your well-being. They will be taken into account as much as possible throughout your hospital stay. Make sure your doctor, your family and your care team know your wishes.

- *Understanding who should make decisions when you cannot.* If you have signed a health care power of attorney stating who should speak for you if you become unable to make health care decisions for yourself, or a "living will" or "advance directive" that states your wishes about end-of-life care; give copies to your doctor, your family and your care team. If you or your family need help making difficult decisions, counselors, chaplains and others are available to help.

- **Protection of your privacy.** We respect the confidentiality of your relationship with your doctor and other caregivers, and the sensitive information about your health and health care that are part of that relationship. State and federal laws and hospital operating policies protect the privacy of your medical information. You will receive a Notice of Privacy Practices that describes the ways that we use, disclose and safeguard patient information and that explains how you can obtain a copy of information from our records about your care.

- **Preparing you and your family for when you leave the hospital.** Your doctor works with hospital staff and professionals in your community. You and your family also play an important role in your care. The success of your treatment often depends on your efforts to follow medication, diet and therapy plans. Your family may need to help care for you at home.

  You can expect us to help you Identify sources of follow-up care and to let you know if our hospital has a financial interest in any referrals. As long as you agree that we can share information about your care with them, we will coordinate our activities with your caregivers outside the hospital. You can also expect to receive information and, where possible, training about the self-care you will need when you go home.

- **Help with your bill and filling insurance claims.** Our staff will file claims for you with health care insurers or other programs such as Medicare and Medicaid. They also will help your doctor with needed documentation. Hospital bills and insurance coverage are often confusing. If you have questions about your bill, contact our business office. If you need help understanding your insurance coverage or health plan, start with your insurance company or health benefits manager. If you do not have health coverage, we will try to help you and your family find financial help or make other arrangements. We need your help with collecting needed information and other requirements to obtain coverage or assistance.

  While you are here, you will receive more detailed notices about some of the rights you have as a hospital patient and how to exercise them. We are always interested in improving. If you have questions, comments, or concerns, please contact _____.

Figure 3-2 (continued)

about an individual's wishes for treatment or no treatment if she is unable or incapable to communicate them. Typically, advance directives apply when end-of-life decisions need to be made.

- Receive continuity of care.

- Be informed of grievance procedures so that any conflicts she may have may be resolved. A **grievance** is a situation in which an individual wishes to file a complaint against the facility where the UAP works, against individuals providing care, or both.

A copy of each of the Bills of Rights is included in this chapter (see Figures 3-1, 3-2, and 3-3).

ETHICAL AND LEGAL STANDARDS

In her role as a caregiver, the UAP will need to make decisions about her actions. Some of these decisions will involve the moral right or wrong of her action. Other decisions will involve the legality of her behavior.

advance directives
Documents stating an individual's wishes for treatment (or no treatment)—completed before it is needed for use when the individual is unable or incapable to communicate.

grievance
A situation in which an individual wishes to file a complaint against the facility where the UAP works, against individuals providing care, or both.

Client's Rights in Home Care

The persons receiving home health care services or their families possess basic rights and responsibilities. As the client, you have:

The right to:

1. be treated with dignity, consideration and respect
2. have your property treated with respect
3. receive a timely response from the agency to requests for service
4. be fully informed on admission of the care and treatment that will be provided, how much it will cost, and how payment will be handled
5. know in advance if you will be responsible for any payment
6. be informed in advance of any changes in your care
7. receive care from professionally trained personnel, and to know their names and responsibilities
8. participate in planning care
9. refuse treatment and to be told the consequences of your action
10. expect confidentiality of all information
11. be informed of anticipated termination of service
12. be referred elsewhere if you are denied services solely based on your inability to pay
13. know how to make a complaint or recommend a change in agency policies and services

The responsibility to:

1. remain under a doctor's care while receiving services
2. provide the agency with a complete health history
3. provide the agency with all requested insurance and financial information
4. sign the required consents and releases for insurance billing
5. participate in your care by asking questions, expressing concerns, and stating if you do not understand
6. provide a safe home environment in which care can be given
7. cooperate with your doctor, the staff, and other caregivers
8. accept responsibility for any refusal of treatment
9. abide by agency policies that restrict the duties our staff may perform
10. advise agency administration of any dissatisfaction or problems with your care

Figure 3-3 Client's Bill of Rights in Home Care *(Delmar/Cengage Learning)*

Two sets of rules help to guide the UAP as she makes decisions. They are:

ethical standards
Guides to moral behavior.

legal standards
Guides to legal behavior.

liable
Being held responsible.

1. **Ethical standards:** These are guides to moral behavior. People who give health care voluntarily agree to live up to these standards. When these rules are not followed, the UAP fails to live up to the promise to give safe, correct care and to do no harm. Failing to live up to ethical standards may result in legal liability.

2. **Legal standards:** These are guides to legal behavior. When laws are not obeyed, the UAP may be prosecuted and found **liable** (held responsible) for injury or damage. Legal liability may result in the payment of fines and/or imprisonment and/or damages (money).

Not following ethical or legal standards could also result in the loss of employment and inability to work in the health care field. Loss of job or inability to work within the health care field can occur whether or not an individual is found responsible for violation of an ethical or legal standard.

The ethical and legal standards were established to guarantee that safe, quality care is given. Following these standards also protects the UAP. The general rule of thumb for a UAP to be protected is to do her job in the manner in which she was trained and consistent with laws and workplace policies and procedures. At times, the rules and principles that govern one's moral actions and the laws that govern one's legal actions cover the same area.

ETHICAL ISSUES

Ethics includes several important principles for the UAP. The first is that life is precious. The main goal of a UAP is to promote health and quality of life for the individuals she serves.

Second, each person has the right to be respected as a unique individual. Our uniqueness is shown in many different ways. At times, this may make caring for an individual challenging or difficult. If the UAP values each individual, though, she will learn to accept and work with each individual in the best possible way.

We all have our own personal, religious, cultural, and other beliefs. A UAP may *never* apply her beliefs when caring for an individual. A UAP should, however, be aware of the beliefs of the individual for whom she is caring. If a UAP's beliefs interfere with her ability to provide care, she should immediately speak with her supervisor or other person of authority.

Ethics Committee

In the health care field, a UAP works with many types of people who provide care to the individuals being served. These people include physicians, nurses, other UAPs, social workers, therapists, family, friends, and others. Many times this team of concerned and caring people do not agree on the care for an individual. How do these disagreements get settled?

In some settings, the disagreements or disputes are presented to an **ethics committee**. An ethics committee is an advisory group that attempts to provide suggestions and alternatives on an issue of concern. Most ethics committees consist of people from various professions, including physicians, lawyers, nurses, social workers, family members, clergy, and other persons.

ethics committee
An advisory group of individuals from multiple professions who are consulted in an attempt to resolve a conflict or issue.

The committee's job is to provide suggestions on what would be the best care for the individual. It is not the job of the ethics committee to solve all problems. Most ethics committees only have the ability to give advice. At an ethics committee meeting, concerned persons present the issue(s) that are in conflict. In certain circumstances, a UAP could have a valuable role at an ethics committee meeting. In some ways, a UAP is the eyes and ears of the workplace.

A UAP works on a day-to-day basis with the individuals being cared for. More often than not, it is the UAP who has a good understanding of the likes and dislikes of an individual. The UAP understands what the individual likes to eat. The UAP understands who the individual likes to have visit her. The UAP knows who upsets an individual. The UAP understands which medications an individual does not mind taking and which medications the individual does not want to take. A UAP may play a very important role in informing members of the ethics committee about the particular individual being served.

An example of an ethical conflict may better explain. For example, an individual whom a UAP serves must take certain medications. What if this individual refuses to take the medication because she does not like how it tastes or does not like the side effects? The **licensed health care provider** wants the individual to take the medication. So do the nurses. The individual does not want to take the medication. Her family just wants the individual to be comfortable and happy. The UAP sees the reaction the individual has to the medication. How may this conflict among the members of the team be resolved?

A consultation with the ethics committee may be helpful. The committee may be able to come up with alternatives on how to give the medication or even recommend that the medication no longer be given. It is hoped that by bringing everyone together in one place, at one time, an agreement may be reached.

The UAP should determine if her workplace has an ethics committee. If it does not, the UAP may wish to consider suggesting to her employer that one be created.

PRIVACY ISSUES

Information about an individual is privileged (private) and must not be shared with others inappropriately. The Health Insurance Portability and Accountability Act of 1996, better known as **HIPAA**, helps to guarantee that an individual's health information is protected. Many individuals believe that HIPAA is a lengthy and complex law. As it relates to UAPs, this is not necessarily true.

The primary purpose of HIPAA is to require health care employees, such as UAPs, not to share health information unless permitted, in writing, by the individual to do so. It is that simple and straightforward. Therefore, when the UAP shares information about the individual(s) for whom she is caring, she needs to be sure that she does so in the appropriate place(s) and only with the proper people.

Remembering the following basic rules when sharing information will assist the UAP in complying with HIPAA regulations:

- Never talk about the individual with one's family, friends, or others in the community.

- Never discuss the individual during lunch or coffee breaks, even with one's coworkers.

- Never discuss information about an individual in a public place, such as a reception or waiting area, elevator, or hallway, or at any time in the presence of the public or people not involved in the care of an individual.

- Never give out documentation or other information on the individual to others. This includes family members, clergy, friends, and members of the public, such as news reporters. Refer all inquiries to one's supervisor.

licensed health care provider
An individual licensed within each state to provide medical care, such as LPN, RN, nurse practitioner, nurse midwife, pharmacist, physician assistant, dentist, podiatrist, physician, and doctor.

HIPAA
The Health Insurance Portability and Accountability Act of 1996; a federal law that guarantees that an individual's health information is protected.

- Discuss the individual(s), the care provided, and their personal concerns *only* with one's supervisor during conference or report. Make sure that the conversation will not be overheard by visitors or others living with the individual.

- Learn to handle questions tactfully. State that all the details of an individual's care or treatment of her condition are known only by that individual's licensed health care providers. Refer the person asking to the supervisor or the individual's licensed health care provider.

- Refer the individual's questions about her care to the supervisor, to her licensed health care provider, or to another appropriate person, such as an assigned liaison or facility administrator.

- Never leave notes, reports, or other documents lying around where others can see them.

- Never leave a computer unattended if it has an individual's information on the computer screen or unprotected.

- Never let anyone bully you or intimidate you into providing information.

- If in doubt whether information may be shared with someone, ask the person to provide proof that she is allowed to receive information. If the person cannot provide the authorization or permission, do not share any medical information. Refer the person to a supervisor.

- Always remember that the individual's sense of hearing is the last sense to fail. Be careful with what is said in the individual's presence even if she is unresponsive. An individual may still be able to hear even if she is in a coma-like state.

A few examples may best illustrate the requirements of HIPAA.

1. While in the elevator of the nursing home, a UAP is discussing the treatment of an individual with the charge nurse. During the conversation, other individuals come onto the elevator. Under such a circumstance, the conversation about the individual should immediately stop. Would it make a difference if the other person(s) knew the individual and asked about the individual's care? No, this would not make a difference. A UAP may not discuss medical treatment with any person who is not authorized to receive it. Even if the additional person had such authorization, such a discussion in an elevator or other public location should not occur.

2. As discussed earlier, a UAP might be asked to participate in an ethics committee meeting. Here various medical information and documents are shared during discussion. After the meeting, could the UAP share information that was discussed at the meeting with other individuals? The answer would be no. In order to share an individual's medical information at the meeting, a consent from the individual would have been obtained. With the individual's consent, HIPAA would permit the use of

medical information in the meeting. It is the responsibility of all involved in the meeting not to share information that was discussed or provided outside the meeting.

3. On leaving the ethics committee meeting discussed previously, the UAP accidently takes documents that were discussed home. Once at home, the documents are put on the counter or table as a reminder to take them back the next day. Would this conduct violate HIPAA? This could be a potential violation since other family members or visitors could read the documents. It is the responsibility of all individuals under any circumstances to make sure that any documents or information they have is kept confidential and stored in a proper manner.

As discussed in more detail later, a UAP needs to remember that not following HIPAA could result in being held legally responsible.

LEGAL ISSUES

Laws are passed by governments (local, state, and federal) to protect individuals. In health care, these laws protect both the individuals who receive care and those who provide the care. The UAP need not fear breaking the laws if she is careful to follow these rules:

- Always works within her scope of function; never oversteps her authority
- Does only those things that she has been trained to do
- Carries out procedures carefully and as she was trained
- Keeps her skills and knowledge up to date
- Asks for help before she takes action in a questionable situation
- Always keeps the safety and well-being of the individual(s) for whom she is caring in mind and acts appropriately
- Makes sure she completely understands directions for the care she is going to give
- Does her job according to her workplace policies
- Does no harm to the individual(s) for whom she is caring
- Respects each individual's belongings and beliefs

The best way to avoid legal issues is to understand the different situations that could create problems for the UAP. Understanding the various ways an individual may be sued or held legally liable (responsible) should serve as guidance on how to go about performing job duties. Following is a discussion on the various legal theories that a UAP should be aware of at all times.

Statutory Violations

The federal government and all states create (enact) various laws (statutes) that must be followed. Breaking these laws (statutes) could result in an individual being sent to jail, being required to pay a fine, or both. This is known as **criminal liability**. An individual who breaks the law may also have **civil liability**. Civil liability may result in an individual being required to pay damages to an injured individual or her family, usually in the form of money. Breaking the law may also result in a UAP losing her job and maybe losing the ability to continue to work in the health care field.

The Nurse Practice Act discussed in Chapter 1 is an example of such a law (statute). Breaking the Nurse Practice Act could result in criminal or civil liability. All states have a Nurse Practice Act or a law that is equal to it. It is a UAP's responsibility to understand that violating the Nurse Practice Act may result in some form of legal responsibility to the individual.

HIPAA, discussed earlier in this chapter, is another example of a law (in this case a federal statute) that was created to provide certain rights to the individuals served by UAPs. Breaking the law (a violation) or standards set forth in HIPAA could result in criminal liability, civil liability, loss of employment, or all three.

Various states also create specific statutes to protect certain individuals. For example, many states make it a crime to abuse or cause injury to elderly individuals, children, or individuals who are disabled. Because many of the individuals served by a UAP are elderly or potentially disabled, the UAP needs to know whether her state has such laws.

Intentional Acts

An intentional act is just what it sounds like: a UAP engages in some form of illegal or improper activity that she "intends" to commit. A good example is committing a crime such as assault, sexual assault, rape, or even murder against an individual for whom a UAP is responsible for providing care. An individual who commits an intentional act can be held criminally or civilly responsible, as discussed previously.

Another example of an intentional act is discriminating against an individual the UAP provides care to. It is illegal to treat an individual differently because of her race, sex, **national origin** (country where an individual comes from), **sexual orientation**, age, or religious beliefs. Discriminating against an individual to whom a UAP provides services could result in a claim being filed for damages (money). A UAP may also lose her job or ability to continue working with her employer if found responsible for **discrimination**.

Any action taken by a UAP that she "intends" to do that may be misconduct could also cause legal problems. For example, if a UAP intentionally administers the wrong medication to an individual, the UAP could be held legally responsible.

Negligence

Negligence is the failure to do that which the UAP was trained to do: failure to provide appropriate care or providing improper or inappropriate care that results in injury or harm, whether physical or emotional, to the individual for whom the UAP is caring. Simply put, negligence is carelessness. It is most often caused by hurrying through tasks or duties or by not focusing on the task one is doing. Another way to look at negligence

criminal liability
Being held legally responsible for illegal conduct; usually results in being sent to jail or prison and/or the payment of a fine issued by the court.

civil liability
Being held legally responsible for inappropriate conduct; usually results in the payment of damages to an injured individual, her family, or her representative.

national origin
Country where an individual comes from.

sexual orientation
The preference of an individual to live a heterosexual (straight), homosexual (gay or lesbian), or bisexual lifestyle.

discrimination
Treating any individual differently because of her race, color, sex, national origin, sexual orientation, age, or religious beliefs.

negligence
Failing to provide appropriate care, or providing improper or inappropriate care that results in injury or harm, whether physical or emotional, to the individual being cared for; carelessness.

is that the action(s) taken by a UAP that resulted in harm to an individual was an accident. Unfortunately, though, even an accident in which an individual gets harmed in some manner may result in a UAP being held legally responsible.

A person trained as a UAP is expected to perform in certain ways. The UAP would be potentially responsible or liable for negligence if the UAP failed to:

1. Perform her work as she was taught. For example, she fails to follow the Six Rights of Medication Administration and gives Joe's medication to Sally.

2. Carry out her job in a conscientious manner. For example, her state regulations and work place policy state that the medication area in her work setting must be kept locked at all times. She leaves the medication area unlocked. Joe enters the area. Joe takes medication that he should not take and becomes ill.

There is no question that in today's world, lawsuits are filed all the time. The health care field is no exception. Most certainly, if an individual receiving care from a UAP or other health care provider is physically or emotionally harmed, a lawsuit could potentially be filed. Unless there is an indication that the caregiver intended to harm the individual, the lawsuit that is filed will most likely be filed using the legal theory of negligence. For that reason, it makes sense for a UAP to fully understand what the elements of negligence are. With such an understanding, the UAP should be able to perform her job responsibilities without the fear or worry of being held legally liable or responsible for negligence.

The most common sources of liability for negligence for the UAP include:

- An individual receiving care who falls or suffers other injury during treatment
- Medication errors
- Failure to properly observe and report changes in an individual receiving care
- Failure to implement plans of care
- Failure to adequately perform care
- Failure to observe policies and procedures
- Improper documentation or alteration of documentation
- Falsification of records or documentation
- Mistaken identification of an individual receiving services

duty
An obligation to provide an established standard of care for an individual receiving care.

breach
A break or violation of a particular duty or standard of care.

Elements of Negligence
There are four elements of negligence. An individual who files a lawsuit claiming negligence has to prove each element to win her case or claim. The four elements are:

- **Duty**
- **Breach**

- **Harm**

- **Causation**

Every UAP has the duty to provide care that meets the proper standard for the individuals to whom they work with. The standard of care is established by the Nurse Practice Act in the state the UAP works in and by the UAP's workplace policies and procedures. For example, a UAP has the duty to administer medications in the proper manner as established by laws, policies, and procedures.

A breach of a UAP's duty happens when she does not follow the established standard of care. A breach occurs when the rules are broken. Using the same example of the duty to administer medications properly, that duty would be breached if a medication were given to the wrong individual (such as administering an ointment or oxygen to the wrong individual) or the medications were administered by an incorrect route (such as administering an eardrop in an individual's eye).

The third and fourth elements of negligence require that as a result of the UAP's breach of a duty, the individual receiving services has been harmed, either physically or emotionally, and that the harm resulted from the breach of duty. For example, an individual suffers physical harm as a result of being given the wrong medication. That harm was the direct result of the UAP breaching the duty to administer medications in a proper manner. The UAP in this example would be considered negligent. If the injured individual brought a legal action, the UAP could be held legally responsible.

To highlight the elements of negligence, here are further examples of negligent conduct:

EXAMPLE 1:

A medication storage area or closet is left unlocked. Such conduct by itself might be considered negligent, but remember that for an individual to "win" a negligence case, all four elements of negligence must exist. In this situation, if an individual got into the unlocked medication storage area, took medication that was not prescribed for her, and suffered harm, negligence exists. Negligence in this situation would exist because:

1. There was a duty to keep the medication storage area locked.

2. That duty was broken (breached) by leaving the storage area unlocked so that the individual took the medication.

3. The individual was harmed by taking the wrong medication.

4. The harm to the individual was caused by the UAP's breach of duty (leaving the storage area unlocked).

EXAMPLE 2:

Other chapters in this text discuss the importance of and need for proper documentation. Failure to document or fraudulent documentation might result in negligence or other types of legal liability. Many tasks within the health care field are repetitive. A UAP has to avoid the temptation to take shortcuts. For example, documenting that a medication was given before it is actually given or documenting that a medication was given when it was never administered could create a problem.

harm
Physical or emotional injury.

causation
A connection between a breach of duty and the harm to the individual resulting from that breach.

If an injury results to the individual being cared for as a result of the fraudulent documentation, the UAP may be legally responsible for negligence or other violations. A UAP should also keep in mind that the more times she fails to follow policies and procedures and/or the more shortcuts she takes to complete a task, the greater her chances are of being held legally responsible for negligence or other inappropriate conduct.

As stated earlier, and as seen in the examples, all four elements of negligence must exist for the UAP to be held legally responsible. What happens if all four elements are not met? A UAP needs to keep in mind that an employer always has the right to discipline the UAP if workplace policies and procedures are broken. In example 1, the failure to lock and safeguard medication was the issue. Whether or not an individual was harmed, the employer has the right to take disciplinary action against the UAP who failed to follow the established procedure of keeping medications locked. The same holds true with regard to fraudulent documentation. Even without an injury to an individual, the employer may take disciplinary action. Depending on the circumstances, an employer may fire the UAP, which would result in the loss of her job and perhaps the inability to work in the health care field in the future.

Defenses to Negligence

The best defense to a claim of negligence is to avoid negligence at all costs. The best way to avoid negligence is for the UAP to perform her duties in the manner she was trained and consistent with the Nurse Practice Act as well as workplace policies and procedures. Performing duties consistent with training, laws, policies, and procedures should protect the UAP from a claim of negligence. If the UAP is faced with a claim of negligence, there are a few other defenses worth discussing that she should be aware of.

statute of limitations
A set time period to bring a legal claim in court.

Statute of Limitations   If an individual being cared for, a family member, or some other person was to make a claim for negligence, the claim must be brought within a certain period of time. That time is set by a **statute of limitations**. The time allowed for filing a claim will be different in each state. In some states, an individual may have up to six (6) years to bring a claim. If a claim for negligence is filed after the time set by the statute of limitations, the claim may be thrown out (dismissed).

Respondeat Superior
A legal doctrine that holds the employer or superior responsible for actions of its employees that are performed in the scope of employment.

Respondeat Superior   ***Respondeat Superior*** is a Latin term that, according to *Black's Law Dictionary* (Garner, 2000), means that an employer or supervisor may be held responsible for the acts of an employee that are committed within the scope of her employment. With regard to a negligence action, this means that if a negligence action is brought against a UAP *and* the UAP was doing what a superior told her to do, then the UAP may not be legally responsible. Instead, the employer or a superior could be legally responsible for the negligent act.

A huge caution has to be stated here. For this defense to work, the employer has to have established, written policies and procedures in place that cover the task(s) the UAP was performing. The UAP has to have followed those policies and procedures. If an individual is harmed as a result of the UAP following the established written policies and procedures, then the UAP may use *Respondeat Superior* as a defense. A UAP should also keep in mind that if asked to do something by a superior that the UAP is not trained to do or is not comfortable doing, the UAP should not do so without the proper training and supervision.

Comparative Negligence   Some states, such as Massachusetts, apply **comparative negligence** theories. Under this theory, more than one person is held responsible for the negligent conduct. Comparative negligence examines who is more responsible for committing an act. For example, if a UAP observes another employee administer an incorrect medication and does not report the medication error, both employees could be found negligent. Because the employee administering the wrong medication directly caused an injury, she may be held more legally responsible than the UAP who observed the medication error and failed to report it.

There are many other defenses to a claim of negligence. These are just a couple that the UAP should be aware of. As stated at the beginning of this section, the best defense is not to engage in negligent conduct. Although the UAP may be able to prove in her defense to a negligence claim that she did nothing wrong, it will be very time consuming and expensive to reach that conclusion. Therefore, the UAP should do whatever she can to avoid being negligent. The UAP should do her job as trained and consistent with laws and policies.

> **comparative negligence**
> A legal rule under which a determination is made as to who is more negligent than another when multiple individuals are involved in a situation.

Malpractice

Malpractice is improper, negligent, or unethical behavior that results in harm, injury, or loss to an individual for whom the UAP is caring. In some ways, the word *malpractice* is a catchall phrase. It is not uncommon for readers of this textbook to have heard the phrase, "I am going to sue for malpractice." What the individual is saying is that she intends to sue using either a theory of negligence, intentional act, statutory violation, or some combination of these. In general, the UAP may avoid a claim or action for malpractice by working within her scope of function, following state laws and regulations, following workplace policies and procedures, and doing things the way she was taught. Respecting the rights of those the UAP cares for, being kind and polite, apologizing when need be, correcting any problems that might arise in the course of her work, and working within the scope of her function will all go a long way toward keeping the UAP safe as she goes about her work.

> **malpractice**
> Improper, negligent, or unethical behavior that results in harm, injury, or loss to an individual.

Theft

Whenever a UAP takes anything that does not belong to her, she becomes guilty or liable for **theft**. The item taken need not be expensive to be considered stolen. The disappearance of the item will most likely trigger or cause an investigation to be conducted. If the UAP is caught, she will be liable (held responsible). Theft may result in criminal prosecution, being sued, loss of employment, or all three.

If the theft involves the loss of medication, the investigation may involve the police and/or a special investigation unit from the state. State regulations may require the reporting of missing medications to

> **theft**
> Stealing.

diversion
Theft of controlled substances (C-II through C-V).

aiding and abetting
To assist or help another individual in the committing of an illegal act, crime, or other inappropriate act, including the failure to report unethical and/or illegal acts that one witnesses.

abuse
Intentional mistreatment or misuse.

a specific department. UAPs must know the specific reporting requirements for their work setting. Theft of controlled substances (C-II through C-V) (**diversion**) is a crime punishable by law.

If a UAP sees someone stealing an item(s) or medication and does not report it, the UAP is guilty of **aiding and abetting**. Aiding and abetting is also a criminal offense punishable by law.

Because of the type of work UAPs perform, they must be honest and dependable. Despite careful screening, however, dishonest people are sometimes hired. The UAP must, therefore, be willing to report any wrongdoing that she observes to the appropriate people. While it may not be pleasant to report a colleague or even a friend, the penalties for failing to report can be severe, including the ending of the UAP's career. When in doubt—report! Remember, the UAP is responsible for her own actions, which can include failing to report. Honesty and integrity are the signs of the sincere and conscientious UAP.

Abuse

Abuse can be either an intentional act or the result of neglignece. An employee who commits abuse and, in certain circumstances, employees who fail to report abuse face significant consequences.

Abuse is defined as follows:

- An act or failure to act that is nonaccidental that *causes* actual harm (physical or emotional) or death to an individual in the UAP's care
- An act or failure to act that is nonaccidental that *may cause* harm (physical or emotional) or death to an individual in the UAP's care
- A deliberate failure to act that *causes* actual harm or death to an individual in the UAP's care
- A deliberate failure to act that *may cause* harm or death to an individual in the UAP's care

Abuse may be difficult to detect, or it may be easily noticed. Nevertheless, abuse causes an individual physical harm and/or mental anguish. Several forms of abuse include verbal abuse, sexual abuse, physical abuse, psychological abuse, financial abuse, and involuntary seclusion. In addition, many states or even separate agencies within a state may define abuse in different ways. For example, some states may include neglect, mistreatment, and/or misappropriation of funds in their definitions.

verbal abuse
Use of communication to cause physical or mental harm.

Verbal Abuse **Verbal abuse** may be directed toward an individual, or it may be expressed about the individual. Several examples are:

- Using profanity (swearing) when caring for an individual
- Raising one's voice in anger at an individual
- Calling an individual unpleasant names or treating an individual in a mean way
- Teasing an individual in a demeaning, insulting, or unwelcomed manner

- Making verbal threats
- Using inappropriate words to describe an individual's race or nationality

Sexual Abuse **Sexual abuse** is the use of physical means or verbal threats to force an individual, or attempt to force an individual to perform sexual acts. Several examples are:

- Teasing an individual in a sexual way
- Touching an individual in a sexual way
- Suggesting sexual activity
- Engaging in unwanted sexual activity with an individual

Physical Abuse **Physical abuse** causes physical harm to an individual. Several examples are:

- Handling an individual roughly or using more force than necessary
- Hitting, slapping, pushing, kicking, and pinching an individual as well as other inappropriate touching
- Performing the wrong treatment on the individual, such as administering the wrong medication

Physical abuse may also result from not properly treating an individual where the result is physical harm.

Psychological, or Emotional, Abuse **Psychological**, or emotional, **abuse** includes:

- Threatening an individual with harm
- Threatening to tell something to others that an individual does not want known
- Threatening to withhold care
- Making fun of an individual
- Taking actions against an individual causing the individual to be upset

Financial Abuse **Financial abuse** is the use of money to control an individual. Several examples are:

- Denying an individual access to her checkbook, bank account, finances
- Demanding the individual's monthly checks, such as a Social Security check

Misappropriation of Funds **Misappropriation of funds** is the unauthorized use of an individual's money or funds for personal use. Several examples are:

- Making personal purchases with an individual's cash or bank card
- Stealing money from an individual
- Paying personal bills with an individual's credit card

sexual abuse
Use of physical, psychological, or verbal means to force an individual to perform sexual acts.

physical abuse
Causing physical harm through hitting, pinching, slapping, biting, or other physical contact.

psychological abuse
Causing mental harm by coercing, threatening, belittling, or by other means; also known as emotional abuse.

financial abuse
Use of money to control an individual.

misappropriation of funds
Unauthorized use of an individual's money or funds for personal use.

involuntary seclusion
The separation from others against the wish of the individual.

Involuntary Seclusion **Involuntary seclusion** is the separation of an individual from others against the individual's will. Several examples of this type of abuse are:

- Shutting the door to an individual's room when the individual is confined to bed and wants the door to remain open

- Placing an individual's wheelchair far from others when she wants to be with other people

- Leaving an individual without a way to communicate, such as without a call bell or a phone

- Blocking an individual's access or ability to exit a particular room or location

Separation may be permitted if it is part of an individual's treatment plan or plan of care, such as a time-out to decrease agitation. The decision, however, has to be made before the seclusion occurs. It also has to be part of the written plan of care and requires accurate documentation. In some settings, the plan of care must also have the approval of the licensed health care provider.

neglect
Failure to do what can be done or should be done.

Neglect **Neglect** is the failure to do what can be done or should be done. Neglect can be considered a form of negligence where there may be a duty to perform that was breached but there was no harm necessarily to the individual. Several examples of neglect are:

- Conducting an improper head count and not accounting for a particular individual

- Leaving an individual in the bathtub for too long of a period of time

- Failing to give a telephone message to an individual

- Failing to clean up an individual's room promptly after something spilled

- Failure to carry through on a promise made to an individual (e.g., "Purchase a pack of gum for me while you are at the store.")

- Failure to reconnect medical equipment

mistreatment
Treating an individual wrongly or badly.

Mistreatment **Mistreatment** is the treating of an individual wrongly or badly. This could be very similar to neglect discussed previously but more often than not will involve some form of medical treatment. Several examples of mistreatment are:

- Not checking the temperature of the water prior to a shower; the water is either too hot or too cold (If an injury results, this could rise to the level of negligence. If done intentionally, it would be considered abuse.)

- Applying ointment or cream in the wrong location

- Conducting a manual lift as opposed to a safe lift with proper equipment

- Requiring an individual to continue walking when she complains that her feet hurt

- Forcing an individual to do something she does not want to do

As can be seen from the previous discussions, there are minor or subtle differences between neglect, negligence, mistreatment, and so on. The best way for a UAP to avoid having to deal with the variations of abuse is to *not* engage in any abusive or inappropriate conduct.

If the UAP observes or suspects that an individual in her care is being abused by others, she must discuss this matter with her supervisor and report the abuse to the proper authorities, if need be. Laws require that a health care provider who suspects or observes abuse must report the situation so that the individual may be protected. This includes UAPs. In some states, health care providers who do not report abuse are held as guilty or liable as the abusing person.

WORKPLACE POLICIES AND PROCEDURES

Although workplace policies and procedures are not necessarily legal standards, they are still important. The UAP needs to understand that not following workplace polices and procedures may have negative consequences. The UAP may be disciplined by an employer for failing to follow rules and procedures. Depending on the situation or the number of times rules are broken, the UAP could be fired. In addition to losing a job, the UAP might also lose the ability to work in other health care settings. Following workplace policies and procedures should be taken as seriously as following the law.

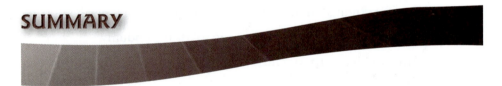

SUMMARY

Regardless of where care is being provided, all individuals have certain rights granted to them by law. Ethical and legal standards exist to protect these individuals and to protect caregivers. It is part of the UAP's role to follow these standards at all times. If for some reason a UAP finds herself in a position where this seems impossible to do, it is then the UAP's responsibility to seek guidance from someone in authority. If the UAP witnesses a situation that is against an individual's right or that breaks a standard, then it is the responsibility of the UAP to report that situation to the appropriate individual and/or agency.

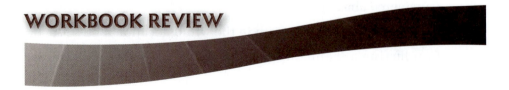

WORKBOOK REVIEW

Go to the workbook and complete the exercises for Chapter 3.

REVIEW QUESTIONS

1. The Omnibus Budget Reconciliation Act (OBRA) was passed by the federal government to:
   a. balance the federal budget
   b. legislate the rights of residents in skilled nursing facilities
   c. legislate the rights of people on a budget
   d. legislate the rights of actors

2. The Resident's Bill of Rights is given to:
   a. any individual admitted to a skilled nursing facility, such as a nursing home
   b. any individual admitted to the hospital, day surgery, or an outpatient clinic
   c. any individual who receives home care services
   d. any individual who is a resident of the United States

3. The Patient Care Partnership: Understanding Expectations, Rights and Responsibilities is given to:
   a. any individual admitted to a skilled nursing facility, such as a nursing home
   b. any individual admitted to the hospital, day surgery, or an outpatient clinic
   c. any individual who receives home care services
   d. any individual who is a resident of the United States

4. The Client's Bill of Rights is given to:
   a. any individual admitted to a skilled nursing facility, such as a nursing home
   b. any individual admitted to the hospital, day surgery, or an outpatient clinic
   c. any individual who receives home care services
   d. any individual who is a resident of the United States

5. Each of the Bill of Rights documents in health care includes:
   a. an individual's right to have visitors whenever she wishes
   b. an individual's right to choose her caregiver daily
   c. an individual's right to freedom
   d. an individual's right to be advised about advanced directives

6. Informed consent means that:
   a. an individual makes a decision about a procedure only after knowing all the information about the procedure, its risks, and its benefits
   b. an individual has to decide on a procedure without understanding it
   c. an individual has to inform her caregiver about her medical history
   d. an individual has to inform her family about her decisions

7. An advance directive is:
   a. a way of advancing in the workplace
   b. a document stating an individual's wishes for treatment or no treatment, completed before it is needed
   c. a document used to file a complaint
   d. a document that identifies an individual's rights

8. A grievance is:
   a. a situation in which an individual is grieving
   b. what happens when an individual complains to her family
   c. a situation in which an individual wishes to file a complaint against the facility where the UAP works, against individuals providing care, or both
   d. what happens when you complain to a coworker

9. Ethical standards are:
   a. guides to legal behavior
   b. guides to moral behavior
   c. problems brought to an ethics committee
   d. suggestions made by an ethics committee

10. Legal standards are:
   a. guides to legal behavior
   b. guides to moral behavior
   c. the promise to do no harm when giving care
   d. fines that are a result of breaking the law

11. Ethical and legal standards were established to guarantee that:
   a. the UAP cannot be fired for negligence
   b. the ethics committee can address issues in an appropriate manner
   c. safe, quality care is given by the UAP
   d. a supervisor can force the UAP to do a task for which she has not been trained

12. A facility's ethics committee is a group of individuals who:
   a. solve every conflict in the facility
   b. provide advice on what would be the best care for an individual
   c. write the facility's policies and procedures
   d. try to convince staff members to get along during work hours

13. The Health Insurance Portability and Accountability Act, or HIPAA, helps to guarantee that:
   a. an individual's health information is protected and kept private
   b. a UAP may share an individual's health information with her coworkers
   c. a UAP may give out an individual's health information to public authorities
   d. a UAP may share an individual's health reports with people who ask

14. To avoid breaking the law, a UAP must:
   a. carry out procedures that she has not been trained to do
   b. proceed with a task even if she does not understand the directions
   c. get her job done in any way possible
   d. work within her scope of function at all times

15. One example of an intentional act is:
   a. discrimination
   b. civil liability
   c. negligence
   d. carelessness

16. Negligence is:
   a. an intent to do harm to an individual
   b. a careless accident that causes harm to an individual
   c. being held responsible for inappropriate behavior
   d. being held responsible for illegal activity

17. The standard of care that a UAP must follow is established by:
   a. the workplace ethics committee
   b. the UAP's clinical supervisor
   c. each state's Nurse Practice Act and workplace policies
   d. federal and state governments

18. For a UAP, the best defense to a claim of negligence is:
   a. to work within her scope of function, following laws and workplace policies
   b. to confide in coworkers and ask them not to report acts of negligence
   c. to leave her job and try to get hired at another facility
   d. to bring her case to the ethics committee

19. Abuse is:
   a. the accidental mistreatment of an individual
   b. an act that causes an individual physical harm and/or mental anguish
   c. carelessness
   d. a situation in which an individual is grieving

CLINICAL SCENARIOS

1. While you are at work, Mrs. Gleason's granddaughter approaches you in the hall with questions about her grandmother's condition. Should you answer them? If so, where would you do this? If not, what should you do?

2. As you are walking toward Mr. Blake's room, you hear yelling. When you get to his door, you see that he is yelling at his caregiver, who then slaps him. What do you do? In what ways is this an ethical issue? In what ways is this a legal issue?

3. Sue Smythe is a UAP employed by Medical Care Services. Her employer has a policy that failure to administer medications may result in discipline, including termination from employment. UAP Smythe is required to administer medications to Bill Juenes, who has a seizure disorder. His licensed HCP has ordered Dilantin 100 mg po three times a day. UAP Smythe fails to administer Bill's Dilantin as ordered for two (2) days. As a result, Mr. Juenes has convulsions, falls out of his bed, and is permanently injured. Mr. Juenes files a complaint in court claiming that Sue Smythe was negligent.

a. Was UAP Smythe negligent in failing to administer Dilantin to Mr. Juenes?

b. What was the duty to Mr. Juenes?

c. What duty, if any, was breached?

d. What harm, if any, was caused to Mr. Juenes?

e. Was there causation between a breach of duty and Mr. Juenes's injury?

f. Did Sue Smythe violate workplace policies and procedures?

g. Could Sue Smythe be disciplined for violating the workplace policies and procedures?

4. Jeff Greene is a UAP employed by Advanced Care Services. His employer has a policy that failure to administer medications may result in discipline, including termination from employment. UAP Greene is required to administer medications to Sally Meade. Sally's licensed HCP has ordered Glucophage 500 mg po twice a day. Give with breakfast and dinner. At 10:00 in the evening, UAP Greene realizes that he failed to administer Sally's dose of Glucophage at dinner. Since Sally is sleeping, he holds the medication without notifying Sally's licensed HCP. Ms. Meade sleeps through the night without any complications due to the missed dose. Ms. Meade's blood glucose level in the morning is 337 mg/dl, much higher than is normal for her. Ms. Meade learns that she did not get her medication at dinner the night before. Ms. Meade tells her brother, who is an attorney, what happened. Her brother files a complaint in court claiming that Jeff Greene was negligent.

a. Was UAP Greene negligent in failing to administer Glucophage to Sally Meade?

b. What was the duty to Sally Meade?

c. What duty, if any, was breached?

d. What harm, if any, was caused to Sally Meade?

e. Did Jeff Greene violate workplace policies and procedures?

f. Could Jeff Green be disciplined for violating the workplace policies and procedures?

MODULE II
Medication Fundamentals

Chapter 4
Introduction to Medications

Learning Objectives

After reading this chapter and completing the review questions, you should be able to:

1. Spell and define terms.
2. Identify four types of medication names.
3. Explain the difference between the brand or trade name and the generic name. Give examples of each.
4. Describe the three basic types of medication preparation.
5. List five types of semisolid and solid medications.
6. List five types of liquid medications.
7. Describe three of the main therapeutic actions of medications.
8. Explain the difference between a side effect, an adverse reaction, and a medication interaction.
9. List the factors a licensed health care provider takes into consideration when prescribing a medication.
10. Choose the medication reference book or material that would be easiest to use.

Key Terms

adverse reaction	caplet	diagnostic use	effervescent tablets
aerosols	capsule	divided dose	elixirs
agonist action	chemical name	dosage	emulsions
antagonist action	chewable tablets	dose	enteric-coated tablets
average dose	curative use	drug	generic equivalents
buccal tablets	depressants	drug substitution laws	generic name

geriatric clients or patients	minimum dose	replacement use	systemic action
idiosyncrasies	mixtures	scored tablets	tablet
initial dose	official name	selective action	therapeutic dose
layered tablets	ointment	side effect	therapeutic use
lethal dose	palliative use	solutions	timed-release medication
liniments	pediatric clients or patients	spansule	tinctures
local action	pharmacodynamics	specific action	topical
lotions	pharmacokinetics	sprays	toxic dose
lozenge	pharmacology	stimulants	trade name
maintenance dose	preventive use	sublingual tablets	troche
maximum dose	prophylactic use	suppository	unit dose
medication interaction	remote action	suspensions	vaginal tablets
		syrups	

INTRODUCTION

According to the American Society for Pharmacology and Experimental Therapeutics (2008), **pharmacology** is the science dealing with the effects of drugs on living things. Pharmacology is made up of two main areas: pharmacodynamics and pharmacokinetics. **Pharmacodynamics** is the study of how drugs act on living things. **Pharmacokinetics** deals with the study of the actions of drugs within the body. There are further subspecialty areas in pharmacology. These areas include, but are not limited to:

> **pharmacology**
> The science dealing with the effects of drugs on living things.
>
> **pharmacodynamics**
> The study of drugs and their actions on living things.
>
> **pharmacokinetics**
> Deals with the study of the metabolism and action of drugs within the body.

1. The study of the effects of drugs on behavior (behavioral pharmacology)

2. The study of the effects of drugs on the heart, the vascular system, and those parts of the nervous and endocrine systems that participate in regulating cardiovascular function (cardiovascular pharmacology)

3. The study of drugs and their relationships to the treatment of disease (clinical pharmacology)

4. The area of pharmacology that deals with drugs used for the treatment of microbial infections and malignancies (cancer) (chemotherapy)

5. The study of actions of drugs that are either hormones or hormone derivatives or drugs that may modify the actions of normally secreted hormones (endocrine pharmacology)

6. The study of drugs that modify the functions of the nervous system, including the brain, the spinal cord, and the nerves that communicate with all parts of the body (neuropharmacology)

7. The study of the adverse or toxic effects of drugs and other chemical agents (toxicology)

A **drug** is a substance used in medicine that may affect how the body works. There are six uses for these drugs, or what are commonly called medications:

- **Therapeutic use:** Medications used in the treatment of diseases, such as insulin to treat diabetes

- **Diagnostic use:** Medications used in radiology (X-ray) to allow a physician to see the location of a tumor or other disease process, such as IVP dye

- **Curative use:** Medications that kill or remove the cause of a disease, such as an antibiotic

- **Replacement use:** Medications, such as hormones and vitamins that are used to replace substances that are normally found in the body, such as calcium and estrogen

- **Preventive or prophylactic use:** Medications, such as immunizations, that are used to prevent or lessen the severity of a disease, such as flu shots

- **Palliative use:** Medications used to promote the quality of life by relieving or soothing the symptoms of a disease or disorder without curing it

IDENTIFYING MEDICATION NAMES

Most medications have the following four types of names:

1. **Generic name:** This is the common or general name used for the medication. It is written with an initial lowercase letter, never capitalized. An example is acetaminophen.

2. **Trade name:** This is the formal name by which a pharmaceutical company identifies and sells its product. The trade name is copyrighted and used only by that company. It is written with a capitalized first letter. The trade name is more commonly called the brand name. The symbol of an "R" with a circle around it—®—is usually found after its name on labels and in references to the medication. This symbol stands for "registered trademark." The trade name for acetaminophen is Tylenol.

3. **Chemical name:** This is usually a very long, difficult name to say and is of little concern to the health care worker. It is the molecular (chemical) formula for the medication. The chemical name for acetaminophen is 4-hydroxyacetanilide.

4. **Official name:** This is the name of the medication as it appears in the official reference, the USP/NF. It is usually the same as the generic name. The official name for acetaminophen is acetaminophen.

Generic names and brand (trade) names for medications can be compared to the various names of grocery products. Two examples of generic names are orange juice and detergent. Brand names for orange

---

drug
A substance used in medicine that may affect how the body works.

generic name
The common or general name used for a medication.

trade name
The brand name of a medication.

chemical name
The molecular (chemical) formula for the medication.

official name
The name of the medication as it appears in the official reference, usually the same as the generic name.

juice are Sunkist, Minute Maid, and Tropicana. Brand names for detergent are Wisk, All, and Tide. While there is only one generic name, there may be many brand names.

When a company develops a new medication, it gives a generic name to the medication. After the FDA has tested and approved the medication, the pharmaceutical company gives the medication a brand name. This is usually something short and easy to remember for marketing purposes.

For seventeen (17) years from the time the company submits an application to the FDA for approval, the company has exclusive rights to sell the medication. Once the medication is approved by the FDA, the medication is listed in the USP/NF under its official name.

Once seventeen (17) years have passed and the patent has expired, other companies may begin to use the same chemical formula to make that specific generic medication for sale. Each company may give the medication its own brand name. For example:

GENERIC NAME	TRADE NAME
Tetracycline hydrochloride	Achromycin V (Lederle Labs)
	Sumycin (Apothecon)
	Tetracycline HCl (Richlyn)*

*Some companies choose to simply market the medication by its generic name.

Most states have passed legislation encouraging licensed health care providers to allow pharmacists to fill prescriptions with **generic equivalents**. Generic equivalents cost less than brand-name medications. Most times the generics are "equivalent," or equal, in effectiveness. The specific **drug substitution laws** that allow this exchange may vary from state to state. The UAP needs to know the laws in his state.

Licensed health care providers often have personal preferences. Even though the basic medication is the same in the generic equivalents, the "fillers," or other ingredients that are used in the medication, may be slightly different. This difference may affect how quickly the medication dissolves or takes effect. Dyes in some generic medications may also change the effects and may even cause an allergic response in some individuals. If a licensed health care provider chooses to have the brand-name medication given to his patient instead of the generic equivalent, the provider need only write "no substitutions" on the prescription.

It should also be noted that a number might be part of the brand name. The number often refers to an amount of one of the generic ingredients and helps to tell it from an almost identical medication. For example:

generic equivalents
Generic medications that cost less than trade- or brand-name medications but that are "equivalent," or equal, in effectiveness.

drug substitution laws
Laws that allow generic medications to be substituted for trade-name medications.

TRADE NAME	GENERIC NAME AND AMOUNT
Empirin	Aspirin, 325 mg
Empirin No. 1	Aspirin, 325 mg Codeine phosphate, 7.5 mg
Empirin No. 2	Aspirin, 325 mg Codeine phosphate, 15 mg

CLASSIFICATION OF MEDICATIONS

Medications may be subclassified or subgrouped in many ways. Two common ways to group medications are by preparation and by therapeutic action (effect). Medications come in three basic types of preparations: semisolids, solids, and liquids. How easily a medication can be dissolved largely determines which form it is in. For example, acetaminophen comes in tablets, caplets, suppositories, and liquid.

Following are some of the different types of semisolid and solid preparations:

Tablet	A small, solid, compressed form of medication (Figure 4-1)
Capsule	A small two-part container usually made of gelatin that contains medication (Figure 4-1)
Caplet	A type of solid medication that has the same size and shape of a capsule but has the consistency of a tablet
Timed-release medication	A medication containing particles of medication that have various coatings that differ in the amount of time needed before the coatings dissolve; made to deliver a dose of medication over an extended period of time; cannot be crushed or chewed
Troche	A hard, circular or oblong piece of medication with a candylike base
Lozenge	A hard, circular or oblong piece of medication with a candylike base
Spansule	A capsule made to release medication at a steady rate over a period of hours
Suppository	A semisolid medication made for administration into the rectum, vagina, or urethra
Ointment	A type of **topical** medication

Following are some of the different types of tablets available:

Buccal tablets	Are placed in the mouth between the cheek and gum, where they dissolve
Chewable tablets	Are made to be chewed and then swallowed
Effervescent tablets	When placed in water, release active ingredients making a solution
Enteric-coated tablets	Are dissolved in the small intestine (Figure 4-1)
Layered tablets	Have two or more layers of medication
Scored tablets	The surface of the tablets have a groove or slit cut into them, making it easy for the tablet to be broken into halves or quarters (Figure 4-1)
Sublingual tablets	Are placed under the tongue, where they dissolve
Vaginal tablets	Are placed into the vagina with an applicator; once placed, they dissolve in the vagina

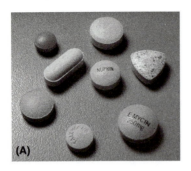
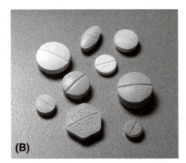
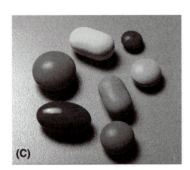
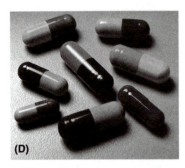
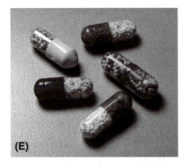
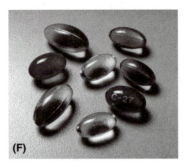

Figure 4-1 Solid dosage forms. A) tablets; B) scored tablets; C) enteric-coated tablets; D) capsules; E) controlled release capsules; F) gelatin capsules *(Delmar/Cengage Learning)*

Liquid preparations contain a medication that has been dissolved or suspended. When prescribed or ordered for internal use, the medication is absorbed through the stomach or intestinal walls. Following are some of the different types of liquid preparations:

Aerosols	May contain medications, ointments, creams, lotions, powders, or liquids; are packaged in pressurized containers; an example is an inhaler used to treat asthma
Elixirs	Medications dissolved in a solution of alcohol and water that has been sweetened and flavored (Note that some elixirs today are nonalcoholic.)
Emulsions	Fine droplets of oil in water or water in oil
Liniments	Medications used externally, with massage, to produce a feeling of heat to an area of the body
Lotions	Medications used externally, without massage, to treat skin conditions; may be a clear solution, suspension, or emulsion
Mixtures and suspensions	Medications that have been mixed with a liquid but are not dissolved in it
Solutions	One or more medications dissolved in an appropriate liquid
Sprays	Medications used mainly to treat nose and throat conditions
Syrups	Medications mixed in a concentrated solution of sugar and water, then flavored with a substance
Tinctures	Medications dissolved in alcohol or alcohol and water

The therapeutic action (effect) of the medication involves the method of treating, relieving, or getting results with the effect of the medication on the body. Table 4-1 is a reference of selected medications with their classification, their definitions with the actions (effects) on the body, and examples of the medications. Medications that affect the body in similar ways are listed under the same classification.

Some medications may have more than one therapeutic effect on the body. These medications are therefore listed under several different classifications. For example, aspirin has a variety of different effects on the body. Aspirin may be given as a blood thinner (anticoagulant), to relieve pain (analgesic), to reduce fever (antipyretic), or to reduce inflammation of tissues (anti-inflammatory). Therefore, aspirin is listed under all multiple classifications in Table 4-1.

Table 4-1 Reference Table of Selected Medications with Classifications and Definitions

CLASSIFICATION	DEFINITION WITH ACTION (EFFECT) ON THE BODY	EXAMPLES OF MEDICATION(S)	
Acne medications	Medications used to treat acne	Benzac Accutane Sotret	
Alpha blockers	Medications that relax the muscles in the neck of the bladder, thereby decreasing the symptoms of BPH and increasing the passing of urine	Cardura Flomax Hytrin	
Analgesics	Medications used to relieve pain caused by many different conditions	Narcotic: Codiene Duragesic Vicodin Dilaudid Morphine	Nonnarcotic: Tylenol Advil Aspirin
Analgesic-antipyretics	Medications that (1) relieve pain and (2) reduce fever	Aspirin Tylenol Excedrin Fioricet	
Androgens	Male hormones that produce male characteristics; also used to treat metastatic breast cancer, endometriosis, and fibrocystic breast disease in women	Danocrine Android Estratest	
Anesthetics	Medications used to (1) prevent pain, (2) relax muscles, and (3) induce lack of sensation during surgery and other procedures	Marcaine HCL Xylocaine HCL Novocain	
Antacids	Medications that neutralize hydrochloric acid in the stomach; used to (1) treat indigestion, heartburn, and pain; (2) to promote healing of ulcers; and (3) to manage esophageal reflux	Tums Riopan Maalox Mylanta	
Antiandrogens	Medications that decrease the size of the prostate, thereby decreasing the symptoms of BPH and the urinary obstruction caused by enlargement of the prostate	Proscar Avodart	
Antianxiety	Medications that counteract or relieve anxiety; also used for sedation before some medical treatments	Xanax Valium Ativan BuSpar	

(continues)

Table 4-1 Reference Table of Selected Medications with Classifications and Definitions—*continued*

CLASSIFICATION	DEFINITION WITH ACTION (EFFECT) ON THE BODY	EXAMPLES OF MEDICATION(S)
Antiarrhythmics	Medications used to treat an arrhythmia (irregular heartbeat)	Verapamil Inderal Pronestyl Norpace
Antibacterials	Medications used to treat bacterial infections	Bactrim Septra
Antibiotics	Medications used to treat infectious diseases	Keflex Erythromycin Amoxicillin Cipro Achromycin
Anticoagulants	Medications that prevent or delay clotting of the blood	Coumadin Aspirin
Anticonvulsants	Medications used to treat seizures in individuals with epilepsy	Tegretol Topamax Dilantin Phenobarbitol
Antidepressants	Medications that elevate mood	Elavil Nardil Celexa Wellbutrin
Antidiabetics (oral)	Medications that are used to manage and treat non–insulin-dependent diabetes mellitus (NIDDM; TYPE 2 diabetes)	Diabinese Glucotrol Diabeta Precose Glucophage
Antidiarrheals	Medications that decrease the number of loose, watery stools an individual is having	Lomotil Kaopectolin Imodium
Antiemetics	Medications that prevent or stop vomiting	Reglan Compazine Tigan Anzemet Zofran
Antiflatulents	Medications used to treat (1) the symptoms of gastric bloating and (2) pain from flatus after surgery	Mylicon
Antifungals	Medications that control conditions caused by fungi	Lotrimin Mycelex Diflucan Monistat
Antiglaucoma medications	Medications used to treat glaucoma	Diamox Isopto Carpine Timoptic Propine Xalatan

Table 4-1 Reference Table of Selected Medications with Classifications and Definitions—*continued*

CLASSIFICATION	DEFINITION WITH ACTION (EFFECT) ON THE BODY	EXAMPLES OF MEDICATION(S)
Antihelmintics	Medications used to treat helminthiasis, an infestation of the intestine with parasitic worms	Stromectrol Vermox Mintezol
Antihistamines	Medications that relieve allergy symptoms	Benadryl Allergy Zyrtec Clarinex Allegra
Antihypertensives	Medications used to treat hypertension (high blood pressure)	Lopressor Norvasc Vasotec Catapres
Anti-infectives	Medications that prevent and treat infections	Trimpex Furadantin Cipro, CiproXR
Anti-inflammatory medications	Medications used to relieve inflammation	Indocin Motrin Acular Aspirin
Antilipidemics	Medications used to lower high blood levels of lipids in the blood	Lipitor Zocor Lopid Zetia
Antimanics (mood stabilizers)	Medications that treat the manic phase of bipolar disorder	Lithium Tegretol Depakote Symbyax
Antimigraine	Medications used to treat migraine headaches	Relpax Maxalt Imitrex
Antineoplastics	Medications that destroy abnormal, damaged, cancer cells (malignant cells)	Cytoxan Oncovin Blenoxane Nolvadex
Antiparkinsonian	Medications used to relieve the symptoms of Parkinson disease; also used to treat Parkinson-like side effects from antipsychotic medications	Sinemet Parlodel Cogentin Symmetrel
Antipruritics	Medications that relieve itching	Solarcaine Benadryl Cortaid
Antiprotozoals	Medications used to treat diseases caused by parasites, such as malaria	Flagyl Mepron Plaquenil

(continues)

Table 4-1 Reference Table of Selected Medications with Classifications and Definitions—*continued*

CLASSIFICATION	DEFINITION WITH ACTION (EFFECT) ON THE BODY	EXAMPLES OF MEDICATION(S)
Antipsychotics	Medications that modify psychotic behavior; also called neuroleptics	Thorazine Navane Prolixin Zyprexa Risperdal
Antispasmodics	Medications that prevent spasms of the urinary bladder	Detrol Ditropan, Ditropan XL Urispas
Antithyroid	Medications used for (1) treatment of hyperthyroidism, (2) preparation for removal of the thyroid, and (3) radioactive iodine therapy	Tapazole PTU Thyro-Block
Antitubercular	Medications used to treat tuberculosis	Seromycin Laniazid Rifadin
Antitussives	Medications that (1) prevent coughing in an individual who does not need to have a productive cough and (2) allow an individual to sleep better, decreasing fatigue	Robitussin AC Tussi-Organidin NR Tessalon Benylin Robitussin DM
Antivirals	Medications used to treat viral infections	Tamiflu Relenza Zovirax Valtrex
Bisphosphonates	Medications that directly act to (1) increase bone thickness at the hip and spine and (2) decrease first fractures and future fractures	Fosamax Boniva Actonel
Bronchodilators	Medications that open an individual's airways, allowing him or her to breathe better	Slophyllin Theo-dur
Burn medications	Medications used to treat burns	Furacin Silvadene
Cardiac glycoside	Medications that (1) strengthen the heartbeat, (2) slow the heart rate (pulse), and (3) improve the contractions of the heart muscle as it pumps blood throughout the body	Lanoxin Lanoxicaps
Cholinesterase inhibitors	Medications that prevent the breakdown of acetylcholine in the brain; used to treat Alzheimer's disease	Cognex Aricept Exelon
Corticosteroids	Medications used to treat asthma and some forms of COPD.	Beconase AQ Azmacort Nasonex Flonase Aerobid

Table 4-1 Reference Table of Selected Medications with Classifications and Definitions—*continued*

CLASSIFICATION	DEFINITION WITH ACTION (EFFECT) ON THE BODY	EXAMPLES OF MEDICATION(S)
Cox 2 inhibitors	Medications that relieve inflammation; pose less risk for GI bleeding and fewer gastric problems than NSAIDs.	Celebrex
Decongestants	Medications that shrink the swollen linings of the respiratory tract and open nasal passages; used to relieve symptoms of nasal congestion	Afrin Allerest Sudafed Neosynephrine
Demulcents	Medications that soothe irritation	A&D Ointment Desitin
Disease-modifying antirheumatics (DMARDs)	Medications used to treat rheumatoid arthritis	Enbrel Humira Arava Rheumatrex
Diuretics	Medications that increase urine output and relieve or prevent edema	Lasix Aldactone Dyazide Bumex
Emollients	Medications that soothe irritation	A&D ointment Desitin
Estrogens	Female hormones that produce female characteristics; used in hormone replacement therapy and contraceptives and to treat various diseases	Estrace Premarin Estratab
Expectorants	Medications that (1) help loosen mucus, (2) liquify bronchial secretions, and (3) remove phlegm (sputum)	Mucinex Robitussin
Gastrointestinal protectants	Medications that protect the lining of the stomach	Carafate Cytotec
Histamine H$_2$ blockers	Medications used for short-term relief of indigestion, heartburn, gastroesophageal reflux disease (GERD), upper GI bleeding, and esophagitis	Tagamet Pepcid Zantac
Hypnotic	A medication that causes sleep	Dalmane Restoril Lunesta Ambien
Keratolytics	Medications that control conditions of abnormal scaling or peeling of the skin	Zetar Tegrin Neutrogena Podophyllin
Laxatives	Medications that aid the body in the elimination of waste	Metamucil Milk of Magnesia Senokot Dulcolox Correctol

(continues)

Table 4-1 Reference Table of Selected Medications with Classifications and Definitions—*continued*

CLASSIFICATION	DEFINITION WITH ACTION (EFFECT) ON THE BODY	EXAMPLES OF MEDICATION(S)
Muscle relaxants	Medications that relax the muscles of the body; used to treat pain, muscle spasms, and other conditions affecting the muscles of the body	Soma Flexeril Dantrium
Mydriatics	Medications used to dilate the pupil	Atropine Cyclogyl Neo-Synephrine
Muscle stimulants	Medications used to treat the symptoms of progressive musculoskeletal disorders, such as myasthenia gravis	Prostigmin
NMDA receptor antagonist	Medications used to treat Alzheimer's disease	Namenda
Nonsteroidal anti-inflammatory medications (NSAIDs)	Medications used to treat inflammation	Motrin, Advil Indocin Naprosyn, Aleve Clinoril
Parasympatholytics	Medications that cause local bronchodilation	Atrovent spiriva
Pediculicides	Medications that treat lice	Acticin Nix Kwell RID
Phosphodiesterase inhibitors	Medications used to treat erectile dysfunction	Viagra Levtitra Cialis
Platelet inhibitors	Medications that stop platelets from sticking together to form clots	Ecotrin Plavix Persantine
Progestins	Synthetic medications that act like the hormone progesterone; used as contraceptives and to treat various diseases	Provera Depo-Provera Megace
Proton pump inhibitors	Medications that decreases secretion of gastric acid; used for short-term relief of GERD, confirmed gastric and duodenal ulcer, erosive esophagitis, and heartburn	Nexium Prevacid Prilosec
Scabicides	Medications that treat scabies	Acticin Nix Kwell RID
Sedative	A medication that calms, soothes, or quiets without causing sleep	Luminal Mebaral Amytal Seconal
Selective estrogen-receptor modifiers	Medications that (1) increase bone thickness and (2) reduce fractures; used to treat osteoporosis	Evista Miacalcin

Table 4-1 Reference Table of Selected Medications with Classifications and Definitions—*continued*

CLASSIFICATION	DEFINITION WITH ACTION (EFFECT) ON THE BODY	EXAMPLES OF MEDICATION(S)
Sympathomimetics	Medications that (1) relieve spasms in the air passages of the lungs and (2) increase the aeration of the lungs; strong bronchodilators with serious side effects	Proventil Volmax Isuprel Alupent
Thyroid medications	Medications used to (1) treat hypothyroidism and for replacement therapy and (2) treatment after the thyroid gland has been surgically removed or the gland has undergone radiological treatment to destroy its cells	Synthroid Levoxyl
Vasoconstrictors	Medications that (1) constrict blood vessels and (2) increase blood pressure	Levophed
Vasodilators	Medications that (1) dilate (enlarge) blood vessels and (2) increase their ability to carry blood; commonly used to treat angina pectoris	Nitrostat Tabs Isordil Nitro-Dur Transderm-Nitro
Wax emulsifiers	Medications used to remove a buildup of wax from an individual's ear(s)	Debrox Murine Earwax Removal System
Xanthines	Medications that cause bronchodilation; used for acute asthma attacks	Uniphyl Theo-24

Source: Based on Deter and Polesky (1999), pp. 65–69.

MAIN THERAPEUTIC ACTIONS OF MEDICATIONS

Medications are prescribed because of the specific action(s) that result when they are administered. The following terms are used to describe medications based on the medication's action(s) on the body:

- **Agonist action**: A medication mixes with special sites on specific cells, causing a response to the medication.

- **Antagonist action**: A medication blocks the effect of a second medication through different actions in the body.

- **Local action**: A term used to describe an external medication that is made to act on an area of the body to which it is applied; for example, hydrocortisone ointment is often applied to areas of poison ivy to control itching and inflammation.

- **Remote action**: A term used to describe a medication affecting a part of the body that is away from the area where it is administered; for example, apomorphine injection is administered in the arm to stimulate the vomiting center in the brain.

- **Selective action**: A medication acts on certain body tissues or on a specific body part; these medications are mainly stimulants and depressants.

local action
A term used to describe an external medication that is made to act on an area of the body to which it is applied.

remote action
A term used to describe a medication affecting a part of the body that is away from the area where it is administered.

- **Stimulants**: Medications that increase actions in the body; an example is Ritalin, which acts to stimulate the cerebrum, a part of the brain.
- **Depressants**: Medications that decrease actions in the body; an example is oxycodone, which acts to slow down the respiratory center in the brain.

- **Specific action**: A term used to describe a medication that has a particular effect on certain bacteria or other pathogens; for example, the action of the medication primaquine on the malarial parasite.

- **Systemic action**: A term used to describe a medication that, once absorbed or injected into the bloodstream, is carried throughout the entire body, affecting all the cells.

Unwanted Actions of Medications

Three common types of unwanted actions by medications are:

1. Side effect
2. Adverse reaction
3. Drug interaction

At times, medications have actions or effects that are not wanted or expected. For example, antibiotics given orally (by mouth) may upset the intestinal tract (bowels) and cause diarrhea. This type of effect is called a **side effect**. A side effect is an unwanted action or effect of a medication. A side effect may limit the usefulness of the medication.

An **adverse reaction** is an unwanted action or effect of a medication that is harmful to the body. For example, the most common adverse reactions for Demerol include light-headedness, dizziness, sedation, nausea, and sweating.

A **medication interaction** may occur when one medication increases or decreases the effect of another medication. This increase or decrease action may or may not be wanted. Medications may also interact with foods, alcohol, tobacco, and/or other substances. It is recommended that UAP consult a pharmacist any time there is the possibility of a medication interaction.

MEDICATION DOSAGE

The **dosage or dose** is the amount of medication that is prescribed (ordered) for administration. When prescribing (ordering) a medication, the licensed health care provider considers the following factors:

1. Weight, sex, ethnicity, and age of the individual
2. Pregnancy and breast feeding
3. The physical and emotional condition of the individual
4. The disease process

systemic action
A term used to describe a medication that, once absorbed or injected into the bloodstream, is carried throughout the entire body, affecting all the cells.

side effect
An unwanted action or effect of a medication.

adverse reaction
An unwanted action or effect of a medication that is harmful to the body.

medication interaction
The interaction between two or more medications that results in the increase, decrease, or cancellation of the effects of one or more of the medications.

dosage or dose
The amount of medication that is prescribed (ordered) for administration.

5. The presence of other disease processes

6. The bacteria causing the infection and the severity of the infection

7. The individual's past medical history, allergies, **idiosyncrasies**, and so forth

8. The safest method, route, time, and amount to get the desired maximum result

idiosyncrasies
Special characteristics of an individual.

Age

The usual adult dose is typically for individuals who are 20 to 60 years old. Infants, children, teenagers (adolescents), and the elderly need individualized doses. Individuals between the ages of 16 and 20 years are transitioning from teenagers to young adults. This group may or may not take the usual adult dose, depending on their individual characteristics, their illness, and their overall medical and health condition.

Infants, children, and teenagers are known as **pediatric clients or patients**. This group is divided into three age-groups:

pediatric clients or patients
Infants, children, and teenagers.

- Newborn: 0 to 4 weeks old

- Infant: 5 to 52 weeks old

- Child: 1 to 16 years old with teenagers being a subgroup of 12 to 16 years old

These individuals require a smaller amount of medication. Their bodies are structured differently and work differently. The dosage is often determined by their body weight rather than their age.

The elderly are known as **geriatric clients or patients**. Because aging occurs differently from individual to individual, this group is not divided into specific age-groups. An individual who is 65 years old may or may not be considered a geriatric client based on his overall condition. A licensed health care provider, therefore, needs to consider all factors when determining medication dosages for an elder, including several special factors, such as:

geriatric clients or patients
Individuals age 65 years old and older; elderly.

- Any changes that may have occurred because of the aging process or disease processes

- Sensitivity to medications

- Number of medications the individual is taking

- Psychosocial changes

- Forgetfulness and/or memory loss

- Cost of the medication

- Individual's living conditions

- Poor fluid and/or nutritional intake

Common Terms Used to Describe Dosages/Doses

The following terms are often used to describe doses of medications:

Average dose	The amount of medication proven most effective with the least amount of side effects
Divided dose	Portions of the dose administered over a period of time
Initial dose	The first dose administered of a medication
Lethal dose	The amount of medication that could kill an individual
Maintenance dose	The amount of medication that will keep medication at a therapeutic level in an individual's bloodstream
Maximum dose	The largest amount of a medication that can be safely administered to an individual
Minimum dose	The smallest amount of medication that can be administered to an individual that will be effective
Therapeutic dose	The amount of medication needed to produce the desired effect
Toxic dose	The amount of medication that causes signs and symptoms of poisoning
Unit dose	A premeasured amount of a medication, individually packaged on a single-dose basis

MEDICATION REFERENCES FOR THE UAP

The *Physician's Desk Reference* (PDR) is one of the most widely used reference books for medications today. It is found in most medical settings. As the name indicates, however, it is mainly for physicians. Today, there are many new reference books and materials available that provide basic, easy-to-understand, and readily accessible information. Several references are in Table 4-2.

Table 4-2 Description of Reference Books

NAME OF BOOK	STRENGTHS	WEAKNESSES
*Physician's Desk Reference** (PDR)	• All medications are cross-referenced by (1) company name, (2) trade names and generic names, and (3) drug classification • Includes pictures of many medications • Includes list of all Poison Control Centers, with addresses and phone numbers • Includes a description of substances used for medical testing, such as barium and X-ray dyes	• Written for physicians and pharmacists • Has lengthy descriptions of medications • Difficult to understand • Difficult to quickly find basic information • Contains only those medications that manufacturers pay to have placed in the book • Does not have information on over-the-counter (OTC) medications

Table 4-2 Description of Reference Books—*continued*

NAME OF BOOK	STRENGTHS	WEAKNESSES
*United States Pharmacopeia/ Dispensing Information (USP/DI)***	• Comes in two volumes: (1) Drug Information for the Health Care Provider and (2) Advice for the Patient • Easy-to-read, practical guidelines • Stresses many tips for the proper use of the medication and precautions to take • Includes a pronunciation key for each medication name	• No pictures of medications
*American Health-System Formulary Service (AHFS Drug Information)****	• Good, exact information • Easy to read • Arranged by classification • Has a general statement about each classification at the beginning of each section	• No pictures of medications • Some parts are not needed for the health care provider

*Published annually by Biomedical Information Corp., New York.
**Published annually by U.S. Pharmacopeial Convention, Inc., Rockville, Maryland.
***Published annually by the American Society of Health-System Pharmacists, Bethesda, Maryland.
Source: Based on Woodrow (2007), pp. 18–19.

Other reference books, such as *The Pill Book, Handbook of Nonprescription Drugs, The PDR Pocket Guide to Prescription Drugs,* and *Delmar's Nurse's Drug Handbook* may be found in bookstores. Many new references that are being printed today are for the general public and the UAP.

In addition, the Internet provides information about medications and the conditions they treat. However, there can be serious dangers with some online sources. Some online sources may not be reliable, professional, or even legitimate. Use only those Web sites that are under the authority of the government and/or supervised by professional groups. Remember that not all Web sites are created equal.

The following Web sites are reliable professional sources of medical information:

www.aphanet.org	Sponsored by the American Pharmaceutical Association
www.cdc.gov/nip	U.S. Centers for Disease Control and Prevention
www.centerwatch.com	Centerwatch
www.fda.gov	U.S. Food and Drug Administration
www.nih.gov	U.S. National Institutes of Health
www.nlm.nih.gov	U.S. National Library of Medicine
www.safemedication.com	Sponsored by the American Society of Health System Pharmacists
www.uspdqi.org	*United States Pharmacopeia/Dispensing Information (USP/DI)*

The UAP must find the reference that is best for him. The most important thing to remember is that whatever reference is used, the reference must always be available. It must also be quickly and easily understood. It is the UAP's responsibility to *never* administer a medication of which he does not have basic knowledge.

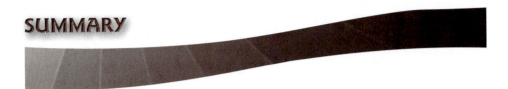

SUMMARY

Reference materials, such as reference books and the Internet, are important tools for the UAP. The materials provide the most up-to-date information on medication names, classifications, therapeutic actions, unwanted actions, dosages, and other important facts. This chapter provides the UAP with an introduction to this information, but it is in no way complete. In addition, it is not expected that the UAP remember all the information about the medications that he will give. What is expected and is part of his scope of function is that the UAP always takes the time to look up the information on a medication before giving it. Under no circumstance should the UAP administer a medication without knowing the basic facts about that medication.

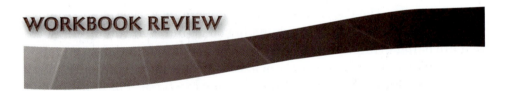

WORKBOOK REVIEW

Go to the workbook and complete the exercises for Chapter 4.

REVIEW QUESTIONS

1. Medications are known by different names. These include:
   a. generic, trade name, and chemical name
   b. trade or brand name and generic name only
   c. chemical and trade name only
   d. official name, chemical name, generic name, and trade or brand name
2. A generic name is given to a new medication:
   a. after it has been tested by the FDA
   b. when the new medication is developed
   c. after seventeen (17) years of approval
   d. once the medication is on the market

3. The trade name of a medication is:

    a. the chemical formula for it

    b. the name used for trading the company's stocks

    c. the brand name used to identify and sell it

    d. the name used as an official reference

4. The three basic types of medication preparation are:

    a. solids, semisolids, and liquids

    b. capsules, tablets, and suppositories

    c. emulsions, syrups, and sprays

    d. lozenges, lotions, and liniments

5. An example of a liquid medication would be:

    a. a capsule

    b. a solution

    c. a lozenge

    d. a buccal tablet

6. An example of a semisolid or solid medication is:

    a. a solution

    b. an elixir

    c. an aerosol

    d. an ointment

7. The therapeutic action of a medication can be described as a:

    a. palliative, treating only the symptoms

    b. diagnostic, when the medication is testing the body

    c. local action, when a medication affects the entire body

    d. systemic action, when a medication affects the entire body

8. An adverse reaction of a medication is:

    a. an unwanted action or effect of a medication

    b. an unwanted action or effect that is harmful to the body

    c. the result of one medication increasing or decreasing the effect of another

    d. the result of one medication interacting with another to make the person irritable

9. When a licensed health care provider prescribes a medication, he must consider:

    a. the water temperature in the individual's home

    b. the pharmacy that delivers the individual's medication

    c. the pharmaceutical company making the medication

    d. the weight, sex, ethnicity, and age of the individual receiving the medication

10. A good medication reference for the UAP would be:

    a. the Physician's Desk Reference (PDR)

    b. any reference that is readily available, reliable, and easily understood by the UAP

    c. any Web site offering information on medications

    d. a good medical dictionary

CLINICAL SCENARIOS

1. You are to administer a lotion to an individual's back. Why would a lotion be prescribed? Is it the same as a liniment? If not, what are the differences?

2. You are asked to give a medication with which you are not familiar. Should you proceed? If not, what should you do before giving the medication?

Chapter 5
Medication Orders

Learning Objectives

After reading this chapter and completing the review questions, you should be able to:

1. Spell and define terms.

2. List the eight parts of a medication order.

3. Briefly describe the five most common types of medication orders.

4. Explain the difference between a written order and a verbal order.

5. List the seven guidelines to follow when taking a telephone order.

6. Describe three of the most common forms used in medication administration.

7. Describe two types of health care provider order forms.

8. Describe CPOE (computerized physician online entry).

9. Describe an electronic Medication Administration Record (eMAR).

10. Explain the difference between the manufacturer's label for a prescription medication, the prescription label from the pharmacy, and the label on an over-the-counter medication.

11. Explain the importance of following a time schedule for medication administration.

Key Terms

abbreviations

Computerized Physician Online Entry (CPOE)

Controlled Substance Count Book

disposal record

electronic Medication Administration Record (eMAR)

faxed orders

medication administration system

medication orders

medication record sheet	pharmacist	prn order	telephone orders (TO)
National Drug Code (NDC) numbers	pharmacy patient profile	routine order	verbal orders (VO)
over-the-counter (OTC) medications	prescriptions	single order	written orders
	progress notes	standing order	
		stat order	

INTRODUCTION

Medication orders are written by the licensed health care provider for a specific individual. The medication ordered by the licensed health care provider is based on the individual's illness or illnesses. The licensed health care provider considers all the factors discussed in Chapter 4, plus other factors that are equally important. Once the medication(s) is prescribed (ordered), it is the UAP's legal responsibility to give the medication as the licensed health care provider prescribed it. If that is not possible, the UAP must notify the licensed health care provider immediately.

> **medication orders**
> Written instructions from the licensed health care provider to the UAP.

THE MEDICATION ORDER

The medication order consists of eight parts:

1. Name of the individual
2. Name of the medication to be administered
3. Dose of the medication to be given
4. Route by which the medication will be administered
5. Frequency and/or time that the medication is to be given
6. Special instructions about the medication, if there are any
7. Date and time when the order was written
8. Signature of the licensed health care provider writing the order

Each medication order should follow a specific pattern or sequence. The name of the medication is written first. The dose, route, and frequency are written next. Here is an example:

Procan SR 500 mg po q6h

1. The name of the medication is *Procan SR.*
2. The dose of the medication is *500 mg.*
3. The route of the medication is *po (by mouth).*
4. The frequency of the medication is *q6h (every six [6] hours).*

This order means "give 500 milligrams of Procan SR by mouth every six (6) hours."

Types of Medication Orders

Depending on the type of setting the UAP works in, there are various types of medication orders that might be used. The following are the most common types of medication orders:

- **Routine order:** This is a detailed order that must be followed regularly. The order includes the name of the medication, dosage, route, and frequency. Some regulations and workplace policies may require that the order also include the reason the medication is being given.
  Example: Digoxin 0.125 mg po (by mouth) every day. Hold for a pulse less than 60 beats per minute.

- **Single order:** This type of order is given for one-time use only. The order includes the name of the medication, dosage, route, time for administration, and the reason the medication is being given.
  Example: Benadryl 50 mg po (by mouth) 1 hour before IVP.

- **Standing order:** This type of order or set of orders are prewritten by the licensed health care provider (or group of licensed health care providers). The order(s) provide specific instructions, guidelines, procedures, treatments, and/or medications for individuals in certain situations.
  Examples: Dulcolax suppository 1 suppository pr (rectally) if no BM (bowel movement) for three days.
  Tylenol 2 tabs po (by mouth) q4h (every 4 hours) for a temperature above 101°F. If fever continues for more than 24 hours, contact the licensed health care provider.

- **Stat order:** This is an order for a medication that is to be given immediately. The licensed health care provider may write to give the medication *now* rather than *stat* to make sure the medication is given right away. The medication order includes the name of the medication, dosage, route, and the order to give the medication *now*.
  Example: Lasix 50 mg po (by mouth) now.

- **prn order:** With this type of medication order, medication is given "as necessary" or "when needed." The order includes the name of the medication, dosage, frequency, route, and the reason the medication is being given.
  Example: Percocet 2 tabs po (by mouth) q4h (every 4 hours) prn (when needed) for back pain.

Note: Depending on state regulations and workplace policies, prn orders for certain controlled substances (such as Schedule II medications) may need to be rewritten (renewed) every three (3) to five (5) days. It is the UAP's responsibility to know and follow all regulations and workplace policies. Remember also all medication orders must be prescribed (ordered) by a licensed health care provider who is registered within the state in which the UAP works.

The UAP may receive medication orders from the licensed health care provider in five main ways:

written orders
Orders that are written by the licensed health care provider.

- **Written orders:** The licensed health care provider will write orders for medications, treatments, guidelines, and other instructions for care onto the health care provider order sheet. Courts usually do not question the legality of a medication order that was written and signed by a licensed health care provider. Written orders are, therefore, the preferred type of order for the UAP to receive. An order that is not readable or that is questionable for some reason requires the UAP to contact the licensed health care provider for an explanation. The UAP may not administer medication until she has received a clear explanation and directions from the licensed health care provider.

- **Faxed orders:** These are written orders that are faxed to the UAP by the licensed health care provider. Not all states permit faxed orders. Refer to state regulations and workplace policies for guidelines about faxed orders. If this is allowed, faxed orders are written instructions to the UAP. These orders are handled in the same manner as all other medication orders.

- **Prescriptions:** A prescription is a written order from the licensed health care provider to the pharmacist. A prescription is *not* written instructions from the licensed health care provider to the UAP. It is not part of an individual's chart or medical record. Its purpose is to control the sale and use of medications safely and effectively under the supervision of a licensed health care provider. A prescription is needed for controlled substances in Schedules II to VI. A prescription may or may not be needed for **over-the-counter (OTC) medications**, depending on the setting in which the UAP works.

- **Verbal orders (VO):** The licensed health care provider speaks or tells the medication order to another health care provider. Licensed health care providers, when taking orders from others, are taught special skills to protect themselves from legal complications. Therefore, it is strongly recommended that UAPs *never* take a verbal order. If a licensed health care provider is present and speaks an order to the UAP, the UAP should *not* take the order verbally but rather should insist that the licensed health care provider write the order on a health care provider order form. If the licensed health care provider insists on giving a verbal order, the UAP should refer the licensed health care provider to her supervisor.

- **Telephone orders (TO):** These are orders given by the licensed health care provider to the UAP over the telephone. Not all states or all work settings permit UAPs to take telephone orders. Once again, it is the UAP's responsibility to know and follow the regulations and policies in the setting where she works.

Note: According to the National Council of State Boards of Nursing, Certified Medication Assistants should not take verbal or telephone orders (National Council of State Boards of Nursing Delegate Assembly, August, 9, 2007).

UAPs who are allowed to take telephone orders should follow seven guidelines when taking a telephone order:

faxed orders
Written orders that are faxed to the UAP by the licensed health care provider.

prescriptions
Written orders from the licensed health care provider to the pharmacist.

over-the-counter (OTC) medications
Nonprescription medications bought and used without medical supervision.

verbal orders
Orders that are given verbally to the staff by the licensed health care provider.

telephone orders
Orders that are told to the UAP over the telephone by the licensed health care provider.

1. Whenever possible, have a second staff person listen on an extension phone to the licensed health care provider giving the telephone order. Have this staff person countersign the telephone order, verifying (confirming) the order received.

2. Write the order down exactly as the licensed health care provider states it.

3. Follow the "Six Rights," which are discussed in Chapter 6.

4. Repeat the order back to the licensed health care provider.

5. Repeat this process until the order is correct.

6. Once the order is correct, document on the health care provider order form that the order has been verified (confirmed) with the licensed health care provider.

7. Have the licensed health care provider sign the order within twenty-four (24) hours.

This may mean taking the order to the licensed health care provider's office the next day or next business day and waiting in the office until it is signed. State regulations may permit the order to be faxed to the licensed health care provider. If so, it is the UAP's responsibility to make sure the order form is signed and faxed back to the UAP within the designated period of time. Check state regulations and workplace policies to see if this is permitted.

Note: States may vary on the length of time permitted for the signing of telephone orders.

Guidelines for Understanding the Medication Order

1. It is the responsibility of the UAP to understand the information on the medications that the licensed health care provider is ordering. Two ways to help the UAP do this are to:

    • Make a list of the medications. Look the medications up in a medication reference book or on an approved Web site.

    • Make a medication reference card for each medication.

2. The UAP is to make sure she understands the medication order completely before giving any medication.

3. If there are any questions about the medication order or the medication, the UAP is to ask them *before* giving the medication. The UAP may ask the licensed health care provider who prescribed the medication, the pharmacist who filled the prescription, or the clinical consultant for her work setting, or she may contact her supervisor for assistance.

4. If the UAP is ever in doubt or is confused about the medication order, the UAP is *not* to administer the medication. She is to immediately contact the individual's licensed health care provider or her supervisor.

5. When the UAP has questions about a specific medication, such as whether the medication may be taken with food, she is to contact her pharmacist. Pharmacists are an excellent source of information on medications.

6. When checking the medication sheet before giving a medication, the UAP is to check for discontinued medications and/or medications that may have been changed. Depending on the UAP's workplace policy, this may be done by highlighting the medication with a colored highlighter, by crossing a section of the order out and making specific notations on the medication record sheet, or by some other method specific to the workplace policy.

FORMS USED IN MEDICATION ADMINISTRATION

The most common forms used in medication administration include:

- The health care provider order form

- A prescription

- A **medication administration system**, a system used in some hospitals, long-term care facilities, and personal care facilities to document medication administration

- A **medication record sheet**, also called a medication sheet, or med sheet

- A **pharmacy patient profile**, a system is used in the pharmacy to document and track an individual's medications

- A **Controlled Substance Count Book**

- A **disposal record**

- **Progress notes**

- Telephone order forms

If the work setting is computerized, the setting may have an electronic medical record. If so, the work setting may use Computerized Physician Online Entry (CPOE) and an electronic Medication Administration Record (eMAR).

Not all of these forms or systems may be used in every work setting. The UAP needs to become familiar with the forms and systems and with the documentation and transcription procedures used in her work setting. For safe and effective medication administration, all staff in a particular work setting *must* use the same forms and systems and *must* document and transcribe the *same* way.

This chapter includes selected examples of typical forms and systems with sample illustrations.

Health Care Provider Order Form

There are many different types of health care provider order forms that are used. The type used will depend on the health care setting. The health care provider (HCP) order form may be a single, duplicate, or triplicate form.

medication record sheet
A form used to document medication administration.

Controlled Substance Count Book
A book used for the documentation of the administration of controlled substances.

disposal record
A form used for the documentation of the disposal of medication(s).

progress notes
Brief notes written by the UAP that provide an explanation of an individual's condition.

Following is a description of two types of health care provider order forms. One form is used in an institutional setting, such as a long-term care facility (nursing home). The second form is used in a community setting, such as a group home.

The first type of HCP order form contains a place for stamping the individual's name and identifying information and for writing the date, time, medication order, and the individual's medication sensitivities (e.g., allergies). This type of form is used more in an institutional setting, such as a hospital or long-term care facility (nursing home) (Figure 5-1).

The licensed health care provider writes the medications to be administered on the HCP order form and signs the form. Each individual has her own form. This is usually a duplicate or a triplicate HCP form. The original form (first copy) is kept in the individual's medical record. The second copy goes to the pharmacy; this is the same as the prescription. If there is a third copy, it is given to the staff person who is administering the medication.

The medication order is then transcribed (copied) onto the medication record sheet. The staff person doing the transcription dates and signs the order form to indicate that the order has been transcribed (copied) onto the medication sheet (Figure 5-2).

The transcriber may be the charge nurse, the medication nurse, a ward secretary, the unit secretary, a medication-certified UAP, or some other individual authorized by the employer to perform this task. The licensed or unlicensed staff person administering the medication is ultimately responsible for making sure the medication is transcribed correctly. This staff person, therefore, needs to check for the accuracy and completeness of the medication order before administering the medication.

The second type of HCP form is commonly used in a community setting. The top portion of the form is completed by the UAP caring for the individual before the individual is seen by the licensed health care provider. The UAP provides the licensed health care provider with recent medical information on the individual.

Once the individual is seen by the licensed health care provider, the licensed health care provider completes the form. The information completed by the licensed HCP includes the results of the licensed health care provider's examination of the individual and her orders. The orders may include an individual's medications but may also include other treatments and orders, such as an order for physical therapy, a special diet, or a wheelchair (Figure 5-3).

This is a single-copy HCP order form. The licensed health care provider will, therefore, provide the staff with copies of prescriptions for each medication ordered for the individual. The UAP will take the prescriptions to the pharmacy. The pharmacist will fill the prescriptions for the UAP.

Once the UAP returns to her work setting, the medication order will need to be transcribed onto the medication record sheet. The transcription process is the same as for all other health care provider forms. One staff person will transcribe the medication order onto the medication record sheet. This staff person will date and sign the

Medical Center Hospital

Health Care Provider Order Form

Instructions:
1. Imprint the patient's identification plate onto the form before placing form into the chart.
2. After each set of orders are written, remove the first yellow copy and send it to the pharmacy.
3. "X" out the remaining unused lines after the last yellow copy is used.

ALLERGIES

Date Ordered	Time Ordered	Time Executed	Time Posted	Use Ball Point Pen Only

Figure 5-1 Example of a Health Care Provider's Order Form. Always remember to include the individual's name and identifying information in the space provided in the upper right-hand corner.

(Delmar/Cengage Learning)

	ENTERED	FILLED	CHECKED	VERIFIED
				—

NOTE: A NON-PROPRIETARY MEDICATION OF EQUAL QUALITY MAY BE DISPENESED - IF THIS COLUMN IS NOT CHECKED!

DATE	TIME WRITTEN	PLEASE USE BALL POINT - PRESS FIRMLY	✓	TIME NOTED	NURSES SIGNATURE
11/3/10	0815	Keflex 250 mg po q6h	✓		
		Codeine 30 mg po q4h prn leg pain	✓	0830	
		Tylenol 650 mg po q4h prn fever > 101°F	✓		L. Despin, R.N.
		Lasix 40 mg po daily	✓		
		Slow-K 8 mEq po bid	✓		
		J. Bolle, M.D.	✓		
			✓		
			✓		

AUTO STOP ORDERS: UNLESS REORDERED, FOLLOWING WILL BE D/C^D AT 0800 ON:

DATE	ORDER		
		☐ CONT ☐ D/C	PHYSICIAN SIGNATURE
		☐ CONT ☐ D/C	PHYSICIAN SIGNATURE
		☐ CONT ☐ D/C	PHYSICIAN SIGNATURE

CHECK WHEN ANTIBIOTICS ORDERED   ☐ Prophylactic   ☐ Empiric   ☐ Therapeutic

Allergies:
Sulfa

PATIENT DIAGNOSIS
Diabetes

HEIGHT 5'10"   WEIGHT 180 lb

McMillan, Joseph P.
#3-11316-7

(1)

FORM 959-708 (6-XX) **HEALTH CARE PROVIDER'S ORDER**   Reynolds + Reynolds LITHO IN U.S.A. K41814 (7-XX) D339360

Figure 5-2 Example of a Health Care Provider's Order Form. *(Delmar/Cengage Learning)*

Health Care Provider Order Form	
Name:	Date:
Licensed Health Care Provider:	Allergies:
Current Medical/Dental Conditions:	
Reason for Visit:	
Current Medications:	
Staff Signature:	Date:
Findings by Licensed Health Care Provider:	
Medications/Orders:	
Instructions:	
Follow-Up Visit:	Lab Work/Tests:
Licensed Health Care Provider Signature:	Date:

Figure 5-3 Example of a Health Care Provider's Order Form. The UAP completes the upper section of the form before the individual sees the licensed health care provider. *(Delmar/Cengage Learning)*

order form to indicate that the transcription has been completed. The staff person administering the medication will check for the accuracy and completeness of the medication order before giving the medication to the individual. Once again, the licensed or unlicensed staff person administering the medication is ultimately responsible for making sure the medication is transcribed correctly.

Medication Administration System

Some hospitals and long-term care facilities use the Bar-Coded Medication Administration System to administer and document medication administration. In this administration system, each medication is marked with its own bar code (label). Staff persons who will administer the medication have bar codes on their identification badges. Each individual who is to receive medication has a wristband with a bar code on it.

When a licensed health care provider writes an order, the order is faxed or hand delivered to the pharmacy. The pharmacist enters the order into a computer system. The pharmacist places a bar code onto the unit dose of medication and delivers the medication to the unit.

When the staff person administers the medication, she uses a handheld device to scan the bar codes on her identification badge, the individual's wristband, and the medication. If the Bar-Coded Medication Administration System is unable to match the medication to be given with the order in the system, it warns the staff person. At that point, the staff person may (1) stop and verify the medication she will administer to make sure she is administering the right medication in the right dose to the right individual at the right time by the right route or (2) override the system and administer the medication. If the staff person overrides the system and administers the medication, the system will evaluate the situation to determine whether a medication error may have occurred. If the staff person does not administer the medication, the system determines whether a medication error was prevented (Medscape Today, 2009).

Medication Administration Record

Medication administration may be documented on paper or on computerized records. When administration is documented on paper, the form is commonly called a medication record sheet or medication sheet (Figure 5-4).

A computerized medication administration record (MAR) may be used by hospitals and other health care facilities that have the proper equipment. There are different medication administration computerized programs and record forms. The licensed health care provider writes the medication on a health care provider order form. This information is then sent to the pharmacy or entered into the computer. A hard copy (paper copy) of the medication administration record (MAR) is kept in the individual's medical record (Figure 5-5).

Documentation of medication administration may be done either on the hard copy in the individual's record or directly on the computer if the health care setting has computer workstations available for the staff.

Controlled Substance Count Book

Because of the potential for addiction and abuse with medications in Schedules II to V, these medications, along with syringes, must be reconciled (counted) at least every twenty-four (24) hours by two staff members. The total numbers of each medication and of syringes are recorded in a bound book called the Controlled Substance Count Book. Often this book is also called the Narcotic Count Book.

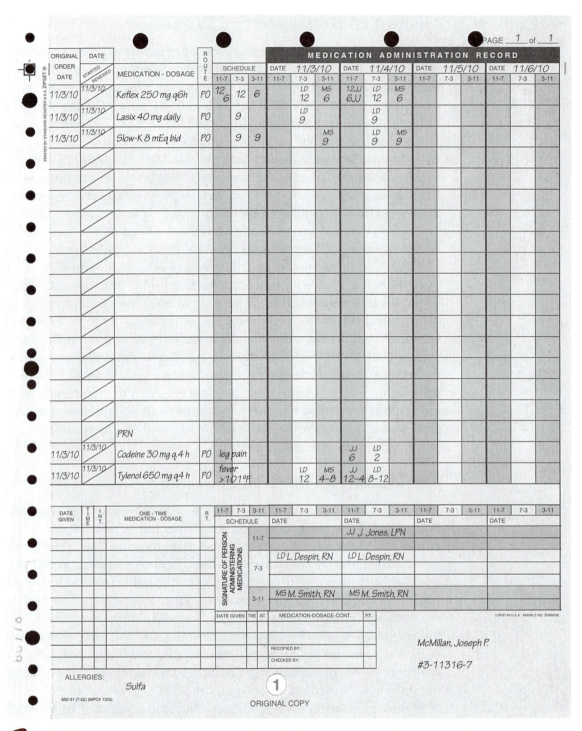

Figure 5-4 Medication Administration Record. It is commonly called a medication record sheet or medication sheet. *(Delmar/Cengage Learning)*

The Controlled Substance Count Book should be bound. In most instances, this book cannot be a three-ring binder or a spiral-bound notebook. Count books may be purchased from a pharmacy or medical supply house.

MEDICATION ADMINISTRATION RECORD

START	STOP	MEDICATION	SCHEDULED TIMES	OK'D BY	0001 HRS. TO 1200 HRS.	1201 HRS. TO 2400 HRS.
08/31/10 1800 SCH		PROCAN SR 500 MG TAB-SR 500 MG Q6H PO	0600 1200 1800 2400	JD	0600 LD 1200 LD	1800 MS 2400 JD
09/03/10 0900 SCH		DIGOXIN (LANOXIN) 0.125 MG TAB 1 TAB EVERY PO OTHER DAY ODD DAYS-SEPT	0900	JD	0900 LD	
09/03/10 0900 SCH		FUROSEMIDE (LASIX) 40 MG TAB 1 TAB DAILY PO	0900	JD	0900 LD	
09/03/10 0845 SCH		REGLAN 10 MG TAB 10 MG AC&HS PO GIVE ONE NOW!!	0730 1130 1630 2100	JD	0730 LD 1130 LD	1630 MS 2100 MS
09/04/10 0900 SCH		K-LYTE 25 MEQ EFFERVESCENT TAB 1 EFF. TAB BID PO DISSOLVE AS DIR START 9-4	0900 1700	JD	0900 LD	1700 LD
09/03/10 1507 PRN		NITROGLYCERIN 1/50 GR 0.4 MG TAB-SL 1 TABLET PRN* SL PRN CHEST PAIN		JD		
09/03/10 1700 PRN		DARVOCET-N 100* 1 TAB Q4-6H PO PRN leg pain		JD		

	NURSE'S SIGNATURE	INITIAL		
7–3	L. Despin, R.N.	LD	ALLERGIES: **NKA**	Patient: Bogue, John D.
3–11	M. Smith, R.N.	MS		Patient # 3-81512-3 Admitted: 08/31/10
11–7	J. Doe, R.N.	JD	DIAGNOSIS: **CHF**	Physician: J. Bolle, MD Room: 231 W

730-13 (12/xx)

Figure 5-5 Computerized Medication Administration Record (MAR). *(Delmar/Cengage Learning)*

Note: Due to a change in some work settings to a computerized medication administration system, the Controlled Substance Count Book may not be used. The need to reconcile (count) Schedules II to V and syringes at least every twenty-four (24) hours by two staff members; however, is still required. It is therefore the responsibility of the UAP to know and follow her workplace policies and state regulations to fulfill this requirement.

Controlled Substance Count Books have three sections:

1. An Index Page gives the name of each medication and lists the page on which the count for each medication is recorded (Figure 5-6).

2. A Count Page provides a rolling log of the medication's usage (Figure 5-7).

INDEX

INDIVIDUAL'S NAME	MEDICATION & STRENGTH	PAGE NUMBER				SIGNATURE OF STAFF RESPONSIBLE FOR REMOVING MEDICATION FROM COUNT

**REMEMBER TO UPDATE INDEX INFORMATION WHEN ITEM IS TRANSFERRED TO ANOTHER PAGE.

Figure 5-6 Index Page of the Controlled Substance Count Book. *(Source: Based on Yoder, M. & Collins, S. (1999). Controlled Substance Count Book. SCRRI: Sturbridge, MA.)*

Name:			( ) Original Entry or ( ) Transferred from Page No.				

Licensed Health Care Provider:	Pharmacy:	Rx No.	Rx Date:

Drug & Strength:	Rx No.	Rx Date:

Directions:	Rx No.	Rx Date:

Date	Time	Amount on Hand	Amount Used	Route	Amount Left	Staff Signature

MEDICATION DISCONTINUED/DISPOSED	**MEDICATION TRANSFERRED**
Discontinue Date: _____ Removal Date: _____ Signature Staff Removing: _____ Signatures of Staff Destroying Medication: (2 signatures required) _____ _____	New Page # _____ Amount Transferred: _____ Signatures of Staff Verification: (2 signatures required) _____ _____

Figure 5-7 Count Page of the Controlled Substance Count Book. *(Source: Based on Yoder, M. & Collins, S. (1999). Controlled Substance Count Book. SCRRI: Sturbridge, MA.)*

3. A Count Verification Page indicates that the count was correct and provides the signature of the *two* staff persons completing the count (Figure 5-8).

CONTROLLED SUBSTANCE COUNT VERIFICATION

DATE	TIME	COUNT CORRECT	STAFF COMING ON DUTY	STAFF GOING OFF DUTY

Figure 5-8 Verification Page of the Controlled Substance Count Book. *(Source: Based on Yoder, M. & Collins, S. (1999). Controlled Substance Count Book. SCRRI: Sturbridge, MA.)*

Disposal Form

Documentation of medication disposal is required in some settings for controlled substances in Schedules II to V. However, a workplace may also require documentation for the destruction of all medications, including

---

Item # _____   Date last filled _____

Name _____   Date _____

Medication/strength _____

Rx # _____   Pharmacy _____

Amount disposed _____   Reason _____

_____

Controlled Substance Book # _____   Page # _____

Signatures: Staff member _____

Supervisor _____

Figure 5-9 Sample Disposal Record. An excerpt from the medication disposal documentation record from the Massachusetts Department of Public Health. The form, titled *Controlled Substance Disposal Record*, is used in the Massachusetts Medication Administration Program. *(Delmar/Cengage Learning)*

over-the-counter medications. The UAP must know the workplace policies and state regulations. Figure 5-9 is an excerpt from the medication disposal documentation record from the Massachusetts Department of Public Health. The form, entitled *Controlled Substance Disposal Record*, is used in the Massachusetts Medication Administration Program.

Telephone Order Form

Not all states or all work settings permit UAPs to take telephone orders. In those workplaces where UAPs are permitted to take telephone orders, a telephone order form is frequently used.

The form serves two purposes. First, the form provides a guideline for the UAP. It lists all of the information the UAP needs to gather from the licensed health care provider during the telephone conversation. Second, the telephone order form may be sent directly to the licensed health care provider for her signature. Once the form is signed, it becomes a legal order (Figure 5-10, shown on next page).

Note: Not all work settings use a telephone order form.

Computerized Physician Online Entry (CPOE)

Computerized Physician Online Entry (CPOE) is a computerized, organized method by which licensed health care providers are able to enter (write) orders for the treatment of individuals. Orders are then communicated over a computer network to staff or to various departments. CPOE is used by all licensed health care providers who have the right to prescribe. In some work settings, staff are able to enter telephone orders provided by licensed staff (Figure 5-11a and b, shown on page 89).

Computerized Physician Online Entry (CPOE)
A computerized, organized method by which licensed health care providers are able to enter (write) orders for the treatment of individuals.

Telephone Order Form	
Date of Telephone Order:	Time of Order:
Name of the Individual:	
Name of Medication: Generic:	Brand:
Strength:	
Amount:	
Frequency:	
Route:	
Reason for Medication Being Ordered or for Change in Medication Order:	
Special Instruction or Precautions:	
Instructions for Refused or Forgotten Medication:	
Discontinue Date (if any):	
Licensed Health Care Provider's Name:	
Staff Signature/Title:	Co-Signature of Staff/Title:
Signature of Licensed Health Care Provider:	Date:

Figure 5-10 Example of a Telephone Order Form. *(Delmar/Cengage Learning)*

A licensed health care provider may:

- Place a new order
- Change or replace an existing order
- Put an order on hold
- Discontinue an order
- Release a held order
- Cancel an existing order (Hebrew Senior Life, 2008a)

Figure 5-12a–c (shown on page 90–91) provide a view of CPOE screens offered to a licensed health care provider as she places a medication(s) order. Figure 5-13 (shown on page 91) is a CPOE edit screen, which allows the licensed HCP to review her orders and make any changes needed.

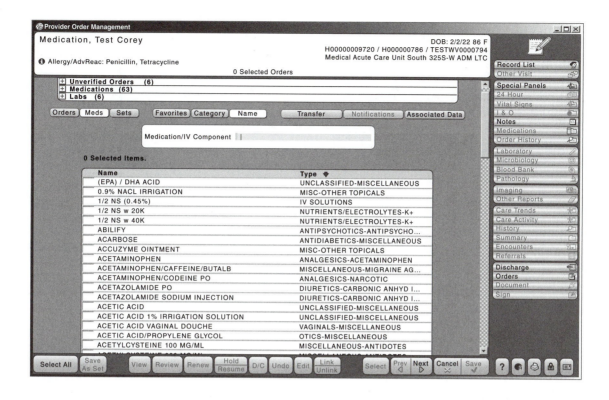

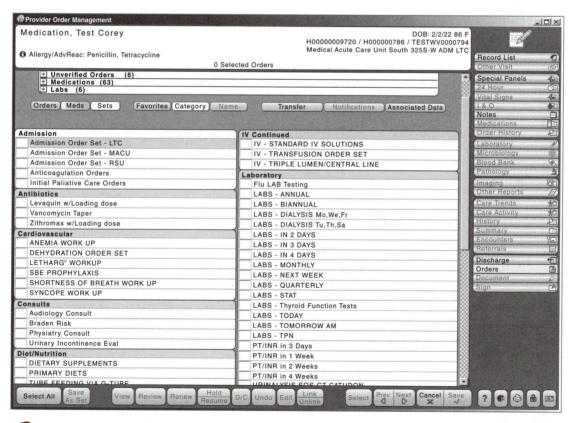

Figure 5-11a and b Computerized Physician Online Entry (CPOE), a computerized, organized method by which licensed health care providers are able to enter (write) orders for the treatment of individuals. Orders are then communicated over a computer network to staff or to various departments. These CPOE screens allow staff to enter telephone orders provided by licensed health care providers. (*Source: Copyright Hebrew Senior Life 2008a*)

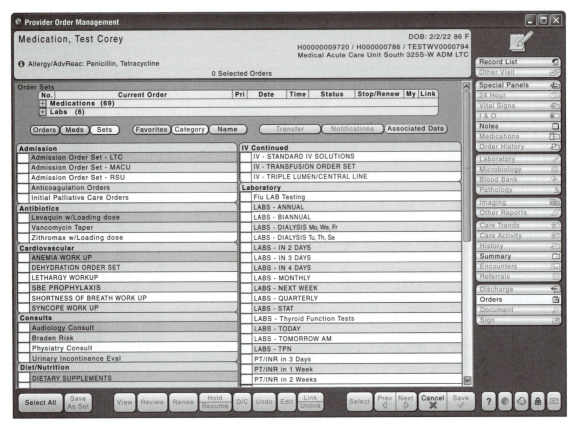

Figure 5-12a An open screen in CPOE ready for ordering. A licensed health care provider enters (writes) her orders on this screen. *(Source: Copyright Hebrew Senior Life 2008a)*

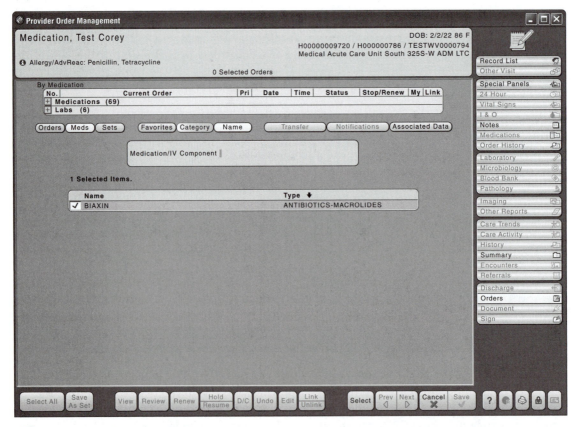

Figure 5-12b A medication selection screen in CPOE. The licensed health care provider makes her initial choice of medications from this screen. *(Source: Copyright Hebrew Senior Life 2008a)*

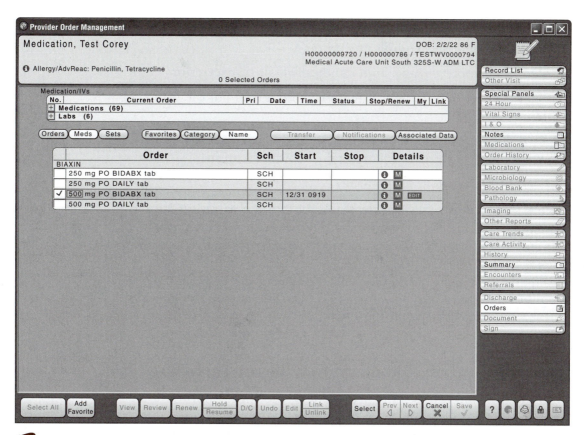

Figure 5-12c Once the licensed HCP chooses a medication, CPOE then offers her a list of times and doses of the medication chosen. The HCP enters (orders) the frequency that she wants the medication to be given and the amount she wants to be given. *(Source: Copyright Hebrew Senior Life 2008a)*

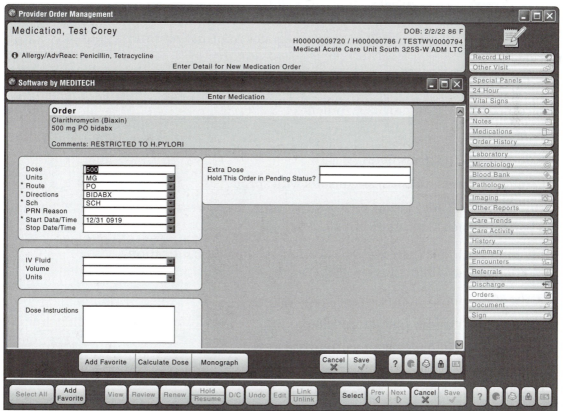

Figure 5-13 An edit screen. On this screen, the licensed HCP can review her orders and make any changes needed. *(Source: Copyright Hebrew Senior Life 2008a)*

CPOE:

1. Decreases delays in completing orders

2. Reduces errors resulting from handwriting or transcription

3. Allows order entry wherever care is being given (in the office, clinic, hospital)

4. Provides a means to check for duplicate or incorrect orders such as for duplicate tests or incorrect doses of medication

5. Simplifies inventory and billing

Clinical studies show that CPOE decreases the rate of medication errors any where from 55% to 88%. In addition, CPOE has reduced (1) length of hospitals stays, (2) hospital charges, and (3) the time it takes to get lab and radiology results. Dr. John Birkmeyer at the University of Michigan estimates that approximately 570,000 to 907,000 serious medication errors could be prevented every year in nonrural U.S. hospitals with CPOE systems (THELEAPFROGGROUP, 2010).

Electronic Medication Administration Record (eMAR)

To prevent medication errors and ensure safety, the Joint Commission and the Institute for Safe Medication Practices (ISMP) recommend that workplaces use the **electronic Medication Administration Record (eMAR)** to document and track medication administration. An eMAR is a computerized record. The eMAR (Figure 5-14) eliminates all paper records and creates an organized system for medication administration (Cerner Corporation, 2008).

electronic Medication Administration Record (eMAR) A computerized record that eliminates all paper records and creates an organized system for medication administration.

This computerized system collects and integrates information from an individual's:

- Admission assessment

- Licensed health care providers' orders

- Care plans

- Nurses' notes/progress notes

- Clinical assessments, such as consults with specialists

- Other clinical information such as lab results, X-rays results, and so on (Medquest Communications, 2008)

All of this information is then available to the UAP during medication administration along with:

- A list of previously administered medications

- A list of medications that are past due

- A list of medications that are currently due

- Alerts (warnings) about medications a UAP may be giving (Cerner Corporation, 2008)

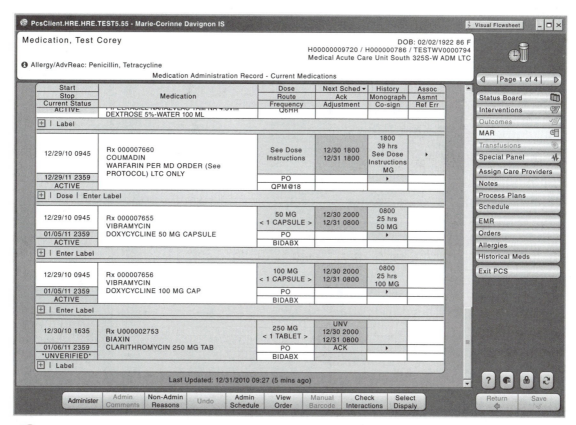

Figure 5-14 An electronic Medication Administration Record (eMAR), a computerized, organized record used to document and track medication administration. The medication Biaxin is displayed as unverified and unacknowledged. *(Source: Copyright Hebrew Senior Life 2008b)*

Note: When the UAP receives an alert, the UAP must hold the medication(s) and immediately notify the individual's licensed health care provider to report the "alert" and obtain follow-up instructions/orders.

The medication administration process for using an eMAR is as follows:

1. The licensed health care provider writes the orders.

2. The order is sent to the pharmacy.

3. The pharmacy enters the order into the computer, if needed (the licensed HCP may have electronically entered the order and sent the order to the pharmacy).

4. The pharmacy "bar codes" the medication and sends it to the individual's place of residence or the unit.

5. When the UAP administers the medication, the UAP reviews the eMAR on the computer screen (Figure 5-15) and then:

   • Reviews the medication list

   • Verifies the medications with the licensed HCP orders

   • Checks for alerts/warnings and cautions

   • If alerts/warnings are present, contacts the licensed HCP for follow-up instructions/orders

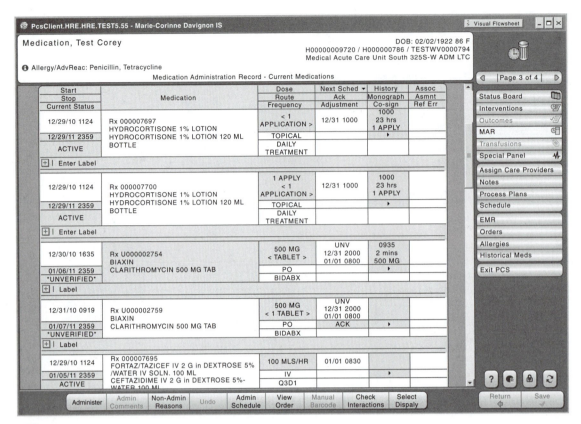

Figure 5-15 An electronic Medication Administration Record (eMAR) with the next scheduled date and time of Biaxin. *(Source: Copyright Hebrew Senior Life 2008b)*

- Following the six rights of medication administration, gives the individual her medications
- If the individual has an electronic wristband, scans the wristband to identify the individual (Doylestown Hospital, 2008)

THE MEDICATION LABEL

The medication label is an important source of information. It does not matter whether the UAP is administering a prescription medication or an over-the-counter (OTC) medication. The medication label provides basic information needed for safe and effective use of a medication. There are three basic types of medication labels that the UAP should become familiar with:

1. The manufacturer's label for a prescription medication
2. The prescription label from the pharmacy
3. A label for over-the-counter medication

The Manufacturer's Label for a Prescription Medication

The UAP administers a prescription medication from a pharmacy-labeled container. This container may or may not have the manufacturer's original label on the container. Even though the UAP does not follow the directions on the manufacturer's label when administering medication, it is good practice to know and understand how to read the manufacturer's label.

The manufacturer's label for a prescription medication includes the following information:

- The name and address of the manufacturer
- The trade or brand name of the medication
- The generic name of the medication (or the listing of active and inactive ingredients)
- The **National Drug Code (NDC) numbers** that can be used to identify the manufacturer, the medication, and the size of the medication container
- The strength in a given amount of the medication (e.g., 250 mg per tablet)
- The usual dose and frequency of administration
- The form in which the medication is supplied
- Any warnings and cautionary statements
- The expiration date for the medication
- The lot or batch code
- The total number or volume (amount) of the medication in the container

National Drug Code (NDC) numbers
Numbers used to identify the manufacturer, the medication, and the size of the medication container.

Understanding the Manufacturer's Label

Figure 5-16 shows a sample medication label for a medication known as Cipro®. While reading the medication information below, follow along on the sample label. The idea is to find this information on the sample label.

1. The trade or brand name for the medication is *Cipro®*.
2. The generic name is ciprfloxacin hydrochloride.
3. The National Drug Code (NDC) numbers are *0028-8512-51*.
4. The strength in a given amount of the medication is 250 *mg*.
5. The usual dose and frequency of administration are *See accompanying literature for complete information on dosage and administration.*
6. The form in which the medication is supplied is *tablets, USP.*
7. The cautionary statement is: *Rx only.*

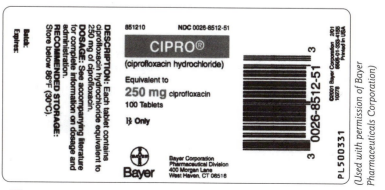

Figure 5-16 Sample of a manufacturer's medication label: Cipro®.

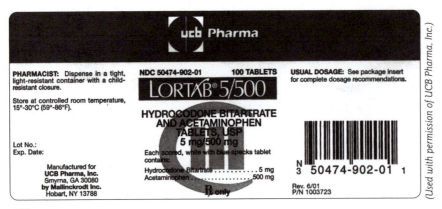

Figure 5-17 Sample of a manufacturer's medication label: Lortab® 5/500.

8. The expiration date for the medication and the lot or batch code number are *expiration date and batch code are not given on the sample label.*

9. The manufacturer's name is *Bayer Corporation.*

10. The total number and/or volume of the medication in the container is *100 tablets.*

Figure 5-17 above is a sample medication label for a medication known as Lortab® 5/500. While reading the medication information below, follow along on the sample label. The idea again is to find this information on the sample label.

1. The trade or brand name for the medication is *Lortab® 5/500.*

2. The generic name is hydrocodone bitartrate and acetaminophen tablet, USP.

3. The National Drug Code numbers are *5047-902-01.*

4. The strength in a given amount of the medication is *hydrocodone bitartrate 5 mg and acetaminophen 500 mg.*

5. The usual dose and frequency of administration are *See package insert for complete dosage recommendations.*

6. The form in which the medication is supplied is *tablets, USP.*

7. The cautionary statement is *Rx only.*

8. The expiration date for the medication and the lot or batch code number are *expiration date and batch code are not given on the sample label.*

9. The manufacturer's name is *UCB Pharma, Inc.*

10. The total number and/or volume of the medication in the container is *100 tablets.*

Prescription Labels

After completing college, a pharmacist becomes licensed in the state where she works. As a licensed **pharmacist**, she prepares prescriptions according

pharmacist
A licensed individual who prepares and dispenses medication according to written instructions of a licensed health care provider.

to a licensed health care provider's order and dispenses the medication. The prescription from the licensed health care provider to the pharmacist includes information about how and when the medication is to be taken. Federal and state regulations provide guidelines to the pharmacist as to how to dispense the medication. When the medication is dispensed, the pharmacist labels the medication with the written instructions from the licensed health care provider and according to the regulations.

A typical prescription will have the following information on the label:

- The prescription number—this number is assigned by the pharmacy
- The name, address, and telephone number of the pharmacy
- The individual's name for whom the medication is ordered
- The date the prescription is filled
- The brand name of the medication
- The generic name of the medication
- The strength of the medication
- The amount of medication in the bottle
- The directions for use
- The lot number—this number is used by the manufacturer to track the medication if there is a problem
- The expiration date of the medication—this should be checked every time the UAP administers the medication
- The name of the licensed health care provider
- If any, the number of refills the prescription may have—this is the number of times that the medication may be refilled by the pharmacy before the licensed health care provider has to write a new prescription for the medication (Figure 5-18)

Rx#	Name of the Pharmacy	Pharmacy Telephone
	Address of the Pharmacy	Number
	Town/City of Pharmacy	
Individual's Name	Date Filled	
Name of Medication & Strength	Amount of Medication in Container	
Generic Name of Medication		
Directions for Use		
Lot Number	Expiration Date	Name of Licensed HCP
		Number of Refills

Figure 5-18 What's on a prescription label? *(Delmar/Cengage Learning)*

0000	Wonders Pharmacy	000-111-2222
	102 Main Street	
	Whits, Massachusetts	
Sue Jones	July 22, 2010	
Ceclor 500 mg	30 tablets	
I/C cefaclor		
Take one tablet three times a day for 10 days.		
3062	July 22, 2011	Dr. S Proctor
		No Refills

Figure 5-19 Sample Prescription Label. *(Delmar/Cengage Learning)*

Understanding a Prescription Label

Figure 5-19 is a sample prescription label for an individual named Sue Jones. Her medication is Ceclor. Read the information below and follow along on the sample prescription label. The idea is to find the information on the sample label.

1. The prescription number is *0000.*
2. The name, address, and telephone number of the pharmacy is Wonders Pharmacy, 102 Main Street, Whits, Massachusetts. The telephone number is 000-111-2222.
3. The individual's name is *Sue Jones.*
4. The date the prescription is filled is *July 22, 2010.*
5. The brand name of the medication is *Ceclor.*
6. The generic name of the medication is *cefaclor.*
7. The strength of the medication is *500 mg.*
8. The amount of medication in the bottle is *30 tablets.*
9. The direction for use is *Take one tablet by mouth three times a day for 10 days.*
10. The lot number is *3062.*
11. The expiration date of the medication is *July 22, 2011.*
12. The name of the licensed health care provider is *Dr. S Proctor.*
13. The number of refills is *0.*

The Label for an Over-the-Counter Medication

Nonprescription medications are commonly called **over-the-counter (OTC) medications**. Individuals routinely buy and take these medications without medical supervision. These medications, therefore, do not need a licensed health care provider's prescription, nor do they need a licensed health care provider's written medication order.

over-the-counter (OTC) medications Nonprescription medications bought and used without medical supervision.

However, when over-the-counter (OTC) medications are administered in some work settings by licensed or unlicensed staff, a licensed health care provider's written medication order is required. In some settings, a prescription may still be needed. Some states require the pharmacist to label over-the-counter (OTC) medications with written instructions when UAPs are administering the medications. The UAP must, therefore, refer to her state regulations and workplace policies to know the guidelines to follow.

OTC medications should always be used cautiously, especially when they are taken with prescription medications. OTC medications may interfere with prescription medications. OTC medications may aggravate a condition or disease that an individual is being treated for. Read the labels on the OTC medications carefully. Call the licensed health care provider if there are any questions.

According to the U.S. Food and Drug Administration (2009), new labels on OTC medications will soon be appearing on store shelves. The FDA has issued a regulation to make sure the labels on all OTC medications have information listed in the same order; are arranged in a simpler eye-catching, consistent style; and may contain easier to understand words. All nonprescription, over-the-counter (OTC) medication labels (Figure 5-20) are to have detailed usage and warning information including:

- Active ingredient: Therapeutic substance in the medication; amount of active ingredient per unit

- Uses: Symptoms or diseases the product will treat or prevent

- Warnings: When not to use the product; conditions that may require advice from a licensed health care provider before taking the product; possible interactions or side effects; when to stop taking the product and when to contact a licensed health care provider; if one is pregnant or breast feeding, seek guidance from a licensed health care provider; keep product out of children's reach

- Inactive ingredients. Substances such as colors or flavors

- Purpose: Medication action or category (such as antihistamine, antacid, or cough suppressant)

- Directions: Specific age categories, how much to take, how to take, and how often and how long to take

- Other information: How to store the product properly and required information about certain ingredients (such as the amount of calcium, potassium, or sodium the product contains)

In addition, the new label is to include information on:

- Expiration date, when applicable (date after which one should not use the product)

- Lot or batch code (manufacturer information to help identify the product)

- Name and address of manufacturer, packer, or distributor

- How much of the product is in the package

- What to do if an overdose occurs

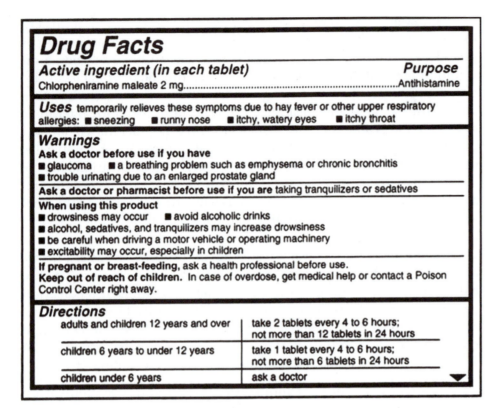

Drug Facts

Active ingredient *(in each tablet)* — **Purpose**

Chlorpheniramine maleate 2 mg...Antihistamine

Uses temporarily relieves these symptoms due to hay fever or other upper respiratory allergies: ■ sneezing   ■ runny nose   ■ itchy, watery eyes   ■ itchy throat

Warnings
Ask a doctor before use if you have
■ glaucoma   ■ a breathing problem such as emphysema or chronic bronchitis
■ trouble urinating due to an enlarged prostate gland

Ask a doctor or pharmacist before use if you are taking tranquilizers or sedatives

When using this product
■ drowsiness may occur   ■ avoid alcoholic drinks
■ alcohol, sedatives, and tranquilizers may increase drowsiness
■ be careful when driving a motor vehicle or operating machinery
■ excitability may occur, especially in children

If pregnant or breast-feeding, ask a health professional before use.
Keep out of reach of children. In case of overdose, get medical help or contact a Poison Control Center right away.

Directions

adults and children 12 years and over	take 2 tablets every 4 to 6 hours; not more than 12 tablets in 24 hours
children 6 years to under 12 years	take 1 tablet every 4 to 6 hours; not more than 6 tablets in 24 hours
children under 6 years	ask a doctor

Drug Facts (continued)

Other Information ■ store at 20-25°C (68-77°F)   ■ protect from excessive moisture

Inactive Ingredients D&C yellow no. 10, lactose, magnesium stearate, microcrystalline cellulose, pregelatinized starch

Figure 5-20 The new over-the-counter medicine label. *(Source: U.S. Food and Drug Administration, 2009)*

MEDICATION ADMINISTRATION TIMES

To make sure individuals get their medications as prescribed and to avoid errors, times of administration for routine medications are scheduled by the UAP's workplace. Table 5-1 shows a sample time schedule. Keep in mind that schedule times may differ. For example, for one individual or in one work setting, every six (6) hours might be 12 a.m., 6 a.m., 12 p.m., and 6 p.m., or it could be 2 a.m., 8 a.m., 2 p.m., and 8 p.m. Whenever possible, the times of medication administration should be scheduled so that an individual's sleep is disturbed as little as possible.

Note that some medications may need to be given with food. Others may need to be given on an empty stomach. Others may require that

Table 5-1 An Example of a Time Schedule

daily	once a day at 10 a.m.	q2h	2 a.m., 4 a.m., 6 a.m., 8 a.m., and so on, OR 1 a.m., 3 a.m., 5 a.m., 7 a.m., and so on.
bid	twice a day at 10 a.m. and 6 p.m.	q3h	3 a.m., 6 a.m., 9 a.m., 12 p.m., and so on.
tid	three times a day at 10 a.m., 2 p.m., 6 p.m.	q4h	4 a.m., 8 p.m., 12 p.m., 4 p.m., and so on.
qid	four times a day at 10 a.m., 2 p.m., 6 p.m., 10 p.m. OR 9 a.m., 1 p.m., 5 p.m., 9 p.m.	q6h	6 a.m., 12 p.m., 6 p.m., 12 a.m. OR 2 a.m., 8 a.m., 2 p.m., 8 p.m.
		q8h	8 a.m., 4 p.m., 12 a.m.
		q12h	12 a.m., 12 p.m. OR 6 a.m., 6 p.m.

Please note that the times stated in the table above are examples only. Your facility or work setting may choose different times to fulfill these schedule requirements.

Source: Delmar/Cengage Learning

an individual drink a large amount of water throughout the day. It is very important that the UAP administers the medication as ordered by the licensed health care provider and according to the directions on the pharmacy label.

ABBREVIATIONS

Abbreviations are a shortened way to write health care orders. Abbreviations are an international language used by professionals and nonprofessionals. They provide a clear and concise way to write an order. Not all abbreviations are used in all work settings. Each workplace decides for itself which abbreviations are approved for its setting.

When determining what abbreviations will be used in a specific work setting, the work setting needs to consider the information published by both the Institute for Safe Medication Practice (ISMP) and the Joint Commission. The ISMP has published a list of problematic abbreviations that are unsafe to use. The list is known as the *ISMP List of Error-Prone Abbreviations, Symbols, and Dose Designations* (Figure 5-21). The Joint Commission has approved a list of "dangerous" abbreviations that are no longer to be used. These abbreviations are highlighted with a double asterisk in the ISMP list (Figure 5-21).

Table 5-2 provides a listing of abbreviations commonly used in the UAP's work setting. The UAP needs to check her workplace policy manual for the approved abbreviations used in her work setting. If the UAP should find an "unapproved" or "problematic" abbreviation on her work setting's approved list, she should report this to her supervisor.

Institute for Safe Medication Practices

ISMP's List of *Error-Prone Abbreviations, Symbols,* and *Dose Designations*

The abbreviations, symbols, and dose designations found in this table have been reported to ISMP through the USP-ISMP Medication Error Reporting Program as being frequently misinterpreted and involved in harmful medication errors. They should NEVER be used when communicating medical information. This includes internal communications, telephone/verbal prescriptions, computer-generated labels, labels for drug storage bins, medication administration records, as well as pharmacy and prescriber computer order entry screens.

The Joint Commission (TJC) has established a National Patient Safety Goal that specifies that certain abbreviations must appear on an accredited organization's do-not-use list; we have highlighted these items with a double asterisk (**). However, we hope that you will consider others beyond the minimum TJC requirements. By using and promoting safe practices and by educating one another about hazards, we can better protect our patients.

Abbreviations	Intended Meaning	Misinterpretation	Correction
μg	Microgram	Mistaken as "mg"	Use "mcg"
AD, AS, AU	Right ear, left ear, each ear	Mistaken as OD, OS, OU (right eye, left eye, each eye)	Use "right ear," "left ear," or "each ear"
OD, OS, OU	Right eye, left eye, each eye	Mistaken as AD, AS, AU (right ear, left ear, each ear)	Use "right eye," "left eye," or "each eye"
BT	Bedtime	Mistaken as "BID" (twice daily)	Use "bedtime"
cc	Cubic centimeters	Mistaken as "u" (units)	Use "mL"
D/C	Discharge or discontinue	Premature discontinuation of medications if D/C (intended to mean "discharge") has been misinterpreted as "discontinued" when followed by a list of discharge medications	Use "discharge" and "discontinue"
IJ	Injection	Mistaken as "IV" or "intrajugular"	Use "injection"
IN	Intranasal	Mistaken as "IM" or "IV"	Use "intranasal" or "NAS"
HS	Half-strength	Mistaken as bedtime	Use "half-strength" or "bedtime"
hs	At bedtime, hours of sleep	Mistaken as half-strength	
IU**	International unit	Mistaken as IV (intravenous) or 10 (ten)	Use "units"
o.d. or OD	Once daily	Mistaken as "right eye" (OD-oculus dexter), leading to oral liquid medications administered in the eye	Use "daily"
OJ	Orange juice	Mistaken as OD or OS (right or left eye); drugs meant to be diluted in orange juice may be given in the eye	Use "orange juice"
Per os	By mouth, orally	The "os" can be mistaken as "left eye" (OS-oculus sinister)	Use "PO," "by mouth," or "orally"
q.d. or QD**	Every day	Mistaken as q.i.d., especially if the period after the "q" or the tail of the "q" is misunderstood as an "i"	Use "daily"
qhs	Nightly at bedtime	Mistaken as "qhr" or every hour	Use "nightly"
qn	Nightly or at bedtime	Mistaken as "qh" (every hour)	Use "nightly" or "at bedtime"
q.o.d. or QOD**	Every other day	Mistaken as "q.d." (daily) or "q.i.d. (four times daily) if the "o" is poorly written	Use "every other day"
q1d	Daily	Mistaken as q.i.d. (four times daily)	Use "daily"
q6PM, etc.	Every evening at 6 PM	Mistaken as every 6 hours	Use "6 PM nightly" or "6 PM daily"
SC, SQ, sub q	Subcutaneous	SC mistaken as SL (sublingual); SQ mistaken as "5 every;" the "q" in "sub q" has been mistaken as "every" (e.g., a heparin dose ordered "sub q 2 hours before surgery" misunderstood as every 2 hours before surgery)	Use "subcut" or "subcutaneously"
ss	Sliding scale (insulin) or ½ (apothecary)	Mistaken as "55"	Spell out "sliding scale;" use "one-half" or "½"
SSRI	Sliding scale regular insulin	Mistaken as selective-serotonin reuptake inhibitor	Spell out "sliding scale (insulin)"
SSI	Sliding scale insulin	Mistaken as Strong Solution of Iodine (Lugol's)	
ī/d	One daily	Mistaken as "tid"	Use "1 daily"
TIW or tiw	3 times a week	Mistaken as "3 times a day" or "twice in a week"	Use "3 times weekly"
U or u**	Unit	Mistaken as the number 0 or 4, causing a 10-fold overdose or greater (e.g., 4U seen as "40" or 4u seen as "44"); mistaken as "cc" so dose given in volume instead of units (e.g., 4u seen as 4cc)	Use "unit"

Dose Designations and Other Information	Intended Meaning	Misinterpretation	Correction
Trailing zero after decimal point (e.g., 1.0 mg)**	1 mg	Mistaken as 10 mg if the decimal point is not seen	Do not use trailing zeros for doses expressed in whole numbers"
"Naked" decimal point (e.g., .5 mg)**	0.5 mg	Mistaken as 5 mg if the decimal point is not seen	Use zero before a decimal point when the dose is less than a whole unit

© ISMP 2007

Figure 5-21 ISMP List of *Error-Prone Abbreviations, Symbols,* and *Dose Designations.* *(Reprinted with the permission of the Institute for Safe Medication Practices)*

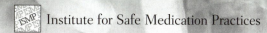
ISMP's List of *Error-Prone Abbreviations, Symbols, and Dose Designations* (continued)

Dose Designations and Other Information	Intended Meaning	Misinterpretation	Correction
Drug name and dose run together (especially problematic for drug names that end in "l" such as Inderal40 mg; Tegretol300 mg)	Inderal 40 mg Tegretol 300 mg	Mistaken as Inderal 140 mg Mistaken as Tegretol 1300 mg	Place adequate space between the drug name, dose, and unit of measure
Numerical dose and unit of measure run together (e.g., 10mg, 100mL)	10 mg 100 mL	The "m" is sometimes mistaken as a zero or two zeros, risking a 10- to 100-fold overdose	Place adequate space between the dose and unit of measure
Abbreviations such as mg. or mL. with a period following the abbreviation	mg mL	The period is unnecessary and could be mistaken as the number 1 if written poorly	Use mg, mL, etc. without a terminal period
Large doses without properly placed commas (e.g., 100000 units; 1000000 units)	100,000 units 1,000,000 units	100000 has been mistaken as 10,000 or 1,000,000; 1000000 has been mistaken as 100,000	Use commas for dosing units at or above 1,000, or use words such as 100 "thousand" or 1 "million" to improve readability

Drug Name Abbreviations	Intended Meaning	Misinterpretation	Correction
ARA A	vidarabine	Mistaken as cytarabine (ARA C)	Use complete drug name
AZT	zidovudine (Retrovir)	Mistaken as azathioprine or aztreonam	Use complete drug name
CPZ	Compazine (prochlorperazine)	Mistaken as chlorpromazine	Use complete drug name
DPT	Demerol-Phenergan-Thorazine	Mistaken as diphtheria-pertussis-tetanus (vaccine)	Use complete drug name
DTO	Diluted tincture of opium, or deodorized tincture of opium (Paregoric)	Mistaken as tincture of opium	Use complete drug name
HCl	hydrochloric acid or hydrochloride	Mistaken as potassium chloride (The "H" is misinterpreted as "K")	Use complete drug name unless expressed as a salt of a drug
HCT	hydrocortisone	Mistaken as hydrochlorothiazide	Use complete drug name
HCTZ	hydrochlorothiazide	Mistaken as hydrocortisone (seen as HCT250 mg)	Use complete drug name
MgSO4**	magnesium sulfate	Mistaken as morphine sulfate	Use complete drug name
MS, MSO4**	morphine sulfate	Mistaken as magnesium sulfate	Use complete drug name
MTX	methotrexate	Mistaken as mitoxantrone	Use complete drug name
PCA	procainamide	Mistaken as patient controlled analgesia	Use complete drug name
PTU	propylthiouracil	Mistaken as mercaptopurine	Use complete drug name
T3	Tylenol with codeine No. 3	Mistaken as liothyronine	Use complete drug name
TAC	triamcinolone	Mistaken as tetracaine, Adrenalin, cocaine	Use complete drug name
TNK	TNKase	Mistaken as "TPA"	Use complete drug name
ZnSO4	zinc sulfate	Mistaken as morphine sulfate	Use complete drug name

Stemmed Drug Names	Intended Meaning	Misinterpretation	Correction
"Nitro" drip	nitroglycerin infusion	Mistaken as sodium nitroprusside infusion	Use complete drug name
"Norflox"	norfloxacin	Mistaken as Norflex	Use complete drug name
"IV Vanc"	intravenous vancomycin	Mistaken as Invanz	Use complete drug name

Symbols	Intended Meaning	Misinterpretation	Correction
ℨ	Dram	Symbol for dram mistaken as "3"	Use the metric system
ℳ	Minim	Symbol for minim mistaken as "mL"	
x3d	For three days	Mistaken as "3 doses"	Use "for three days"
> and <	Greater than and less than	Mistaken as opposite of intended; mistakenly use incorrect symbol; "< 10" mistaken as "40"	Use "greater than" or "less than"
/ (slash mark)	Separates two doses or indicates "per"	Mistaken as the number 1 (e.g., "25 units/10 units" misread as "25 units and 110" units)	Use "per" rather than a slash mark to separate doses
@	At	Mistaken as "2"	Use "at"
&	And	Mistaken as "2"	Use "and"
+	Plus or and	Mistaken as "4"	Use "and"
°	Hour	Mistaken as a zero (e.g., q2° seen as q 20)	Use "hr," "h," or "hour"

**These abbreviations are included on TJC's "minimum list" of dangerous abbreviations, acronyms and symbols that must be included on an organization's "Do Not Use" list, effective January 1, 2004. Visit www.jointcommission.org for more information about this TJC requirement.

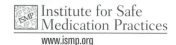
Institute for Safe Medication Practices
www.ismp.org

Table 5-2 Abbreviations and Their Meanings

ABBREVIATION	MEANING	ABBREVIATION	MEANING
ac	before meals	s̄	without
ad lib	as desired, as much as needed	stat	immediately
am	morning	tid	three times a day
bid	two times a day, twice daily	TO	telephone order
		VO	verbal order
c̄	with	WA	while awake
cap	capsule		
hr	hour	**Measurements**	
H₂O	water		
L/min	liters per minute	cm	centimeter
ml, mL	milliliter	mcg	microgram
O₂	oxygen	mg	milligram
OTC	over the counter	g	gram
pc	after meals	kg	kilogram
pm	afternoon	mL	milliliter
pr	per rectum	L	liter
prn	as necessary, when needed	oz	ounce
q2h	every two (2) hours	lb	pound
q3h	every three (3) hours	gtt	drops
q4h	every four (4) hours	t, tsp	teaspoon
qid	four times a day	T, tbs	tablespoon
Rx	treatment	tab	tablet
		C	Celsius
		F	Fahrenheit

Source: Delmar/Cengage Learning

SUMMARY

The health care provider order form gives written instructions to the UAP. The order form needs to list specific directions. The prescription contains the written instructions from the licensed health care provider to the pharmacist. The pharmacist prepares and dispenses the medication to the UAP according to the licensed health care provider's instructions and federal and state regulations. The UAP follows the instructions on the order form and the directions of the pharmacist when she gives medication(s) to an individual(s). The medication label helps the UAP to identify the medication(s) she is giving to the individual(s). The label provides important information so that the individual receives the right medication and that medication errors do not occur. The medication forms discussed in this chapter provide the UAP with a place to document the medication(s) that she has administered. The forms used in medication administration differ in each work setting. It is the responsibility of the UAP to know and follow the state regulations and workplace policies in the setting in which she works.

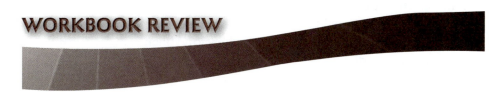

WORKBOOK REVIEW

Go to the workbook and complete the exercises for Chapter 5.

REVIEW QUESTIONS

1. A medication order includes the following information:
   a. the lot or batch code
   b. the name of the manufacturer
   c. the name of the pharmacist
   d. the medication dose, route, and frequency
2. A routine medication order is:
   a. given for one time use
   b. a detailed order that must be followed regularly
   c. an order for a medication to be given "as needed"
   d. given over the telephone
3. A stat order is:
   a. for a medication that is to be given immediately
   b. an order prewritten by the licensed health care provider
   c. given verbally by the licensed health care provider
   d. also called a prescription
4. A written order is:
   a. told by the licensed health care provider to a staff member, who writes it down
   b. instructions for care taken over the telephone and written down
   c. written on the order sheet by the licensed health care provider
   d. also called a prescription
5. When taking a telephone order from the licensed health care provider, it is important to:
   a. repeat the order only once—the licensed HCP's time is limited
   b. have the licensed health care provider sign the order within seventy-two (72) hours
   c. take the order yourself because staff are busy
   d. have another staff person listen on an extension phone then countersign the phone order

6. A prescription is:
   a. a written order to the UAP so she may administer medication
   b. needed for OTC medications but not for controlled substances
   c. needed for the disposal of medications
   d. a written order from the licensed health care provider to the pharmacist
7. To document medication administration, a UAP should use:
   a. a health care provider order form
   b. a medication record sheet or medication sheet
   c. a written order
   d. a piece of lined paper
8. The manufacturer's label for a medication:
   a has a prescription number
   b. has the name of the individual who will take it
   c. includes National Drug Code numbers to identify the manufacturer, the medication, and the container size
   d. contains instructions from the licensed health care provider to the pharmacist
9. The prescription label for a medication:
   a. is the same as the manufacturer's label
   b. contains specific instructions for administration written by the licensed health care provider
   c. can be removed from the bottle and thrown away
   d. includes National Drug Code numbers
10. Following a time schedule for medication administration is important because:
    a. it allows the UAP to better plan her work day
    b. it helps staff plan the individual's daily activities
    c. it aids in the inventory and reordering of medications
    d. it helps to make sure that an individual gets her medications as ordered
11. The eMAR:
    a. delivers medication to an individual's home
    b. electronically disposes of unused medication
    c. tracks the storage of medications in the pharmacy
    d. is a computerized, organized record used for the documentation and tracking of medication administration
12. The eMar provides the UAP with the following information:
    a. a list of medications that cannot be crushed
    b. a copy of the most recent monthly review
    c. a list of medications that are due to be given
    d. a list of the licensed health care providers in the immediate area

CLINICAL SCENARIOS

1. What information would you expect to find in a medication order? List the eight parts.
2. You go with Sally on a trip to her licensed health care provider. During the visit she writes an order that says, "Lasix 50 mg po stat." What do you do?
3. An individual's licensed health care provider visits the group home you work in, to perform an exam. As she is leaving, she tells you what medication changes she wants and states that she doesn't have time to write them down. How would you respond?

Chapter 6
Principles of Medication Administration

Learning Objectives

After reading this chapter and completing the review questions, you should be able to:

1. Spell and define terms.
2. Define the "Six Rights" of medication administration.
3. Describe the Three Checks.
4. Explain the formula "dose = strength × amount."
5. List five of the basic guidelines for medication administration.
6. List seven occasions when the UAP should wash his hands.
7. Describe three situations when gloves are worn for medication administration.
8. Describe the four steps in the procedure for medication administration.
9. Provide a description of a medication room and storage area.
10. Complete documentation for a Controlled Substance Count.
11. State three reasons for disposing of medication.
12. State acceptable methods of disposing of medication.
13. Complete documentation for disposing of a medication.

Key Terms

amount	dose	internal medications	route
contraindications	external medications	medication cart	strength
Controlled Substance Count Book	implication(s) for administration	medication loss	

INTRODUCTION

Medicating oneself is an easy and simple task. One listens to the instructions given to him by his licensed health care provider, reads the label on the pharmacy container, and then takes his medication. No one else is involved in the process. No paperwork (documentation) is needed.

However, giving medication to another individual may be much more complicated. Usually many other staff are involved. The UAP does not always have the opportunity to talk directly to the licensed health care provider. The medication containers and the paperwork (documentation) are handled by many different people.

To assist the UAP with the task of medication administration, this chapter provides the UAP with the basic steps and guidelines for medication administration. When followed, these steps and guidelines help to make the process as simple and easy as possible. The UAP who follows the steps and guidelines will be able to administer medications safely and effectively. Remember always that it is the UAP's legal responsibility to administer medications as he has been trained and according to the policies and regulations within the setting where he works.

THE SIX RIGHTS OF MEDICATION ADMINISTRATION

Giving medication to an individual is a big responsibility. Medication administration involves giving an individual a substance that will, in some way, change his body chemistry. Giving the wrong medication to an individual is a violation of his rights. Doing so may also cause the individual to become very sick. Making sure that the correct medication is given in the correct amount and the correct way, to the correct individual, is very important.

Every time the UAP gives an individual a medication, he needs to follow the **"Six Rights."** In this instance, when we say "right," we mean "correct" rather than referring to a individual's "legal rights."

The UAP needs to make sure that the:

1. Medication is given to the right *individual*

2. UAP is giving the right *medication*

3. UAP is measuring the right *dose (amount) of medication*

4. UAP is giving the medication at the right *time*

5. UAP is giving the medication by the right *route*

6. UAP is completing the right *documentation in a timely fashion*

A good way to remember the "Six Rights" is to use the use the phrase "*I* *M*ust *D*o *T*his *R*ight," where *I* stands for individual, *M* stands for medication, *D* stands for dose, *T* stands for time, and *R* stands for route. Of course, the UAP always has to remember to document. Figure 6-1 provides an illustration to assist the UAP in remembering the "Six Rights".

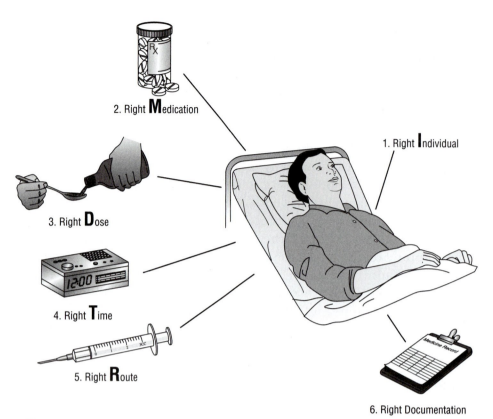

2. Right **M**edication

1. Right **I**ndividual

3. Right **D**ose

4. Right **T**ime

5. Right **R**oute

6. Right Documentation

Figure 6-1 The Six Rights of Medication Administration. Using the phrase "I Must Do This Right" will help the UAP to remember the Six Rights of medication administration. Of course, the UAP always has to document! *(Delmar/Cengage Learning)*

Right Individual

The UAP must make sure that he is medicating the *right individual.* If he does not know the individual or is unsure of who the individual is, he is not to give the medication. He may ask another staff person to identify the individual for him. He may use a photograph (picture) if there is one available to identify the individual. Photographs (pictures) are often kept with the medication sheet or in the individual's record. The UAP may not identify the individual by simply asking the individual what his name is.

The UAP is to compare the individual's name on the licensed health care provider's order with the individual's name on the medication sheet and the individual's name on the pharmacy label. If all three names match, the UAP may give the medication. If all three names do not match, the UAP cannot give the medication. The UAP must then contact his supervisor at once. The supervisor will be able to tell him what to do next.

Right Medication

The UAP needs to check that he is giving the *right medication.* He does this by making sure that the name or names of the medication match in three places:

1. The licensed health care provider's order

2. The pharmacy label

3. The medication sheet

The UAP must be sure all three of these match! The UAP will then check the name or names of the medications again to make sure that the medication ordered is the one he is about to give. If the names of the medications all match, the UAP will give the medication. If the names do not match, even on just one of the above, the UAP will not give the medication. He will contact his supervisor immediately!

Note: **The UAP never administers a medication that has been prepared (poured) by another licensed or unlicensed staff person. The UAP never prepares or administers a medication from a container that is unlabeled.**

Right Dose

The *right dose* of medication is how much an individual is getting at one time. In order to determine the dose, the UAP needs to know the strength of the medication and the amount to be given. In this chapter, the UAP will learn where he can quickly find the dosage information he needs to use the formula "**dose = strength × amount.**"

The *dose* is found in the licensed health care provider's order. Usually the dose is written right after the name of the medication. For example, in the order below,

dose
The amount of medication ordered by the licensed health care provider.

strength
The measurement in which each unit of medication is available.

amount
The number of units of medication to be given.

Depakote 500 mg po bid

the dose is *500 mg.*

The *strength* is found on the pharmacy label, after the name of the medication. The strength is the measurement in which each unit of medication is available. For example, on a pharmacy label stating,

Depakote 250 mg

the strength is *250 mg.* This means that each pill in the bottle has 250 mg of Depakote in it. Therefore, two pills would be needed to satisfy the licensed health care provider's order calling for 500 mg of Depakote.

The licensed health care provider's order gives the UAP the written instructions for administering or giving a medication(s). The pharmacy label provides the UAP with a way to identify the medication he is giving. The *amount* to be given is found in the licensed health care provider's order, as well as on the pharmacy label. The amount is the number of units of medication that are to be given. The amount may be the number of pills, tablets, capsules, and so on. For example, in the order below,

Depakote two tablets by mouth twice a day

the amount given each time the medication is given is *two tablets.*

Before the UAP gives an individual a medication, he must compare the dose on the licensed health care provider's order with the dose on the medication sheet and with the dose on the pharmacy label. To avoid errors, the UAP must be sure to double-check the doses. If any of the doses do not match or if he has any questions about the information, he is not to give the medication. He is to contact his supervisor immediately for help or clarification.

Right Time

The *right time* for giving a medication can mean a few different things. It can mean:

- A specific time of day
- The number of times per day a medication is given
- The time between doses
- A portion of the day

The time of day can be either morning (a.m.) or afternoon, evening, or night (p.m.). The time may also be specific—10 a.m., 4 p.m., and so on. The number of times per day is how many times in one day the individual gets that medication—once a day, twice a day, and so on. The UAP will usually see the following abbreviations for the number of times per day:

- "bid" = twice a day
- "tid" = three times a day
- "qid" = four times a day

The time between doses is based on how often an individual is supposed to get a medication.

The UAP will usually see the following abbreviations to express the time between doses:

- "q4h" = every four (4) hours
- "q6h" = every six (6) hours
- "q8h" = every eight (8) hours

Remember that medications *must* be given within a one (1)-hour time period. The UAP has *from half an hour (1/2) before it is due to half an hour (1/2) after it is due* to give the medication. Otherwise, the UAP is not following the licensed health care provider's order. For example, if the UAP is to give a medication at 4:00 p.m., he can give it any time between 3:30 p.m. and 4:30 p.m. He cannot give it before 3:30 p.m. or after 4:30 p.m. The UAP should try, however, to administer the medication as close to the designated time as possible.

> *Note:* Some community settings permit a two (2)-hour time period for administration of medication. If this is the rule, the UAP would have from one (1) hour before the medication is due to one (1) hour after the medication is due to give the medication. It is the responsibility of the UAP to know and follow his state regulations and workplace policy.

Again, before the UAP gives an individual a medication, he must check the time on the licensed health care provider's order, the medication sheet, and the pharmacy label. To avoid errors, the UAP must be sure to double-check the administration times in all three places to make sure the times match. If the time in any of the places does not match or if he has any questions about the time, he is not to give the medication. The UAP is to then contact his supervisor right away. Giving a medication at the wrong time may result in the individual having a bad reaction or becoming ill, especially if he is taking more than one medication daily.

Right Route

route
The way the medication enters the body.

The *right route* for giving medication means how and where the medication enters the body. The most common way, or **route**, to give medication is by mouth. However, medications may also be given in the ear, the eye, the nose, the skin, the rectum, or the vagina or by injection.

Before giving a medication, the UAP needs to check the route on the licensed health care provider's order, the medication sheet, and the pharmacy label. To avoid errors, the UAP must double-check the route in all three places to make sure the route matches. If the information does not match, even in one place, the UAP is not to give the medication. He is to contact his supervisor right away for help or clarification.

Note: The medication may only be administered by the route ordered by the licensed health care provider.

Right Documentation

To prevent medication errors, documentation of medication administration should be done when the medication is given to the individual. After administering an individual's medication(s), the UAP needs to document on the appropriate medication forms in the individual's record the:

- Name of the medication(s) given
- Amount of medication(s) given
- Time the medication(s) was actually given
- Route the medication(s) was given
- Location the medication(s) was applied (if applicable), for instance, where a patch was placed or ointment was applied
- Effectiveness of a PRN medication(s)
- Individual's response to the medication(s) administered
- Individual's complaints, if any, to the medication(s)
- Any side effects or adverse effects the individual may experience from the medication(s)

Medication documentation also includes the completion of the **Controlled Substance Count Book**, disposal forms if medication has been discarded or destroyed, and medication error forms if an error has been made during administration of the medication.

Accurate documentation of medication administration is a very important legal responsibility of the UAP. The individual's medication records may be examined in court to seek a legal judgment or may be used in an investigation.

Note: Never document a medication as given before administering the medication.

THREE CHECKS

Medication administration involves Three Checks. The checks are made to go together with the Six Rights discussed earlier. Together, the Three Checks and Six Rights help the UAP to make sure that he is preparing and giving the right medication in the right dose to the right individual.

Below is an explanation of the Three Checks:

- Check #1: When removing the medication from the storage area, compare the pharmacy label to the medication sheet. Make sure the Six Rights match.

- Check #2: When removing the medication from package/container it is kept in, compare the pharmacy label to the medication sheet again. Make sure the Six Rights match.

- Check #3: When returning the package to where it is stored, compare the pharmacy label to the medication sheet again. Make sure the Six Rights match.

Whenever the UAP is checking one record against the other, such as the medication sheet with the pharmacy label, he must make sure to use the Six Rights—*right individual*, *right medication*, *right dose*, *right time*, *right route*, and *right documentation*.

BASIC GUIDELINES FOR MEDICATION ADMINISTRATION

1. *Put the safety of the individual first.* This is the UAP's number one priority when giving medication. In addition to following the Three Checks and using the Six Rights, it is the UAP's responsibility to contact a supervisor for any unusual situation. The UAP should never try to handle a situation that he has not been trained to handle or has not had experience with. Holding a medication, contacting a supervisor or a licensed health care provider, and administering a medication late are better than causing harm to an individual.

2. Remember the Three Checks and Six Rights at all times.

3. Always check the expiration date to make sure the medication has not expired.

4. Compare the medication on the pharmacy label to the individual's allergies on his medication sheet. Make sure that the individual is not allergic to the medication you are going to administer.

5. Always ask questions when unsure about a medication.

6. Wash hands before handling medications.

7. Make sure that there is enough time to complete the task.

8. Work in an area that has enough light. Be able to read labels and records clearly.

9. Check the name, dose, and instructions for the medication *every time* the medication is given. The licensed health care provider's order may have changed since the last time the medication was given. *Remember, the information on the licensed health care provider's order, medication sheet, and pharmacy label must all match. If these do not match exactly, do not give the medication. Contact the supervisor right away.*

10. Know why the individual is getting the medication; this includes knowing each medication's:
    a. **Implication(s) for administration**
    b. Precautions
    c. **Contraindications**
    d. Interactions
    e. Side effects and when they might happen.

11. Before leaving the medication area to administer a medication, make sure the medications are replaced in the storage area and locked as required by policy and regulation.

implication(s) for administration
The medical conditions that are treated by the medication; the reason why the medication is being used.

contraindications
Conditions making medication dangerous to use.

PRECAUTIONS

In the UAP's daily care of people, there will be times when he is expected to use precautions to prevent the spread of infection. These precautions apply to every individual for whom the UAP cares and are meant to protect the UAP as well as the individual with whom he is working. In medication administration, there are two primary precautions that are commonly used: handwashing and, at times, gloves.

Procedure 6-1
Hand Washing

The single most important way to keep an infection from spreading is to *wash your hands*.

1. Check that there is an adequate supply of soap and paper towels. A waste container lined with a plastic bag should be in the area near you.

2. Remove rings, if possible, or be sure to lather soap underneath.

3. Remove watch, or push up over wrist.

4. Turn on the faucet with a dry paper towel held between your hand and the faucet (Figure 6-2).

5. Adjust the water to a warm temperature. Drop the towel in the waste container. Stand back from the sink so you do not contaminate your uniform. Wet your hands, keeping your fingertips pointed downward (Figure 6-3).

6. Apply soap and lather over your hands and wrists, between fingers, and under rings. Use friction and interlace your fingers (Figure 6-4). Work lather over every part of your hands and wrists. Clean your fingernails by rubbing them against the palm of the other hand to force soap under the nails for 15 to 20 seconds (Figure 6-5).

7. Rinse your hands with your fingertips pointed down. Do not shake water from your hands.

8. Dry your hands thoroughly with a clean paper towel(s).

9. Turn off the faucet with another paper towel (Figure 6-2); drop the towel in the waste container.

10. Apply lotion to your hands.

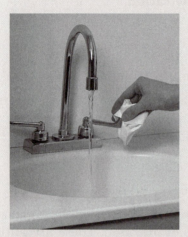

Figure 6-2 Use a clean, dry paper towel to turn *on* and *off* the faucets. *(Delmar/Cengage Learning)*

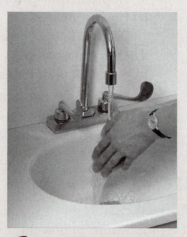

Figure 6-3 Keep your fingertips pointed down when washing your hands. *(Delmar/Cengage Learning)*

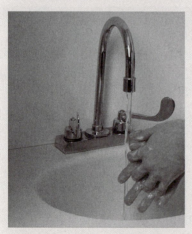

Figure 6-4 Interlace the fingers to clean between them. *(Delmar/Cengage Learning)*

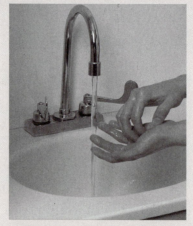

Figure 6-5 Rub your nails against the palms of your hands to clean under the nails. *(Delmar/Cengage Learning)*

Handwashing is the most effective way to prevent the spread of infection. The UAP should wash his hands:

- At the start of his shift
- Before handling food or drink items or medication
- After handling food, drinks, or medication
- After using the bathroom
- After coughing or sneezing
- After blowing his nose
- After touching any item or surface that is soiled
- Before and after caring for each individual on his assignment
- Before putting on and after removing gloves
- After smoking
- At the end of his shift

According to the CDC, the use of waterless (alcohol-based) hand rubs may also be used by health care workers for hand hygiene. Health care workers, however, should continue to wash their hands if:

- Hands are visibly soiled (dirty)
- Hands are visibly contaminated with blood or body fluids
- Before eating
- After using the restroom
- When caring for individuals with C-Diff or other diseases that are spread by spores

When using a waterless (alcohol-based) hand rub, apply the solution to the palm of one hand, then rub hands together, covering all surfaces of hands and fingers until hands are dry (St. Mary's Medical Center, retrieved March 14, 2009, from http://www.stmaryhealthcare .org).

In addition to handwashing, the UAP will at times also need to wear gloves. Gloves are worn any time the UAP comes into contact with blood, body fluids, mucous membranes, or open areas of the skin. In medication administration, gloves are worn for such things as applying ointments to rashes on an individual's skin, inserting vaginal and rectal suppositories, and giving an enema. Gloves are also worn whenever the UAP needs to clean up body fluid spills or clean equipment that may be contaminated and for hands that are cut, scratched, or chapped or that have a rash.

Gloves need to be changed:

- After working with each individual
- Before touching clean items or clean surfaces
- Between tasks with the same individual if the UAP is in contact with any infectious material

PROCEDURE FOR MEDICATION ADMINISTRATION

Now that the Six Rights—handwashing, use of gloves, general guidelines for giving medication, and the Three Checks—have all been reviewed, the next topic for discussion is the procedure for administering medication. The procedure for administering medications is broken down into specific steps that must be followed in order to do this safely and correctly.

1. Preparation

   - *Right Individual:* Identify the individual to whom the medication is being given.

   - Wash hands thoroughly.

   - Gather all the equipment needed—gloves, water, spoon, reading glasses, and so on.

   - Unlock the storage area.

   - Review the medication sheet for any noted allergies, any special measures such as pulse or blood pressure measurement before administration, or the requirement to administer medication with or without food.

2. Begin Pouring the Medication

   - Compare the medication sheet with the licensed health care provider's order.

   - From the medication sheet, identify the *Right Medication.* Take the medication out of the storage area.

   - Compare the pharmacy label to the medication sheet.

   - Prepare the *Right Dose.*

   - Sign the count sheet for countable medications (see section on "Handling and Counting Controlled Substances").

   - Compare the pharmacy label to the medication sheet again.

   - Double-check the medication sheet to make sure that the medication is being given to the individual at the *Right Time.*

   - If the UAP must leave the storage area to give the medication, he must remember to *lock the medications back up before leaving the area.*

3. Administration

   - Give the medication to the individual by the *Right Route.*

   - Make sure the individual takes the medication.

   - If it is given by mouth, watch the individual swallow the medication. *Never leave the medication at the bedside or on the table for the individual to take later.*

4. Documentation

   - As the UAP documents the medication he gave, he must compare the pharmacy label to the medication sheet again.

- Return the medication to the storage area.

- Lock the storage area.

- Wash hands.

- Observe the individual for any unpleasant or harmful effects from the medication.

Note: Some medications may be double packed. For instance, a labeled bottle of eyedrops or eardrops may come from the pharmacy in a second, labeled container. In addition, bubble packs or bingo cards may at times have two labels on them. The upper left side of the card may have the original pharmacy label, while a second label may have been placed by the pharmacy in the upper right-hand corner of the card for the specific individual stating the medication name and directions for use. The UAP needs to read all of the labels to make sure he is giving the right medication.

PROPER STORAGE OF MEDICATIONS

Whenever a medication is not being given, it must be safely stored. A work setting may choose to use a **medication cart** (Figure 6-6), a medication room, or another arrangement that meets their state regulation. Although the place to store it may change from one work setting to another, certain precautions and guidelines should be followed wherever the UAP works. These precautions and guidelines are as follows:

1. It is preferable that one room be identified as the medication room. It should be set up in the following ways:

   - It should be away from the flow of general traffic.

   - It should be well lighted.

   - It should be kept clean, neat, cool, and dry.

   - It should have a sink and a refrigerator.

   - It should have enough cabinet space so that **internal medications** can be kept separate from **external medications**.

   - It should have a cabinet, drawer, or metal lockbox with a double lock for storing controlled substances.

   - The room should be kept locked when no one is using it.

   - There should be emergency supplies and medications easily available whenever a medication is being given to a individual.

2. Medications must be stored in their original containers. A medication may need to be stored in an opaque or glass container; always leave medications in the original containers they are in when delivered from the pharmacy.

3. Refrigerate unopened insulin, sera, vaccines, liquid vitamins, suppositories, and certain liquid antibiotics. The pharmacy

internal medications
Medications that are taken into the body.

external medications
Medications that are applied or put onto the outside of the body.

label should indicate if a medication needs to be stored in the refrigerator.

4. Check medications, supplies, and equipment regularly. Make sure there is an adequate amount of everything available and that everything is in working order. Check for expiration dates on a regular basis. Follow the workplace policy and regulations for destruction and disposal of outdated medications and supplies.

5. Controlled substances must be kept separate from other medications. They must be placed in a double-locked storage area such as a securely locked box and then placed in a locked safe or a substantially constructed, locked cabinet. Access to the controlled substances must be kept to only a minimum number of staff. The staff person responsible for the administration of controlled substances must keep the controlled substance keys, sometimes referred to as "narcotic keys," protected from possible misuse.

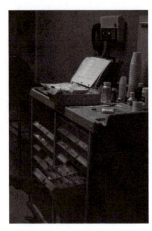

Figure 6-6 In some work settings, medications are stored in and administered from a medication cart.
(Delmar/Cengage Learning)

HANDLING AND COUNTING CONTROLLED SUBSTANCES

Because of their potential for addiction and abuse, medications in Schedules II to V must be reconciled (counted) at least every twenty-four (24) hours by two staff members. It is preferable that the medications, along with syringes, be counted at the end of each shift by two staff members. The count is typically done by one staff person who is ending his shift and another staff person who is starting his shift. As previously discussed in Chapter 5, the total numbers of each medication and number of syringes are recorded in a Controlled Substance Count Book or may be completed in a computerized medication administration system. UAPs should make sure they check and understand their workplace policies and state regulations to determine how the count should be completed.

If using a Controlled Substance Count Book, the UAP may follow the guidelines below for counting controlled substance medications:

1. Medications in Schedules II to V, along with syringes, should be counted at least every twenty-four (24) hours, preferably at the end of each shift. Depending on a facility's particular procedures, all medications, including Schedule VI medications, may require these guidelines.

   • There must always be two staff present to conduct the count, one individual to count and the other to witness the count, One of these individuals is ending his shift. The other individual is starting his shift.

   • In the count section of the Controlled Substance Count Book, compare the actual amount of medication left in the pharmacy container with the number in the "amount left" column in the Controlled Substance Count Book. These must match for the count to be correct (see Figure 6-7).

					( ) Original Entry or
Name:					( ) Transferred from Page No.

Licensed Health Care Provider:	Pharmacy:	Rx No.	Rx Date:

Drug & Strength:	Rx No.	Rx Date:

Directions:	Rx No.	Rx Date:

Date	Time	Amount on Hand	Amount Used	Route	Amount Left	Staff Signature

MEDICATION DISCONTINUED/DISPOSED	**MEDICATION TRANSFERRED**
Discontinue Date: _____ Removal Date: _____ Signature Staff Removing: _____ Signatures of Staff Destroying Medication: (2 signatures required) _____ _____	New Page # _____ Amount Transferred: _____ Signatures of Staff Verification: (2 signatures required) _____ _____

Figure 6-7 Count Page of the Controlled Substance Count Book. *(Source: Yoder, M. & Collins, S. (1999) Controlled Substance Count Book. SCRRI: Sturbridge, MA.)*

- If the count is not correct, first check the addition and subtraction to make sure the math is correct.

- If the count is still not correct and the UAP is not able to account for the missing medication, he is to notify his supervisor immediately. If the staff members who handled those medications on that shift are still present, the work setting may wish for those staff members to account for any differences noted.

- If a medication cannot be accounted for, it is considered a **medication loss**. Medication losses are discussed in Chapter 30.

2. If the UAP finds a documentation error in the Count Book, he should draw a single line through the error and write his initials next to the line. He must also write in the correct information and write his initials next to that correction. When correcting an error in the Controlled Substance Count Book, follow these guidelines:

   - *Do not* use correction fluids, such as Wite Out, or correction tape.

   - *Do not* erase or scribble over the error.

   - The Count Book is a legal document, just like documentation sheets and progress notes are legal documents. See Chapter 28 for a review of the ten (10) guidelines for documentation as needed.

3. The staff member who counts and the staff member who witnesses the count must indicate if the count is correct, or incorrect. Both must sign their names in the verification section of the Count Book (see Figure 6-8).

Reminder: Count pages in the Controlled Substance Count Book are completed as medications are being administered.

Note: For examples of the Controlled Substance Count and additional worksheets, refer to Chapter 6 of the accompanying workbook.

DISPOSAL OF MEDICATIONS

Disposal of medications is one of the tasks the UAP may be asked to perform. This includes destruction of the medication so that it is unusable as well as documentation of the destruction of controlled substances. Although documentation is only required for controlled substances, a facility may also expect documentation of destruction of all medications, including over-the-counter medications. The UAP needs to be aware of state regulations and his workplace policy.

Reasons for Disposal of Medications

All unused or discontinued medications must be destroyed. Depending on state and workplace policies, medications may be destroyed at the work site or at a central location. Some reasons for medication disposal include:

- The medication has been refused by the individual after it was poured or prepared.

- The medication has been dropped on the floor.

CONTROLLED SUBSTANCE COUNT VERIFICATION

DATE	TIME	COUNT CORRECT	STAFF COMING ON DUTY	STAFF GOING OFF DUTY

Figure 6-8 Verification Page of the Controlled Substance Count Book. *(Source: Yoder, M. & Collins, S. (1999) Controlled Substance Count Book. SCRRI: Sturbridge, MA.)*

- The medication has expired—the UAP must check the expiration date every time he gives a medication.
- The individual for whom it was prescribed has left the facility or program.
- The medication has been discontinued by the licensed health care provider.

Rules of Medication Disposal

When disposing of medications, remember the following do's and don'ts:

Do:

- Do dispose of medication according to state and federal regulations and workplace policy.
- It is strongly recommended that two staff members be present when the medication is being disposed of.
- Do complete the documentation for disposal required by workplace policy and/or state regulations.

Don't:

- Unless permitted by state regulation, do not use any medication brought back to the facility or site.
- Unless permitted by state regulation, do not return medications to a pharmacy for disposal.
- Do not leave any blank spaces on disposal documentation records.

The Office of National Drug Control Policy, in conjunction with the U.S. Food and Drug Administration, has established federal guidelines for the disposal of "Unused Medicines." Figure 6-9 provides the UAP with a copy of the guidelines published by the Office of National Drug Control Policy. Figure 6-10 provides the UAP with a copy of the guidelines published by the U.S. Food and Drug Administration.

Documentation of Medication Disposal

As noted in Chapter 5, documentation of medication disposal is required in some settings for controlled substances in Schedules II to V. However, a workplace may also require documentation for destruction of all medications, including over-the-counter medications. The UAP must know the workplace and state regulations. Figure 6-11 is an excerpt from the medication disposal documentation record from the Massachusetts Department of Public Health. The form, titled *Controlled Substance Disposal Record*, is used in the Massachusetts Medication Administration Program.

Proper Disposal of Prescription Drugs

Office of National Drug Control Policy   February 2007

Federal Guidelines:

- Take unused, unneeded, or expired prescription drugs out of their original containers and throw them in the trash.

- Mixing prescription drugs with an undesirable substance, such as used coffee grounds or kitty litter, and putting them in impermeable, non-descript containers, such as empty cans or sealable bags, will further ensure the drugs are not diverted.

- Flush prescription drugs down the toilet *only* if the label or accompanying
- patient information specifically instructs doing so (see box).

- Take advantage of community pharmaceutical take-back programs that allow the public to bring unused drugs to a central location for proper disposal. Some communities have pharmaceutical take-back programs or community solid-waste programs that allow the public to bring unused drugs to a central location for proper disposal. Where these exist, they are a good way to dispose of unused pharmaceuticals.

> The FDA advises that the following drugs be flushed down the toilet instead of thrown in the trash:
>
> **Actiq** (fentanyl citrate)
> **Daytrana Transdermal Patch** (methylphenidate)
> **Duragesic Transdermal System** (fentanyl)
> **OxyContin Tablets** (oxycodone)
> **Avinza Capsules** (morphine sulfate)
> **Baraclude Tablets** (entecavir)
> **Reyataz Capsules** (atazanavir sulfate)
> **Tequin Tablets** (gatifloxacin)
> **Zerit for Oral Solution** (stavudine)
> **Meperidine HCl Tablets**
> **Percocet** (Oxycodone and Acetaminophen)
> **Xyrem** (Sodium Oxybate)
> **Fentora** (fentanyl buccal tablet)
>
> ---
>
> Note: Patients should always refer to printed material accompanying their medication for specific instructions.

Office of National Drug Control Policy
ONDCP, Washington, D.C. 20503
p (202) 395-6618   f (202) 395-6730

Figure 6-9 Proper Disposal of Prescription Drugs. (*Source: Office of National Drug Control Policy, 2007*)

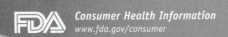

Consumer Health Information
www.fda.gov/consumer

www.fda.gov/consumer/updates/drug_disposal062308.html

How to Dispose of Unused Medicines

I s your medicine cabinet filled with expired drugs or medications you no longer use? How should you dispose of them?

Most drugs can be thrown in the household trash, but consumers should take certain precautions before tossing them out, according to the Food and Drug Administration (FDA). A few drugs should be flushed down the toilet. And a growing number of community-based "take-back" programs offer another safe disposal alternative.

Guidelines for Drug Disposal

FDA worked with the White House Office of National Drug Control Policy (ONDCP) to develop the first consumer guidance for proper disposal of prescription drugs. Issued by ONDCP in February 2007, the federal guidelines are summarized here:

• Follow any specific disposal instructions on the drug label or patient information that accompanies the medication. Do not flush prescription drugs down the toilet unless this information specifically instructs you to do so.

• If no instructions are given, throw the drugs in the household trash, but first:

  • Take them out of their original containers and mix them with an undesirable substance, such as used coffee grounds or kitty litter. The medication will be less appealing to children and pets, and unrecognizable to people who may intentionally go through your trash.

  • Put them in a sealable bag, empty can, or other container to prevent the medication from leaking or breaking out of a garbage bag.

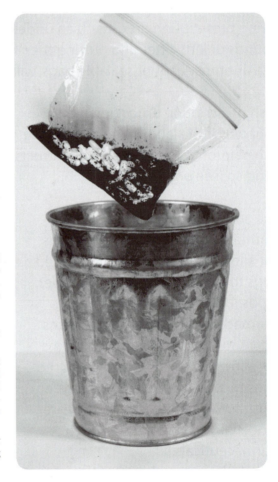

Take drugs out of their original containers and mix them with an undesirable substance, such as used coffee grounds ...

Photo Illustration: FDA/Michael Ermarth

Figure 6-10   How to Dispose of Unused Medications. *(Source: U.S. Food and Drug Administration, 2008)*

FDA *Consumer Health Information*
www.fda.gov/consumer

www.fda.gov/consumer/updates/drug_disposal062308.html

- Take advantage of community drug take-back programs that allow the public to bring unused drugs to a central location for proper disposal. Call your city or county government's household trash and recycling service (see blue pages in phone book) to see if a take-back program is available in your community.

FDA's Director of Pharmacy Affairs, Ilisa Bernstein, Pharm.D., J.D., offers some additional tips:

- Before throwing out a medicine container, scratch out all identifying information on the prescription label to make it unreadable. This will help protect your identity and the privacy of your personal health information.

- Do not give medications to friends. Doctors prescribe drugs based on a person's specific symptoms and medical history. A drug that works for you could be dangerous for someone else.

- When in doubt about proper disposal, talk to your pharmacist.

Bernstein says the same disposal methods for prescription drugs could apply to over-the-counter drugs as well.

Why the Precautions?

Disposal instructions on the label are part of FDA's "risk mitigation" strategy, says Capt. Jim Hunter, R.Ph., M.P.H., Senior Program Manager on FDA's Controlled Substance Staff. When a drug contains instructions to flush it down the toilet, he says, it's because FDA, working with the manufacturer, has determined this method to be the most appropriate route of disposal that presents the least risk to safety.

About a dozen drugs, such as powerful narcotic pain relievers and other controlled substances, carry instructions for flushing to reduce the danger of unintentional use or overdose and illegal abuse.

For example, the fentanyl patch, an adhesive patch that delivers a potent pain medicine through the skin, comes with instructions to flush used or left-over patches. Too much fentanyl can cause severe breathing problems and lead to death in babies, children, pets, and even adults, especially those who have not been prescribed the drug. "Even after a patch is used, a lot of the drug remains in the patch," says Hunter, "so you wouldn't want to throw something in the trash that contains a powerful and potentially dangerous narcotic that could harm others."

Environmental Concerns

Despite the safety reasons for flushing drugs, some people are questioning the practice because of concerns about trace levels of drug residues found in surface water, such as rivers and lakes, and in some community drinking water supplies. However, the main way drug residues enter water systems is by people taking medications and then naturally passing them through their bodies, says Raanan Bloom, Ph.D., an Environmental Assessment Expert in FDA's Center for Drug Evaluation and Research. "Most drugs are not completely absorbed or metabolized by the body, and enter the environment after passing through waste water treatment plants."

A company that wants FDA to approve its drug must submit an application package to the agency. FDA requires, as part of the application package, an assessment of how the drug's use would affect the environment. Some drug applications are excluded from the assessment requirement, says Bloom, based on previous agency actions.

"For those drugs for which environmental assessments have been required, there has been no indication of environmental effects due to flushing," says Bloom. In addition, according to the Environmental Protection Agency, scientists to date have found no evidence of adverse human health effects from pharmaceutical residues in the environment.

Nonetheless, FDA does not want to add drug residues into water systems unnecessarily, says Hunter. The agency is in the process of reviewing all drug labels with disposal directions to assure that the recommended methods for disposal are still appropriate.

Another environmental concern lies with inhalers used by people who have asthma or other breathing problems, such as chronic obstructive pulmonary disease. Traditionally, many inhalers have contained chlorofluorocarbons (CFC's), a propellant that damages the protective ozone layer. The CFC inhalers are being phased out and replaced with more environmentally friendly inhalers.

Depending on the type of product and where you live, inhalers and aerosol products may be thrown into household trash or recyclables, or may be considered hazardous waste and require special handling. Read the handling instructions on the label, as some inhalers should not be punctured or thrown into a fire or incinerator. To ensure safe disposal, contact your local trash and recycling facility. FDA

This article appears on FDA's Consumer Health Information Web page (*www.fda.gov/consumer*), which features the latest on all FDA-regulated products. Sign up for free e-mail subscriptions at *www.fda.gov/consumer/consumernews.html*.

For More Information
Proper Disposal of Prescription Drugs Fact Sheet and Video Clip
www.ondcp.gov/drugfact/factsht/proper_disposal.html

SMARxT Disposal Campaign
www.smarxtdisposal.net

Albuterol Inhalers: Time to Transition
www.fda.gov/consumer/updates/albuterol053008.html

Figure 6-10 (continued)

Item # _____   Date last filled _____

Name _____   Date _____

Medication/strength _____

Rx # _____   Pharmacy _____

Amount disposed _____   Reason _____

_____

Controlled Substance Book # _____   Page # _____

Signatures: Staff member _____

Supervisor _____

Figure 6-11 A sample disposal record. An excerpt from the medication disposal documentation record from the Massachusetts Department of Public Health. The form, titled *Controlled Substance Disposal Record*, is used in the Massachusetts Medication Administration Program. *(Delmar/Cengage Learning)*

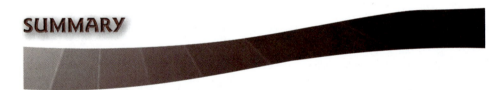

SUMMARY

Safe and effective medication administration is based on a series of simple yet critical procedures and guidelines. These include the Six Rights, the Three Checks, the basic guidelines for medication administration, the four-step procedure for medication administration, handwashing, and the use of gloves. These principles of medication administration provide the UAP with a strong foundation on which he will be able to develop his skills.

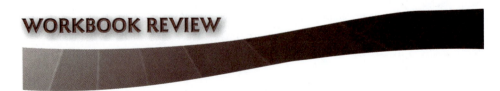

WORKBOOK REVIEW

Go to the workbook and complete the exercises for Chapter 6.

REVIEW QUESTIONS

1. The Six Rights of medication administration involve checking for all of the following *except*:
   a. individual
   b. medication
   c. dose, time, and route
   d. reason

2. When using the Six Rights, information is checked on the:
   a. health care provider order, pharmacy label, and medication sheet
   b. progress notes from the last week
   c. list in the storage area
   d. facility's communication board

3. The dose of a medication is:
   a. how much an individual gets at one time
   b. the quantity of medication in a manufacturer's bottle
   c. the amount of medication a pharmacist places in the prescription bottle
   d. all of the above

4. If a medication is to be given at 4:00 p.m., you can:
   a. only give it at 4:00 p.m.
   b. give it any time after 2:00 p.m.
   c. give it any time between 3:30 p.m. and 4:30 p.m.
   d. give it when you have time

5. The Three Checks are:
   a. times when the UAP compares the health care provider order, the pharmacy label, and the medication sheet during medication administration
   b. times when the UAP makes sure an individual is available to take his medications
   c. times when the UAP makes sure the storage area is locked
   d. times when the UAP checks the medical supplies during his shift

6. The number one priority of the UAP when giving medication is:
   a. to work in an area with enough light for reading
   b. to ask questions whenever he is unsure about a medication
   c. to wash his hands before giving medications
   d. to put the safety of the individual first

7. The single most important way to keep an infection from spreading is to:
   a. wear gloves at all times when working
   b. wash your hands
   c. blow your nose only when in the bathroom
   d. only eat in the kitchen

8. Gloves need to be changed:
   a. after gathering all of the dirty linens
   b. before blowing one's nose
   c. before beginning one's tasks for the day
   d. between tasks with the same individual if there is contact with any infectious material
9. When administering a medication, the UAP should:
   a. use the Six Rights and Three Checks to ensure accuracy
   b. offer the individual his choice of a drink for taking pills
   c. tell everyone around to be quiet so the UAP can concentrate
   d. give pills in applesauce if the individual wants it
10. The medication room in a workplace should:
    a. be near the bathroom to have access to water
    b. be near the kitchen to have access to the refrigerator
    c. be kept unlocked so staff have easy access to medications
    d. have a secure, locked storage area for controlled substances

CLINICAL SCENARIOS

1. The UAP is doing temporary coverage at a facility. Part of the UAP's assignment is to give Mrs. Chikowski her medications. How does the UAP figure out who Mrs. Chikowski is?
2. After the UAP identifies Mrs. Chikowski, the UAP needs to give Mrs. Chikowski's medications to her. Describe the procedure for medication administration.

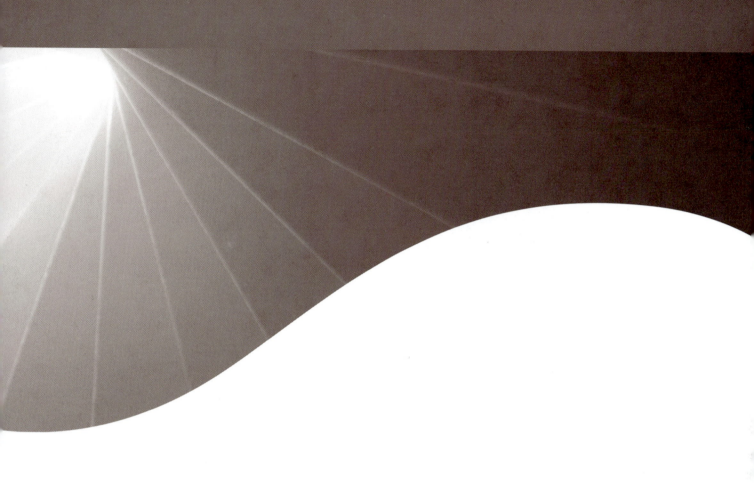

MODULE III
Medication Administration

Chapter 7
Administration of Nonparenteral Medications

Learning Objectives

After reading this chapter and completing the review questions, you should be able to:

1. Spell and define terms.
2. List three advantages and five disadvantages of taking medications orally.
3. Prepare medications for administration.
4. Demonstrate the administration of oral medications.
5. Demonstrate the administration of eye medications.
6. Demonstrate the administration of ear medications.
7. Demonstrate the administration of nasal medications.
8. Demonstrate the administration of transdermal medications.
9. Demonstrate the administration of rectal medications.
10. Demonstrate the administration of vaginal medications.
11. Demonstrate the application of medications to the skin and hair.
12. Demonstrate the use of a handheld inhaler (MDI).
13. Demonstrate the use of a small-volume nebulizer and IPPB machine.
14. Write a clinical progress note for an individual receiving aerosol therapy.

Key Terms

buccal medications

COPD (Chronic Obstructive Pulmonary Disease)

douche

enema

handheld inhaler

herpes

inhalant medications

inhalation

intermittent positive-pressure breathing (IPPB) machine

menopausal symptoms

nasal medications

nebulizer

nonparenteral
medications

nostrils

ophthalmic
medications

oral

otic medications

parenteral medications

pediculosis

perforated eardrum

pulmonary medications

rebound bronchospasm

rebound nasal
congestion

rectal medications

rectum

scabies

sterile

sublingual medications

suppository

tolerance

topical medications

transdermal system

unit dose container

vagina

vaginal medications

INTRODUCTION

As discussed in Chapter 6, the way a medication enters the body is called
the route of administration. Routes of administration are grouped into
two main categories:

1. Parenteral medications

2. Nonparenteral medications.

Parenteral medications are those medications that are injected into
the body. This may be done intravenously directly into the bloodstream or
by injection though the skin, fatty tissue, and/or muscle into the body.

Nonparenteral medications are those medications that enter the
body through any route other than injection. This chapter describes
the following nonparenteral routes of administration:

- Oral (by mouth)

- Sublingual (under the tongue)

- Buccal (in a pouch between the cheek and the gum at the back of
  the mouth)

- Topical, including:
  - Ophthalmic (eye)
  - Otic (ear)
  - Nasal (nose)
  - Transdermal (patches)
  - Skin and hair
  - Rectal
  - Vaginal
  - Pulmonary inhalant (medication breathed in through the nose
    or mouth)

Nonparenteral medications may also be administered by enemas,
gastrostomy tubes, and jejunostomy tubes. These routes are discussed in
Chapters 9 and 10.

The licensed health care provider chooses the route of administration to be used. Her decision is based on several factors. These factors
include the following:

- The condition of the individual

- The individual's disease or illness

- How fast the licensed health care provider wants the medication to be absorbed (used) by the body
- The form of the medication that is available for use

ORAL MEDICATIONS

oral
By mouth.

The most common way to administer a medication is **orally** (by mouth). Advantages of the oral route include:

1. Comfort for the individual
2. Convenience for the individual and/or staff
3. Safety—administration of the medication can be stopped if an error is discovered during adminsitration
4. Financial—the most cost-effective route of adminsitration.

Disadvantages of the oral route include:

1. Oral medications cannot be used for an unconscious individual.
2. Oral medications cannot be used if the individual is NPO (fasting).
3. Oral medications may have a foul or bad taste.
4. Oral medications may cause an individual's teeth, mouth, or tongue to change color.
5. Oral medications may irritate the stomach causing nausea or heartburn.
6. The body may not absorb the medication well.
7. The oral medication may come in a form that is too large for the individual to swallow.
8. The individual may be unable to take the medication because she is having nausea or vomiting.
9. The individual may refuse to take the oral medication.
10. The effect of an oral medication on the body may be less predictable than when the medication is given by injection.

As discussed in Chapter 4, oral medications are available in solid and liquid forms. Solid forms, such as tablets, caplets, and capsules, are usually swallowed with a glass of water. Other forms, such as lozenges and troches, cannot be swallowed. Once lozenges and troches are administered, these must dissolve in the mouth. Solid medications can be measured by weight in micrograms, milligrams, grams, grains, milliequivalents, or units.

Liquid medications, such as suspensions, elixirs, and syrups, are absorbed more quickly. They are used more readily by the body than solid medications. Liquid medications are often artificially colored and flavored to hide their true appearance and taste.

Liquid medication is measured in milliliters, cubic centimeters, minims, drams, ounces, and such household measures as teaspoons and tablespoons. Liquid medications may also be measured by weight in micrograms, milligrams, grams, grains, milliequivalents, or units. The licensed health care provider determines the amount of medication an individual will receive.

Equipment and Supplies Used in the Administration of Oral Medications

The following equipment and supplies may be used in the administration of oral medications:

- Medication sheet

- Electronic medication adminstration record (eMAR)

- The medication(s) ordered by the licensed health care provider

- Medicine cup (paper or plastic)

- Medicine dropper

- Water cup (plastic, glass, or paper)

- Drinking straws

- Syringes

- Tablet crusher

- Medication cart (used mainly in an institutional setting) (Figure 7-1)

- Computer on Wheels

- Medication room that includes a medication cabinet, a refrigerator, a sink, Controlled Substance Count Book, computer

Note: Use of medication sheets, eMAR, and Controlled Substance Count Books are discussed in Chapters 5, 6, and 29.

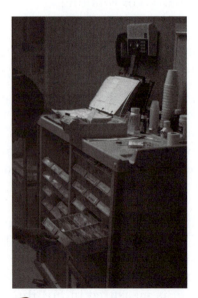

Figure 7-1 Medication cart.
(Delmar/Cengage Learning)

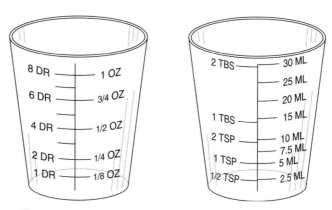

Figure 7-2 Medicine cup with approximate equivalent measures. *(Delmar/Cengage Learning)*

The medicine cup comes in different sizes and shapes, depending on its use and manufacturer. In Figure 7-2, note that the medicine cup is marked off in fluid ounces, fluidrams, milliliters (mL), teaspoons (tsp), and tablespoons (Tbs).

The water cup is usually a three (3)-ounce, disposable cup made of plastic or paper. The cup, however, may be made of glass if the UAP is working in a home care setting.

The medicine dropper may be marked off in milliliters, minims, or drops (Figure 7-3). Many times, the droppers are provided as part of a prescription package with many medications. Unmarked droppers may be provided when the medication is being administered only in drops. The size of the drops differs according to the size of the opening of the dropper, the angle at which the dropper is held, the thickness of the medication, and the amount of force used to squeeze the rubber top of

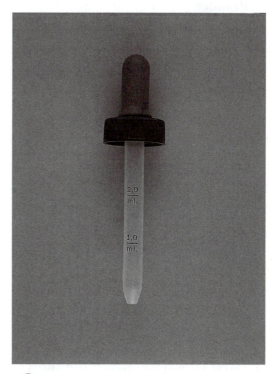

Figure 7-3 Calibrated dropper.
(Delmar/Cengage Learning)

the dropper. It is, therefore, important that the UAP use the dropper that comes with the prescribed medication.

To measure the dose of medication correctly, it is important that the UAP choose the right container to measure the medication that she is administering.

Principles and Procedures for Medication Administration

Chapter 6 lists the Six Rights of Medication Administration, the Three Checks, and the procedure for administering medications safely and effectively. As a brief review, read the procedure for administering medications:

1. Preparation

   - *Right Individual:* Identify the individual to whom the medication is being given.

   - Wash hands thoroughly.

   - Gather all the equipment needed—gloves, water, spoon, reading glasses, and so on.

   - Unlock the storage area.

   - Review the medication sheet for any noted allergies, any special measures such as pulse or blood pressure measurement before administration, or the requirement to administer medication with or without food.

2. Begin Pouring the Medication

   - Compare the medication sheet with the licensed health care provider's order.

   - From the medication sheet, identify the *Right Medication.* Take the medication out of the storage area.

   - Compare the pharmacy label to the medication sheet.

   - Prepare the *Right Dose.*

   - Sign the count sheet for countable medications (see "Handling and Counting Controlled Substances" in Chapter 6).

   - Compare the pharmacy label to the medication sheet again.

   - Double-check the medication sheet to make sure that the medication is being given to the individual at the *Right Time.*

   - If the UAP must leave the storage area to give the medication, she must remember to *lock the medications back up before leaving the area.*

3. Administration

   - Give the medication to the individual by the *Right Route.*

   - Make sure the individual takes the medication.

   - If it is given by mouth, watch the individual swallow the medication.

4. Documentation

- As the UAP documents the medication she gave, she must compare the pharmacy label to the medication sheet again.
- Return the medication to the storage area.
- Lock the storage area.
- Wash hands.
- Observe the individual for any unpleasant or harmful effects from the medication.

Remember that these basic principles and procedures are followed for all medications. In addition, however, each route has special considerations that must be followed.

Procedure 7-1
Administration of Oral Medications

The principles and procedures for administering medications are always the same and always followed. However, the actual steps to administering a medication will differ depending on the route that the medication is given. For oral medications, use the following steps:

1. Complete steps 1 and 2 as per the procedure for giving medications.

2. To administer oral medications, do the following:

   A. Have the individual take a drink of water to moisten her mouth.

   B. Administer the medication with water.

   C. Watch the individual swallow the medication.

3. Complete step 4 as per the procedure for giving medications.

Special Considerations for the Administration of Oral Medication

- If an individual says she has not had this medication before or that it is different from what she usually takes, call the licensed health care provider *before* giving the medication.
- If giving more than one solid medication to an individual at the same time, put all of the medications in the same medicine cup.

Note: If the UAP must check an individual's pulse or blood pressure before administering a medication, the UAP should place the medication in a separate medicine cup in case the medication needs to be held.

- If giving a solid medication and a liquid medication at the same time, give the solid medication first and then give the liquid medication.

- Do not mix medication with food or liquids such as juice or milk without first consulting with the licensed health care provider who wrote the medication order. Once permission is received to mix the medication with food or liquid, have the licensed health care provider write an order to do so. Transcribe this information under the section on the medication sheet entitled "Special Instructions/Precautions."

- If giving two liquid medications at one time and one of the liquid medications is a cough syrup, give the cough syrup last. The cough syrup coats and soothes the throat.

Note: When giving medications, the UAP should never change the form of a medication without a licensed health care provider's written order unless her state regulations and workplace policy permit her to do so. This means:

- Do not crush or dissolve a tablet, caplet, capsule, or other form of solid medication.

- Do not take the medication out of a capsule or tablet.

- Do not mix a solid medication with a liquid medication.

- Do not mix two liquids together.

- Do not mix medication with food unless ordered by the licensed health care provider.

These are guidelines for liquid medications:

- Unless otherwise instructed *not* to do so, shake the bottle well before pouring the medication.

- Take the cap or top of the container off the bottle and place it upside down on the countertop or table.

- Use a marked medicine cup when measuring or pouring medication.

- Place the liquid medicine cup at eye level. It might be helpful to place the medicine cup on the countertop or table. Or hold the cup at eye level and fill the cup to the right level. Use the markings on the medicine cup as a guide to the right measurement (Figure 7-4).

- Measure the medicine at the lowest level of the liquid in the medicine cup. This point is called the meniscus.

- When pouring the medication, the UAP should hold the bottle so that the label is covered with her hand. Then she should wipe off the top of the bottle after pouring the medication. This keeps the label from getting soiled.

- When pouring the medication into the medicine cup, do not let the bottle touch the medicine cup.

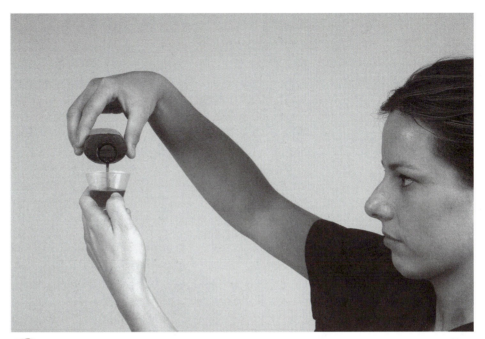

Figure 7-4 Hold the medication bottle with the label side up. Keep the medicine cup at eye level. Use the thumbnail to mark the measurement. *(Delmar/Cengage Learning)*

- If too much medication is poured into the medicine cup, throw the extra amount of medication away. Do not pour the extra amount back into the bottle.

- Ask the licensed health care provider if the liquid medication may be given with juice or water. Ask if it may be mixed with juice, water, or another liquid.

- Store the liquid medications in the refrigerator if the pharmacy label states to do so. If unsure, call the pharmacist and ask if refrigeration is needed.

- After administering the liquid medication, if the UAP needs to reuse the medicine cup, she must wash the medicine cup with soap and warm water, then rinse and dry it well.

- Remember, *never* mix two liquid medications together in the same cup. Each medication gets its own medication cup.

Administering Unit Dose Medication

When administering medication using unit dose containers, the UAP should open the **unit dose container** when she is at the individual's side. This way, if the individual refuses the medication, the medication will not have to be wasted. Once the medication container is opened, place the medication in the individual's hand (Figures 7-5a and 7-5b). Be sure not to touch the medication. If more than one medication is being administered, the UAP may find it easier to open and pour all of the medications into a medication cup while at the individual's side, then administer them to the individual.

unit dose container
A container that holds a single dose of medication.

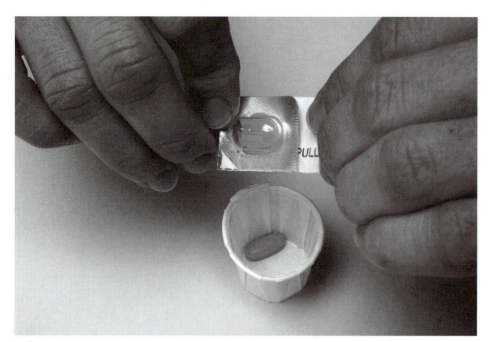

Figure 7-5a Open the unit-dose packet of medication. Drop the medication into the medicine cup. *(Delmar/Cengage Learning)*

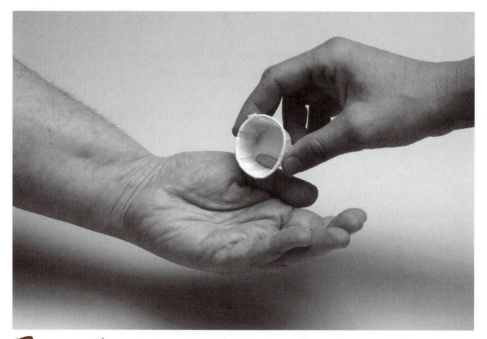

Figure 7-5b Place the medicine cup containing the medication in the individual's hand. *(Delmar/Cengage Learning)*

Crushing a Medication for Administration

There are times when a medication will need to be crushed. Certain individuals may have difficulty swallowing tablets, capsules, and other solid forms of medications. These medications will not be available in a liquid form. Once the UAP has consulted with the licensed health care provider and has received a written order to crush a medication, the medication may be crushed and mixed with food or liquid as per the licensed health care provider's order. Remember that even with a licensed HCP order, certain medications cannot be crushed because they are made to be long acting.

How the UAP crushes the tablet will depend on the the equipment available in her work setting. There are specially designed pieces of equipment that may be purchased to crush medication (Figure 7-6). These are called a mortar and pestle (Figure 7-7). If these are not available, the UAP may use two spoons to crush the medication (Figure 7-8). The UAP needs to pay special attention to make sure that none of the medication is lost during the crushing of the medication.

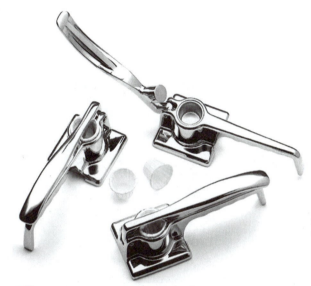

Figure 7-6 Pill and tablet crusher. *(Reprinted with permission from www.pillcrusher.com 1-888-622-6522)*

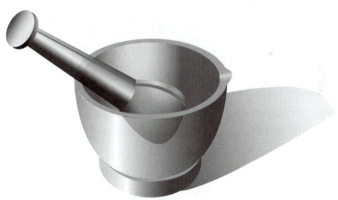

Figure 7-7 Mortar and pestle. *(Delmar/Cengage Learning)*

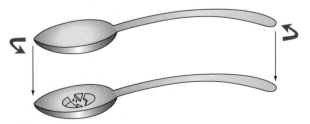

Figure 7-8 Crushing a tablet between two spoons. *(Courtesy of James Russell, Jr.)*

If the licensed health care provider orders it, the UAP may use small amounts of food (applesauce, strained fruit, vanilla pudding, or vanilla ice cream) as a way to administer the crushed medicine. The individual needs to be told that the food has crushed medicine in it. All of the food has to be eaten for the individual to take the medication, which is why only a small amount of food is used.

Devices Used to Administer Oral Liquid Medications

When an individual is unable to drink a liquid medication from a cup or other container, the UAP may use a syringe to administer the liquid medication into the individual's mouth. The UAP must make sure she has the correct amount of medication measured (milliliters, minims, or teaspoons) in the right syringe (Figures 7-9a and 7-9b).

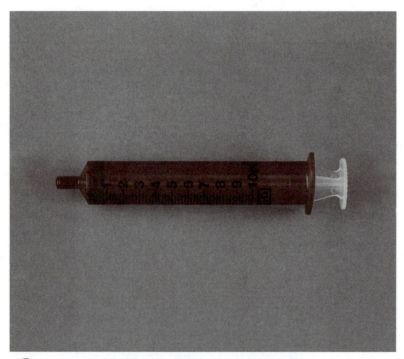

Figure 7-9a A syringe with the safety feature of color to indicate it is used only to adminster oral liquid medications. *(Delmar/Cengage Learning)*

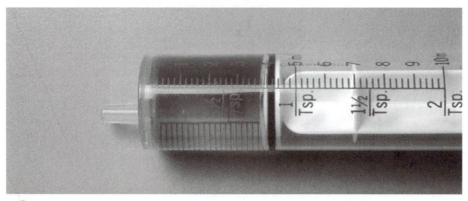

Figure 7-9b An eccentric syringe. Tip is off-center. Used only to administer oral liquid medications. *(Delmar/Cengage Learning)*

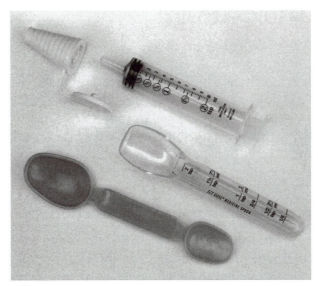

Figure 7-10 Devices for administering liquid medications. *(Delmar/Cengage Learning)*

In addition to the use of a syringe, the UAP may use other forms of equipment to administer a liquid medication. These pieces of equipment are readily available in most pharmacies and other department stores. See Figure 7-10 for examples of these pieces of equipment.

Figure 7-10 has a picture of a double-ended spoon. This double-ended spoon has one end for teaspoons and the other end for tablespoons.

It is very important when using these tools that the UAP accurately and correctly measure the prescribed dose of medication that is to be administered. The marked tools are in teaspoons and milliliters. There are five (5) milliliters to a teaspoon. There are three (3) teaspoons to a tablespoon.

Special Considerations for the Administration of Sublingual Medication

sublingual medications
Medications administered under the tongue where they dissolve and are absorbed into the body.

Sublingual medications are a form of oral medication in that they are taken into the body through the mouth. Sublingual medications, however, are not swallowed. These medications are placed under the tongue and are allowed to dissolve slowly. The medication is then absorbed directly from the mouth into the body. Sublingual medications are used for the treatment of heart (cardiac) and seizure (convulsive) disorders.

Special Considerations for the Administration of Buccal Medication

buccal medications
Tablets that are dissolved in the mouth in a pouch between the cheek and gum at the back of the mouth.

Buccal medications are a form of oral medication in that they are taken into the body through the mouth. Buccal medications, like sublingual medications, are not swallowed. These medications are placed in the pouch between the cheek and the gum at the back of the mouth. Medications placed here are rapidly absorbed directly into the body. Buccal medications are used when a quick response is required.

TOPICAL MEDICATION

In medicine, the word *topical* means "local." Medications that are called **topical medications** are those that are applied to a local area of the body and have their effect there. These medications include ophthalmic (eye), otic (ear), nasal (nose), hair, skin, rectal, and vaginal. Because transdermal medications (patches) are applied to a local area of the body, they are being included in this section. Note, though, that these patches often do not have a local effect. Instead, they have a remote and/or systemic effect on the body.

topical medications
Medications applied to and having effect on a local area of the body.

Administration of Ophthalmic Medication

Ophthalmic medications are medications for the eye. These medications are usually administered to treat eye infections, glaucoma, or dryness. Eye medications commonly come in two forms: eyedrops and eye ointment. The eyedrops are administered by slowly pouring or dropping a liquid medication into the lower pocket of the eye (Figure 7-11). The eye ointment is administered in the same way as the eyedrops, by applying or placing a small portion of the ointment into the lower pocket of the eye. The medication has a local effect, which is why it is a type of topical medication.

ophthalmic medications
Medications for the eye.

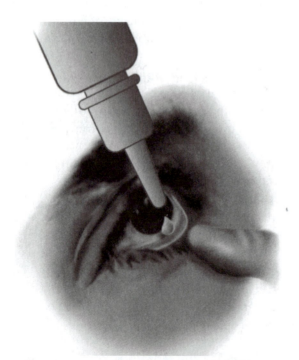

Figure 7-11 Administering eye medication. Gently pull the lower lid of the eye down and have the individual look upward. Place the ophthalmic medication into the lower lid of the eye. *(Delmar/Cengage Learning)*

Equipment and Supplies Used in the Administration of Ophthalmic Medications

The following equipment and supplies may be used in the administration of ophthalmic medications:

- Medication sheet

- Electronic medication administration record (eMAR)

- The individual's eyedropper; in some settings this may need to be a sterile eyedropper

- The medication ordered by the licensed health care provider

- Clean paper tissue (unscented, no aloe); in some settings, sterile cotton balls may be used

- Gloves; in some settings, these may be sterile gloves

Procedure 7-2
Administration of Ophthalmic Medications

The principles and procedures for administering medications are always the same and are always followed. However, the actual steps to administering a medication will differ, depending on the route that the medication is given. For ophthalmic medications, use the following steps:

1. Complete steps 1 and 2 as per the procedure for giving medications.

2. To administer eyedrops, do the following:

    A. Put on gloves.

    B. Make sure the medication is at room temperature.

    C. Use a clean tissue or sterile cotton ball to wipe the eye and eyelid.

    D. Wipe from the inside of the eye (nose side) to the outside of the eye and eyelid to remove any drainage.

    E. If an eyedropper is being used, check the eyedropper to make sure that it is not chipped or cracked.

    F. Do not touch the eyedropper or the bottle of medication against the eye or against anything else. The medication is sterile and must be kept sterile at all times.

    G. If using an eyedropper, always hold the eyedropper with the tip (opening) end down to prevent the medication from running back into the rubber end (bulb) of the eyedropper.

H. Check the eye medication. If the medication looks cloudy, shake the bottle for about ten (10) seconds. Counting to ten (10) is one way to estimate the ten (10) seconds.

I. Have the individual sit down and tilt her head back. If it is more comfortable for the individual, she may lie down on her back. The UAP may need to help the individual stay in the position.

J. If using an eyedropper, squeeze the rubber tip (bulb) of the dropper to draw the medication up into the dropper. Be sure to draw up just the amount of medication that will be administered.

K. The UAP uses her index finger to pull the individual's lower eyelid down to form a "pocket" (see Figure 7-11).

L. Hold the eyedropper in the other hand.

M. Place the eyedropper as close to the pocket of the eye as possible without touching the eye, eyelid, eyelashes, or anything else. Support the remaining fingers of the hand holding the eyedropper against the individual's cheek or nose.

N. Gently drop the prescribed number of drops into the pocket of the lower lid. Do not drop the medication onto the surface of the eyeball. To do so may cause discomfort or even injure the eye.

Note: If the medication should accidentally drop onto the surface of the eye, the UAP should immediately rinse the eye with water and contact the licensed health care provider and her supervisor.

O. Replace the dropper into the bottle of medication right away. Do not wipe the dropper off. Do not rinse the dropper off.

P. Press a finger against the inner corner (nose side) of the eye for one (1) minute (Figure 7-12). Note that the individual will most likely close her eye at this point. If not, the UAP should suggest that the individual gently close her eyes for comfort.

Note: If more than one drop of the same medication needs to be administered, the UAP needs to wait at least thirty (30) seconds to one (1) minute before applying the second drop. If a second eye medication needs to be administered, the UAP needs to wait three (3) to five (5) minutes before administering the second eye medication.

Q. Wipe off any excess medication with a clean paper tissue or sterile cotton ball.

R. Remove gloves. Wash hands.

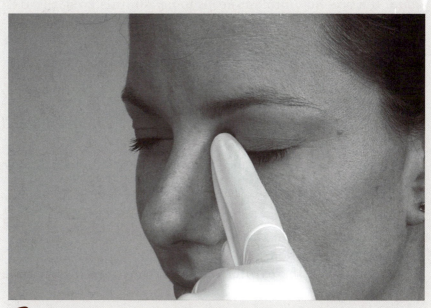

Figure 7-12 Apply gentle pressure on the inner corner of the eye after administering eye medications. This prevents the medication from entering the body through the tear duct of the eye. *(Delmar/Cengage Learning)*

3. To administer eye ointment, do the following:

   A. Follow the same preparation and positioning as for the administration of eyedrops.

   B. When preparing to administer an eye ointment, place the cap and the tube of the ointment container on a clean paper towel or tissue to decrease the chance of contamination.

   C. Squeeze a small amount of the eye ointment from the tube onto the clean paper towel or clean tissue. Throw this portion of medication away.

   D. Gently make the "pocket" with the individual's lower eyelid as was done for the administration of eyedrops.

   E. Apply or place a thin line of the eye ointment into the "pocket" in the lower eyelid. Start from the inner corner of the eye (nose side) and work toward the outer side of the eye. Do not allow the tube of ointment to touch the eye, eyelid, or eyelashes. Note that the licensed HCP may order the amount of eye ointment to be given in fractional amounts, for example, ¼ inch.

   F. The body's temperature will melt the ointment. Allow the ointment to spread over the eye. Encourage the spread of the ointment by asking the individual to roll (rotate) her eye from side to side. If the individual is unable to roll her eye, the UAP may gently massage the closed lower lid in a circular motion to spread the eye ointment.

Note: If a second ointment needs to be administered, the UAP needs to wait at least fifteen (15) minutes before applying the second ointment.

    G. Inform the individual that her vision may be blurry from the medication.

    H. Remove gloves. Wash hands.

    I. Watch the individual closely. Assist with mobility and other activities as needed.

  4. Complete step 4 as per the procedure for giving medications.

Special Considerations for the Administration of Ophthalmic Medication

- Always check the expiration date *before* administering eye medications.
- All eye medications *must* be **sterile**.
- All containers of eye medications *must* have the word *ophthalmic* or *eye* written on the label.
- Eye medication may *never* be shared between people.
- When the treatment is over, all eye medication *must* be discarded, or thrown away, properly. Workplace policies will provide directions on how to dispose of medications.
- When administering medications, *never* touch the eyeball.
- *Never* put pressure on the eyeball.
- *Never* let the medication from one eye run into the other eye. This may spread infection.
- If more than one drop of the same medication needs to be administered, the UAP needs to wait at least thirty (30) seconds to one (1) minute before applying the second drop.
- If a second eye medication needs to be administered, the UAP needs to wait three (3) to five (5) minutes before administering the second eye medication.
- If a second ointment needs to be administered, the UAP needs to wait at least fifteen (15) minutes before applying the second ointment.
- Remember to wash hands well *before* and *after* giving eye medication.
- Remember to wear gloves when giving eye medication.

sterile
Being free from bacteria.

Administration of Otic Medication

Otic medications are medications for the ear. These medications are usually administered to treat ear infections and inflammation, treat pain, and soften earwax to make it easier to remove. Eardrops are usually

otic medications
Medications for the ear.

perforated eardrum
A hole in the eardrum.

herpes
An acute viral disorder of which there are many different types.

not given if an individual has a **perforated eardrum**, is hypersensitive to any ingredient in the medication, or has certain conditions such as **herpes** or other viral infections or certain types of fungal infections. The medication has a local effect, which is why it is a type of topical medication. Ear medication is usually administered by ear dropper.

Equipment and Supplies Used in the Administration of Otic Medications

The following equipment and supplies may be used in the administration of otic medications:

- Medication sheet
- Electronic medication administration record (eMAR)
- The individual's ear dropper; in some settings, this may need to be a sterile ear dropper
- The medication ordered by the licensed health care provider
- Clean paper tissue (unscented, no aloe) or cotton balls
- Gloves

Procedure 7-3
Administration of Otic Medications

The principles and procedures for administering medications are always the same and are always followed. As stated earlier, the actual steps to administering a medication will differ, depending on the route that the medication is given. For otic medications, follow these steps:

1. Complete steps 1 and 2 as per the procedure for giving medications.

2. To administer eardrops, do the following:

   A. Put on gloves.

   B. Make sure the medication is at room temperature.

   C. Have the individual lie on her side with the unaffected ear (side of the head) facing downward and the affected ear (side of the head) facing upward. Or the individual may be seated and tilt her head so that the unaffected ear (side of the head) is facing downward and the affected ear (side of the head) is facing upward (Figure 7-13).

   D. Using the tissue or cotton ball, wipe any secretions or drainage on the outside of the ear. *Do not use a cotton swab or any other sharp object!*

   E. Squeeze the rubber tip (bulb) of the ear dropper to draw up the medication into the dropper. Be sure to draw up just the amount of medication that will be administered.

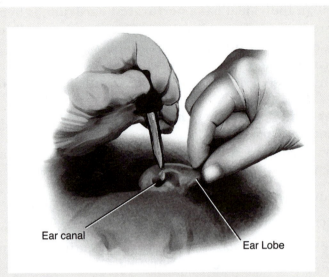

Ear canal

Ear Lobe

Figure 7-13 When administering ear drops into the individual's ear, have the individual tilt her head so that the affected ear is facing upward. *(Delmar/Cengage Learning)*

F. For an adult, straighten out the ear canal by gently pulling the ear up and outward (toward the top and back of the head).

G. Drop the medication onto the outer part of the ear canal and let it gently roll into the ear canal. *Never drop the medication directly into the ear.*

H. Do not put the dropper into the ear canal. The dropper might become contaminated.

I. Remove any extra medication by wiping the outer ear with a tissue or cotton ball.

J. Help the individual keep her head tilted for approximately five (5) minutes to keep the medication from rolling back out of the ear.

K. If the written instructions from the licensed health care provider instruct the UAP to do so, place a cotton ball in the individual's ear. If there are no written instructions to do so, do not place a cotton ball in the individual's ear. If the UAP is unsure, she must call the licensed health care provider to clarify the instructions.

L. Remove gloves. Wash hands.

3. Complete step 4 as per the procedure for giving medications.

Special Considerations for the Administration of Otic Medication

- Always check the expiration date *before* administering eardrops.

- Be careful when administering eardrops. *Do not force air into the ear when administering ear medication.* Forcing air into the ear causes pain.

- Remove any discharges or drainage from the ear frequently using clean tissues or cotton balls each time.

- If there is a lot of drainage or discharge from the ear, apply petroleum jelly to the outer ear to protect the skin.

- *Never* plug the ear if it is draining or has a discharge.

- *Never* apply heat to an ear without a licensed health care provider's written order.

- Remind the individual not to touch her ear if the ear is draining or has a discharge.

- Observe the amount of drainage or discharge from the ear. Note what the drainage or discharge looks like and the amount. Document those observations.

- If there is any change in the drainage or discharge, report it immediately to the individual's licensed HCP.

- If the drainage or discharge is being noticed for the first time, report it immediately to the individual's licensed HCP.

- Make sure the individual does *not* use cotton swabs, toothpicks, matchsticks, a pen, a pencil, or other sharp object to clean her ears.

- Do not use any sharp objects to clean an individual's ears. A cotton swab may be used for cleaning *only* the outside of an individual's ears.

Administration of Nasal Medication

nasal medications
Medications for the nose.

Nasal medications are medications for the nose. These medications are administered to treat sinus infections and symptoms of seasonal allergies, to treat pain, and to relieve nasal congestion due to colds. Nasal medications are usually not given if an individual is hypersensitive to any ingredient in the medication. Nasal medications may be used as a topical medication and, therefore, have a local effect. These medications may also be used for systemic treatments. When administered for systemic treatment, the medication is administered into the nose but then spreads to other parts of the body. Nasal medication is usually administered by nasal spray, nose dropper, or nasal inhaler.

Many times, nasal medications are best administered by the individual herself. However, if the individual is to self-administer the medication, the UAP needs to advise her of several important facts:

1. Instruct the individual to clear her nose before using nasal medication.

2. Warn the individual *not* to use over-the-counter (OTC) medications without the advice of her licensed health care provider. Her nasal medication may interact with or affect her other medications.

3. Instruct the individual on the proper way to self-administer the nasal medications.

4. Instruct the individual that, as with all medications, nasal medications must be used as directed. The individual must not exceed the recommended daily dose.

5. Warn the individual that continued long-term use of nasal sprays may lead to a chronic problem called **rebound nasal congestion**, which is swelling and congestion of the lining of the nose.

rebound nasal congestion
The swelling and congestion of the lining of the nose due to the overuse of nasal sprays.

Equipment and Supplies Used in the Administration of Nasal Medications

The following equipment and supplies may be used in the administration of nasal medications:

- Medication sheet

- Electronic medication administration record (eMAR)

- If it is going to be used, the individual's nose dropper; in some settings, this may need to be a sterile dropper

- The medication ordered by the licensed health care provider

- Clean paper tissue (unscented, no aloe)

- Gloves

Procedure 7-4
Administration of Nasal Medications

The principles and procedures for administering medications are always the same and are always followed. As stated earlier, the actual steps to administering a medication will differ, depending on the route that the medication is given. For nasal medications, follow the steps below:

1. Complete steps 1 and 2 as per the procedure for giving medications.

2. To administer nasal spray, do the following:

   A. Put on gloves.

   B. Assist the individual to blow her nose. Wipe the outside of the individual's nose with a clean paper tissue.

   C. Have the individual sit with her head in an upright position.

   D. Hold the bottle of medication under the first nostril.

   E. Hold the nostril closed that is not receiving the medication.

   F. Instruct the individual to inhale (breathe in) as the UAP squeezes the bottle of medication. Repeat for the second nostril.

Note: If a second nasal medication needs to be administered, the UAP needs to wait at least thirty (30) seconds to one (1) minute before applying the second nasal medication.

 3. To administer nose drops, do the following:

  A. Put on gloves.

  B. Wipe the outside of the individual's nose with a clean paper tissue.

  C. Have the individual sit with her head tipped back or lie with her shoulders raised up on a pillow and her head tipped back.

  D. Squeeze the rubber tip (bulb) of the nose dropper to draw up the medication into the dropper. Be sure to draw up the amount of medication that will be administered into both **nostrils** (openings of the nose).

  E. Hold the nose dropper at the opening of the first nostril (opening to the nose). Slowly drop the prescribed number of drops of medication into the first nostril. Then drop the prescribed number of drops of medication into the second nostril.

  F. Help the individual hold her head back for three (3) to five (5) minutes.

 4. For a nasal inhaler, follow the written instruction on the package drug insert carefully.

 5. Complete step 4 as per the procedure for giving medications.

Note: Some nasal medications may be administered daily using alternate nostrils. The UAP should check the licensed HCP order carefully before administering nasal medications to ensure proper and safe medication administration.

Special Considerations for the Administration of Nasal Medication

- *Be gentle.* Even a small injury can cause a nosebleed.

- *Do not allow the tip of the nose dropper to enter the nostril of the nose.* This can cause contamination.

- Nasal medications should be dated when opened.

Important Points to Remember When Using Droppers

When using an eye, ear, or nose dropper:

- Always hold the rubber tip (bulb) end of the dropper up so that the medication cannot enter the rubber tip (bulb) or come in contact with the rubber tip (bulb).

- Do not touch the tip (open end) of the dropper to the eyes, ears, or nose. It must remain free of bacteria (germs).

- Draw only the amount of medication into the dropper that will be administered.

- If any medication is left in the dropper after administering the medication, throw the medication away. Do not return it to the bottle of medication.

- Relax when administering the medication. Sudden or jerky movements may make the individual feel uncomfortable or frightened.

- Speak in a calm and soothing voice. Breathe deeply and steadily. Playing calm and quiet music may be helpful. When the UAP is relaxed and calm, it is easier for others to be comfortable.

- Droppers are *never* shared between individuals. Each individual *must* have her own dropper.

Medications for Skin and Hair

Medications applied to the skin and hair are done so to treat infections, inflammation, skin irritation, sore muscles and joints, rashes, dry skin, itching, body lice (**scabies**), or head lice or nits (**pediculosis**). These medications include creams, ointments, lotions, tinctures, solutions, suspensions, powders, and shampoos. These medications are applied locally to the specific area of the body requiring treatment and are, therefore, called topical medications. Medications may be applied (1) directly to the skin, (2) as a dressing by spreading the medication on a piece of gauze, (3) with a cotton swab, (4) with a glove, (5) with medicated or wet dressings, or other similar methods.

scabies
Body lice.

pediculosis
Head lice or nits.

Equipment and Supplies Used in the Administration of Medications for the Skin and Hair

The following equipment and supplies may be used in the administration of medications for the skin and hair:

- Medication sheet
- Electronic medication administration record (eMAR)
- The medication ordered by the licensed health care provider
- Gloves

Procedure 7-5
Administration of Medications for Skin and Hair

The principles and procedures for administering medications are always the same and are always followed. As stated earlier, the actual steps to administering a medication will differ, depending on the route that the medication is given. For medications for the skin and hair, follow the steps on the next page:

1. Complete steps 1 and 2 as per the procedure for giving medications.

2. To administer powders, do the following:

   A. Put on gloves.

   B. Unless there is a specific reason that the UAP should not do so, wash the area to be treated with mild soap and warm water. Rinse well.

   C. Gently pat dry with a clean dry cloth. Make sure that the area is completely dry before applying the medication.

   D. If the skin is broken and open, use a soft disposable material for drying. Some work settings may use sterile materials for drying the skin. Throw away the material properly once the area is dry.

   E. Apply powder to the skin.

   F. Do not shake the powder in the air. The individual may breathe the powder into her lungs.

   G. Apply the powder directly onto her skin. Gently cover the area with a light layer of the powder.

   H. Use only as much powder as needed. See the licensed health care provider's written orders for specific instructions.

   I. Remove gloves. Wash hands.

3. To administer lotions, tinctures, solutions, and suspensions, do the following:

   A. Put on gloves.

   B. Unless there is a specific reason that the UAP should not do so, wash the area to be treated with mild soap and warm water. Rinse well.

   C. Gently pat dry with a clean dry cloth.

   D. If the skin is broken and open, use a soft disposable material for drying. Some work settings may use sterile materials for drying the skin. Throw away the material properly once the area is dry.

   E. Shake the medication container well.

   F. Apply the medication with a gauze pad or a gloved hand. Gently pat the medication on the area.

   G. Do not rub or massage the area unless specifically instructed to do so in the licensed health care provider's written order.

   H. Remove gloves. Wash hands.

4. To administer ointments and creams, do the following:

   A. Put on gloves.

   B. Unless there is a specific reason that the UAP should not do so, wash the area to be treated with mild soap and warm water. Rinse well.

C. Gently pat dry with a clean dry cloth.

D. If the skin is broken and open, use a soft disposable material for drying. Some work settings may use sterile materials for drying the skin. Throw away the material properly once the area is dry.

E. Apply the ointment or cream with a gauze pad or a gloved hand.

F. Apply with light, smooth, gentle strokes.

G. Apply sparingly. See the licensed health care provider's order for specific instructions.

H. Do not rub or massage the area unless specifically instructed to do so in the licensed health care provider's written order.

I. Do not put any pressure on the skin.

J. Do not apply a bandage unless specifically instructed to do so in the licensed health care provider's written order.

K. Remove gloves. Wash hands.

5. To administer shampoos, do the following:

A. Put on gloves. The UAP may also want to wear a waterproof apron.

B. If required, wash the individual's hair with a nonmedicated shampoo and/or hair rinse (conditioner) before administering the medication.

C. Make sure the individual's eyes, nose, and mouth are protected when applying shampoo.

D. Follow the specific instructions for applying the medicated shampoo.

E. Shampoo the hair. Rinse well. Repeat if instructed to do so.

F. Towel dry the individual's hair. If instructed to do so, dry the individual's hair with a hair dryer.

Note: Not all individuals may use a hair dryer to dry their hair.

G. Remove gloves. Wash hands.

6. Complete step 4 as per the procedure for giving medications.

Special Considerations for the Administration of Medication for the Skin

- Inspect the condition of the individual's skin frequently. If there is any blistering or if the condition of the skin appears to get worse, report this at once to the licensed health care provider.

- Never directly touch an individual's skin with the tube of medication. Bacteria from the skin may enter the tube of medication and contaminate the medication.

- Be sure to always wear gloves when applying topical medications.

Special Considerations for the Administration of Medication for the Hair

- Some medicated shampoos are available by prescription only. These shampoos must be stored and locked as any other medication.

- Do not use one individual's medicated shampoo for another individual, even if they both have the same condition.

- Properly dispose of the medicated shampoo or rinse when the treatment is finished.

- Treatments with a medicated shampoo or rinse are documented the same as any other medication.

Administration of Transdermal Medication

transdermal system
A small adhesive patch or disk filled with medication that is applied directly to the body near the area to be treated.

Today, medications can be delivered to a specific targeted area by a special delivery system. The system is known as a **transdermal system**. The system is a small adhesive patch or disk that is applied directly to the body near the area to be treated. The patch or disk usually consists of four layers:

1. A backing that keeps the medication from leaking out of the system

2. A reservoir or area that stores the medication

3. A membrane or material with tiny holes in it that controls the amount of medication that is released into the body over time

4. An adhesive layer or gel that holds the patch or disk in place

Transdermal medications are used to treat hormonal problems, heart (cardiac) problems, and motion sickness; to help people quit smoking; and for birth control, pain control, and other reasons. The patches or disks provide a constant, controlled amount of medication that is slowly released through the skin into the body, usually over a period of twenty-four (24) hours (Figure 7-14). Some patches or disks, however, may release medication for much longer periods of time.

Equipment and Supplies Used in the Administration of Transdermal Medications

The following equipment and supplies may be used in the administration of transdermal medications:

- Medication sheet

- Electronic medication administration record (eMAR)

- The medication ordered by the licensed health care provider

- Gloves

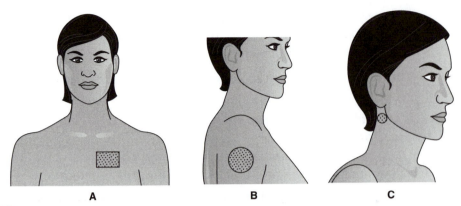

Figure 7-14 Transdermal patches vary in size and shape. (A, B) for prevention of angina pectoris; (C) for prevention of motion sickness. Analgesic patches for pain are also available. *(Delmar/Cengage Learning)*

Procedure 7-6

Administration of Transdermal Medications

The principles and procedures for administering medications are always the same and are always followed. As stated earlier, the actual steps to administering a medication will differ, depending on the route that the medication is given. For transdermal medications, follow the steps below:

1. Complete steps 1 and 2 as per the procedure for giving medications.

2. To administer a patch or disk, do the following:

   A. Put on gloves.

   B. Following the licensed health care provider's order and the instructions from the drug insert, apply the new patch (or disk) to a new area of the body.

   C. Date and initial the new patch to indicate the date the patch was changed. *Never* apply the new patch (or disk) to the same area of the body where the old patch or disk is (Figure 7-15).

   D. Remove the old patch (or disk). Fold the old patch in half and discard it in the trash. Unless instructed otherwise, clean the area with mild soap and warm water. Rinse and dry the skin well.

   E. Remove gloves. Wash hands.

3. Complete step 4 as per the procedure for giving medications.

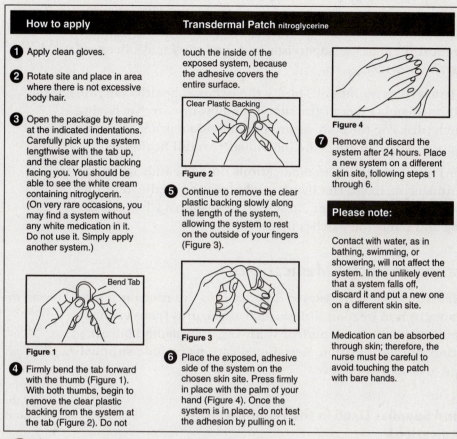

How to apply   **Transdermal Patch** nitroglycerine

1. Apply clean gloves.

2. Rotate site and place in area where there is not excessive body hair.

3. Open the package by tearing at the indicated indentations. Carefully pick up the system lengthwise with the tab up, and the clear plastic backing facing you. You should be able to see the white cream containing nitroglycerin. (On very rare occasions, you may find a system without any white medication in it. Do not use it. Simply apply another system.)

Figure 1

4. Firmly bend the tab forward with the thumb (Figure 1). With both thumbs, begin to remove the clear plastic backing from the system at the tab (Figure 2). Do not

touch the inside of the exposed system, because the adhesive covers the entire surface.

Clear Plastic Backing

Figure 2

5. Continue to remove the clear plastic backing slowly along the length of the system, allowing the system to rest on the outside of your fingers (Figure 3).

Figure 3

6. Place the exposed, adhesive side of the system on the chosen skin site. Press firmly in place with the palm of your hand (Figure 4). Once the system is in place, do not test the adhesion by pulling on it.

Figure 4

7. Remove and discard the system after 24 hours. Place a new system on a different skin site, following steps 1 through 6.

Please note:

Contact with water, as in bathing, swimming, or showering, will not affect the system. In the unlikely event that a system falls off, discard it and put a new one on a different skin site.

Medication can be absorbed through skin; therefore, the nurse must be careful to avoid touching the patch with bare hands.

Figure 7-15 Application of a transdermal patch: how to administer transdermal medications. *(Delmar/Cengage Learning)*

Special Considerations for the Administration of Transdermal Medication

- Instruct the individual to keep the patch (disk) dry unless instructions from the pharmacist and/or the licensed health care provider state that the patch (disk) may get wet. Some patches (disks) may be worn during swimming, showering, and so on.

- Avoid applying patches (disks) to hairy areas of the body.

- Unless otherwise ordered by the licensed health care provider, change the patch (disk) at the same time every day. This allows the body to keep a constant level of the medication at all times.

- Inspect the individual's skin daily for rashes, blisters, scratching, or other signs of skin irritation or allergic reaction. Listen for complaints about itching. Immediately report any changes in the skin to the individual's licensed health care provider.

- Watch for possible side effects from the medication. Transdermal medications may affect many systems in the body in many different ways. If any side effects are noted, the UAP needs to immediately report them to her supervisor and the individual's licensed health care provider.

- If the patch (disk) comes off, notify the licensed health care provider immediately to get instructions for follow-up care. Not having the patch (disk) on the body means the individual is not receiving medication. This can affect the individual's overall health.

- The UAP *must not* get these medications on her hands when she is administering them. Her hands might take the medication into her own body and affect her. Be sure to wear gloves when administering and removing patches (disks).

Administration of Rectal Medications

Rectal medications are administered directly into the **rectum**. These medications are given to treat an illness, such as seizures (convulsions); for fever; to relieve pain, nausea and/or vomiting, itching and burning, and constipation; and for sedation. Rectal medications include **suppositories**, creams, gels, and **enemas**.

Equipment and Supplies Used in the Administration of Rectal Medications

The following equipment and supplies may be used in the administration of rectal medications:

- Medication sheet
- Electronic medication administration record (eMAR)
- The medication ordered by the licensed health care provider
- Water-soluble lubricating gel; *do not use* a petroleum-based gel
- A towel or disposable pad for the bed
- Clean paper tissue
- Gloves

rectal medications
Medications administered directly into the rectum.

rectum
The opening of the body that leads into the bowel.

suppository
Form of semisolid medication that, when placed into the rectum, vagina or urethra dissolves and has an effect on the surrounding area.

enema
A way to administer a liquid solution or liquid medication into the rectum and colon (part of the bowel); may also be used to clean the bowel.

Procedure 7-7
Administration of Rectal Medications

The principles and procedures for administering medications are always the same and are always followed. As stated earlier, the actual steps to administering a medication will differ, depending on the route that the medication is given. For rectal medications, follow the steps below:

1. Complete steps 1 and 2 as per the procedure for giving medications.

2. To administer a rectal suppository, do the following:

    A. Have the individual urinate and/or move her bowels, if possible, before giving the suppository.

    B. Provide privacy.

    C. Encourage the individual to relax. Speak calmly. Playing soothing music may be helpful.

    D. Put on gloves.

    E. If the suppository is soft, holding it under cold water while it is still in its wrapper will make it harder and therefore easier to insert.

    F. Have the individual lie down on her side, with the lower leg straightened out. The upper leg should be bent at the hip, with the knee bent forward and upward toward the stomach.

    G. Lower the individual's pants.

    H. Remove the wrapper of the suppository.

    I. Do not flush the wrapper down the toilet. Throw the wrapper in the trash.

    J. Lubricate the tip of the suppository with the water-soluble gel. *Do not use* petroleum gel.

    K. Separate the buttocks with one hand. Insert the suppository into the rectum with a finger, until it passes the sphincter muscle—about one (1) inch for adults. If the suppository is not inserted past the sphincter muscle, it will pop back out of the rectum. Do not place the suppository into stool or against the wall of the rectum (Figure 7-16).

    L. Wipe the buttocks with a tissue.

    M. Hold the individual's buttocks together for three (3) to five (5) minutes. Have the individual hold the medication in her rectum (without moving her bowels) for as long as possible, or according to the licensed health care provider's directions.

    N. Remove gloves. Wash hands.

    O. Help the individual to the bathroom, if needed.

3. To administer a rectal cream or gel, do the following:

    A. Have the individual urinate and/or move her bowels, if possible, before giving the medication.

    B. Provide privacy.

    C. Encourage the individual to relax. Speak calmly. Playing soothing music may be helpful.

    D. Put on gloves.

    E. Have the individual lie down on her side, with the lower leg straightened out. The upper leg should be bent at the hip, with the knee bent forward and upward toward the stomach.

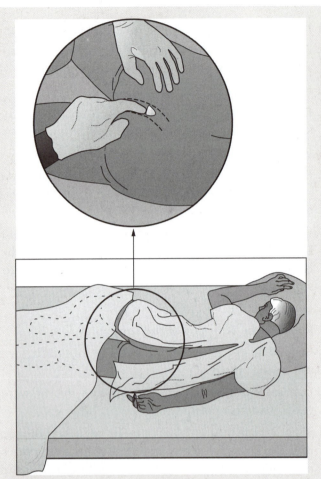

Figure 7-16 Administration of a rectal suppository. Lubricate the tip of the suppository. Insert the suppository into the rectum past the sphincter muscle. *(Delmar/Cengage Learning)*

F. Lower the individual's pants.

G. Open the container or wrapper of the medication.

H. Do not flush the container or wrapper down the toilet. Throw the container or wrapper in the trash.

I. If the applicator for the cream or gel is not prefilled, fill the applicator with the prescribed amount of medication.

J. Lubricate the tip of the applicator with the water-soluble gel. *Do not use* petroleum gel.

K. Separate the buttocks with one hand. Insert the applicator gently into the rectum until it passes the sphincter muscle— about one (1) inch for adults. If the applicator is not inserted past the sphincter muscle, the medication will ooze back out of the rectum.

L. To insert the medication, push the plunger of the applicator. Tell the individual that the medication may feel cold.

M. Wipe the buttocks with a tissue.

N. Hold the individual's buttocks together for three (3) to five (5) minutes. Have the individual hold the medication in her rectum (without moving her bowels) for as long as possible, or according to the licensed health care provider's directions.

O. Throw the applicator in the trash. Do not flush it down the toilet.

P. Remove gloves. Wash hands.

4. Complete step 4 as per the procedure for giving medications.

Special Considerations for the Administration of Rectal Medication

- Store suppositories in a cool place to avoid melting. Refrigerate the suppositories if the label says to do so.

- Remember that a suppository, if soft, may be run under cold water in its wrapper. This hardens the suppository and makes it easier for insertion into the rectum.

- Once a suppository is administered, if it pops out, do not reuse the suppository. Open a new suppository and readminister the medication. Dispose of the used suppository according to regulations and workplace policy.

- Follow the instructions that accompany the creams and gels to make sure those medications are stored and handled properly.

Administration of Vaginal Medication

Vaginal medications are administered directly into the **vagina**. These medications are given to treat infection, relieve itching, relieve vaginal dryness, for **menopausal symptoms**, and for birth control. Vaginal medications include suppositories, creams, ointments, and **douches**. Being a topical medication, these medications have a local effect on the body.

Equipment and Supplies Used in the Administration of Vaginal Medications

The following equipment and supplies may be used in the administration of vaginal medications:

- Medication sheet
- Electronic medication administration record (eMAR)
- The medication ordered by the licensed health care provider
- Water-soluble lubricating gel; *do not use* a petroleum-based gel
- A towel or disposable pad for the bed

vaginal medications
Medications administered directly into the vagina.

vagina
The opening of the body that leads to the cervix and uterus.

menopausal symptoms
The symptoms that occur as a normal result of aging when a woman's ovaries stop functioning and her menstrual cycle stops.

douche
An irrigation of the vaginal canal with medicated or normal saline solution.

- A sanitary pad
- Clean paper tissue
- Gloves

Procedure 7-8
Administration of Vaginal Medications

The principles and procedures for administering medications are always the same and are always followed. As stated earlier, the actual steps to administering a medication will differ, depending on the route that the medication is given. For vaginal medications, follow the steps below:

1. Complete steps 1 and 2 as per the procedure for giving medications.

2. To administer a vaginal suppository, do the following:

   A. Have the individual urinate and/or move her bowels, if possible, before giving the suppository.

   B. Provide privacy.

   C. Encourage the individual to relax. Speak calmly. Playing soothing music may be helpful.

   D. Put on gloves.

   E. Have the individual lie down on her back.

   F. Lower the individual's pants. Have her spread her legs apart (Figure 7-17).

   G. Inspect the area around the vagina (Figure 7-18). If there are any signs of increased irritation, such as redness or swelling, do not insert the medication. Call the licensed health care provider instead and report those observations.

   H. Open the wrapper of the suppository.

   I. Do not flush the wrapper down the toilet. Throw the wrapper in the trash.

   J. Lubricate the tip of the suppository with water-soluble gel. *Do not use* petroleum gel.

   K. Spread the labia apart with one hand and gently insert the tip of the suppository into the vagina with the other hand. Gently move the suppository forward into the vagina about two (2) inches (see Figure 7-18).

   L. The suppository should stay in the body so the medication can melt into the body. Once a suppository is administered, if it pops out, do not reuse the suppository. Open a new suppository and readminister the medication.

M. Dispose of the used suppository according to regulations and workplace policy.

N. Follow the instructions that accompany the suppositories to make sure vaginal medications are stored and handled properly.

O. Remove gloves. Wash hands.

P. Have the individual remain lying down for half an hour after inserting the medication. Then check the vaginal area for signs of allergic reaction.

Q. Immediately report any signs of an allergic reaction to the licensed health care provider and one's supervisor.

R. Explain to the individual that she is not to use tampons because the tampons will absorb the medication. Have her wear a sanitary pad if she wants to. This pad will absorb any vaginal drainage or discharge.

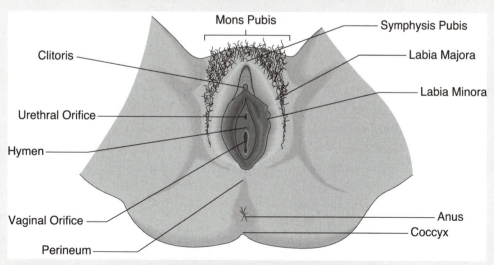

Figure 7-17 Position to administer vaginal medications. *(Delmar/Cengage Learning)*

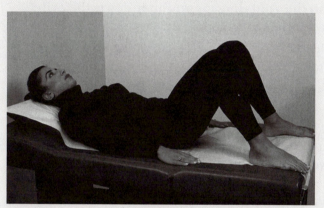

Figure 7-18 External female reproductive organs. *(Delmar/Cengage Learning)*

3. To administer a vaginal cream or ointment, do the following:

A. Have the individual urinate and/or move her bowels, if possible, before giving the medication.

B. Provide privacy.

C. Encourage the individual to relax. Speak calmly. Playing soothing music may be helpful.

D. Put on gloves.

E. Have the individual lie down on her back.

F. Lower the individual's pants. Have her spread her legs apart (see Figure 7-17).

G. Inspect the area around the vagina (see Figure 7-18). If there are any signs of increased irritation, such as redness or swelling, do not insert the medication. Call the licensed health care provider instead and report those observations.

H. Open the container or wrapper of the medication.

I. Do not flush the container or wrapper down the toilet. Throw the container or wrapper in the trash.

J. If the applicator for the cream or gel is not prefilled, fill the applicator with the prescribed amount of medication.

K. Lubricate the tip of the applicator with the water or water-soluble gel. *Do not use* petroleum gel.

L. Spread the labia apart with one hand and gently insert the applicator tip into the vagina with the other hand. Gently move the applicator forward into the vagina about two (2) inches. Tip the applicator slightly backward toward the tailbone.

M. To insert the medication, push the plunger of the applicator. Tell the individual that the medication may feel cold.

N. Remove the applicator. If the applicator is disposable, throw it in the trash. Do not flush it down the toilet. If it is reusable, wash the applicator thoroughly with soap and warm water, rinse and dry it well, and return it to its original container for storage.

O. If the licensed health care provider orders it, apply a light layer of the cream or ointment to the vulva (the area around the vagina, including the area around the vaginal opening, labia majora, and labia minora).

P. Follow the instructions that accompany the creams and gels to make sure vaginal medications are stored and handled properly.

Q. Remove gloves. Wash hands.

R. Have the individual remain lying down for half an hour after inserting the medication. Then check the vaginal area for signs of allergic reaction.

S. Immediately report any signs of an allergic reaction to the licensed health care provider and one's supervisor.

T. Explain to the individual that she is not to use tampons because the tampons will absorb the medication. Have her wear a sanitary pad if she wants to. This pad will absorb any vaginal drainage or discharge.

4. Complete step 4 as per the procedure for giving medications.

Note: The administration of a douche requires additional knowledge, skills, and clinical practice that are not addressed in this textbook.

Special Considerations for the Administration of Vaginal Medication

- It is best to administer the medication after the individual bathes and just before bedtime.

- Additional information about the way to administer the medication can usually be found on the package drug insert directions included in the medication package or on the pharmacy label.

Some workplace settings may require that only female staff administer vaginal medications or, if vaginal medications are administered by male staff, that a female staff member be present during administration of the medication. It is the responsibility of the UAP to know and follow her state regulations and workplace policy.

ADMINISTRATION OF MEDICATIONS BY INHALATION

inhalant medications
Medications used to treat diseases of the respiratory tract; also called pulmonary medications.

COPD
Chronic obstructive pulmonary disease; a condition that interferes with normal breathing over a long period of time, such as emphysema or bronchitis.

Inhalation is the act of breathing. During inhalation therapy, oxygen, water vapor, and inhalant medications may be administered. **Inhalant medications**, also called **pulmonary medications**, are usually used to treat asthma or other respiratory (breathing) conditions like **COPD** (chronic obstructive pulmonary disease). Inhalant medications are taken into the body through the mouth and/or nose. Inhalant medications are administered by a handheld inhaler, small-volume aerosol nebulizer, or intermittent positive-pressure breathing (IPPB) machine.

Equipment and Supplies Used in the Administration of Medications by Inhalation

The following equipment and supplies may be used in the administration of medications by inhalation:

- Medication sheet

- Electronic medication administration record (eMAR)

- The medication ordered by the licensed health care provider
- If ordered, the nebulizer or IPPB machine
- Gloves

Use of a Metered Dose Inhaler (MDI)

A **handheld inhaler** is a container of medication that is under pressure. The container has a "button" on it. When the "button" is pushed, the container releases the medication as a fine mist or spray. This mist or spray is sometimes called a "puff." The handheld inhaler is used to deliver medications to the lungs.

The handheld inhaler may be held in the individual's hand allowing the individual to self-administer. At times a special chamber will need to be used along with the handheld inhaler to get the most benefit from the inhaler (Figure 7-19). Other times, the handheld inhaler has its own chamber built into it.

When a larger amount of medication needs to be delivered to the lungs, a small-volume aerosol **nebulizer** (Figure 7-20) or **intermittent positive-pressure breathing (IPPB) machine** (Figure 7-21) may be ordered by the licensed HCP. The medication used with these machines comes in a liquid form and is measured into the machine. The mist may be heated or cooled. The medication is delivered to the individual through a face mask or mouthpiece.

handheld inhaler
A sealed container of medication that is under pressure.

nebulizer
A machine that is used to administer a fine mist of liquid medication deep into the lungs.

intermittent positive-pressure breathing (IPPB) machine
A machine that combines an aerosol that administers a fine mist of liquid medication deep into the lungs with a mechanical breather to assist patients who are unable to take a deep breath on their own.

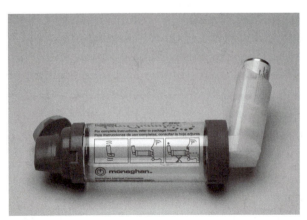

Figure 7-19 Metered dose inhaler (MDI) with spacer. *(Delmar/Cengage Learning)*

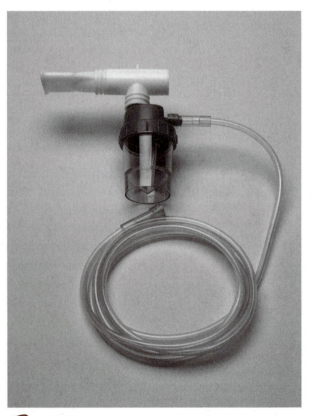

Figure 7-20 Small-volume aerosol nebulizer delivers moisture or medication deep into the lungs. *(Delmar/Cengage Learning)*

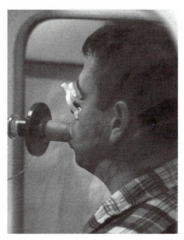

Figure 7-21 Administration by intermittent positive-pressure breathing (IPPB) machine.
(Delmar/Cengage Learning)

Procedure 7-9
Administration of Medications by Inhalation

The principles and procedures for administering medications are always the same and are always followed. As stated above, the actual steps to administering a medication will differ, depending on the route that the medication is given. For medications by inhalation, follow the steps below:

1. Complete steps 1 and 2 as per the procedure for giving medications.

2. To administer a medication by an inhaler, do the following:

   A. Assemble the inhaler properly. If unsure, read the package insert directions or call the pharmacist for assistance.

   B. Remove or ask the individual to remove her upper dentures if the dentures are loose. Loose dentures may fall down during the administration of the medication and block the sprayed medication from entering her lungs.

   C. Remind the individual to keep her tongue flat in her mouth. Otherwise, the medication will spray onto her tongue and not into her lungs.

   D. Have the individual take a drink of water to moisten her mouth.

   E. Shake the cartridge of the inhaler well to mix the medication.

   F. Place the opening of the inhaler at the individual's mouth. Instruct the individual to breathe out through her nose. *Important:* Remind the individual to breathe out only the stale air that is in her lungs. Do not have her empty *all* the air out of his lungs. Forcing all the air out of her lungs will collapse the airways in the lungs and not allow the medication into the airways.

    G. Have the individual press down firmly on the inhaler while at the same time she takes a deep breath.

    H. Have the individual hold her breath for a count of ten (10) before breathing out.

    I. Have the individual brush her teeth and rinse well with an oral rinse after the administration of the medication.

3. Complete step 4 as per the procedure for giving medications.

Special Considerations for the Administration of Medications by Inhalation

- The UAP must know how to use the inhaler and its chamber *before* giving the medication. If unsure as to how they work, she needs to seek assistance from her supervisor, the pharmacist, or the licensed health care provider *before* giving the medication.

- The same rule applies to the nebulizer and the IPPB machine. If the UAP has never used one of these machines, she will need training on how to use them *before* giving the medication.

- Pulmonary inhalant medications are stored and documented like all other medications.

- The UAP should warn individuals to avoid the overuse of the inhaler. Side effects from overuse include **tolerance**, **rebound bronchospasm**, and adverse cardiac effects.

- Inhalers should not be used past the total number of doses indicated on the prescription label.

- The UAP should notify the licensed health care provider if the prescribed dose of medication does not have the desired effect. In other words, the licensed health care provider is to be notified if the medication is not helping the individual.

- The UAP is to instruct the individual to brush her teeth well, including rinsing her mouth, after each use of the inhaler or after each inhalation therapy treatment. This prevents the growth of fungi in her mouth.

- *Before* beginning a nebulizer treatment, the UAP should:

  - Place the individual in an upright position.

  - Obtain a resting pulse—Count the pulse for a full sixty (60) seconds.

  - Turn on the nebulizer before applying the mask to the individual's nose and mouth or before placing the mouthpiece into the individual's mouth. The UAP needs to check to make sure the nebulizer is providing a mist to the individual.

tolerance
A condition in which the individual's body adjusts to the dose of a medication and a larger amount of the medication is needed to achieve the desired or wanted effect.

rebound bronchospasm
A spasm in the airways that is a response to overuse of an inhalant medication.

- *During* a nebulizer treatment, the UAP should:

  - Stay with the individual during the breathing treatment or check on the individual every five (5) minutes to monitor for side effects from the treatment, including, but not limited to, increased pulse rate of twenty (20) beats per minute or more, palpitations, dizziness, shakiness, nausea, chest pain, and uncontrollable coughing.

SUMMARY

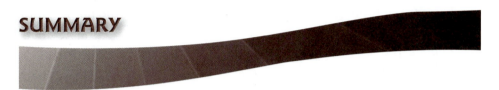

When administering medications, remember the following:

1. Always follow the Six Rights of medication administration, the Three Checks, and the procedure for administering medications safely and effectively.

2. When in doubt, ask—ask the supervisor, the pharmacist, and/or the individual's licensed health care provider—*but* always know the answer *before* giving a medication.

3. *Never* use equipment until proper training has been received.

4. Always report any changes that are observed in an individual to the supervisor and the individual's licensed health care provider. The UAP will most likely be the first person to notice a change in an individual.

WORKBOOK REVIEW

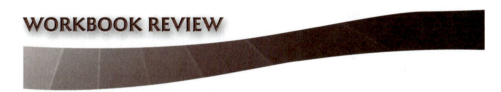

Go to the workbook and complete the exercises for Chapter 7.

REVIEW QUESTIONS

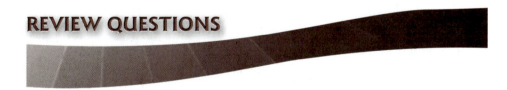

1. Nonparenteral medications:
   a. do not require the use of gloves
   b. go only on the skin, not into the body
   c. enter the body through any route other than injection
   d. can be shared among individuals who have the same symptoms
2. Giving medication orally is:
   a. the safest way to give medications
   b. the fastest way to give medications
   c. the least expensive way to give medications
   d. all of the above

3. When giving medications, the UAP should never change the form of a medication without:
   a. a licensed health care provider's written order
   b. first checking with one's supervisor
   c. first checking a medication reference book
   d. consulting with the individual's pharmacist

4. When measuring liquid medication:
   a. pour extra liquid medication back into the bottle
   b. multiple liquid medications for an individual may be poured into the same cup
   c. place the medicine cup at eye level and measure at the lowest level of the meniscus
   d. all of the above

5. When giving a crushed medication mixed with food:
   a. the UAP may crush it with the bottom of a drinking glass
   b. the UAP must tell the individual there is medicine in the food and that she needs to eat all of it
   c. the UAP may mix the medication in the food with her finger
   d. it does not matter if some of the medication is lost while crushing it

6. Topical medications:
   a. are applied to an area of the body and have an effect on that area
   b. are applied to an area of the body and have an effect on a different area
   c. are only applied to the skin
   d. are layered on top of an ointment or lotion

7. When giving eye medication:
   a. it is okay to share medications between individuals if they have the same diagnosis
   b. it is okay if the medication runs from one eye into the other eye
   c. all eye medications must have the word "ophthalmic" or "eye" on the label
   d. make sure you touch the eyeball with the medication when giving it

8. When using a dropper to give a medication:
   a. hold the rubber tip up so that the rubber tip serves as a reservoir for the medication
   b. do not touch the tip to the eye, ear, or nose
   c. if you draw too much medication into the dropper, simply place the dropper back into the medication bottle
   d. all of the above

9. When applying a transdermal patch:
   a. it is OK to change the patch whenever the UAP has the time
   b. if the UAP notices skin irritation, she is to observe the skin for twenty-four (24) hours
   c. if the patch comes off, it is OK to leave it off for that day
   d. do not get the medication on your hands while applying the patch

10. When an individual is using a handheld inhaler, she may benefit:
    a. by standing upright when using the handheld inhaler
    b. using a special chamber with the handheld inhaler
    c. using the handheld inhaler after she eats
    d. using the handheld inhaler outdoors

CLINICAL SCENARIOS

1. Jerry has an infection in his right eye. His licensed HCP has ordered an anitbiotic eye ointment to be administered three times a day in his right eye.
   a. List the equipment and supplies that you will need to administer Jerry's eye ointment.
   b. What special considerations will you need to take when administering Jerry's eye ointment?
   c. Describe how you will administer Jerry's eye ointment.
2. You are asked to help Mrs. Berkowitz with her new handheld inhaler. Describe what you would do to administer an inhalant medication.

Chapter 8
Administration of Oxygen

Learning Objectives

After reading this chapter and completing the review exercises, you should be able to:

1. Spell and define terms.

2. Explain the responsibilities of the UAP in regard to the administration of oxygen.

3. List five conditions that may require the administration of oxygen.

4. List eight signs and symptoms of an inadequate oxygen supply (hypoxemia).

5. Perform a pulse oximetry reading.

6. List six basic guidelines for the care of an individual who is receiving pulse oximetry.

7. List the four items that are to be included in the written licensed health care provider order for oxygen.

8. Describe the two most common methods of oxygen delivery.

9. Describe four types of oxygen administration equipment.

10. Demonstrate the changing of a prefilled humidifier bottle and a refillable humidifier bottle.

11. List ten basic guidelines for the care of an individual who is receiving oxygen.

12. Describe the four basic respiratory positions.

13. List five symptoms of oxygen toxicity.

14. Demonstrate the use of an incentive spirometer.

15. Demonstrate the use of a CPAP device.

16. Write a clinical progress note for an individual receiving:
- Pulse oximetry
- Incentive spirometer
- CPAP

17. List six oxygen safety precautions.

Key Terms

atelectasis

congestive heart failure

continuous positive airway pressure (CPAP) device

COPD

cyanosis

dyspnea

hemoglobin

humidifier

hypoxemia

incentive spirometer

kyphoscoliosis

liquid oxygen canister

Lou Gehrig's disease

malaise

mask

minimum oxygen saturation level

multiple sclerosis

myocardial infarction (MI)

nasal cannula

obesity

oxygen

oxygen concentrator

pneumonia

pulse oximeter

pulse oximetry

rales

shock

sleep apnea

tachycardia

tracheostomy

INTRODUCTION

oxygen
An odorless, colorless, tasteless gas.

According to *Webster's New World Dictionary and Thesaurus*, **oxygen** is an odorless, colorless, tasteless gas. The body requires oxygen to live. Without it, the body dies. Oxygen is taken into the body when an individual breathes. When an individual is not able to take in enough oxygen to meet his body's needs, oxygen is prescribed by the licensed health care provider. Once the order for oxygen has been written, the UAP administers the oxygen just as he would administer any other medication.

ADMINISTRATION OF OXYGEN

pneumonia
An infection of the lungs.

COPD
Chronic obstructive pulmonary disease; a condition that interferes with normal breathing over a long period of time, such as emphysema or bronchitis.

myocardial infarction (MI)
A heart attack.

sleep apnea
A period of time during sleep when respirations stop for ten (10) seconds or more.

Oxygen is administered to individuals for many different reasons. Conditions that may require oxygen administration include the following:

- Conditions caused by diseases within the lungs—pulmonary diseases such as asthma, **pneumonia**, and **COPD**

- Respiratory problems as a result of complications from other conditions—lung cancer, severe curvature of the spine (**kyphoscoliosis**), and neuromuscular diseases such as **multiple sclerosis** and **Lou Gehrig's disease**

- During and after surgery (postoperatively)

- Cardiac disease, such as **congestive heart failure** and **myocardial infarction (MI)**

- **Sleep apnea**

- Decreased level of consciousness

- **Obesity**

- Immobility
- Being on prolonged bed rest
- Carbon monoxide poisoning
- Drowning
- **Shock**

SIGNS AND SYMPTOMS OF AN INADEQUATE OXYGEN SUPPLY (HYPOXEMIA)

An individual who has an inadequate amount of oxygen in his blood (**hypoxemia**) may show certain signs and symptoms. These signs and symptoms may include one or more of the following:

- Cool, clammy skin
- Slow, rapid, or irregular breathing
- Shortness of breath or difficulty breathing (**dyspnea**)
- Noisy breathing
- Gasping for breath
- Rattling in the lungs, or "wet" respirations (**rales**)
- Changes in skin color, such as paleness, or blue or gray discoloration (**cyanosis**)
- Changes in the color of the lips, mucous membranes, nail beds, or lining of the roof of the mouth
- Choking on saliva
- Changes in mental status, such as confusion or an increase in confusion, a decrease in responsiveness, drowsiness, sleepiness for no special reason, or restlessness
- Pulse of more than 100 beats per minute (**tachycardia**)

Observations of the skin, nail beds, mucous membranes in the mouth, and the lips can alert the UAP early to possible problems. In a light-skinned individual, the skin, nail beds, mucous membranes in the mouth, and lips should all be pink. The pink coloring of these areas means the individual is receiving an adequate supply of oxygen.

In a dark-skinned individual, the UAP needs to look at the nail beds, the mucous membranes of the mouth, and the lips. As with the light-skinned individual, these areas should all be pink. Because the dark coloring of the skin prevents the UAP from seeing any discoloration of the skin, observation of the skin is not reliable in a dark-skinned individual.

PULSE OXIMETRY

Blood enters the lungs from the heart through the pulmonary artery. Once in the lungs, the blood passes through tiny structures called alveoli. In these tiny areas, the blood rids itself of the waste product called

shock
A state in which the circulation of the body is disrupted and the blood pressure is dangerously low.

hemoglobin
A part of the blood that carries oxygen from the lungs to the cells.

pulse oximetry
A reliable method used to determine the amount of oxygen in the blood.

pulse oximeter
A device used to measure the amount of oxygen in the blood.

carbon dioxide and picks up oxygen. Oxygen is then carried to the cells of the body through the arteries by a part of the blood called **hemoglobin**.

Pulse oximetry is a reliable method used to determine the amount of oxygen in the arteries of the body. This simple test is quick, painless, and easy to perform. The instrument used to perform the test, a **pulse oximeter**, measures the amount of oxygen in the hemoglobin.

The pulse oximeter has an external sensor that is attached to the individual's skin. Several types of sensors are available, including the following:

- Finger-clip sensor (Figure 8-1)
- Toe sensor
- Earlobe sensor
- Foot sensor
- Forehead sensor
- Nasal sensor, attached to the bridge of the nose (Figure 8-2)

The most commonly used sensors are the finger-clip sensor and the earlobe sensor. Both of these sensors are attached in a clothespin-like fashion to the finger or ear. For dark-skinned individuals, the finger-clip sensor and toe sensor work best. For all individuals, poor circulation will interfere with the use of the pulse oximeter. The pulse oximeter is not used for an individual with known or suspected carbon monoxide poisoning.

There are two sides to the sensor clip. One side of the clip is made up of two light-emitting diodes (LEDs). One LED is red. The other LED is infrared. The other side of the clip contains a photodetector.

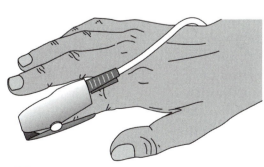

Figure 8-1 The finger-clip sensor.
(Delmar/Cengage Learning)

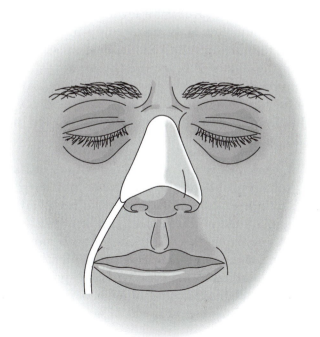

Figure 8-2 The nasal sensor. *(Delmar/Cengage Learning)*

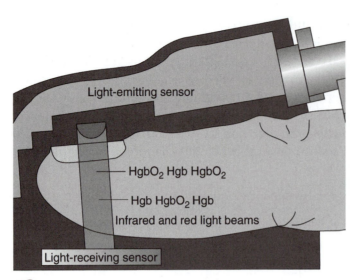

Figure 8-3 The pulse oximeter uses light to measure the amount of oxygen in the blood in an artery. *(Delmar/Cengage Learning)*

When a pulse oximeter reading is being performed, a beam of light passes from the LEDs through the tissue and blood to the photodetector. The photodetector receives the light and measures the amount of light absorbed by the oxygenated and unoxygenated hemoglobin (Figure 8-3). Unoxygenated hemoglobin absorbs more red light. Oxygenated hemoglobin absorbs more infrared light. The amount of each light and, therefore, the amount of oxygen in the blood is determined by the spectrum of light.

The pulse oximeter then changes this information into a percentage. The percentage is shown on the digital display screen of the pulse oximeter unit. Based upon the reading(s), the licensed health care provider will write an order for the **minimum oxygen saturation level**.

A normal saturation level is between 95% and 100%. A saturation level below 90% may mean complications. Reading levels below 90% need to be reported to the individual's licensed health care provider. Readings below 70% are life threatening and require immediate emergency action. For readings below 70%, the UAP must immediately call 911 or his local emergency medical services. Once the individual is cared for, the UAP must notify his supervisor and the individual's licensed health care provider.

Note: **Nail polish and artificial nails will interfere with observation of the nail beds and with the use of the pulse oximeter. Nail polish must be removed for accurate observation and to get an accurate reading on the pulse oximeter. Some workplaces will choose to remove nail polish from only one finger or toe. Other workplaces will remove nail polish from all nails. It is the UAP's responsibility to know his workplace policy and to follow it. Nonacetone polish remover is to be used for the removal of acrylic and sculptured nails.**

The pulse oximeter has an alarm. The manufacturer usually presets the alarm to normal limits. The UAP should always ask the individual's

minimum oxygen saturation level
The minimum level of oxygen to be maintained in an individual's blood.

licensed health care provider (HCP) if the alarm settings need to be changed. If so, a licensed health care provider must write an order stating the specific settings desired. Before leaving the individual, the UAP must make sure that the alarm is turned on and is set as ordered by the licensed HCP. The alarm must *NEVER* be turned off!

Pulse oximetry is usually done continuously. However, the test may be done at periodic intervals. Pulse oximetry detects important changes in the individual's condition that occur before any visible changes may be observed by the UAP, such as a change in skin color. This early detection allows for quick and early treatment, improved quality of care, and better outcomes for the individual.

Equipment and Supplies

The following equipment will be needed to accurately perform pulse oximetry:

- Pulse oximeter unit
- Appropriate external sensor
- Tape, if needed
- Alcohol wipe or soap and water
- Nail polish remover and/or nonacetone polish remover if necessary

Procedure 8-1
Use of a Pulse Oximeter

When using a pulse oximeter, follow these steps:

1. Identify the individual for whom the oxygen saturation level is needed.
2. Verify the licensed health care provider order for the test.
3. Wash hands.
4. Gather all the equipment needed. (See the previous section "Equipment and Supplies.")
5. Explain the procedure to the individual.
6. Per the licensed health care provider order, locate the sensor site to be used. If necessary, remove nail polish or artificial nails. Cleanse the site with the alcohol wipe or soap and water.
7. Apply the sensor (Figure 8-4a). If the sensor has position markings, place them opposite each other. Correctly positioning the sensor will ensure an accurate reading.
8. Using the sensor cable, attach the sensor to the pulse oximeter unit.

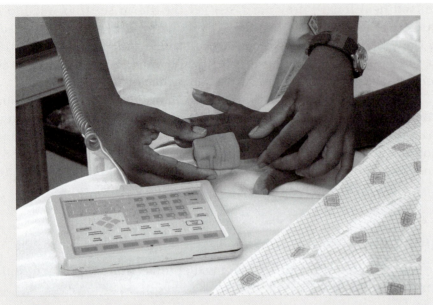

Figure 8-4a Apply the sensor to the finger. *(Delmar/Cengage Learning)*

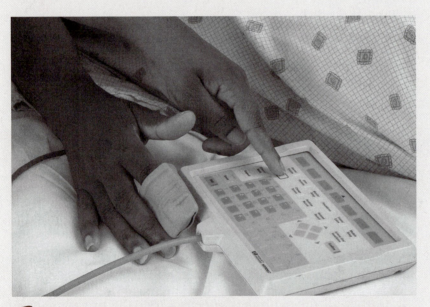

Figure 8-4b Turn the unit on. Adjust the volume of the unit to the desired volume. *(Delmar/Cengage Learning)*

9. Turn the unit on. A beep should be heard with each pulse beat of the individual. Adjust the volume of the unit to the desired volume (Figure 8-4b).

Note: Some pulse oximeter units do not make a sound; instead, the unit has light bars that indicate the strength of the individual's pulse.

10. Adjust the alarm limits for high and low oxygen saturation levels, according to the licensed HCP order.

11. Compare the pulse rate on the unit to the individual's actual pulse rate to make sure the unit is accurately measuring the individual's pulse rate.

12. Cover the sensor with a towel or sheet to block bright light and make sure the readings are accurate.

13. Note the percentage of oxygen saturation. Notify the licensed health care provider of the initial reading. Document per workplace policy.

14. If the pulse oximeter is being used for continuous monitoring, move clothespin-like sensors every two (2) hours and taped sensors every four (4) hours.

15. Monitor the individual's pulse rate, respiratory rate, and general appearance.

16. Notify the licensed health care provider of abnormal readings (those readings falling outside the range provided by the licensed HCP).

17. Document per workplace policy.

18. If the individual's condition changes, notify the licensed health care provider.

Special Considerations

- Clean the individual's nails or skin properly before attaching sensors.

- Always plug in the pulse oximeter between uses to make sure it is charged and ready when needed.

- Do not use the pulse oximeter if its battery light shows that the battery is low.

- Always compare the individual's pulse rate with the pulse rate being monitored by the pulse oximeter unit. If these rates are not the same, notify the supervisor immediately and/or the individual's licensed HCP.

- Always compare the oxygen saturation readings with readings previously taken. If an important difference is noted, contact the individual's licensed HCP immediately.

Caring for an Individual Receiving Pulse Oximetry

An individual who is receiving pulse oximetry needs ongoing monitoring on a regular basis. Follow these basic guidelines when caring for an individual who is receiving pulse oximetry:

- Before applying the pulse oximeter, check to see if the individual is receiving oxygen. If so, document the liter flow rate.

- Always be sure to report the initial pulse oximeter reading and vital signs to the individual's licensed health care provider.

- If the individual's vital signs and/or appearance change, notify his licensed health care provider immediately.

- Notify the licensed HCP if the individual's reading falls below the minimum oxygen saturation level ordered by the licensed HCP.

- If the individual is receiving oxygen, monitor his oxygen use. Keep the oxygen at the level ordered by the licensed health care provider.

- Change the position of the sensor at least every four (4) hours. A clothespin-like sensor should be changed every two (2) hours. Changing the position of the sensor helps to prevent skin breakdown and complications due to pressure.

- If tape is used to hold the sensor in place, check frequently for signs and symptoms of allergic reaction to the tape. If signs or symptoms of an allergic reaction are noted, remove the sensor immediately. Apply a clothespin-like sensor.

- Individuals with thickened nails may have inaccurate readings. Inaccurate readings may lead to improper treatment. Other sensor sites, such as the earlobes or the nose, may need to be used for these individuals.

Guidelines for Documentation

When documenting information on pulse oximetry, the UAP needs to document the following:

- Date and time the sensor was attached
- Type of sensor
- Location of the sensor
- Initial oxygen saturation reading
- Pulse, respiratory rate, and general appearance of the individual when the sensor was initially attached
- Alarm settings of the pulse oximeter unit
- Oxygen with liter flow rate if the individual is receiving oxygen
- Dates, times, and oxygen saturation readings when monitored
- Dates and times of rotation of sensor sites, with condition of skin
- Any changes noted in the individual

OXYGEN THERAPY

To administer oxygen, the UAP needs a written licensed health care provider order and, in some work settings, a prescription. The medication order written by the licensed health care provider will include the following:

- The oxygen flow rate (the amount of oxygen to be administered) written as liters per minute (L/min)

- The concentration of the oxygen to be administered written as a percentage (%) of oxygen to be delivered
- The method of delivery
- The length of time for administration

The dose of oxygen prescribed by the licensed health care provider for an individual is based upon the individual's need at the time the oxygen is ordered. As with all medications, it is the UAP's responsibility to follow the licensed HCP's order and to follow the principles of medication administration as discussed in Chapter 6.

Methods of Delivery

The method used to deliver oxygen to an individual will be determined by the licensed health care provider. Several different methods exist today. The most common methods used are (1) nasal cannula and (2) mask.

Nasal Cannula

nasal cannula
A device used to administer oxygen to an individual.

A **nasal cannula** is the simplest and most convenient method of delivery to use. It is used to administer low concentrations of oxygen to an individual. A cannula is a long, plastic tube that has two hollow short tubes called prongs (Figure 8-5). The prongs are placed in the openings of the nose. A strap may hold the cannula on the individual's head. Oxygen passes through the tube and prongs into the individual's nose (Figure 8-6). If the

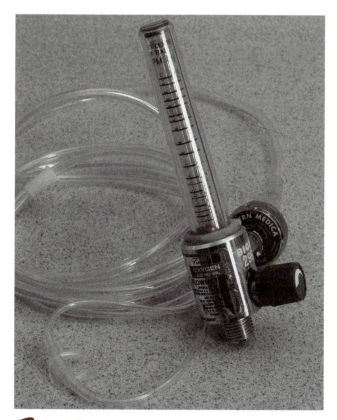

Figure 8-5 Nasal cannula and oxygen tubing attached to a flow meter. *(Delmar/Cengage Learning)*

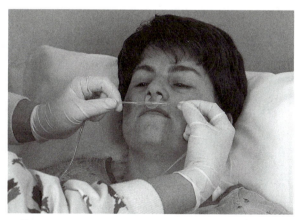

Figure 8-6 Oxygen administered by a nasal cannula. *(Delmar/Cengage Learning)*

flow rate exceeds more than two (2) liters per minute (L/min), the oxygen may need to go through a bottle of water for humidification.

Special Considerations

- Check for signs of irritation at the points where the cannula tubing or strap touches the individual's ears and face.

- Check for signs of irritation at the point where the prongs of the cannula enter the openings of the nose.

- If the cannula has a strap, make sure the strap is secure but is not too tight.

- Never use a petroleum-based lubricant or gel on irritated areas of the nostrils.

- Check to be certain that mucus does not block the prongs of the cannula. If need be, clean the prongs.

- When the cannula is not being used, store the cannula safely to prevent contamination of the cannula.

Oxygen Masks

A **mask** is a cuplike, plastic object that fits over an individual's nose, mouth, and chin. Like a nasal cannula, the mask is held in place on an individual's head by a strap. A tube connects the mask to the oxygen supply (Figure 8-7). Masks come in several different sizes and different styles. Each style serves a different purpose. There is a special mask to fit over a **tracheostomy** (Figure 8-8). The style of mask used depends on the oxygen needs of the individual. To be effective, the mask must fit well to the individual's face.

mask
A device used to administer oxygen to an individual.

tracheostomy
An opening made into the trachea (windpipe) through which an individual may breathe.

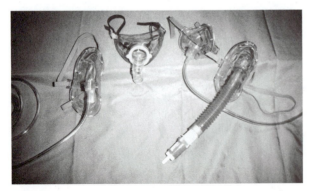

Figure 8-7 Various types of oxygen masks with tubing. *(Delmar/Cengage Learning)*

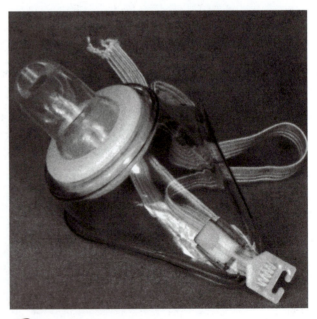

Figure 8-8 An adult tracheostomy mask. *(Delmar/Cengage Learning)*

Masks are used when:

- An individual breathes through his mouth

- An individual has a tracheostomy

- An individual needs to receive a precise amount of oxygen

- The individual needs a higher moisture content with the oxygen

- High liter flows of oxygen are ordered by the licensed health care provider

Special Considerations

- Never use a mask with a liter flow rate of less than five (5) liters per minute (L/min). Doing so may cause an individual to rebreathe carbon dioxide, having a smothering effect.

- Be sure the mask is placed over the individual's mouth and nose.

- Be sure the mask fits snugly but is not too tight. Adjust the fit of the mask by pulling gently on the ends of the elastic strap.

- For a tight fit around the nose, adjust the metal strip over the bridge of the nose.

- On a regularly scheduled basis, remove the mask. Wash, rinse, and dry the area under the mask well. Reapply the mask.

- When an individual has a nonrebreathing mask, the bag should be fully inflated at all times (Figure 8-9). Notify the licensed HCP if the bag collapses more than halfway during inspiration (when the individual breathes in).

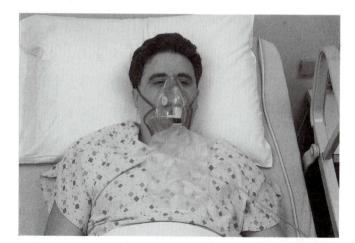

Figure 8-9 The nonrebreathing mask provides very high amounts of oxygen. The individual's exhaled air escapes through the one-way flaps on the sides, but room air cannot enter because of the one-way design. The bag at the bottom increases the amount of oxygen delivered to the individual. The bag should not collapse more than halfway when the individual inhales. *(Delmar/Cengage Learning)*

Note: A nonrebreathing mask is a combination of a bag and mask. This mask provides very high amounts of oxygen by increasing the amount of oxygen delivered to the individual. The mask should not be used for more than twenty-four (24) hours without an evaluation by a licensed HCP.

OXYGEN ADMINISTRATION EQUIPMENT

Oxygen is available in cylinders (oxygen tanks), in liquid oxygen canisters, by oxygen concentrators, and by piped-in oxygen systems (Figure 8-10).

Oxygen Cylinders

In the United States, oxygen cylinders (tanks) are always colored green. The UAP needs to transport the cylinders carefully. A chain holds the cylinder securely in place during transport. Cylinders must not be dropped. If dropped, the cylinder's valve may be damaged. The cylinder may explode. Once at the proper location, the UAP is to secure the cylinder in a proper base or to the wall with a chain. Before use, the UAP must identify the contents of the cylinder.

Liquid Oxygen Canisters

Liquid oxygen is made by cooling oxygen gas. The liquid oxygen is then stored in large canisters. The canisters allow large amounts of liquid oxygen to be easily and conveniently stored. UAPs are then able to fill small containers with the liquid oxygen as needed for use by individuals (Figure 8-11).

Note: Liquid oxygen cannot be stored for long periods of time. It will evaporate.

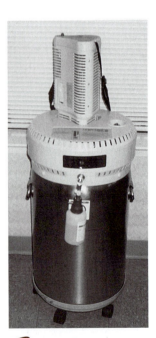

Figure 8-11 The liquid oxygen canister. The portable tank on top is filled from the large tank, then detached.
(Delmar/Cengage Learning)

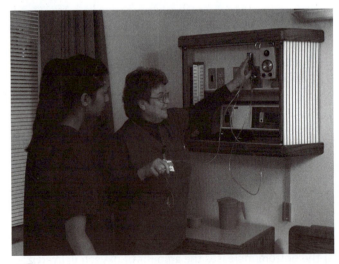

Figure 8-10 A piped-in oxygen system. *(Delmar/Cengage Learning)*

liquid oxygen canister
A type of oxygen administration equipment that makes liquid oxygen by cooling oxygen gas.

The **liquid oxygen canister** delivers a higher concentration of oxygen than an oxygen concentrator. The canister is portable and convenient. Electricity is not required. The canister, however, is more expensive than an oxygen concentrator.

Special Considerations

- Avoid opening, touching, or spilling a liquid oxygen container. Although liquid oxygen is nontoxic, it will cause severe burns upon direct contact. If liquid oxygen touches one's skin or clothing, immediately rinse the area with large amounts of water.

- Be sure to follow oxygen safety precautions. The use of liquid oxygen results in a rapid buildup of high concentrations of oxygen. Sparks, fires, and the presence of highly flammable materials may cause a dangerous situation.

- *Never* seal or close the cap or the vent port on the liquid oxygen canister. This will increase the pressure in the system and may cause a dangerous situation.

- If a tank or canister filled with liquid oxygen falls or tips over, the UAP is to *immediately* remove himself and all individuals from the room. Close the door to the room. Follow the emergency procedures per workplace policy. Notify the supervisor.

Oxygen Concentrators

oxygen concentrator
A type of oxygen administration equipment that provides low liter flows of oxygen.

An **oxygen concentrator** provides low liter flows of oxygen, usually at a flow rate of two (2) liters per minute (L/min). The individual receives the oxygen by nasal cannula. The cannula is connected to the concentrator by tubing (Figure 8-12 shown on next page).

The concentrator takes in room air, removes impurities and other gases, and leaves oxygen. The remaining oxygen becomes concentrated in the unit. The concentrator provides the individual with air that is more than 90% oxygen. The oxygen may or may not be humidified to increase the amount of moisture content in the oxygen.

Special Considerations

- Place the concentrator at least five (5) feet away from any source of heat and at least four (4) inches away from the wall, drapes, or bedding.

- Be sure the concentrator is plugged in and grounded.

- Notify the appropriate individual if the alarm sounds.

- Do not use a mask with a concentrator. The concentrator has a low liter flow. The carbon dioxide the individual breathes out cannot leave the mask. The individual may rebreathe the carbon dioxide, having a smothering effect.

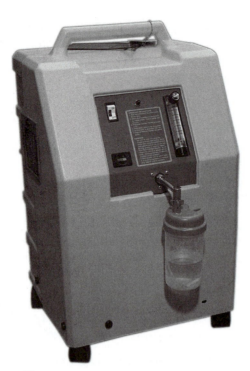

Figure 8-12 The oxygen concentrator provides low liter flows of oxygen. Most concentrators have an attachment for a humidifier, but humidification is not needed at low liter flows. *(Delmar/Cengage Learning)*

- Clean the surfaces of the concentrator with a damp cloth only.
- Remove the filter from the concentrator weekly. Wash the filter in warm soapy water, rinse well, squeeze dry, and replace in the concentrator.

Humidifiers

Some workplaces, but not all, add a humidifier to the oxygen administration equipment when the liter flow rate is more than five (5) L/min. If the liter flow rate is less than five (5) L/min, a humidifier is not necessary but may still be used.

A **humidifier** is a bottle of water that is attached to the oxygen administration equipment (Figure 8-13). The bottle attaches to an adapter on the flow meter (Figures 8-11 and 8-12). The cannula or mask connects to the opposite side of the humidifier.

Oxygen passes from the oxygen administration equipment, such as the liquid oxygen canister, through the water in the bottle. As the oxygen passes through the water, it picks up moisture. The oxygen then passes through the tubing to the individual. The added moisture in the oxygen prevents drying of the mucous membranes of the nose, mouth, and lungs and provides comfort.

There are two common types of humidifier bottles: (1) prefilled bottles and (2) refillable bottles. The prefilled humidifier bottle is commonly

humidifier
A bottle of water that is attached to the oxygen administration equipment.

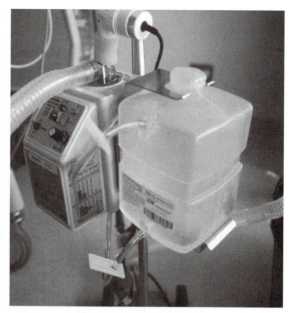

Figure 8-13 A humidifier. *(Delmar/Cengage Learning)*

used in an acute care setting such as a hospital or an acute rehabilitation center. In these settings the bottle is usually changed:

- When it empties
- Weekly
- According to the manufacturer's directions
- Per workplace policy

Once the new bottle is replaced, the used bottle is discarded per workplace policy. It is recommended that the new bottle be labeled with the date and time that it was changed and with the initials of the staff person who changed the bottle.

When a refillable humidifier bottle is being used, the bottle should be washed with soap and warm water, rinsed well, and then sterilized every twenty-four (24) hours. A 2% alkaline gluteraldehyde solution may be used in place of soap and warm water. Once sterilized, the bottle is to be filled with sterile distilled water to the fill line on the bottle. Again, it is recommended that the bottle be labeled with the date and time the bottle was changed and with the initials of the staff person who changed the bottle.

Procedure 8-2
Changing a Humidifier Bottle

When changing a humidifier bottle, follow these steps:

1. Identify the individual who is receiving oxygen.
2. Verify the licensed health care provider order for the oxygen flow rate.
3. Wash hands.

4. Gather the equipment:
    - Humidifier bottle—a refillable humidifier bottle or a sterile prefilled disposable bottle
    - Sterile distilled water, if needed

5. Explain the procedure to the individual.

6. Remove the humidifier bottle from its package.

7. If using a sterile, prefilled disposable bottle, skip to step 10.

8. If using a refillable humidifier bottle, make sure the bottle has been washed and sterilized. Remove the bottle cover. Place the cover of the bottle on the table with the sterile side up.

9. Fill the bottle with sterile water to the fill line on the bottle. Replace the cover. *Do not touch the inside of the bottle or its cover. These are sterile.*

10. Connect the humidifier bottle to the flow meter on the oxygen administration equipment. Tighten securely.

11. Connect the cannula or mask to the side of the humidifier bottle.

12. Turn on the oxygen. Set the oxygen flow rate to the flow rate ordered by the individual's licensed health care provider. Check the pressure relief valve by pinching the tubing. The safety valve should pop off.

13. Write the date and time the bottle was changed and one's initials on a sticker. Place the sticker on the bottle.

14. Document per workplace policy.

Special Considerations

- Before caring for humidifiers, the UAP needs to check his workplace policy to make sure this task is permitted. In most workplaces, *but not all*, UAPs are responsible for the care of humidifiers.

- *Do not use tap water in humidifier bottles.* Use of tap water is associated with an increase in Legionnaires' disease. *Sterile distilled water is to be used at all times.*

- *Always* keep the water level in the humidifier bottle at or above the "minimum fill" line on the bottle.

- *Always* check the pressure relief valve when setting up a humidifier. Once the humidifier bottle is attached to the oxygen administration equipment, turn on the oxygen and pinch the connecting tubing. If the humidifier bottle is connected properly, the safety valve should pop off.

- Frequently check the oxygen tubing on the mask or cannula to make sure the tubing is not twisted or blocked. Oxygen cannot pass through the tubing to the individual if this happens.

Note: When the oxygen administration equipment is working correctly and the individual is receiving oxygen, the water in the humidifier bottle will bubble constantly.

PROVIDING CARE FOR AN INDIVIDUAL RECEIVING OXYGEN

When providing care for an individual who is receiving oxygen, the UAP should follow these basic guidelines:

1. If the plan of care permits it, elevate the head of the individual's bed. This makes it easier for the individual to breathe.

2. If the individual is wearing an oxygen mask, contact the licensed HCP to get an order for use of a cannula at mealtimes. An individual wearing a mask is unable to eat.

3. Offer reassurance and support frequently. Being unable to breathe tends to be very frightening. Check on the individual often. Whenever possible, spend time with the individual.

4. Shortness of breath and difficulty breathing make it very difficult for an individual to speak. If the individual is having trouble talking, ask "yes" and "no" questions. Spend additional time with the individual. Just being with the individual has a calming effect and is reassuring.

5. Observe the skin under the oxygen delivery devices (mask, cannula) for signs of skin irritation. Report any changes in the skin to the individual's licensed HCP immediately.

6. Offer extra fluids to drink. Oxygen is very drying.

7. Provide frequent mouth and nose care.

8. Change the individual's clothing and bedding often. Extra changes may be needed because the individual may sweat heavily.

9. Adjust the room temperature if necessary.

10. Wear gloves and follow the principles of standard precautions when coming into contact with the individual's oral and/or nasal secretions.

11. Know the oxygen flow rate ordered by the individual's licensed HCP.

12. Have a basic understanding of how to read a flow meter.

13. Notify the licensed HCP if there is a change in the flow rate.

14. Make sure the oxygen tubing is not kinked or twisted in any way. Kinked or twisted tubing will block the flow of oxygen to the individual.

15. Check often for proper positioning of the mask or cannula.

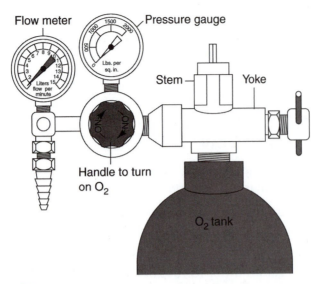

Figure 8-14 The flow meter shows the amount of oxygen being delivered. The pressure gauge shows the amount of oxygen remaining in the tank.
(Delmar/Cengage Learning)

16. Use a portable oxygen tank to transport the individual to other areas.

   • Check to be sure there is enough oxygen in the tank. Check the gauge each time you visit the individual (Figure 8-14).

   • Check to be sure the oxygen is turned on.

   • Keep an extra oxygen tank nearby to exchange for the tank in use when it is empty.

   • Be sure the tank is in the upright position and is secure on its carrier or in the stand.

Oxygen Safety Precautions

Oxygen does not cause a fire, but it does support burning. There is, therefore, the danger of a fire being started when oxygen is in use. Since fire may be started by friction, static electricity, or a lighted cigar or cigarette, people must be careful when around the use of oxygen. For this reason, UAPs must follow these guidelines when caring for an individual on oxygen:

1. Place an *"Oxygen in Use—No Smoking"* sign clearly on the door to the room and over the head of the bed of the individual who is using oxygen.

2. Do not use electrical equipment such as heating pads, electric blankets, electric razors, and so on while oxygen is in use.

3. Suction machines, X-ray machines, and EKG equipment are to be used with caution while administering oxygen.

4. Check the individual's room for safety before beginning the administration of oxygen. When possible, replace electrical devices with nonelectrical ones.

5. In a home setting, there are to be no open flames such as the use of candles, a gas stove, and so on.

6. Explain safety measures to the individual, friends, and family members.

Respiratory Positions

There are four basic respiratory positions:

1. High Fowler's position

2. Orthopneic position

3. Tripod position

4. Dangling at the bedside

When an individual is sitting in the high Fowler's position, the individual's back is lying against the elevated head of the bed (Figure 8-15). To place an individual in the high Fowler's position, follow these steps:

1. Position three pillows behind the individual's head and shoulders.

2. Adjust the knee rest.

3. Keep the feet in proper position.

Note: **Check the skin often for signs of skin breakdown due to shearing.**

The orthopneic position is an alternative position to the high Fowler's position. In the orthopneic position, the individual sits up as straight as possible, leans slightly forward, and uses his forearms for support (Figure 8-16 shown on next page).

The tripod position offers another alternative. To place an individual in the tripod position, follow these steps:

1. Elevate the head of the bed as far as it will go.

2. Place the bedside table across the bed.

3. Place a pillow or two on the bedside table.

4. Help the individual to lean across the bedside table with his arms placed on or beside the pillows (Figure 8-17 shown on next page).

Having the individual dangle his legs on the side of the bed will also provide an alternative position. With the bed in the lowest horizontal

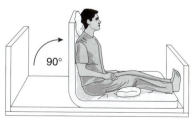

Figure 8-15 The individual is in the high Fowler's position.
(Delmar/Cengage Learning)

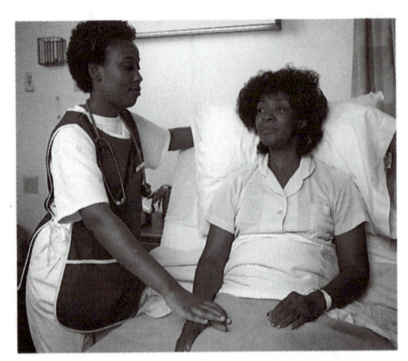

Figure 8-16 The individual is sitting straight up in the orthopneic position, supported on her arms. *(Delmar/Cengage Learning)*

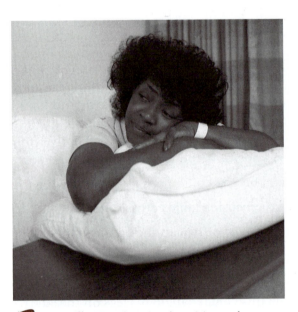

Figure 8-17 The tripod position enlarges the chest cavity, making breathing easier.
(Delmar/Cengage Learning)

position, have the individual sit on the side of the bed. Make sure the individual's legs are supported on the floor or on a stool. Use the bedside table in the same fashion as for the tripod position discussed earlier. The individual is to lean across the bedside table with his arms placed on or beside pillows.

These positions allow the lungs to expand and the airway to be kept straight. The positions may be helpful to an individual with respiratory distress.

Oxygen Toxicity

As with any medication, oxygen may reach a toxic (poisonous) level in the body. Toxicity depends upon the dose, time, and the individual's response to the oxygen he is receiving. The higher the dose or flow rate of the oxygen, the shorter the time required for toxicity to develop. The symptoms of toxicity are as follows:

- Chest pain located under the sternum
- Nausea/vomiting
- **Malaise** (a feeling of illness)
- Fatigue
- Numbness and tingling in extremities (arms, hands, legs, and feet)

If the individual complains of any of these symptoms, it is important that the UAP contact the individual's licensed health care provider immediately. Once the licensed HCP is notified, the UAP needs to contact his supervisor.

ADDITIONAL EQUIPMENT
Incentive Spirometer

incentive spirometer
A device used to help an individual breathe deeply.

atelectasis
A collapse of a lung.

An **incentive spirometer** may be used to help an individual breathe deeply. Breathing deeply will expand an individual's lungs and prevent pneumonia (an infection of the lungs) and **atelectasis** (a collapse of a lung). The use of an incentive spirometer requires a written licensed health care provider order.

Procedure 8-3
Use of an Incentive Spirometer

When assisting an individual to use an incentive spirometer, follow these steps:

1. Identify the individual.
2. Verify the licensed health care provider order.
3. Wash hands.
4. Gather the equipment:
   - Incentive spirometer with appropriate mouthpiece
   - Tissue
   - Emesis basin
   - Pillow, if needed
5. Explain the procedure to the individual.
6. Demonstrate deep breathing.
7. Assist the individual into a sitting position. See the section "Respiratory Positions" for different positions that may be used.

8. Set the pointer on the incentive spirometer at the level or point where the disk or ball should reach, per the licensed health care provider order.

9. Have the individual use the incentive spirometer.

   - Have the individual inhale (breathe in) and exhale (breathe out) completely before using the incentive spirometer.

   - Have the individual place his lips tightly around the mouthpiece.

   - Instruct the individual to breathe in slowly and deeply until the disk or ball reaches the ordered level or point (Figure 8-18).

   - Instruct the individual to hold his breath at this point for at least three (3) seconds, or as long as he is able.

   - Have the individual remove the mouthpiece and breathe out slowly.

   - If needed, have the individual cough any sputum into the emesis basin.

10. Repeat this action per the licensed HCP order.

11. Dispose of soiled tissue. Clean the emesis basin, if needed.

12. Clean the mouthpiece with soap and warm water. Rinse and dry the mouthpiece well. Store the mouthpiece in a plastic bag in a safe place.

13. Provide mouth care as needed.

14. Wash hands.

15. Return the individual to a comfortable position.

16. Document per workplace policy.

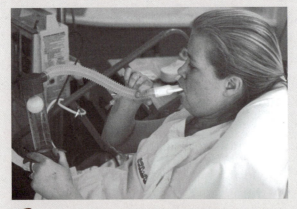

Figure 8-18 The individual inhales through the mouth, raising the level of the ball inside the plastic chambers. *(Delmar/Cengage Learning)*

Special Considerations

- Observe the individual closely during use of the incentive spirometer to make sure he is using it correctly.

- Instruct the individual not to take in too many deep breaths in a row because this may make him dizzy.

- Be sure the individual does not become overly tired during use of the incentive spirometer.

- Encourage the individual to cough and clear his throat when needed.

- Report to the licensed health care provider if the individual gets overly tired during use of the spirometer or has any other difficulties or complaints.

- Carefully observe and report any unusual reactions, such as dizziness, lightheadedness, pain, or throat or airway irritation, to the licensed health care provider.

Guidelines for Documentation

When documenting information on the use of the incentive spirometer, the UAP needs to document the following:

- The individual's respiratory rate and depth before and after use of the incentive spirometer

- The lung volume in milliliters (mL) or cubic centimeters (cc)

- The type and amount of sputum (phlegm) expectorated (coughed up)

Continuous Positive Airway Pressure (CPAP)

Some individuals have a condition called sleep apnea. Sleep apnea occurs when an individual is sleeping. When the individual falls asleep, his muscles relax, and a blockage or obstruction occurs in his airway. The blockage or obstruction stops his breathing. An individual who has sleep apnea may stop breathing hundreds of times a night. When the individual starts to breathe again, he snores loudly. The snoring interrupts his sleep. The frequent interruptions in an individual's sleep cause him to be very tired during the day.

continuous positive airway pressure (CPAP) device
A device that delivers pressure to the individual's airway while the individual sleeps.

Treatment of sleep apnea involves a device called a **continuous positive airway pressure (CPAP)** (Figure 8-19). The device delivers pressure to the individual's airway while the individual sleeps. The pressure holds the individual's airway open.

A mask is placed on the individual's face and held in place with a head strap. Tubing connects the mask to the device. The mask must fit tightly against the face. The amount of pressure is controlled by an adjustment on the device. The amount of pressure may range from two (2) cm H_2O to twenty (20) cm H_2O. A written order for the amount of pressure is needed from the individual's licensed health care provider.

A licensed health care provider, such as a respiratory therapist, usually sets up the CPAP device initially for the individual. The licensed

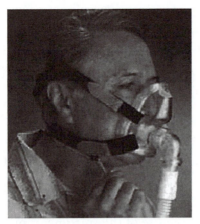

Figure 8-19 The CPAP mask applies pressure to keep the airway open while the individual sleeps, preventing sleep apnea.
(Delmar/Cengage Learning)

HCP works with the individual to determine the type of equipment the individual needs, including the type of mask that will be the most effective and most comfortable for him.

Special Considerations

- Before applying the individual's mask, wash and dry the individual's face thoroughly. If the individual puts on his own mask, remind him to wash and dry his face. This prevents skin oil from getting on the mask.

- Check to make sure the mask fits tightly but fits comfortably.

  - Check for air leaks around the top of the mask and adjust the mask as needed. Air blowing from the CPAP device into the individual's eyes may be very irritating.

  - If the mask is too tight, loosen it until it is snug but comfortable. A mask that is too tight may cause pain and/or skin breakdown on the nose.

- Monitor the individual while he is using the CPAP device.

- Do not use petrolatum products in the nasal passages (nose). If the individual complains of nasal dryness, notify the licensed HCP. The licensed HCP may order saline spray or nose drops to decrease the nasal dryness and irritation.

- Elevate the head of the individual's bed, if need be, to prevent or reduce air swallowing. If an individual swallows large amounts of air, he will belch frequently and/or feel pressure in his abdomen.

- Wash the mask each morning after the individual takes it off. Wash the mask with soap and warm water or according to workplace policy.

- Store the mask in a clean plastic bag until the individual uses it again at bedtime.

Guidelines for Documentation

When documenting information on the CPAP device, the UAP needs to document the following:

- Date and time the CPAP device was attached and removed
- Pulse, respiratory rate, and general appearance of the individual when the CPAP device was initially attached and during its use
- Alarm settings of the CPAP device
- Any changes noted in the individual during or after use of the CPAP device

STORAGE OF OXYGEN

In many states, oxygen is a Schedule VI controlled substance. Storage of oxygen, therefore, follows the same guidelines and principles as for other Schedule VI medications, such as antibiotics and heart medications. Oxygen may also require a written prescription from the licensed health care provider.

SUMMARY

In most settings, oxygen is a Schedule VI controlled substance. As such, a written licensed health care provider order is required for use of oxygen, and, in some settings, a prescription is also needed. When administering oxygen, the UAP follows the same medication administration principles as for all other medications. In addition, individuals receiving oxygen require continuous monitoring. Changes in an individual's status during oxygen administration must be reported to the individual's licensed health care provider and the UAP's supervisor per workplace policy.

REVIEW QUESTIONS

1. Conditions that may require oxygen administration include:
   a. COPD, sleep apnea, and immobility
   b. sleeplessness, anxiety, and hypertension
   c. before surgery, fatigue, and shock
   d. diabetes, COPD, and hypotonia
2. An early indicator of hypoxemia is:
   a. color changes of lips and nail beds
   b. hot, dry skin
   c. a pulse rate of less than sixty (60) beats per minute
   d. quiet, even breathing

3. Blood gets rid of carbon dioxide and picks up oxygen in the:
   a. bronchi   c. alveoli
   b. bronchioles   d. arteries

4. The most commonly used pulse oximeter sensors are the:
   a. nasal and toe sensors
   b. toe and forehead sensors
   c. earlobe and foot sensors
   d. finger-clip and earlobe sensors

5. A normal oxygen saturation level is:
   a. 90% to 100%   c. below 90%
   b. 95% to 100%   d. below 70%

6. Which oxygen saturation level is life threatening?
   a. below 95%   c. below 80%
   b. below 90%   d. below 70%

7. If an individual receiving pulse oximetry is using oxygen, the UAP needs to:
   a. plug the pulse oximeter into the oxygen concentrator
   b. shut off the oxygen concentrator before attaching the pulse oximeter
   c. document the liter flow rate
   d. contact the individual's licensed HCP to clarify the order for pulse oximetry

8. The two most common methods of oxygen delivery are by:
   a. nasal cannula and mask
   b. nasal cannula and tracheostomy
   c. mask and nebulizer
   d. mask and IPPB machine

9. When using a mask for oxygen therapy, the flow rate should never be less than:
   a. 2 L/min   c. 4 L/min
   b. 3 L/min   d. 5 L/min

10. In the United States, oxygen tanks are always colored:
    a. red   c. green
    b. blue   d. yellow

11. When providing care to an individual receiving oxygen therapy, the UAP may help by:
    a. asking "yes" and "no" questions and providing frequent mouth and nose care
    b. checking on the individual only once or twice per shift, so that the individual does not have to talk too much
    c. folding up the oxygen tubing so it is not lying on the floor
    d. keeping the individual's room warm to make the individual more comfortable

12. Two of the four basic respiratory positions include:
    a. high Folk's and triangle positions
    b. high Fowler's and orthopneic positions
    c. tripod and orthopedic positions
    d. standing-at-bedside and triangle positions

13. Use of an incentive spirometer will help to prevent:
    a. fatigue and chest pain
    b. numbness and tingling
    c. pneumonia and atelectasis
    d. dizziness and lethargy
14. A CPAP device is used to treat an individual who has:
    a. pneumonia   c. atelectasis
    b. sleep apnea   d. sleep deprivation

CLINICAL SCENARIOS

1. You are asked to do a pulse oximetry reading on Mrs. Cavanaugh.
   a. As with any procedure, what are the first five steps you must do to begin the pulse oximetry reading?
   b. What must you do to prepare Mrs. Cavanaugh after you locate the sensor site ordered by her licensed HCP?
   c. Write a note documenting Mrs. Cavanaugh's pulse oximetry test. Use today's date and the time you are completing this assignment. Presume the following:

      - Initial pulse rate of eighty-four (84) and respiratory rate of eighteen (18)
      - Use of a finger-clip sensor on Mrs. Cavanaugh's right fifth finger
      - Initial oxygen saturation rate of 91%, monitored rate of 93%
      - Mrs. Cavanaugh is not receiving oxygen therapy
      - The licensed HCP has not specified alarm settings

      Use what you have learned in the textbook, as well as class discussion and/or your own work experience, to document Mrs. Cavanaugh's general appearance and any changes that may be observed.

2. You are asked to give care to Mr. Humphrey, who is receiving oxygen therapy.
   a. One of your tasks is to change the refillable humidifier bottle on Mr. Humphrey's oxygen concentrator. How often is the bottle cleaned, and with what cleaning agents?
   b. Describe the steps you would take to change the humidifier bottle.
   c. List five guidelines you may follow when giving care to Mr. Humphrey.

3. Mr. Calloway has used oxygen therapy according to the licensed HCP order for the past few months. When you are assisting him one day, he says he is not feeling well. His symptoms include fatigue, tingling in his legs and feet, and pain right in the middle of his chest. He points to his sternum when describing the pain in his chest. What could this be? What do you do?

Chapter 9
Administration of Enemas

Learning Objectives

After reading this chapter and completing the review exercises, you should be able to:

1. Spell and define terms.
2. List three reasons enemas are administered.
3. Describe three types of enemas.
4. List five types of enema solutions.
5. Describe a cleansing enema.
6. Describe a ready-to-use (prepackaged) enema.
7. Describe an oil retention enema.
8. Demonstrate the administration of a cleansing enema.
9. Demonstrate the administration of a ready-to-use (prepackaged) enema.
10. List seven guidelines for documenting the administration of an enema.

Key Terms

colon	enema	peristalsis	rectum
constipation	feces	proctoscopy	sigmoidoscopy
endoscopy	flatus		

INTRODUCTION

An **enema** is a way to administer a liquid solution or liquid medication into the **rectum** and **colon** (part of the bowel). An enema may be used to:

1. Clean the bowel by removing **feces** (stool) and/or **flatus** (gas)

2. Administer rectal medications

3. Prepare an individual for diagnostic tests such as X-rays, **sigmoidoscopy**, **proctoscopy**, or **endoscopy** and for surgery and other special procedures

Each individual has her own routine for moving her bowels. One individual may have a bowel movement (BM) every day. Another individual may have a bowel movement (BM) every two (2) to three (3) days. Bowel movements (stool, BM) are normally soft and formed. The stool usually moves through the body at a regular pace.

If the stool passes through the body too slowly, the stool will become hard, dry, sticky, and/or pasty, resulting in a condition called **constipation**. Aging, disease, surgery, immobility, diet, stress, and medications all may cause an individual to become constipated. One way to treat constipation is to administer an **enema**.

Medications are given by many different routes. Medications may be given rectally for the following reasons:

1. When the rectum is the area to be medicated

2. When an individual is unable to take medications orally

3. When the provider wants the medication to be absorbed quickly

Rectal medications may be given by suppository, cream, gel, or enema.

When preparing an individual for diagnostic tests, surgery, or other procedures, enemas may be part of the preparation. The enema cleans the bowel. The licensed health care provider is then able to see the bowel clearly on examination or during surgery.

TYPES OF ENEMAS

Licensed health care providers frequently order three basic types of enemas. These are:

1. Cleansing enema

2. Ready-to-use (prepackaged) enema

3. Return-flow enema

Many different types of solutions are used for enemas. These solutions include:

- Tap water

- Normal saline (considered to be a safe solution because it is similar to the body's own fluids)

- Soap solutions (known to be very irritating to the bowel and rarely ordered anymore)

rectum
The opening of the body that leads into the bowel.

colon
Part of the large intestine (bowel).

feces
Stool; semisolid waste passed out of the body through the rectum; bowel movement or BM.

flatus
Gas or air in the stomach or intestines; commonly passed out of the body by belching or through the rectum.

- Oil
- Solutions used to provide relief from gas
- Other solutions as determined by the licensed health care provider

Cleansing Enemas

Cleansing enemas are probably the most common type of enema. This type of enema irritates the bowel and causes distention (stretching) of the bowel. The feces or stool in the rectum and bowel are then passed out of the body. Depending on the purpose for the enema and the age and condition of the individual, the amount of fluid to be ordered may range from 500 mL to 1,000 mL.

When ordering a cleansing enema, the licensed health care provider order will specify:

1. The type of solution to be used

2. The amount of solution to be given

3. The length of time the individual is to retain (hold) the enema solution

4. Any special instructions

When a cleansing enema is ordered before a diagnostic procedure or surgery, the licensed health care provider may order "enemas until clear." This means that the cleansing enemas are to be repeated until the fluid that is passed from the individual's body is clear and has no feces or stool in the fluid.

Note: Most workplaces have written guidelines stating the maximum number of cleansing enemas that may be administered to an individual at one time. If the UAP's workplace does not have such guidelines, the UAP is to contact the licensed health care provider for written instructions before administering the cleansing enema.

Ready-to-Use (Prepackaged) Enemas

Ready-to-use, prepackaged enemas are commonly used in many settings, including the home. Each package holds approximately four (4) ounces of solution. The solution may be saline, oil, phosphosoda, or another solution.

These enemas are available over-the-counter in most drugstores, grocery stores, pharmacies, and general department stores (such as Wal-Mart and Target). However, as with all medications, the UAP needs a licensed health care provider order before she may administer an enema. Ready-to-use enemas, such as the Fleet® Enema, are easily administered. In fact, if ordered by the licensed health care provider, an individual may self-administer this enema under the supervision of the UAP.

When administering the prepackaged oil-retention enema, the individual holds the oil in her bowel for up to an hour. This allows the oil to soften the hard stool in the bowel. Once the hour passes—or sooner if the individual is unable to hold the oil in her bowel for the full hour—the individual passes the solution and stool. A cleansing enema may be administered after the oil-retention enema is completed to remove the remaining stool from the bowel.

Return-Flow Enemas

peristalsis
Involuntary, wave-like contractions of the bowel.

Return-flow enemas are used to remove flatus (gas) from the bowel and to increase the involuntary wavelike contractions of the bowel known as **peristalsis**. These enemas are used often after abdominal surgery to help restart bowel activity and to decrease abdominal distention (bloating). For this reason, these enemas are most commonly used in acute care settings.

Note: As stated earlier, return-flow enemas are often administered in the acute care setting. For this reason, UAPs administering return-flow enemas may require additional knowledge, skills, and clinical practice that are not addressed in this training manual.

PROPER POSITIONING FOR ADMINISTRATION OF AN ENEMA

When receiving an enema, an individual is usually most comfortable when lying on her left side with her left leg out straight. The upper (right) leg should be bent at the hip, with the knee bent forward and upward toward the stomach (Figure 9-1). The enema solution will enter

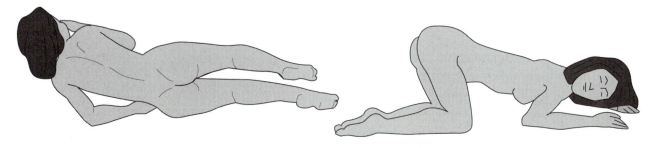

Left-Lateral Position   Knee-Chest Position

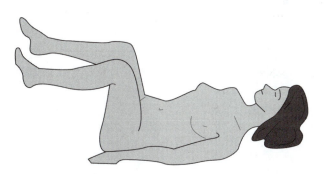

Position for Self-Administration

Figure 9-1 Alternative positions for the administration of an enema. *(Delmar/Cengage Learning)*

the body most easily in this position. This is the most common position used in the administration of an enema.

However, there are times when this position may not be able to be used. Figure 9-1 shows two additional positions that may be used. First, the individual may lie on her back, either to self-administer the enema, if so ordered by the licensed health care provider, or sit on a bedpan (bedpan not shown) to aid in the administration of the enema by the UAP. This position is often used when the individual is unable to hold the enema solution in her bowel or is unable to lie in the position on her left side (left-lateral position). Second, the individual may use the knee-chest position for comfort.

EQUIPMENT AND SUPPLIES USED IN THE ADMINISTRATION OF ENEMAS

The following equipment may be used in the administration of a cleansing enema:

- Disposable enema kit that includes a plastic container, tubing with a clamp, and water-soluble lubricating gel; *do not use* a petroleum-based gel (Figure 9-2)
- A towel or disposable pad for the bed
- Clean paper toilet tissue
- Paper towel
- Liquid enema solution as ordered by the licensed health care provider
- Gloves
- Towel, soap, and a basin
- Bedpan with cover or a bedside commode if the individual is unable to walk to the bathroom (Figure 9-3)
- Trash bag

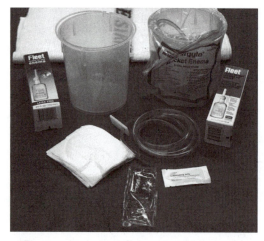

Figure 9-2 Various types of enema equipment and solutions. *(Delmar/Cengage Learning)*

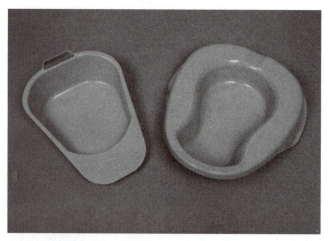

Figure 9-3 Fracture (orthopedic) bedpan (left) and regular bedpan (right). *(Delmar/Cengage Learning)*

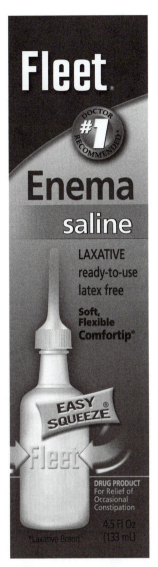

Figure 9-4
Disposable Fleet® Ready-to-Use Enema. *(Courtesy of Fleet Company, Inc.)*

The following equipment may be used in the administration of a ready-to-use (prepackaged) enema:

- Disposable prepackaged enema as ordered by the licensed health care provider (Figure 9-4)
- Water-soluble lubricating gel if the tip is not prelubricated; *do not use* a petroleum-based gel
- A towel or disposable pad for the bed
- Clean paper toilet tissue
- Gloves
- Towel, soap, and a basin
- Bedpan with cover or a bedside commode if the individual is unable to walk to the bathroom
- Warm water (if the enema solution is to be warmed)
- Trash bag

Procedure 9-1
Administration of a Cleansing Enema

To administer a cleansing enema, follow these steps:

1. Identify the individual to whom the enema is being given.
2. Verify the licensed HCP order.
3. Wash hands.
4. Gather all the equipment needed. (See the section "Equipment and Supplies Used in the Administration of Enemas.")
5. Prepare the equipment in the utility room or the individual's bathroom.
   A. If necessary, connect the tubing to the solution container (Figure 9-5A shown on page 211).
   B. Adjust the clamp on the tubing. Close the clamp (Figure 9-5B shown on page 211).
   C. Fill the container with the type and amount of solution ordered by the licensed health care provider.
   D. If the solution needs to be warmed, use a bath thermometer to make sure the temperature is 105°F (Figure 9-5C shown on page 211).
   E. If necessary, using the tip of the tubing, mix the solution gently or gently rotate the container. Do not shake the container.
   F. Run a small amount of the solution through the tubing to remove the air in the tubing. Clamp the tubing closed (Figures 9-5D and 9-5E shown on page 211).
   G. Wash hands.
   H. Take the equipment to the individual's bedside.

6. Place a chair at the foot or at the side of the bed. Cover the chair with a disposable pad or towel. Place the equipment, including a bedpan if one will be used, on the covered chair.

7. Explain the procedure to the individual. Tell the individual that she may have a feeling of fullness or the need to move her bowels during administration of the enema. Instruct the individual to report any feelings of cramping or abdominal pain if they occur.

8. Have the individual urinate, if possible, before giving the enema.

9. Provide privacy.

10. If possible, raise the bed to a comfortable and safe working height.

11. Encourage the individual to relax. Speak calmly. Playing soothing music may be helpful.

12. Put on gloves.

13. Cover the individual with a towel or blanket. Lower the individual's pants.

14. Have the individual lie down on her left side, with her left leg out straight. Her right leg should be bent at the hip, with the knee bent forward and upward toward the stomach. If need be, assist the individual with positioning.

15. Place a disposable pad on the bed under the individual.

16. If the tubing is not already lubricated, lubricate the tip of the tubing with water-soluble gel. *Do not use* petroleum-based gel.

17. Separate the buttocks with one hand. Ask the individual to breathe deeply and bear down. Gently insert the tube into the rectum two (2) to four (4) inches. *Never force the tube into the rectum. If the tube cannot be easily inserted into the rectum, stop administering the enema and notify the supervisor and the individual's licensed HCP.*

18. Open the clamp. Raise the container twelve (12) to eighteen (18) inches above the level of the opening of the rectum (anus). Be sure the enema solution flows slowly into the rectum and bowel (Figure 9-5F shown on next page).

    A. Instruct the individual to take deep breaths. This relaxes her abdomen and provides comfort.

    B. If the individual complains of cramping, clamp the tube. Wait until the cramping stops, then unclamp the tube and continue administering the enema. Repeat this process if needed.

19. When the solution has been administered or when the individual cannot hold any more solution, clamp the tubing.

Note: Be sure to clamp the tubing before all of the solution drains out of the container. A small amount of solution should be left in the container to prevent air from entering the rectum and bowel.

20. Instruct the individual to hold her breath while the tubing is being removed from her rectum.

21. Wipe the buttocks with toilet tissue. Discard the tissue in the trash.

22. Wrap the tubing in a paper towel. Place the wrapped tubing on the covered chair.

23. If the bed is elevated, lower the bed.

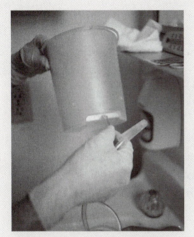

Figure 9-5a Attach the tubing to the enema container. *(Delmar/Cengage Learning)*

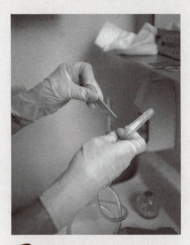

Figure 9-5b Slip the clamp over the tubing. *(Delmar/Cengage Learning)*

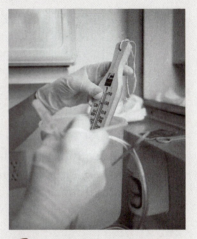

Figure 9-5c Use a bath thermometer to make sure the temperature of the enema solution is 105°F. *(Delmar/Cengage Learning)*

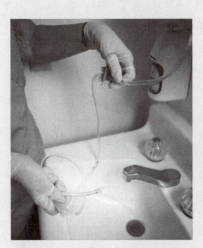

Figure 9-5d Run a small amount of the enema solution through the tubing to remove the air in the tubing. *(Delmar/Cengage Learning)*

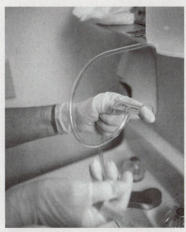

Figure 9-5e Once all the air has been removed from the tubing, clamp the tubing closed. *(Delmar/Cengage Learning)*

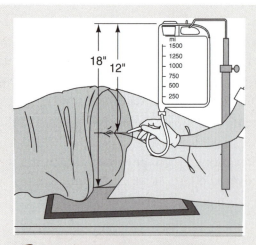

Figure 9-5f Raise the container twelve (12) to eighteen (18) inches above the level of the opening of the rectum (anus) so that the enema solution flows slowly into the rectum and bowel.
(Delmar/Cengage Learning)

24. Remove gloves.

25. When the individual has held the enema solution for the ordered amount of time or for as long as possible, help the individual to the bathroom. If she is unable to use the bathroom, help her to the commode or onto the bedpan.

26. Provide privacy.

27. Maintain the individual's safety.

28. If the individual is using the bathroom, instruct the individual not to flush the toilet.

29. When the individual is finished, assist with perineal care.

30. Return the individual to a comfortable position.

31. Put on gloves.

32. Care for the equipment and supplies. Throw all disposable materials in the trash as per workplace policy.

33. Observe the results of the enema.

34. Remove gloves.

35. Wash hands.

36. Document administration of the enema correctly.

37. Observe the individual for any unpleasant or harmful effects from the enema. If need be, contact the individual's licensed health care provider to report an adverse reaction(s), complaints of cramping or pain, poor results or no results from the enema, rectal bleeding, or other observation.

Note: If the enema solution to be used is a medication, follow steps 1 and 2 of the procedure for administering medications, then follow steps 4 through 37.

Procedure 9-2
Administration of a Ready-to-Use (Prepackaged) Enema

To administer a ready-to-use enema, follow these steps:

1. Identify the individual to whom the enema is being given.
2. Verify the licensed HCP order.
3. Wash hands.
4. Gather all the equipment needed. (See the section "Equipment and Supplies Used in the Administration of Enemas.")
5. Prepare the equipment in the utility room or the individual's bathroom.
   A. Open the enema package and remove the container of enema solution.
   B. If the enema solution needs to be warmed, place the container in a basin of warm water.
   C. Wash hands.
   D. Take the equipment to the individual's bedside.
6. Place a chair at the foot or at the side of the bed. Cover the chair with a disposable pad or towel. Place the equipment, including a bedpan if one will be used, on the covered chair.
7. Explain the procedure to the individual. Tell the individual that she may have a feeling of discomfort or the need to move her bowels during administration of the enema. Instruct the individual to report any feelings of cramping or pain if they occur.
8. Have the individual urinate, if possible, before giving the enema.
9. Provide privacy.
10. If possible, raise the bed to a comfortable and safe working height.
11. Encourage the individual to relax. Speak calmly. Playing soothing music may be helpful.
12. Put on gloves.
13. Cover the individual with a towel or blanket. Lower the individual's pants.
14. Have the individual lie down on her left side, with her left leg out straight. Her right leg should be bent at the hip, with the knee bent forward and upward toward the stomach. If need be, assist the individual with positioning.
15. Place a disposable pad on the bed under the individual.
16. Remove the cover from the tip of the enema container. Gently squeeze the container to make sure the tip is not damaged. The solution should easily pass out of the tip of the container (Figure 9-6A shown on page 215).

17. Check to make sure the tip has enough lubricant on it. If need be, lubricate the tip of the container with water-soluble gel. *Do not use* petroleum-based gel.

18. Separate the buttocks with one hand. Ask the individual to breathe deeply and bear down. Gently insert the tip of the container two (2) inches into the rectum (Figure 9-6B). *Never force the tip into the rectum. If the tip cannot be easily inserted into the rectum, stop administering the enema and notify the supervisor and the individual's licensed HCP.*

19. With the tip of the container in the rectum, gently squeeze and roll the enema container from the bottom. This will gently push the enema solution into the rectum. Squeeze until the ordered amount of solution has been administered. A small amount of solution will remain in the bottle (Figure 9-6C). *Do not release the pressure on the enema container.* Doing so will cause the enema solution to leak back into the container.

20. Slowly remove the tip of the container from the individual's rectum. Place the container back in its original box and put the box on the covered chair.

21. Wipe the buttocks with toilet tissue. Discard the tissue in the trash.

22. Remove gloves.

23. If the bed is elevated, lower the bed.

24. When the individual has held the solution for the ordered amount of time or for as long as possible, help the individual to the bathroom. If she is unable to use the bathroom, help her to the commode or onto the bedpan.

25. Provide privacy.

26. Maintain the individual's safety.

27. If the individual is using the bathroom, instruct the individual not to flush the toilet.

28. When the individual is finished, assist with perineal care.

29. Return the individual to a comfortable position.

30. Put on gloves.

31. Care for the equipment and supplies. Throw all disposable materials in the trash as per workplace policy.

32. Observe the results of the enema.

33. Remove gloves.

34. Wash hands.

35. Document administration of the enema correctly.

36. Observe the individual for any unpleasant or harmful effects from the enema. If need be, contact the individual's licensed health care provider to report an adverse

reaction(s), complaints of cramping or pain, poor results or no results from the enema, rectal bleeding, or other observation.

Note: If the enema solution to be used is a medication, follow steps 1 and 2 of the procedure for administering medications, then follow steps 4 through 36.

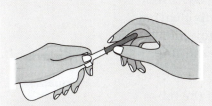

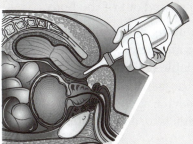

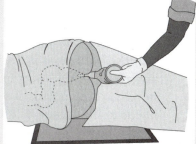

Figure 9-6a Remove the cover from the tip of the ready-to-use (prepackaged) enema bottle. *(Delmar/Cengage Learning)*

Figure 9-6b Insert the tip of the enema bottle two (2) inches into the rectum. *(Delmar/Cengage Learning)*

Figure 9-6c Squeeze the enema bottle from the bottom. A small amount of enema solution will remain in the container. *(Delmar/Cengage Learning)*

SPECIAL CONSIDERATIONS IN THE ADMINISTRATION OF ENEMAS

- *Before* administering an enema, the UAP needs to make sure that administering an enema is an approved procedure according to her state regulations and her workplace policies and procedures.

- UAPs administer enemas only under the orders of a licensed health care provider. The licensed HCP needs to provide clear instructions to the UAP about (1) the type of enema to be given, (2) the amount and type of solution(s) to use, (3) the length of time the individual is to hold the enema solution, and (4) any special instructions. If the UAP does not understand these instructions, she must call the licensed HCP with any questions *before* giving the enema to the individual.

- The UAP is to immediately notify her supervisor and the licensed health care provider if (1) any difficulty occurs during administration of the enema, such as the individual's inability to hold the enema solution in her bowel; (2) the individual receiving the enema has an adverse reaction, such as severe cramping, pain, or dizziness; or (3) the individual has little or no results from the enema.

- When administering an enema, the UAP follows standard precautions.

- When possible, administer an enema before breakfast or before an individual takes a bath or shower.

- Do not administer an enema within an hour after an individual eats a meal. The individual will have a more difficult time holding the solution in her bowel.

- Do not administer an enema to an individual who is sitting on the toilet. The enema solution will not enter high enough into the bowel, will cause the rectum to become enlarged, and will cause the solution to be quickly passed out of the body.

- If the individual will be using the bathroom (not a bedpan or commode) after receiving an enema, the UAP needs to make sure that the bathroom is available (not in use by another individual) and that the pathway to the bathroom is clear. If the individual needs to use an assistive device such as a cane or walker, the UAP needs to make sure that this is also available.

- If the UAP meets any resistance when inserting the tip of the tubing or prepackaged enema into the rectum or when administering the enema solution, the UAP must *immediately* stop administering the enema, remove the tubing or prepackaged enema, and *immediately* notify her supervisor and the individual's licensed health care provider.

- Do not administer an enema to an individual who has a bowel obstruction, inflammation of the bowel, infection of the abdomen, or dehydration or to an individual who has had recent rectal surgery or anal surgery. Contact the licensed health care provider before administering the enema to report the individual's condition and obtain additional orders.

Note: NEVER force the tip of the enema tubing, the tip of the prepackaged enema, or the enema solution into an individual's rectum. Forcing the enema may result in injury to the individual, including perforation and/or abrasion of the rectum!

Guidelines for Documentation of the Administration of an Enema

The final steps in the administration of an enema involve proper documentation of the procedure. By accurately communicating important information to staff members caring for the individual, medication errors are prevented. The individual is kept safe. The best care is provided.

For the administration of an enema, the UAP needs to document the following:

- The date and time the enema was given

- The type and amount of enema solution given

- The results of the enema, including the amount and description of the feces (BM, stool) the individual passed and the amount of the enema solution she passed

- Any complaints by the individual or unusual events that may have happened with the individual during administration of the enema

- If the licensed health care provider and/or the supervisor were notified and, if so, the reason for the notification and the instructions and orders received

If the enema was a medication, the UAP needs to document in the appropriate place on the medication sheet and medication progress note.

If the enema was not a medication, the UAP needs to document on the treatment sheet, progress note, and/or other document per regulation and workplace policy.

SUMMARY

As with the administration of all medications, the administration of enemas requires the UAP to follow basic steps. Following the steps outlined in this chapter will assist the UAP in administering enemas safely. In addition, the UAP must remember to do the following:

- Contact the individual's licensed health care provider if needed *before* administering the enema to clarify orders and to answer any questions

- *Never* force the tip of the enema tubing, the tip of the prepackaged enema, or the enema solution into an individual's rectum

- *Immediately* notify her supervisor and the licensed health provider if (1) any difficulty occurs during administration of the enema; (2) the individual receiving the enema has an adverse reaction, such as severe cramping, pain, or dizziness; or (3) the results of the enema are not those expected by the licensed health care provider.

WORKBOOK REVIEW

Go to the workbook and complete the exercises for Chapter 9.

REVIEW QUESTIONS

1. An enema is used to:
   a. administer a colonoscopy
   b. clean the bowel
   c. irrigate the bladder
   d. administer vaginal medications

2. An endoscopy is:
   a. a visual inspection of the inside of a body cavity using special instruments
   b. a visual inspection of the rectum using a proctoscope
   c. a visual inspection of the sigmoid colon using special instruments
   d. a surgical procedure done on the bowel and intestines

3. Types of rectal medications include:
   a. suppositories, creams, and enemas
   b. creams, lotions, and powders
   c. gels, lotions, and solutions
   d. suppositories, tablets, and powders

4. The three basic types of enemas are:
   a. clean, ready-to-mix, and return
   b. clear, premixed, and through-flow
   c. cleansing, prepackaged, and return-flow
   d. clear, unmixed, and full-flow

5. A cleansing enema:
   a. removes feces from the bowel and slows peristalsis
   b. softens any hard stool in the bowel
   c. removes flatus from the bowel and increases peristalsis
   d. irritates the bowel and causes bowel distention

6. An oil-retention enema:
   a. irritates the bowel and causes bowel distention
   b. softens any hard stool in the bowel
   c. removes flatus from the bowel and increases peristalsis
   d. removes feces from the bowel and slows peristalsis

7. A return-flow enema:
   a. softens any hard stool in the bowel
   b. removes feces from the bowel and slows peristalsis
   c. removes flatus from the bowel and increases peristalsis
   d. irritates the bowel and causes bowel distention

8. The most common position for administration of an enema is with the individual:
   a. sitting upright on a bedpan or on the toilet
   b. lying on her back with a bedpan underneath her buttocks
   c. lying on her back with both knees pulled up toward her chest
   d. lying on her left side with her left leg straight and right leg bent at the hip and knee pulled up toward the stomach

9. Before administering an enema, the UAP should have the individual:
   a. urinate if possible
   b. move his bowels if possible
   c. call her licensed HCP with any questions
   d. take a nap for around twenty (20) to thirty (30) minutes

CLINICAL SCENARIOS

1. Today you are giving care to Mrs. Adams. In report, you hear that she has had no BM for three (3) days and that her licensed HCP has ordered the administration of an enema. When you check the communication book, you see a note stating that the licensed HCP ordered an enema; however, there are no specific instructions. The licensed HCP order form and the medication sheet for Mrs. Adams do not show an order for an enema.
   a. To administer an enema, what information do you need to know?
   b. What is the best way to get this information?
   c. By the time you get the information you need, breakfast has already been served. Will you give Mrs. Adams her enema now? If not, why not? If not, when will you give the enema to Mrs. Adams?
   d. After giving the enema to Mrs. Adams, what information should you document?

2. Today you are giving care to Mr. Smith. His licensed HCP has ordered a Fleet® enema to relieve constipation. You are instructed to give him the enema before his shower.
   a. Before preparing the enema, what steps will you take?
   b. When you tell Mr. Smith that you will be giving him an enema, he says, "I can't lie on my left side, you know—I've got pretty bad arthritis in that shoulder. Can I sit on the toilet while you do it?" How would you respond to Mr. Smith's request?

Chapter 10
Care and Use of Gastrostomy and Jejunostomy Tubes

Learning Objectives

After reading this chapter and completing the review exercises, you should be able to:

1. Spell and define terms.
2. Describe three types of feeding tubes.
3. Explain the differences between a nasogastric tube, a gastrostomy tube, and a jejunostomy tube.
4. Describe the difference between a continuous tube feeding and an intermittent tube feeding.
5. List four advantages of a continuous feeding.
6. Demonstrate the administration of a continuous tube feeding.
7. Describe the difference between the bolus method and the gravity drip method.
8. List two advantages and two disadvantages of an intermittent tube feeding.
9. Demonstrate the administration of an intermittent feeding by bolus.
10. Demonstrate the administration of an intermittent feeding by the gravity drip method.
11. List three contraindications for a tube feeding.
12. Demonstrate the care of gastrostomy and jejunostomy tubes.
13. Demonstrate the procedure for flushing gastrostomy and jejunostomy tubes.
14. Demonstrate the procedure for checking for residual feeding.
15. List six basic guidelines for caring for gastrostomy and jejunostomy equipment.

16. List ten guidelines to follow when caring for an individual with a gastrostomy or jejunostomy tube.

17. Demonstrate the administration of medication via gastrostomy and jejunostomy tube when the individual is receiving a continuous tube feeding.

18. Demonstrate the administration of medication via gastrostomy and jejunostomy tube when the individual is receiving an intermittent tube feeding.

Key Terms

aspiration	gastrostomy tube	jejunum	pancreatitis
bolus	GI ischemia	nasogastric (NG) tube	paralytic ileus
diffuse peritonitis	incision	navel	sternum
enterocutaneous fistulae	jejunostomy tube		

nasogastric (NG) tube
A tube that is placed through the nose into the stomach.

gastrostomy tube
A tube that is placed directly into the stomach through a surgical incision (cut) in the skin.

jejunostomy tube
A tube that is placed directly into the individual's jejunum (small bowel) through a surgical incision (cut) in the skin.

aspiration
The entrance of stomach contents, liquids, or other substances into the respiratory tract; may cause pneumonia.

INTRODUCTION

If an individual cannot swallow, has trouble swallowing, or cannot take foods by mouth, a licensed health care provider may order a **nasogastric (NG) tube**, **gastrostomy tube**, or **jejunostomy tube**. These tubes, known as feeding tubes, allow the individual to receive feedings, liquids, and medications.

The tubes are available in different types and sizes (diameters and lengths). The licensed health care provider (HCP) will determine the tube to be used depending upon several factors, including:

1. The physical condition and nutritional needs of the individual

2. The reason for placement of the tube

3. The length of time the tube will remain in place (will be used)

4. The potential risk of **aspiration**

NASOGASTRIC (NG) TUBE

The nasogastric (NG) tube is inserted through the nose into the stomach by a licensed health care provider (Figure 10-1 shown on next page). Once inserted, an X-ray is taken to make sure the tube is positioned correctly.

NG tubes are usually used for short periods of time to administer feedings, liquids, and medications. Unlike gastrostomy and jejunostomy tubes, NG tubes may easily become dislodged. When this occurs, the tube often lodges itself in an individual's lungs, resulting in aspiration. Serious complications may result if a NG tube becomes dislodged.

Note: Because of the complications that may arise during the administration of tube feedings, liquids, and/or medications via nasogastric (NG) tubes, the UAP may not be permitted to

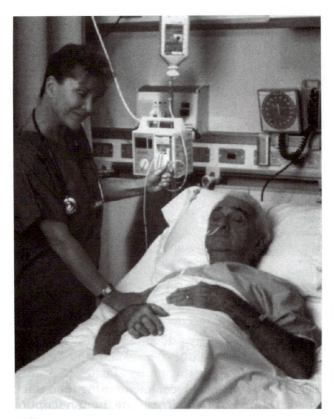

Figure 10-1 A nasogastric (NG) tube is inserted through the individual's nose into the stomach.
(Delmar/Cengage Learning)

administer these substances by the nasogastric tube. State regulations and workplace policies may differ on the role of the UAP regarding this task. It is the UAP's responsibility to know his state regulations and workplace policy regarding this issue.

GASTROSTOMY AND JEJUNOSTOMY TUBES

To maintain life, the body must receive basic nutrients on a daily basis. When an individual is unable to take in these nutrients on his own, a gastrostromy or jejunostomy tube provides a way for the individual to receive these basic nutrients, liquids, and medications over a long period of time. As with NG tubes, these tubes are inserted by a licensed health care provider. Once inserted, an X-ray is taken to make sure the tube is positioned correctly.

A gastrostomy tube (G-tube) is a twelve (12)- to fifteen (15)-inch-long, flexible tube. The tube has one opening leading into the stomach. The remainder of the tube stays outside the body. G-tubes are held in place with a balloon inside the stomach and a soft piece of rubber that fits against the skin on the outside of the body. The piece of rubber on the outside of the stomach may be called a "bumper" or a "skin disk" (Figure 10-2).

The gastrostomy tube is placed directly into the individual's stomach through a surgical **incision** (cut) in the skin by the licensed health

incision
A cut or wound in the body.

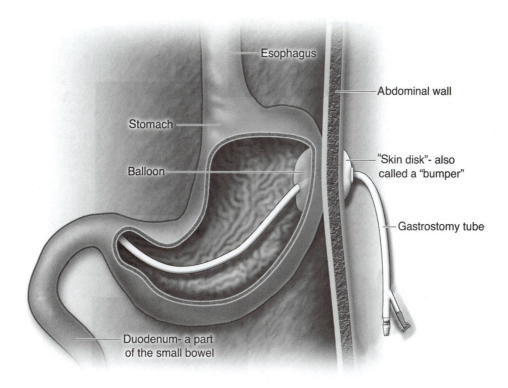

Figure 10-2 Gastrostomy tubes are held in place with a balloon inside the stomach and a soft piece of rubber that fits against the skin on the outside of the body. The rubber piece is known as a "skin disk" or "bumper." *(Delmar/Cengage Learning)*

sternum
Breastbone.

navel
Belly button.

care provider. The gastrostomy tube is located below the **sternum** (breastbone) and above the **navel** (belly button) (Figures 10-3A and 10-3B).

A percutaneous endoscopic gastrostomy tube (PEG tube) may be used in place of the longer G-tube. This tube sits flush with the skin (Figure 10-4). The licensed health care provider can insert a PEG tube at the bedside or in a treatment room without the use of general anesthesia. Because surgery is not required, the PEG tube is less risky for the individual and less costly for the insurance carrier. The PEG tube is, therefore, more commonly used.

The jejunostomy tube (J-tube) is very similar to a G-tube but is used when an individual cannot have a G-tube for some special reason. Instead of placing the tube into the stomach, the tube is placed into the jejunum, also called the small bowel (Figure 10-5).

The jejunostomy tube is placed directly into the individual's **jejunum**, a part of the small bowel (colon), through a surgical incision (cut) in the skin by the licensed health care provider. The jejunostomy tube is located below the navel (belly button) on the abdomen (Figure 10-6).

jejunum
A part of the small bowel (colon).

Once a gastrostomy tube or jejunostomy tube is placed by the licensed HCP, the tube is clamped, held in place by sutures, and covered with a dressing. As the area heals, a pathway or tract is formed. With a gastrostomy and PEG tube, the tract is between the stomach and the skin. With a jejunostomy tube, the tract is between the jejunum (small bowel) and the skin.

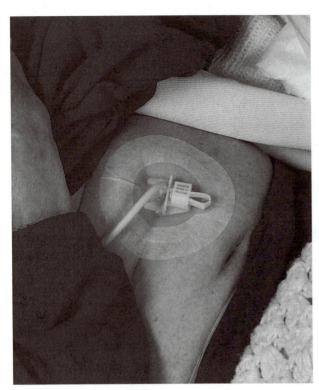

Figure 10-3a Gastrostomy tubes are surgically inserted through the abdominal skin into the stomach. This type of tube is used when an individual needs long-term feeding. *(Delmar/Cengage Learning)*

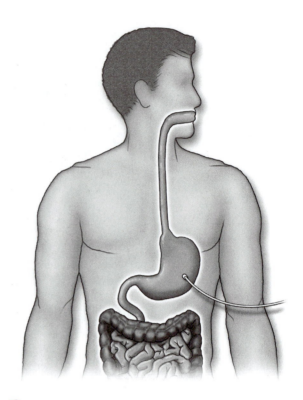

Figure 10-3b Placement of a gastrostomy tube into the stomach. *(Delmar/Cengage Learning)*

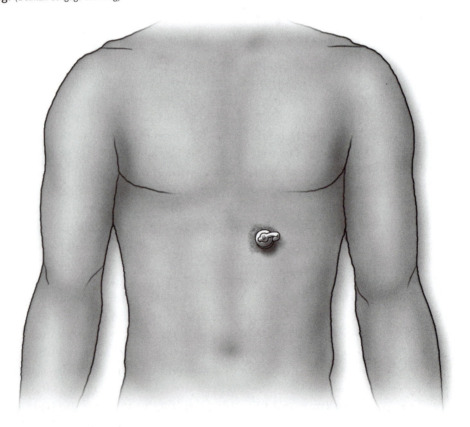

Figure 10-4 A percutaneous endoscopic gastrostomy tube (PEG Tube). *(Delmar/Cengage Learning)*

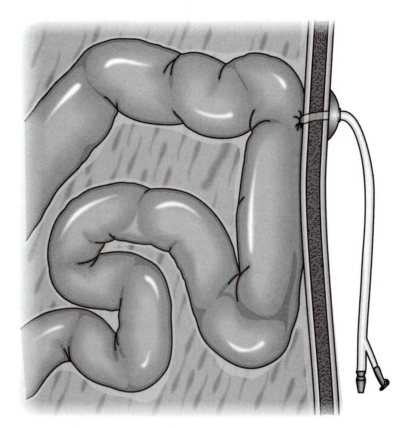

Figure 10-5 The jejunostomy tube is placed into the jejunum (small bowel). *(Delmar/Cengage Learning)*

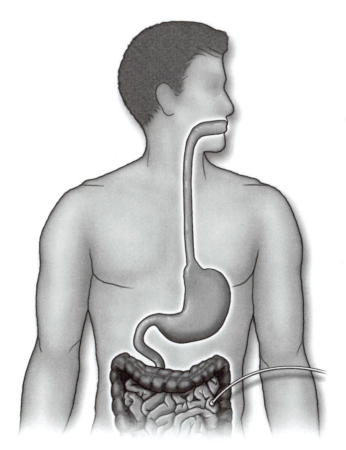

Figure 10-6 The jejunostomy tube is located on the abdomen below the navel. *(Delmar/Cengage Learning)*

Feedings by Gastrostomy and Jejunostomy Tubes

A specially prepared liquid solution, commonly called formula, contains the basic nutrients needed daily by an individual (Figure 10-7). Formula is administered according to the individual's licensed health care provider order. The licensed health care provider will order:

- The type of formula to be administered

- The total amount of formula to be administered in a twenty-four (24)-hour period

- The amount of formula to be given per hour or in a **bolus**

- If needed, any substances to be added to the formula

The feeding may be administered continuously or intermittently (stopping and starting at different times) by bolus. The feeding container is usually hung from a pole, such as an IV (intravenous) pole. The tubing that extends down from the feeding container may be attached to a mechanical pump that automatically controls the amount of formula the individual receives over a given period of time (Figure 10-8).

Continuous Tube Feeding

With a continuous tube feeding, a mechanical pump is used to administer a specific amount of formula per hour (Figure 10-9). The feeding may run constantly, or the feeding may run for a set number of hours each day, such as six (6) hours every day. The UAP sets the pump at a specific rate per hour as written in the licensed health care provider order. The pump provides a level of safety by preventing the formula from flowing into the individual too quickly.

The advantages of a continuous feeding with a mechanical pump are:

- There is only a small amount of formula in the stomach or small bowel at one time

- The residual volume is kept at a minimum

> **bolus**
> A large amount of liquid instilled into the stomach or small intestine.

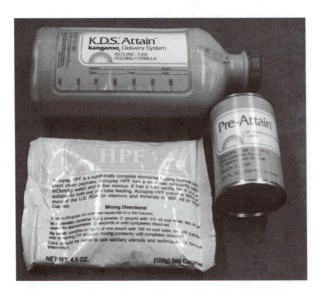

Figure 10-7 Feeding formulas. *(Delmar/Cengage Learning)*

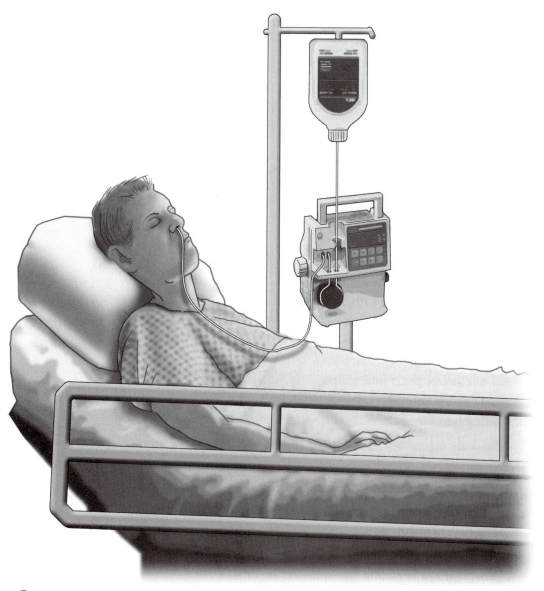

Figure 10-8 Tube feedings are usually administered through a mechanical pump. *(Delmar/Cengage Learning)*

- The risk of aspiration pneumonia is less
- Side effects (bloating, nausea, abdominal distention, and diarrhea) are less likely

Continuous feeding is recommended for individuals who are seriously ill or in a coma.

Equipment and Supplies. The following equipment and supplies will be needed to safely administer continuous tube feedings:

- Formula as ordered by the licensed HCP
- 60-mL syringe
- Warm water
- Nonsterile gloves

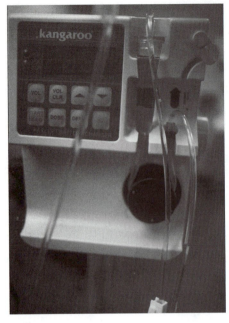

Figure 10-9 A feeding pump.
(Delmar/Cengage Learning)

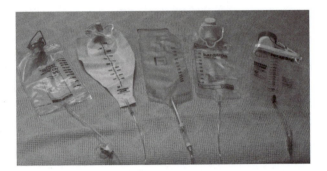

Figure 10-10 Formula bags. *(Delmar/Cengage Learning)*

- Emesis basin
- Paper towel(s)
- Formula bag (Figure 10-10)

Note: As discussed in Chapter 1, the UAP's scope of function is determined by federal and state regulations and workplace policies. It is the UAP's responsibility to know if administering basic nutrients, liquids, and/or medications by NG tube, G-tube and/or J- tube is permitted before doing so.

Procedure 10-1
Administration of a Continuous Tube Feeding

When administering a continuous tube feeding, follow these guidelines:

1. Identify the individual.
2. Verify the licensed health care provider order for the:
   - Type of formula
   - Amount of formula to be given, along with the rate per hour or total amount to be given in a twenty-four (24)-hour period
   - Time(s) of day the formula is to be administered; for example, 6:00 a.m. to 6:00 p.m. (12 hours) or 6:00 a.m. to 6:00 a.m. (24 hours)

3. Wash hands.

4. Gather equipment. (See the section "Equipment and Supplies.") Make sure the formula is given at room temperature. If using formula in a can, wash the top of the formula can with soap and warm water, rinse well, and dry.

5. Provide privacy.

6. Explain the procedure to the individual.

7. Assist the individual into a Fowler's position. See Chapter 8.

8. If possible, raise the working area to a safe and comfortable working height.

9. Check the G-tube or J-tube to make sure the tube is in the correct position. The tube should have a permanent mark on it indicating the correct length. If the tube does not have a mark or a bumper, measure the length of the tube. Compare this measurement to the original measurement to ensure that the tube is still in its correct position. If the tube is a PEG tube, this step is not necessary. *If the G-tube or J-tube is not in the correct position, DO NOT administer the feeding. Immediately notify the individual's licensed health care provider and the supervisor.*

10. Shake the can of formula well.

11. Clamp the tubing of the formula bag closed. Fill the formula bag with the amount of formula ordered by the licensed HCP (Figure 10-11).

12. Unclamp the tubing of the formula bag. Allow the formula to flow slowly through the tubing, removing all of the air from the tubing. Once all of the air is removed, clamp the tubing closed.

13. Put on nonsterile gloves.

14. At the beginning of each feeding, check the area around the tube for the following:
    • Redness
    • Drainage
    • Pain
    • Swelling

    If any of these signs or symptoms is noted, contact the individual's licensed health care provider.

15. If there is a licensed health care provider order to do so, rotate the tube.

16. Remove the plug from the G-tube or J-tube. Place the plug on a clean paper towel or in the emesis basin.

17. Pinch the G-tube or J-tube.

18. Remove the plunger from the 60-mL syringe. Insert the syringe without the plunger into the G-tube or J-tube.

19. Pour 50 mL of warm water into the syringe. Unpinch the G-tube or J-tube. Allow the warm water to flow slowly through the tube and into the stomach or small bowel by gravity.

20. Repinch the G-tube or J-tube before the syringe completely empties of the warm water. This prevents air from entering the stomach or small bowel. *NEVER allow the syringe to completely empty!*

21. Remove the syringe from the G-tube or J-tube. Insert the tip of the tubing from the formula bag into the G-tube or J-tube. Unpinch the tube.

22. Set up the pump. Thread the tubing from the formula bag through the pump, following the manufacturer's directions (Figure 10-12). Set the flow rate per the licensed health care provider order. Make sure the alarm is set as ordered.

23. Open the clamp on the tubing.

24. Turn on the pump. Press the start/run button. Check to be sure the feeding is flowing properly.

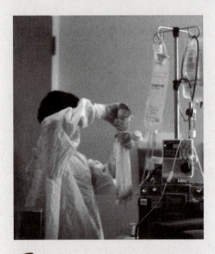

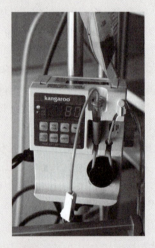

Figure 10-11 Fill the bag with the amount of formula ordered by the individual's licensed health care provider. *(Delmar/Cengage Learning)*

Figure 10-12 Following the manufacturer's directions, thread the tubing from the formula bag through the pump. *(Delmar/Cengage Learning)*

Note: The UAP should be trained in the use of the pump before he uses the pump. Just as there are different manufacturers and types of cars, there are also different manufacturers and types of pumps. It is the UAP's responsibility to use only that equipment on which he has been trained and with which he is knowledgeable. Depending on the setting in which the UAP is working, a licensed health care provider or a representative from the medical supply company that sells the pump may train the UAP in the use of the pump.

25. Once the correct amount of formula has been administered, turn off the pump. Close the clamp on the tubing. Pinch the

G-tube or J-tube. Remove the tubing of the formula bag. Cap the end of the tubing.

26. Insert the syringe without the plunger into the G-tube or J-tube.

27. Pour 50 mL of warm water into the syringe. Unpinch the G-tube or J-tube. Allow the warm water to flow through the tube into the stomach or small bowel. This time, allow the syringe to empty. This clears the G-tube or J-tube of formula and prevents the tube from blocking.

28. Once all of the warm water has entered the body, pinch the G-tube or J-tube. Remove the syringe from the tube. Reinsert the plug into the tube.

29. Keep the individual in the Fowler's position at all times when he is receiving a continuous tube feeding. Do not lower the head of the individual's bed! This will prevent the individual from aspirating the formula into his lungs.

30. Lower the working area.

31. Care for equipment and supplies. *Before storing leftover formula, be sure to write the date and time the formula was opened or mixed on the container's cover. All unused formula must be stored in a covered container in a refrigerator. All opened or mixed formula must be discarded within twenty-four (24) hours even if it has been refrigerated!*

32. Remove gloves.

33. Wash hands.

34. Document per workplace policy.

Intermittent Tube Feeding by Bolus

Intermittent feedings by bolus are given every four (4) to six (6) hours. The rate at which the feeding is administered is determined by the height of the syringe or container used. Usually, adults are given 250 to 400 mL of formula each time. A large syringe that fits into the end of the G-tube or J-tube is used. The feeding is then poured into the syringe and allowed to flow slowly into the individual. This feeding, given all at one time, is called a bolus.

A gravity drip method may be used instead of administering a feeding by bolus. A container holding the feeding is hung on a pole above the individual. The feeding then slowly drips into the individual over a twenty (20)- to thirty (30)-minute period of time.

The intermittent method is often used in a home care setting. The method requires a minimum amount of equipment. It is the easiest method to perform. However, it is not the preferred method. This method places a large amount of formula in the stomach at one time. This method often causes cramping, vomiting, aspiration, flatus (gas), and/or diarrhea. Individuals with a normal and healthy gastrointestinal system are people who do best with this type of feeding.

Equipment and Supplies. The following equipment and supplies will be needed to safely administer intermittent tube feedings:

- Formula as ordered by the licensed HCP
- 60-mL syringe
- Warm water
- Nonsterile gloves
- Emesis basin
- Paper towel(s)
- Formula bag (if administering by gravity drip method)

Procedure 10-2

When administering an intermittent feeding by bolus, follow these guidelines:

1. Identify the individual.
2. Verify the licensed health care provider order for the:
   - Type of formula
   - Amount of formula to be given
   - Time(s) of day the formula is to be administered
3. Wash hands.
4. Gather equipment. See the previous section "Equipment and Supplies." Make sure the formula is given at room temperature. If using formula in a can, wash the top of the formula can with soap and warm water, rinse well, and dry.
5. Provide privacy.
6. Explain the procedure to the individual.
7. Assist the individual into a Fowler's position. See Chapter 8.
8. If possible, raise the working area to a safe and comfortable working height.
9. Check the G-tube or J-tube to make sure the tube is in the correct position. The tube should have a permanent mark on it indicating the correct length. If the tube does not have a mark or a bumper, measure the length of the tube. Compare this measurement to the original measurement to ensure that the tube is still in its correct position. If the tube is a PEG tube, this step is not necessary. *If the G-tube or J-tube is NOT in the correct position, DO NOT administer the feeding. Immediately notify the individual's licensed health care provider and the supervisor.*
10. Shake the can of formula well.

11. If using a powdered formula, mix the formula as directed. Follow the licensed HCP order for directions. Be sure to mix well.

12. Put on nonsterile gloves.

13. At the beginning of each feeding, check the area around the tube for the following:

    - Redness
    - Drainage
    - Pain
    - Swelling

    If any of these signs or symptoms is noted, contact the individual's licensed health care provider.

14. If there is a licensed HCP order to do so, rotate the tube.

15. Remove the plug from the G-tube or J-tube. Place the plug on a clean paper towel or in the emesis basin.

16. Pinch the G-tube or J-tube.

17. Remove the plunger from the 60-mL syringe. Insert the syringe without the plunger into the G-tube or J-tube.

18. Pour 50 mL of warm water into the syringe. Unpinch the G-tube or J-tube. Allow the warm water to flow slowly through the tube and into the stomach or small bowel by gravity.

19. Repinch the G-tube or J-tube before the syringe completely empties of the warm water. This prevents air from entering the stomach or small bowel. *NEVER allow the syringe to completely empty!*

20. Fill the syringe with formula. Unpinch the G-tube or J-tube. Allow the formula to flow slowly through the tube and into the stomach or small bowel by gravity. *NEVER push the formula into the stomach or small bowel!*

21. Control the flow of formula into the body by raising or lowering the syringe. Raising the syringe will speed up the flow of the formula. Lowering the syringe will slow down the flow of the formula.

22. When the syringe is about one-quarter (1/4) empty, pour more formula into the syringe. Continue to allow the formula to flow through the tube into the individual. Continue to slowly add more formula until the amount of formula ordered by the individual's licensed HCP has been administered. *Once again, NEVER allow the syringe to completely empty!*

23. Once all of the formula has been administered, repinch the G-tube or J-tube.

24. Pour 50 mL of warm water into the syringe. Unpinch the G-tube or J-tube. Allow all of the water to flow into the stomach or small bowel. This time, allow the syringe to empty.

This clears the G-tube or J-tube of formula and prevents the tube from blocking.

25. Once all of the warm water has entered the body, pinch the G-tube or J-tube. Remove the syringe from the tube. Reinsert the plug into the tube.

26. Leave the individual in the Fowler's position for forty-five (45) to sixty (60) minutes. This will prevent the individual from aspirating the formula into his lungs.

27. Lower the working area.

28. Care for equipment and supplies.

29. Remove gloves.

30. Wash hands.

31. Document per workplace policy.

Procedure 10-3

Administration of an Intermittent Feeding by Gravity Drip Method

When administering an intermittent feeding by gravity drip, follow these guidelines:

1. Identify the individual.

2. Verify the licensed health care provider order for the:
   - Type of formula
   - Amount of formula to be given
   - Time(s) of day the formula is to be administered

3. Wash hands.

4. Gather equipment. See the section "Equipment and Supplies" before Procedure 2. Make sure the formula is given at room temperature. If using formula in a can, wash the top of the formula can with soap and warm water, rinse well, and dry.

5. Provide privacy.

6. Explain the procedure to the individual.

7. Assist the individual into a Fowler's position. See Chapter 8.

8. If possible, raise the working area to a safe and comfortable working height.

9. Check the G-tube or J-tube to make sure the tube is in the correct position. The tube should have a permanent mark on it indicating the correct length. If the tube does not have a mark or a bumper, measure the length of the tube. Compare this measurement to the original measurement to ensure that the tube is still in its correct position. If the tube is a PEG tube, this step is not necessary. *If the G-tube or J-tube is NOT*

in the correct position, DO NOT administer the feeding. Immediately notify the individual's licensed health care provider and the supervisor.

10. Shake the can of formula well.

11. Clamp the tubing of the formula bag closed. Fill the formula bag with the amount of formula ordered by the licensed HCP.

12. Unclamp the tubing of the formula bag. Allow the formula to flow slowly through the tubing, removing all of the air from the tubing. Once all of the air is removed, clamp the tubing closed.

13. Put on nonsterile gloves.

14. At the beginning of each feeding, check the area around the tube for the following:
    - Redness
    - Drainage
    - Pain
    - Swelling

    If any of these signs or symptoms is noted, contact the individual's licensed HCP.

15. If there is a licensed health care provider order to do so, rotate the tube.

16. Remove the plug from the G-tube or J-tube. Place the plug on a clean paper towel or in the emesis basin.

17. Pinch the G-tube or J-tube.

18. Remove the plunger from the 60-mL syringe. Insert the syringe without the plunger into the G-tube or J-tube.

19. Pour 50 mL of warm water into the syringe. Unpinch the G-tube or J-tube. Allow the warm water to flow slowly through the tube and into the stomach or small bowel by gravity.

20. Repinch the G-tube or J-tube before the syringe completely empties of the warm water. This prevents air from entering the stomach or small bowel. *NEVER allow the syringe to completely empty!*

21. Remove the syringe from the G-tube or J-tube. Insert the tip of the tubing from the formula bag into the G-tube or J-tube. Unpinch the tube.

22. Regulate the flow of formula into the stomach or small bowel by adjusting the tightness of the clamp on the tubing of the formula bag. Set the flow rate so that the formula enters the body in fifteen (15) to thirty (30) minutes.

23. Hang the bag approximately eighteen (18) inches above the abdomen. Place it on an intravenous (IV) pole or on a wall hook near the individual.

24. Once all of the formula has been administered, repinch the G-tube or J-tube. Remove the tubing of the formula bag from the G-tube or J-tube.

25. Reinsert the syringe without the plunger into the G-tube or J-tube.

26. Pour 50 mL of warm water into the syringe. Unpinch the G-tube or J-tube. Allow all of the water to flow into the stomach or small bowel. This time, allow the syringe to empty. This clears the G-tube or J-tube of formula and prevents the tube from blocking.

27. Once all of the warm water has entered the body, pinch the G-tube or J-tube. Remove the syringe from the tube. Reinsert the plug into the tube.

28. Leave the individual in the Fowler's position for forty-five (45) to sixty (60) minutes. This will prevent the individual from aspirating the formula into his lungs.

29. Lower the working area.

30. Care for equipment and supplies. *Before storing leftover formula, be sure to write the date and time the formula was opened or mixed on the container's cover. All unused formula must be stored in a covered container in a refrigerator. All opened or mixed formula must be discarded within twenty-four (24) hours even if it has been refrigerated!*

31. Remove gloves.

32. Wash hands.

33. Document per workplace policy.

Contraindications for Tube Feedings

Not all individuals are able to receive tube feedings. Tube feedings are contraindicated (not recommended) in individuals with the following conditions:

- **Diffuse peritonitis**
- Intestinal obstruction that prevents normal bowel function
- Uncontrollable vomiting
- **Paralytic ileus**
- Severe diarrhea

In addition, tube feedings are to be used with caution in individuals with the following conditions:

- Severe **pancreatitis**
- **Enterocutaneous fistulae**
- **GI ischemia**

diffuse peritonitis
Widespread inflammation of the lining of the abdominal cavity.

paralytic ileus
Slowing or absence of intestinal peristalsis (involuntary contractions that move food through the intestine).

pancreatitis
Inflammation of the pancreas.

enterocutaneous fistulae
Abnormal passages or pathways from the intestines to the skin.

GI ischemia
Decreased blood supply to the gastrointestinal system.

Guidelines for Documentation of Tube Feedings

When documenting information on tube feedings, the UAP needs to document the following information:

- Time and date feeding was administered
- Type of formula and amount of formula administered
- That the tube placement was checked, what method was used, and the findings
- Condition of the area around the tube
- Total amount of formula and water; document this total on the intake and output sheet
- The individual's response to the feeding
- Any complaints from the individual or adverse effects, including bloating, nausea, vomiting, diarrhea, or constipation
- Whether the individual's licensed health care provider and/or the supervisor was contacted; if so, why they were contacted and the result(s) of the contact

Additional Procedures

Care of Gastrostomy and Jejunostomy Tubes

Gastrostomy and jejunostomy tubes require daily care. The area around the tube is washed with warm water and soap, then rinsed well and patted dry. At times the licensed HCP may order medication or a treatment for this area. The UAP needs to be certain that he follows the licensed HCP orders.

Some individuals may wear a dressing (bandage) over the area. Many individuals with a gastrostomy or jejunostomy tube, however, do not wear a dressing. If a dressing is to be used, the UAP needs to make sure that the dressing is changed daily or whenever the dressing is wet and/or soiled. If the licensed HCP has not written orders for the care of the dressing, the UAP needs to contact the licensed HCP to get written orders to do dressing care.

Equipment and Supplies. The following equipment and supplies will be needed to care for gastrostomy and jejunostomy tubes:

- A clean washcloth and towel
- Mild soap and warm water
- Cotton swabs
- Gloves (nonsterile if incision is healed; if incision is not healed, sterile gloves are needed)
- If a dressing is needed, sterile gauze pads: two sterile 4″ × 4″ gauze pads cut halfway down the center and two sterile 4″ × 4″ sterile gauze pads uncut
- Hypoallergenic one (1)-inch tape

Procedure 10-4
Care of Gastrostomy and Jejunostomy Tubes

When caring for a gastrostomy tube or jejunostomy tube, follow these guidelines:

1. Identify the individual.

2. Verify the licensed health care provider order.

3. Wash hands.

4. Gather equipment. See the previous section "Equipment and Supplies."

5. Provide privacy.

6. Explain the procedure to the individual.

7. Assist the individual into a comfortable position.

8. If possible, raise the working area to a safe and comfortable working height.

9. Check the G-tube or J-tube to make sure the tube is in the correct position. The tube should have a permanent mark on it indicating the correct length. If the tube does not have a mark or a bumper, measure the length of the tube. Compare this measurement to the original measurement to ensure that the tube is still in its correct position. If the tube is a PEG tube, this step is not necessary. *If the G-tube or J-tube is NOT in the correct position, DO NOT give care. Immediately notify the individual's licensed health care provider and the supervisor.*

10. Put on nonsterile gloves.

11. If an old dressing is present, remove the old dressing. Check for drainage.

Note: Some drainage is normal. The UAP needs to check with the individual's licensed health care provider(s) for guidelines regarding the amount and type(s) of drainage that are acceptable.

12. Check for any of the following:
    - Unusual redness
    - Tenderness
    - Warmth
    - Yellow-green drainage
    - Foul-smelling or thick drainage
    - A displaced tube (tube is not in its correct position)
    - Bleeding around the tube
    - Blood in the individual's stool or bowel movement

Note: If the UAP observes any of these, the UAP is to notify the supervisor and the individual's licensed health care provider.

13. If there is a licensed HCP order to do so, rotate the tube.

14. If the incision is not healed, remove nonsterile gloves and put on sterile gloves. Follow sterile technique to clean the area and apply a new dressing. Otherwise, follow the steps as listed.

15. Using the washcloth, carefully wash the area around the G-tube or J-tube with warm water and soap. Rinse the area well. Be sure to clean under the soft piece of rubber (disk) that is against the skin.

16. Using the cotton-tipped swab, thoroughly clean any crust or drainage. Make sure to be gentle.

17. If the G-tube or J-tube has a disk, turn the disk one-quarter (1/4) of the way around every day.

18. Be sure to clean under the disk every day.

19. If the disk moves away from the skin and up the tube, notify the individual's licensed HCP.

20. If the individual needs to have the dressing replaced, place the two sterile 4″ × 4″ cut gauze pads around the tube. The slits are to overlap each other. When applying the dressing, be sure the dressing is on top of the disk and never underneath the disk (Figure 10-13A).

21. Cover the slit pads with the two uncut sterile 4″ × 4″ gauze pads. Hold the pads in place with the one (1)-inch tape (Figure 10-13B).

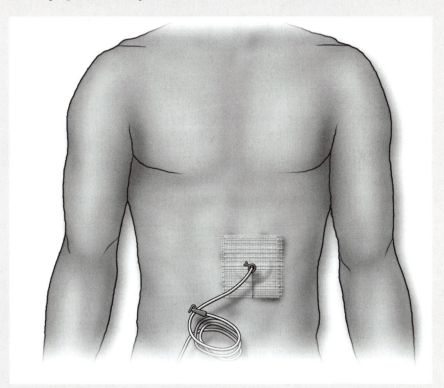

Figure 10-13a Place two sterile 4″ × 4″ cut gauze pads around the tube. The slits are to overlap each other. Be sure the dressing is on top of the disk and never underneath the disk. *(Delmar/Cengage Learning)*

22. If the G-tube or J-tube is twelve (12) inches or longer, secure it by gently looping the tube and taping it to the abdomen (Figure 10-13B).

23. Lower the working area.

24. Care for equipment and supplies.

25. Remove gloves.

26. Wash hands.

27. Document per workplace policy.

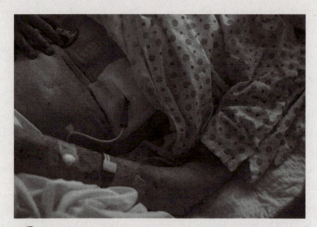

Figure 10-13b Cover the slit pads with two (2) uncut sterile 4″ × 4″ gauze pads. Tape the pads in place. Secure the tube by gently looping the tube and taping it to the abdomen. *(Delmar/Cengage Learning)*

Guidelines for Documentation of Care of Gastrostomy and Jejunostomy Tubes. When documenting information on the care of G-tubes and J-tubes, the UAP needs to document the following information:

- That the tube placement was checked, what method was used, and the findings

- Condition of the area around the tube—if drainage is present, be sure to describe the amount, color, odor, and thickness of the drainage

- Care provided (cleansing and dressing change)

- Whether the tube was rotated

- Any complaints from the individual or adverse effects, including bloating, nausea, vomiting, diarrhea, or constipation

- Whether the individual's licensed health care provider and/or the supervisor was contacted; if so, why they were contacted and the result(s) of the contact

Flushing Gastrostomy and Jejunostomy Tubes

To prevent blocking of a gastrostomy or a jejunostomy tube, the tubes are flushed on a regular basis. Usually 50 mL of warm water is used to flush the tubes. There may be times, however, when a licensed health care provider orders a tube flushed with other types of liquids, such as a carbonated beverage or cranberry juice.

Gastrostomy and jejunostomy tubes are usually flushed at the following times:

- After checking the residual feeding
- Before and after administration of a tube feeding
- Before and after administration of medication
- At regularly set intervals for a tube that is not actively being used
- According to the licensed health care provider order (there are times when the licensed HCP may want the tube flushed in addition to the times listed here)

Note: Because PEG tubes are small in diameter, PEG tubes require frequent flushing to prevent blockage.

Equipment and Supplies. The following equipment and supplies will be needed to flush gastrostomy and jejunostomy tubes:

- 60-mL syringe
- Warm water
- Nonsterile gloves
- A paper towel
- Emesis basin

Procedure 10-5
Flushing Gastrostomy and Jejunostomy Tubes

When flushing a gastrostomy tube or jejunostomy tube, follow these steps:

1. Identify the individual.
2. Verify the licensed health care provider order.
3. Wash hands.
4. Gather equipment. See the previous section "Equipment and Supplies."
5. Provide privacy.
6. Explain the procedure to the individual.
7. If possible, raise the working area to a safe and comfortable working height.
8. Place the individual in a Fowler's position. See Chapter 8.

9. Check the G-tube or J-tube to make sure the tube is in the correct position. The tube should have a permanent mark on it indicating the correct length. If the tube does not have a mark or a bumper, measure the length of the tube. Compare this measurement to the original measurement to ensure that the tube is still in its correct position. If the tube is a PEG tube, this step is not necessary. *If the G-tube or J-tube is NOT in the correct position, DO NOT flush the tube. Immediately notify the individual's licensed health care provider and the supervisor.*

10. Put on nonsterile gloves.

11. At the beginning of each tube flushing, check the area around the tube for the following:

    • Redness

    • Drainage

    • Pain

    • Swelling

    If any of these signs or symptoms is noted, contact the individual's licensed HCP.

12. If there is a licensed health care provider order to do so, rotate the tube.

13. Using fingers, pinch off the G-tube or J-tube.

14. Remove the plug from the G-tube or J-tube. Place the plug on a clean paper towel or in the emesis basin.

15. Remove the plunger from the 60-mL syringe. Insert the 60-mL syringe without the plunger into the opening of the G-tube or J-tube.

16. Fill the syringe with warm water.

17. Unpinch the G-tube or J-tube.

18. Allow the warm water to flow slowly through the G-tube or J-tube into the stomach or small bowel. *Do not force the water through the G-tube or J-tube into the body!*

19. When the G-tube or J-tube is almost empty, pinch the tube again. Remove the syringe from the opening of the tube. Replace the plug.

20. Have the individual remain in the Fowler's position for at least forty-five (45) to sixty (60) minutes.

21. Lower the working area.

22. Care for the equipment and supplies.

23. Remove gloves.

24. Wash hands.

25. Document per workplace policy.

Note: If the warm water does not flow through the G-tube or J-tube into the stomach or small bowel, contact the individual's licensed health care provider and the supervisor immediately.

Guidelines for Documentation of Flushing Gastrostomy and Jejunostomy Tubes

When documenting information on the flushing of G-tubes and J-tubes, the UAP needs to document the following information:

- Time and date flushing was completed

- Amount of water used to flush the tube

- That the tube placement was checked, what method was used, and the findings

- Condition of the area around the tube

- Whether the tube was rotated

- Total amount of water used; document this on the intake and output sheet

- The individual's response to the flushing

- Any complaints from the individual or adverse effects, including bloating, nausea, vomiting, diarrhea, or constipation

- Whether the individual's licensed health care provider and/or the supervisor was contacted; if so, why they were contacted and the result(s) of the contact

Checking for Residual Feeding

From time to time the UAP will need to check to make sure the formula that is being administered through the feeding tube is passing through the stomach or small bowel as it should. When the formula is not digested but remains in the stomach or small bowel, a residual occurs. This is especially true with continuous feedings.

The licensed HCP will, therefore, order the UAP to check for residual feeding on a regular basis. The licensed HCP may also order the UAP to check the residual at other times, such as when the individual starts to vomit or cough uncontrollably, or if the formula is leaking anywhere.

Equipment and Supplies. The following equipment and supplies will be needed to check for residual feeding:

- 60-mL syringe

- Clean bowl or emesis basin

- Warm water

- Nonsterile gloves

- Paper towel

Procedure 10-6
Checking for Residual Feeding

When checking for residual feeding, follow these steps:

1. Identify the individual.
2. Verify the licensed health care provider order.

3. Wash hands.

4. Gather equipment. See the previous section "Equipment and Supplies."

5. Provide privacy.

6. Explain the procedure to the individual.

7. If possible, raise the working area to a safe and comfortable working height.

8. Place the individual in a Fowler's position. See Chapter 8.

9. Check the G-tube or J-tube to make sure the tube is in the correct position. The tube should have a permanent mark on it indicating the correct length. If the tube does not have a mark or a bumper, measure the length of the tube. Compare this measurement to the original measurement to ensure that the tube is still in its correct position. If the tube is a PEG tube, this step is not necessary. *If the G-tube or J-tube is NOT in the correct position, DO NOT continue with the residual check. Immediately notify the individual's licensed health care provider and the supervisor.*

10. Put on nonsterile gloves.

11. At the beginning of each residual check, check the area around the tube for the following:

    • Redness

    • Drainage

    • Pain

    • Swelling

    If any of these signs or symptoms is noted, contact the individual's licensed health care provider.

12. If there is a licensed health care provider order to do so, rotate the tube.

13. Stop the feeding.

14. Remove the tubing of the formula bag from the G-tube or J-tube opening. Cap the tubing. Place the tubing on the paper towel or hang it over the pump.

15. Put the 60-mL syringe with the plunger into the opening of the G-tube or J-tube.

16. Gently pull back the plunger of the syringe.

17. The contents of the stomach or small bowel will enter the syringe.

18. *If the amount that enters the syringe is less than one syringe full, immediately push the fluid back into the stomach or small bowel.*

19. Remove the plunger from the syringe. Fill the syringe with 50 mL (cc) of warm water. Allow the warm water to flow through the G-tube or J-tube into the stomach or small bowel.

20. Remove the syringe from the G-tube or J-tube. Insert the tubing from the formula bag into the G-tube or J-tube. Start the pump.

21. If you are able to fill the syringe, pinch off the G-tube or J-tube. Remove the syringe from the tube. Empty the contents from the syringe into the bowl or emesis basin.

22. Reconnect the syringe to the G-tube or J-tube. Repeat the filling of the syringe until you are unable to remove any more fluid from the stomach or small bowel. The stomach or small bowel is now empty.

23. Add up the amount of the fluid in the bowl or emesis basin. This is the residual.

24. *If the total removed is more than 100 mL, return all of the contents back into the stomach or small bowel. Flush the G-tube with 50 mL of warm water.*

25. Remove the syringe from the G-tube or J-tube. Insert a plug or cap. *Do NOT restart the feeding! Wait thirty (30) to sixty (60) minutes.*

26. Check the residual again after thirty (30) to sixty (60) minutes. Follow the same instructions.

27. *If there is less than 100 mL of fluid, return the contents back into the stomach or small bowel. Flush the tube with 50 mL of warm water as in step 19.*

28. Remove the syringe. Insert the tubing from the formula bag into the G-tube or J-tube. Start the pump.

29. *If the residual is still more than 100 mL, return the contents to the stomach or small bowel. Flush the G-tube with 50 mL of warm water.*

30. Remove the syringe. Insert the plug or cap.

31. *Do not restart the feeding!* Notify the individual's licensed HCP and the supervisor.

32. Have the individual remain in the Fowler's position.

33. Lower the working area.

34. Care for the equipment and supplies.

35. Remove gloves.

36. Wash hands.

37. Document the amount of the residual and the action taken in the individual's record per workplace policy.

Guidelines for Documentation When Checking for Residual Feeding. When documenting information on checking residual feeding, the UAP needs to document the following information:

- Date and time residual was checked
- Amount of residual obtained

- That the tube placement was checked, what method was used, and the findings

- Condition of the area around the tube

- Whether the tube was rotated

- Total amount of water used for flushing; document this on the intake and output sheet

- The individual's response to the procedure

- Any complaints from the individual or adverse effects, including bloating, nausea, vomiting, diarrhea, or constipation

- Whether the individual's licensed health care provider and/or the supervisor was contacted; if so, why they were contacted and the result(s) of the contact

Cleaning of Gastrostomy and Jejunostomy Equipment

Gastrostomy and jejunostomy equipment needs to be as clean as possible. Each individual is to have his own equipment. Sharing equipment poses a risk of cross contamination and the spread of infection.

When cleaning equipment, follow these basic guidelines:

- Wash hands before handling equipment.

- Establish a regular schedule for cleaning and replacing the formula bags, tubing, and syringes.

- Always label the new equipment with the date and the individual's name.

- Change all equipment at least every thirty (30) days or if it becomes discolored or if the UAP is unable to clean the equipment thoroughly between feedings.

- Follow the workplace policy regarding the frequency for changing the formula bag. Some workplaces change the formula bags daily. Other workplaces reuse formula bags.

- If the formula bag needs to be used for more than one day, do the following:

  - Once a day, wash the formula bag with warm water (no soap) and rinse it thoroughly.

  - Clean the corners of the bag to remove old formula. This prevents bacterial growth.

  - Hang the bag to dry with the clamp open.

  - Wash the syringe with warm water (no soap). Dry the syringe.

- If the feedings are continuous (run over twenty-four [24] hours) and the formula bags are not discarded daily, use two formula bags and two tubing sets. Alternate the sets each day so that a clean one is used every day. After seven (7) days, discard the two sets. Open two new formula bags and two new tubing sets. Label each bag and tubing set with the date they were opened and the name of the individual.

- If the feeding comes in a prepackaged container, use the container for only twenty-four (24) hours. These containers are not safe for use after twenty-four (24) hours. Label the container with the date and time it was opened. *Be sure to discard the container after twenty-four (24) hours!*

Special Considerations

- At times it is difficult for the licensed health care provider to adjust the rate and strength of the feeding formula. The formula may cause constipation or diarrhea. Keep the licensed HCP informed of any changes in the individual's bowel patterns, such as constipation or diarrhea.

- Most individuals with a feeding tube are NPO (take nothing by mouth). Some, however, are permitted to have certain foods or liquids by mouth. Before giving an individual anything to eat or drink, check the licensed health care provider orders. *Written licensed HCP orders are needed for individuals with G-tubes and J-tubes to take foods, liquids, medications, or other substances by mouth.*

- *Always* know the location of the feeding tube. Avoid pulling on the tube. Serious complications may result if the tube is dislodged.

- G-tubes and J-tubes may crack and wear when used over long periods of time. The UAP should check for damage and wear to the tube each and every time he administers a feeding, performs a flushing, or checks for residual. If the UAP notes that the tube is worn or damaged, the UAP should immediately contact his supervisor and the individual's licensed health care provider.

- *ALWAYS check the date on the formula before administering a feeding.* Formulas do spoil! Discard formula that is outdated, not labeled properly, or not stored correctly.

- A UAP should *never* attempt to replace a G-tube or J-tube if the tube falls out.

- A UAP should *never* attempt to readjust the position of a G-tube or J-tube when the tube is either too short or too long.

- The UAP is to *immediately* contact the individual's licensed health care provider if a change in the position of the G-tube or J-tube is noted.

Caring for an Individual with a Gastrostomy or Jejunostomy Tube

- *ALWAYS* keep the head of the bed elevated 45 to 60 degrees during the feeding and for thirty (30) to sixty (60) minutes after the feeding, to prevent aspiration.

- Monitor the individual closely for signs of respiratory distress:
  - Unusual skin color, such as pale, blue, gray, or dusky skin
  - Unusual color of the lips, mucous membranes, nail beds, lining or roof of the mouth
  - Cool, clammy skin
  - A respiratory rate of less than twelve (12) or more than twenty-four (24) breaths per minute
  - Noisy breathing, "gurgling"
  - Coughing
  - Choking
  - A change in breathing pattern, or irregular breathing
  - Difficulty breathing or labored breathing
  - Tachycardia (a pulse over 100 beats per minute)
  - Changes in mental status (confusion, sleepiness for no known reason, drowsiness, decreased responsiveness, restlessness)

Note: If the UAP observes signs and symptoms of respiratory distress, the UAP is to immediately notify the individual's licensed health care provider. If the licensed HCP does not respond in a timely fashion, the UAP is to contact the emergency medical services in his community by calling 911 or the local EMS number.

- Keep the skin around the feeding tube clean and dry *at all times!* If there is a dressing at the tube site, change the dressing as needed, following the licensed HCP orders provided.

Note: After the tube's incision site is healed, most tube sites do not need a dressing. This varies, however, from one individual to another.

- Once the tube's incision site is healed, clean the skin around the tube site daily with a clean washcloth, soap, and warm water. Report any signs of redness, irritation, drainage, or gastric leakage to the individual's licensed HCP and the supervisor.
- PEG tubes require daily rotation to relieve pressure on the skin. If the UAP is unable to rotate the PEG tube, the UAP is to notify the individual's licensed HCP. The PEG tube may have become internally imbedded in the wall of the stomach.
- Flush the PEG tube frequently as ordered. If the licensed HCP orders are not available, the UAP needs to contact the individual's licensed HCP for specific orders on the care of the PEG tube, including orders for flushing of the tube should it become blocked.

- If the individual has an NG tube:
  - Clip the NG tube to his clothing to prevent pulling.
  - Check the skin around the NG tube frequently, at least every two (2) hours. If the tape that holds the NG tube in place loosens or pulls the skin causing irritation, notify the supervisor and the individual's licensed health care provider.

- Monitor the individual's skin integrity, especially on the hips and buttocks, for redness and irritation. The elevation of the head of the bed increases the risk of damage to the skin. Report any signs of skin irritation or breakdown immediately to the individual's licensed HCP and the supervisor.

- Report nausea, vomiting, or dry heaves immediately to the individual's licensed health care provider and the supervisor.

- Check the G-tube or J-tube and the container's tubing for kinking. Be sure the individual is not lying or sitting on the tubing. This will stop the flow of the feeding.

- Provide frequent mouth care. For individuals with an NG tube, be sure to provide nasal care also.

- Notify the supervisor, the workplace's clinical consultant, and the individual's licensed health care provider if the mechanical pump's alarm sounds and cannot be reset per the instructions for the pump.

- Keep the perineal area clean and free from stool. Wash the individual after each bowel movement.

- *Always* have the assistance of at least one other person when moving the individual in bed and when transferring the individual. Caution has to be taken at all times to avoid dislodging the feeding tube!

- Make sure the individual's clothing is not too tight. Tight clothing may pull on the G-tube or J-tube. Tight clothing may also interfere with the individual's feedings or medications by causing blockage of the tube. In addition, tight clothing may cause pressure on the individual's skin, resulting in irritation, redness, and/or soreness.

- Record the total amount of formula and water administered on the individual's record. An intake and output form is commonly used.

Medication Administration by Gastrostomy and Jejunostomy Tubes

All medications administered through gastrostomy or jejunostomy tubes must be in the form of a liquid or crushed and dissolved in a liquid. All liquids administered through a G-tube or J-tube must be at room temperature.

Note: State regulations and/or workplace policy may require the UAP to obtain a written licensed health care provider order to crush or dissolve medication. If a licensed HCP order is not available, the UAP may need to contact the licensed health care provider to obtain a written order before administering the medication.

Special Considerations

- Whenever possible, it is best to use the liquid form of a medication.

- Not all medications may be crushed.

- Whenever possible, use a commercial pill crusher to crush medication. If a commercial pill crusher is not available, the UAP may place the medication in a plastic bag. Close the bag tightly. Roll a glass or a rolling pin over the bag to crush the medication.

- Once crushed, the medication should be mixed with approximately three (3) tablespoons of warm water, dissolved, and then administered.

- *Never* mix medication with formula.

- *Never* crush enteric-coated or time-release tablets or capsules.

- If the UAP is unable to administer a medication or flush a G-tube or J-tube, he is to contact the individual's licensed health care provider. *Under no circumstances is the UAP to force any liquid or medications through the G-tube or J-tube into the individual's stomach or small bowel!*

- When administering the medication Dilantin, *always* shut off the tube feeding for one (1) hour before and for one (1) hour after administration of the medication.

- When administering medications by G-tube or J-tube, the UAP must follow the Six Rights and the Three Checks.

- A UAP should *never* attempt to replace a G-tube or J-tube if the tube falls out.

- A UAP should *never* attempt to readjust the position of a G-tube or J-tube when the tube is either too short or too long.

- The UAP is to *immediately* contact the individual's licensed health care provider if a change in the position of the G-tube or J-tube is noted.

Equipment and Supplies

The following equipment and supplies will be needed to administer medications through a gastrostomy or jejunostomy tube:

- Medication(s)
- 60-mL syringe
- Warm water

- Nonsterile gloves
- Paper towel(s)
- Emesis basin

When administering medication through a gastrostomy or jejunostomy tube, the UAP must first determine the type of feeding the individual is receiving. Although the steps for administering medication remain the same, the procedure for administering medication through a G-tube or J-tube will differ depending upon the type of feeding the individual is receiving.

Note: According to the National Council of State Boards of Nursing, medication administration through nasogastric, gastrostomy, or jejunostomy routes shall not be delegated to certified medication assistants (MA-C) (National Council of State Boards of Nursing Delegate Assembly, August, 9, 2007).

Procedure 10-7

Administration of Medication through a Gastrostomy or Jejunostomy Tube with a Continuous Feeding

When administering medication with a continuous feeding, follow these steps:

1. Identify the individual.
2. Verify the licensed health care provider order.
3. Wash hands.
4. Gather equipment. See the previous section "Equipment and Supplies."
5. Prepare the medications per the licensed HCP orders.
6. Provide privacy.
7. Explain the procedure to the individual.
8. If possible, raise the working area to a safe and comfortable working height.
9. Keep the individual in Fowler's position. See Chapter 8.
10. Check the G-tube or J-tube to make sure the tube is in the correct position. The tube should have a permanent mark on it indicating the correct length. If the tube does not have a mark or a bumper, measure the length of the tube. Compare this measurement to the original measurement to ensure that the tube is still in its correct position. If the tube is a PEG tube, this step is not necessary. *If the G-tube or J-tube is NOT in the correct position, DO NOT administer the medication. Immediately notify the individual's licensed health care provider and the supervisor.*
11. Put on nonsterile gloves.

12. At the beginning of each medication administration, check the area around the tube for the following:
    - Redness
    - Drainage
    - Pain
    - Swelling

    If any of these signs or symptoms is noted, contact the individual's licensed health care provider.

13. Stop the feeding. Shut off the pump.

14. Pinch the G-tube or J-tube. Remove the tubing of the formula bag from the G-tube or J-tube. Cap the tubing. Place the tubing on the paper towel or hang it over the pump.

15. Insert the plug into the G-tube or J-tube. Unpinch the tube.

16. If administering Dilantin, wait one (1) hour before administering the medication. If administering other medications, continue with the steps of this procedure.

Note: There are other medications that require a waiting period between administration of the medication and administration of the feeding. The UAP needs to check with the individual's licensed HCP or pharmacist to determine if a waiting period is needed.

17. Pinch the G-tube or J-tube again.

18. Remove the plunger from the 60-mL syringe. Put the 60-mL syringe without the plunger into the opening of the G-tube or J-tube.

19. Unpinch the G-tube or J-tube. Pour 50 mL of warm water into the syringe. Allow the warm water to flow slowly through the tube into the stomach or small bowel. *Do not force the water through the G-tube or J-tube! If the water does not flow, call the individual's licensed health care provider and the supervisor.*

20. When the syringe is almost empty, pinch the G-tube or J-tube.

21. Pour in the first medication. Unpinch the G-tube or J-tube. Allow the medication to flow slowly into the stomach or small bowel.

22. When the medication has drained out of the syringe, pinch off the G-tube or J-tube.

23. If another medication is to be administered, pour 5 to 10 mL of warm water into the syringe. Unpinch the tube. Allow the warm water to flow through the tube. This cleans the tube.

24. Repeat this procedure until all the medications have been administered.

25. After administering the final medication, pinch the G-tube or J-tube again.

26. Pour 50 mL of warm water into the syringe. Allow the warm water to flow through the G-tube or J-tube until the syringe is completely empty.

27. Pinch the G-tube or J-tube. Remove the syringe.

28. Remove the cap from the tubing. Connect the tubing to the G-tube or J-tube. Unpinch the tube.

29. Restart the pump. *If administering Dilantin, wait one (1) hour before restarting the pump.*

30. Keep the individual in the Fowler's position at all times when he is receiving a continuous tube feeding. Do not lower the head of the individual's bed!

31. Lower the working area.

32. Care for the equipment and supplies.

33. Remove gloves.

34. Wash hands.

35. Document the administration on the medication sheet per workplace policy.

Procedure 10-8

Administration of Medication through a Gastrostomy or Jejunostomy Tube with an Intermittent Feeding

When administering medication with an intermittent feeding, follow these steps:

1. Identify the individual.

2. Verify the licensed health care provider order.

3. Wash hands.

4. Gather equipment. See the section "Equipment and Supplies" prior to Procedure 10-7.

5. Prepare the medications per the licensed HCP orders.

6. Provide privacy.

7. Explain the procedure to the individual.

8. If possible, raise the working area to a safe and comfortable working height.

9. Place the individual in Fowler's position. See Chapter 8.

10. Check the G-tube or J-tube to make sure the tube is in the correct position. The tube should have a permanent mark on it indicating the correct length. If the tube does not have a mark or a bumper, measure the length of the tube. Compare this measurement to the original measurement to ensure that the tube

is still in its correct position. If the tube is a PEG tube, this step is not necessary. *If the G-tube or J-tube is NOT in the correct position, DO NOT administer the medication. Immediately notify the individual's licensed health care provider and the supervisor.*

11. If the medications are ordered at the same time(s) as the feedings, give the medications at either the beginning or at the end of the feeding.

12. If administering Dilantin, either administer the Dilantin one (1) hour before administering the feeding or administer the Dilantin one (1) hour after administering the feeding.

Note: There are other medications that require a waiting period between administration of the medication and administration of the feeding. The UAP needs to check with the individual's licensed HCP or pharmacist to determine if a waiting period is needed.

13. Put on nonsterile gloves.

14. At the beginning of each medication administration, check the area around the tube for the following:

- Redness
- Drainage
- Pain
- Swelling

If any of these signs or symptoms is noted, contact the individual's licensed health care provider.

15. Pinch the G-tube or J-tube. Remove the plug from the G-tube or J-tube. Place the plug on the paper towel or in the emesis basin.

16. Remove the plunger from the 60-mL syringe. Put the 60-mL syringe without the plunger into the opening of the G-tube or J-tube.

17. Unpinch the tube. Pour 50 mL of warm water into the syringe. Allow the warm water to flow slowly through the tube into the stomach or small bowel. *Do not force the water through the tube! If the water does not flow, call the individual's licensed health care provider and the supervisor.*

18. When the syringe is almost empty, pinch the G-tube or J-tube.

19. Pour in the first medication. Unpinch the tube. Allow the medication to flow slowly into the stomach or small bowel.

20. When the medication has flowed through the syringe, pinch off the tube.

21. If another medication is to be administered, pour 5 to 10 mL of warm water into the syringe. Unpinch the G-tube or J-tube. Allow the warm water to flow through the syringe. This cleans the tube.

22. Repeat this procedure until all the medications have been administered.

23. After administering the final medication, pinch the G-tube or J-tube again.

24. Pour 50 mL of warm water into the syringe. Allow the warm water to flow through the tube until the syringe is completely empty.

25. Pinch the G-tube or J-tube. Remove the syringe. Reinsert the plug into the G-tube or J-tube.

26. *If administering Dilantin, wait one (1) hour before administering the feeding.*

27. Keep the individual in the Fowler's position for at least forty-five (45) to sixty (60) minutes. Do not lower the head of the individual's bed!

28. Lower the working area.

29. Care for the equipment and supplies.

30. Remove gloves.

31. Wash hands.

32. Document the administration on the medication sheet per workplace policy.

SUMMARY

Medication administration and feedings by gastrostomy and jejunostomy tubes may appear to be complex procedures; however, if the UAP follows the step-by-step instructions described in this chapter, these tasks may be performed safely and effectively. If any questions or concerns arise during the performance of these procedures, the UAP needs to call the individual's licensed health care provider for additional instructions and assistance. When in doubt, the UAP should *not* administer the medications or feeding until he has contacted the individual's licensed health care provider.

WORKBOOK REVIEW

Go to the workbook and complete the exercises for Chapter 10.

REVIEW QUESTIONS

1. A feeding tube is used to give an individual:
   a. feedings, liquids, and medications
   b. oxygen, liquids, and medications
   c. vitamins, minerals, and water
   d. medications, oxygen, and feedings

2. A gastrostomy tube is placed:
   a. into the stomach through the nose
   b. into the small bowel through a surgical incision
   c. into the stomach through a surgical incision
   d. into the small bowel through the navel

3. A jejunostomy tube is placed:
   a. into the stomach through a surgical incision
   b. into the small bowel through a surgical incision
   c. into the stomach through the nose
   d. into the small bowel through the navel

4. Aspiration is:
   a. the entrance of stomach contents into the mouth
   b. the entrance of stomach contents into the respiratory tract
   c. the entrance of stomach contents into the intestine
   d. the entrance of liquids into the stomach

5. The licensed HCP order for a feeding by G-tube or J-tube includes:
   a. the type and amount of formula to be given
   b. the formula for calculating the flow rate
   c. the procedure for giving a bolus feeding
   d. instructions for reinserting a G-tube or J-tube if needed

6. A continuous tube feeding is recommended for an individual who:
   a. is using an NG tube for short-term tube feeding
   b. is seriously ill or in a coma
   c. is given a G-tube in the hospital
   d. has a normal and healthy normal gastrointestinal system

7. Any time the UAP administers a tube feeding, gives care, flushes a feeding tube, or checks a residual amount, he must check the area around the tube for:
   a. the initials of the last UAP to check the tube
   b. shrinking of the skin around the tube
   c. pain, redness, drainage, and swelling
   d. risk of dislodging

8. If there is no permanent mark on an individual's G-tube or J-tube, to check that the tube is in the correct position, the UAP must:
   a. pull on the tube to see if it moves
   b. measure the length of the tube and compare it with the initial measurement
   c. ask the individual if his tube has moved at all
   d. call the individual's licensed HCP

9. Adverse effects of a tube feeding include:
   a. bloating, vomiting, and diarrhea
   b. fever, malaise, and constipation
   c. choking, dehydration, and nausea
   d. headache, fever, and weight gain

10. G-tubes and J-tubes require care:
    a. once per shift
    b. daily
    c. weekly
    d. twice weekly

11. When caring for an individual's G-tube or J-tube, the UAP rotates the tube:
    a. once per shift
    b. once per hour
    c. if there is a licensed HCP order to do so
    d. if his supervisor tells him to do so

12. The UAP must flush an individual's G-tube or J-tube:
    a. to prevent dehydration
    b. to prevent residual feeding
    c. to prevent constipation
    d. to prevent blocking

13. When checking a residual feeding, if the amount of fluid that enters the syringe is less than 100 mL (cc), the UAP must:
    a. immediately contact the individual's licensed HCP and the supervisor
    b. empty the syringe into a bowl and repeat filling the syringe from the feeding tube
    c. pour 100 mL (cc) of warm water into the feeding tube to flush it
    d. immediately push the fluid back into the stomach or small bowel and flush the tube

14. If a residual check results in more than 100 mL (cc) being drawn from the stomach or small bowel, the UAP must:
    a. wait thirty (30) to sixty (60) minutes, then check the residual again
    b. wait thirty (30) minutes, then restart the feeding
    c. wait sixty (60) minutes, then restart the feeding
    d. immediately contact the individual's licensed HCP and the supervisor

15. If an individual with a feeding tube asks for a glass of water, the UAP needs to:
    a. bring him a fresh glass of water
    b. check for a written licensed HCP order to give the individual fluids by mouth
    c. tell the individual he cannot have a glass of water because he has a feeding tube
    d. immediately contact the individual's licensed HCP and the supervisor

CLINICAL SCENARIOS

1. Your assignment today includes giving a continuous tube feeding to Mr. Berg, a man who is unfamiliar to you.
   a. When you verify the licensed HCP order, what specific information are you looking for?
   b. When you check the area around Mr. Berg's tube site, you notice some redness and swelling. What should you do?
   c. After the licensed HCP gives his approval for you to proceed with Mr. Berg's tube feeding, you successfully start Mr. Berg's feeding. How should he be positioned when you leave his room?
   d. Approximately thirty (30) minutes after you leave him, you go back to check on Mr. Berg. When you enter his room, you see that the head of his bed is flat. Is this appropriate? If not, why not? What should you do?

2. Your assignment today includes giving daily care to Mrs. Condon. This includes caring for her feeding tube. She had a feeding tube inserted seven days ago. The site is covered with a dressing.
   a. When you remove the old dressing, you smell an unusual odor and observe thick, yellow-green drainage. What should you do?
   b. As you are giving care, you notice that the permanent mark on Mrs. Condon's feeding tube is approximately one (1) inch away from her abdomen. What should you do?

Chapter 11
Administration of Epinephrine by EpiPen Auto-Injector

Learning Objectives

After reading this chapter and completing the review exercises, you should be able to:

1. Spell and define terms.
2. List five causes of anaphylaxis.
3. List five initial signs and symptoms of anaphylaxis.
4. List four life-threatening signs and symptoms of anaphylaxis.
5. Explain why anaphylaxis is life threatening.
6. List four items that must be included in the licensed health care provider order for the administration of epinephrine.
7. List three possible side effects of epinephrine.
8. List two classes of medications that may interact with epinephrine.
9. Describe five requirements for the proper storage and handling of epinephrine.
10. Describe the emergency procedure to be followed when epinephrine is administered.
11. Demonstrate the use of an EpiPen Auto-Injector.

Key Terms

allergen

anaphylaxis

bronchodilator

EpiPen Auto-Injector

hives

INTRODUCTION

Anaphylaxis (anaphylactic reaction) is a rapid, severe allergic reaction. Anaphylaxis occurs in response to exposure to an allergy-causing substance known as an **allergen**. When an allergen enters the bloodstream, the body releases chemicals to protect itself from the allergen. These chemicals may cause dangerous signs and symptoms of anaphylaxis.

An anaphylactic reaction involves the whole body. If left untreated, it will eventually result in death. Anaphylaxis can happen to anyone. Anaphylaxis may happen to individuals with no known allergies as well as to those with known allergies. According to Dey (2009), anaphylaxis "is a health threat to as many as 40.9 million Americans."

anaphylaxis
A rapid, severe allergic reaction; an anaphylactic reaction.

allergen
An allergy-causing substance.

ANAPHYLAXIS
Causes of Anaphylaxis

The most common cause of an anaphylactic reaction is medication. Penicillin alone is responsible for an estimated 75% of the known deaths from anaphylaxis each year in the United States (Dey, 2009). Those individuals most likely to have an anaphylactic reaction are those who receive penicillin by parenteral administration or for long-term therapy. A reaction to penicillin may occur after an individual has received multiple doses of penicillin rather than on administration of the first dose of penicillin.

Other medications that are commonly known to cause allergic reactions are:

- Sulfa antibiotics
- Allopurinol
- Seizure and antiarrhythmia medications
- Nonsteroidal anti-inflammatory drugs (NSAIDS, such as aspirin and ibuprofen)
- Muscle relaxants
- Certain postsurgery fluids
- Vaccines
- Radio-contrast media
- Antihypertensives
- Insulin
- Blood products

Additional causes of anaphylaxis include:

- Insect stings (particularly bee, wasp, hornet, yellow jacket, and fire ant stings)
- Foods (particularly peanuts and other nuts, milk, eggs, fish, shellfish, and some additives)
- Food dyes and preservatives

- Latex, such as that found in sterile and nonsterile gloves, elastic waistbands, kitchen cleaning gloves, balloons, and other house-hold items
- Exercise—in rare cases
- Unknown causes

Signs and Symptoms of Anaphylaxis

An anaphylactic reaction may happen very quickly (within a few seconds) once an individual is exposed to or eats that which she is allergic to, or the reaction may not occur for up to two (2) hours after the exposure to the allergen. The initial signs and symptoms of anaphylaxis may include:

- Flushing of the skin
- A rash followed by **hives** (red, raised bumps on the skin)
- Sneezing
- Swelling of the lips and tongue
- Hoarseness
- Headache
- Wheezing
- Nausea and/or vomiting
- Abdominal cramps
- A feeling of doom or fright

However, if treatment does not begin *immediately* with the onset of the initial symptoms, other, more dangerous signs and symptoms may rapidly follow, creating a life-threatening situation. These more dangerous, life-threatening signs and symptoms include:

- Weakness
- Dizziness
- Swelling of an individual's airway, causing difficulty breathing
- Collapse due to low blood pressure
- Shock
- Seizures
- Death

Because death may result in only a few minutes, the UAP must always know the allergies and types of reactions that individuals in her care may have. Providing emergency care in a timely fashion may save an individual's life.

Treatment of Anaphylaxis

bronchodilator
A medication that opens the airway, allowing an individual to breathe.

Epinephrine is the medication of choice when caring for an individual who is having an anaphylactic reaction. Epinephrine is classified as a **bronchodilator**. This medication opens the airway of an individual who is having an anaphylactic reaction so that she may breathe. In addition, epinephrine reverses swelling and increases the heartbeat.

Epinephrine is a prescription medication. The UAP follows the guidelines for administration and storage of medications when handling and administering epinephrine. Epinephrine is an injectable medication that is available in a prefilled syringe-needle unit known as an **EpiPen Auto-Injector**. An EpiPen Auto-Injector comes in two strengths: (1) 0.3 mg for individuals weighing over sixty-six (66) pounds and (2) 0.15 mg for individuals weighing thirty-three (33) to sixty-six (66) pounds (Figures 11-1 and 11-2).

EpiPen Auto-Injector
A syringe-needle unit prefilled with the medication epinephrine.

Note: There may be times when an individual's licensed health care provider orders more than one dose of epinephrine (more than one EpiPen) to be administered at one time because the individual needs a larger dose.

An EpiPen requires a licensed health care provider order for administration. The licensed HCP order should clearly state:

1. Permission for the individual to carry the EpiPen with her at all times.

2. Permission for the UAP to carry the EpiPen with her at all times if the individual is unable to do so.

3. Specific instructions for the administration of the EpiPen, including an order for multiple EpiPen Auto-Injectors.

4. Specific instructions for care after administration of the EpiPen. *Individuals must go to an emergency medical care center for evaluation and follow-up after receiving an injection of epinephrine. After transporting the individual to the emergency medical care center, the UAP needs to contact her supervisor and the individual's licensed health care provider, then complete the needed documentation.*

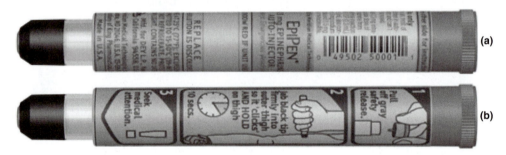

Figure 11-1 Epipen® Auto-Injector for individuals weighing over sixty-six (66) pounds. a) front; b) back. *(Courtesy of Dey, LP, Napa, California)*

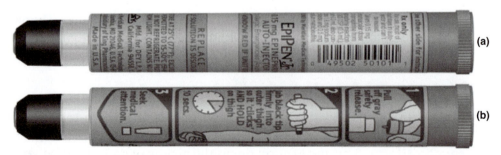

Figure 11-2 Epipen Junior® Auto-Injector for individuals weighing thirty-three (33) to sixty-six (66) pounds. a) front; b) back. *(Courtesy of Dey, LP, Napa, California)*

Anaphylaxis requires immediate treatment. The sooner an individual is treated, the better her chance for survival. The UAP, therefore, has to be able to administer an EpiPen within seconds of an individual having an anaphylactic reaction. For this reason, the licensed health care provider order must include permission for the individual and/or caregiver to carry the EpiPen with them at all times.

In addition, when ordering an EpiPen Auto-Injector for an individual, the licensed health care provider should order multiple EpiPen Auto-Injectors for the individual. One EpiPen should be kept with the individual or UAP at all times. Another EpiPen should be stored with the remainder of the individual's medication as a backup. If the EpiPen the individual or UAP is carrying breaks or the date for use expires, the UAP should have a backup EpiPen(s) on hand for an emergency. Other EpiPens should be placed in locations where the individual spends a great deal of time, such as at a day program, school, and/or the gym.

The EpiPen Auto-Injectors at the UAP's workplace need to be accounted for with each shift change or change in staff. It is the UAP's responsibility to follow her workplace policy for the storage, handling, and tracking of EpiPen Auto-Injectors.

Side Effects of Epinephrine

EpiPen Auto-Injectors must be used with extreme caution in individuals with heart disease or diabetes and with individuals who are taking certain medications. The UAP needs to consult with the individual's licensed health care provider to see if any special precautions need to be taken with administration of the EpiPen to a specific individual. Special precautions need to be written by the individual's licensed HCP in the licensed HCP orders and communicated in writing to other staff.

Common side effects of epinephrine are:

- Nervousness

- Headache

- Palpitations

- Angina

- Hyperglycemia (high blood glucose level)

Epinephrine may interact with many medications, including:

- Cardiac medications, such as digoxin and Inderal

- MAO inhibitors, such as Marplan and Parnate

- Tricyclic antidepressants, such as Asendin and Elavil

- Antihistamines, such as Benadryl

- Thyroid hormones, such as Synthroid

Note: Because of the possible interactions with various medications, the UAP must call the emergency medical response system (911) and the individual's licensed health care provider immediately after administering an EpiPen.

ADMINISTRATION OF AN EPIPEN AUTO-INJECTOR

The EpiPen Auto-Injector is an easy-to-use, prefilled, disposable syringe-needle unit. It is developed for self-administration. For use in an emergency situation, the EpiPen may be administered through an individual's clothing. For ease of use in an emergency situation, instructions for use of the EpiPen Auto-Injector and EpiPen Auto-Injector Junior accompany the EpiPens from the manufacturer. Figures 11-3a and 11-3b show a copy of the patient insert from the manufacturer.

PATIENT INSERT

PHARMACIST, PLEASE DISPENSE WITH PRODUCT

NDC 49502-500-01 (EpiPen®)
NDC 49502-500-02 (EpiPen 2-Pak®)
NDC 49502-501-01 (EpiPen® Jr)
NDC 49502-501-02 (EpiPen Jr 2-Pak®)

EPIPEN®
(Epinephrine) Auto-Injector 0.15/0.3mg

For allergic emergencies (anaphylaxis)

Amount of epinephrine delivered
EpiPen® = one dose of 0.30 mg epinephrine (USP, 1:1000, 0.3 mL)
EpiPen® Jr = one dose of 0.15 mg epinephrine (USP, 1:2000, 0.3 mL)

1323

MANUFACTURED FOR DEY®
NAPA, CA 94558, U.S.A.
by Meridian Medical Technologies, Inc.,
a subsidiary of King Pharmaceuticals, Inc.,
Columbia, MD 21046, U.S.A.
03-535-04 2/06
0001323

IMPORTANT INFORMATION

Please be prepared! Read both sides of this insert before an emergency occurs!
EpiPen® and EpiPen® Jr are disposable, prefilled automatic injection devices for use during allergic emergencies. They contain a single dose of epinephrine which you inject into your outer thigh. EpiPen® and EpiPen® Jr contain **no latex.**

It's important that you have this emergency medicine with you at all times. If you need additional units to keep at work, school, etc, please talk to your doctor.

WHEN TO USE

EpiPen® and EpiPen® Jr auto-injectors are used to treat severe allergic reactions (anaphylaxis). You should use this medication only if your doctor has prescribed it for allergic emergencies. Such emergencies may occur from insect stings or bites, foods, drugs, latex, other allergens, exercise-induced anaphylaxis, or unknown causes.

CARE AND STORAGE

- Keep the EpiPen® or EpiPen® Jr auto-injector nearby and ready for use at all times.
- Store at 25°C (77°F); excursions permitted to 15°C-30°C (59°F-86°F) (See USP Controlled Room Temperature). Contains no latex. Protect from light.
- **Do NOT** store in refrigerator.
- **Do NOT** expose to extreme cold or heat. For example, do NOT store in your vehicle's glove box.

Your auto-injector has an expiration date

- Example: "DEC 05" = December 31, 2005.
- Replace it before the expiration date.

To dispose of expired units

Expired auto-injectors must be disposed of properly.
To dispose of an expired auto-injector and carrier, take it to your doctor's office or to a hospital for proper disposal.

Examine contents in clear window of auto-injector periodically

- If the solution is discolored or contains solid particles (precipitate), replace the unit. Solution should be clear.

EPIPEN® CENTER FOR ANAPHYLACTIC SUPPORT™

Take advantage of the EpiPen® Center for Anaphylactic Support™—your FREE information resource for severe allergic reactions.
You'll receive expiration reminders, information about managing your severe allergic reactions, resource listings and valuable offers. To enroll please complete and mail the form below.

Mail to:
EpiPen® Center for Anaphylactic Support™
DEY®
P.O. BOX 2000
Napa, CA 94558-9956

EpiPen® Center for Anaphylactic Support™ Enrollment Form
Please fill in the information below.
To ensure accuracy, please PRINT neatly in uppercase letters in black or dark-blue ink.

Your Name

Child's Name (if child is allergy sufferer)

Address

City State ZIP

E-mail Address

Opt-In: I would prefer to receive communications via e-mail: ❑ Yes ❑ No

EpiPen®/EpiPen® Jr Lot # (on unit, example 2ST059) □□□□□□

Exp. Date (on unit, example DEC05) □□□□□

Is this your first EpiPen® prescription or a refill? ❑ First Prescription ❑ Refill

For what type of allergy was this EpiPen® prescribed?
Check all that apply.

❑ Food ❑ Insect bite or sting
❑ Latex ❑ Medication
❑ Other________

EPIPEN® CENTER FOR ANAPHYLACTIC SUPPORT™

Figure 11-3a Patient insert for Epipen® and Epipen, Jr.® gives general information on the use, storage, and administration of the Epipen® and Epipen Junior® Auto-Injectors. *(Courtesy of Dey, LP, Napa, California)*

DIRECTIONS FOR USE

- NEVER PUT THUMB, FINGERS, OR HAND OVER BLACK TIP.
- DO NOT REMOVE GRAY SAFETY RELEASE UNTIL READY TO USE.
- DO NOT USE IF SOLUTION IS DISCOLORED OR RED FLAG APPEARS IN CLEAR WINDOW.
- DO NOT PLACE PATIENT INSERT OR ANY OTHER FOREIGN OBJECTS IN CARRIER WITH AUTO-INJECTOR, AS THIS MAY PREVENT YOU FROM REMOVING THE AUTO-INJECTOR FOR USE.

Clear Window

Black Tip
(needle comes out during use)   Expiration Date and Lot Number   Gray Safety Release
(do **NOT** remove until ready to use)

1. Unscrew the yellow or green cap off of the EpiPen® or EpiPen® Jr carrying case and remove the EpiPen® or EpiPen® Jr auto-injector from its storage tube.

2. Grasp unit with the black tip pointing downward.

3. Form fist around the unit (black tip down).

4. With your other hand, pull off the gray safety release.

5. Hold black tip near outer thigh.

6. Swing and **jab firmly** into outer thigh until it clicks so that unit is perpendicular (at a 90° angle) to the thigh. (Auto-injector is designed to work through clothing.)

7. Hold **firmly against thigh** for approximately 10 seconds. (The injection is now complete. Window on auto-injector will show red.)

8. Remove unit from thigh and massage injection area for 10 seconds.

9. Call 911 and seek immediate medical attention.

10. Carefully place the used auto-injector (without bending the needle), needle-end first, into the storage tube of the carrying case that provides built-in needle protection after use. Then screw the cap of the storage tube back on completely, and take it with you to the hospital emergency room.

Note: Most of the liquid (about 90%) stays in the auto-injector and cannot be reused. However, you have received the correct dose of the medication if the red flag appears in window.

⚠ WARNING

- **NEVER** put thumb, fingers, or hand over black tip. The needle comes out of black tip. Accidental injection into hands or feet may result in loss of blood flow to these areas. If this happens, go immediately to the nearest emergency room.
- EpiPen® and EpiPen® Jr should be injected only into the outer thigh (see "Directions for Use").
- Do NOT remove gray safety release until ready to use.

IMMEDIATELY AFTER USE

- **Go immediately to the nearest hospital emergency room or call 911.** You may need further medical attention. Take your used auto-injector with you.
- Tell the doctor that you have received an injection of epinephrine in your thigh.
- Give your used EpiPen®/EpiPen® Jr to the doctor for inspection and proper disposal.

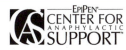

EpiPen®
CENTER FOR ANAPHYLACTIC SUPPORT™

Join the Free EpiPen® Center for Anaphylactic Support™ Today!

Because it's important that you always have an up-to-date EpiPen® or EpiPen® Jr with you at all times, we started an expiration reminder program as part of the *EpiPen® Center for Anaphylactic Support*™. Every time you purchase a new EpiPen®, be sure to register it with us, and we'll send you reminders so you can have an up-to-date EpiPen®. *This important program is a FREE service!*

See other side for more details.

Figure 11-36 Patient insert for Epipen® and Epipen, Jr.® gives general information on the use, storage, and administration of the Epipen® and Epipen Junior® Auto-Injectors. *(Courtesy of Dey, LP, Napa, California)*

Note: As discussed in Chapter 1, the UAP's scope of function is determined by federal and state regulations and workplace policies. It is the UAP's responsibility to know if administering an Epi-Pen Auto-Injector is permitted before doing so.

Procedure 11-1
Administration of an EpiPen Auto-Injector

When administering an EpiPen Auto-Injector, follow these steps:

1. When arriving at work and before the emergency occurs:

    A. Compare the medication sheet, pharmacy label, and licensed HCP order for use of the EpiPen

    B. Check the expiration date on the EpiPen

    C. Check the medication for discoloration

2. When an emergency arises, identify the right individual.

3. Obtain the EpiPen.

4. Grasp the EpiPen with the black tip pointing downward.

5. Form a fist around the EpiPen. Make sure the black tip of the EpiPen is down.

6. With the other hand, pull the gray activation cap off the EpiPen.

7. Hold the black tip near the individual's thigh. Swing the EpiPen and jab it firmly into the individual's outer thigh at a 90-degree angle to the thigh (Figure 11-4).

8. Hold the EpiPen firmly in place for ten (10) seconds.

9. Remove the EpiPen. Massage the area for several seconds.

10. Check the black tip. If the needle is showing, the medication has been administered. If the needle is not showing, the medication was not administered. Repeat steps 7 through 9.

11. Bend the needle back against a hard surface. Put the needle-syringe unit back into its carrying case. Recap the carrying case. Discard the unit at the earliest possible time into a sharps container.

12. Call 911. Keep the individual warm and avoid unnecessary movement. Immediately transport the individual to the nearest emergency medical care center.

13. Inform the health professionals that the individual has had an injection of epinephrine.

14. If the EpiPen has not yet been discarded, give the EpiPen to the staff at the emergency medical care center to discard.

15. Contact the individual's licensed health care provider and the supervisor.

16. Once back at work, document per workplace policy.

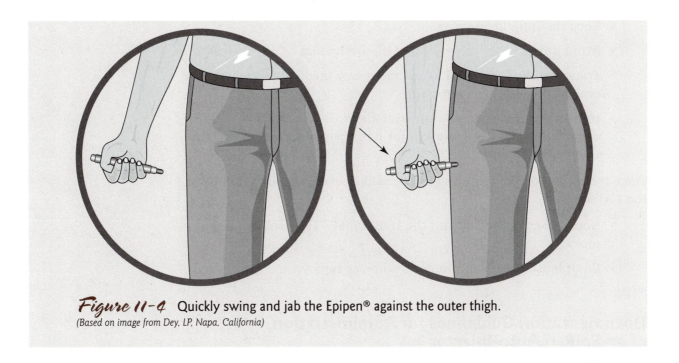

Figure 11-4   Quickly swing and jab the Epipen® against the outer thigh.
(Based on image from Dey, LP, Napa, California)

Special Considerations

Points to remember when administering an EpiPen include:

- Never remove the safety cap from the EpiPen until ready to administer the injection.
- Never place one's fingers over the black tip of the EpiPen when removing the safety cap or after the safety cap has been removed.
- Never place one's thumb over the end of the EpiPen.
- When administering, quickly swing and jab the EpiPen against the outer thigh (Figure 11-4).
- *Never administer an EpiPen in any other part of the body. EpiPens are administered only in the thigh!*
- Immediately after administering the injection, place the EpiPen into a sharps container.
- After injection, a small amount of medication will remain in the EpiPen. This is normal.

Important: Accidental injection of the EpiPen into the hands or feet of the individual, staff, or other person may result in the loss of blood flow to the area injected and needs to be avoided. If there is an accidental injection of epinephrine into these areas, the individual injected by accident must immediately go to the nearest emergency medical care center for emergency treatment.

Immediately after administering the EpiPen Auto-Injector, the UAP needs to:

- Call 911 or the local emergency medical services phone number

- Keep the individual warm
- Avoid unnecessary movement of the individual
- Transport the individual to an emergency medical care center for evaluation and follow-up care
- Inform the health care professionals at the emergency medical care center that the individual has received an epinephrine injection

Once the individual has received the needed treatment and is stabilized, the UAP needs to:

- Notify the supervisor and the individual's licensed health care provider
- Complete documentation per workplace policy

Documentation Guidelines for Administration of an EpiPen Auto-Injector

When documenting administration of an EpiPen, the UAP needs to document the following information:

- Time and date administered
- Route
- Site of injection
- Condition of the injection site
- Reason the EpiPen was administered
- Individual's response to the EpiPen
- Any complaints from the individual or adverse effects from the EpiPen
- Emergency medical care center the individual was transported to
- Time at which the individual's licensed health care provider and the workplace supervisor were notified
- Orders, if any, received from the licensed HCP

Storage and Handling of EpiPen Auto-Injectors

- Always replace the EpiPen before the EpiPen expires.
- Store EpiPens at room temperature. Do not refrigerate!
- Do not expose EpiPens to direct sunlight.
- Do not keep EpiPens in a vehicle during hot weather.
- Store EpiPens in the plastic tube they come in. An EpiPen must be stored in a light-resistant, airtight container, or the medication will become ineffective.

- Inspect EpiPens regularly with each shift change or change of staff. Make sure the EpiPens have not expired and that the medication is clear and colorless. If the medication turns brown, discard the EpiPen per workplace policy. Replace the EpiPen with a new EpiPen.

- Be sure to have multiple EpiPens available in case a hospital cannot be reached within a few minutes.

- If an EpiPen expires and is discarded because the medication has turned brown, immediately replace the EpiPen. If refills are needed, immediately contact the individual's licensed health care provider. Have the licensed HCP contact the pharmacist to reorder the EpiPens. Obtain the EpiPens from the pharmacy as soon as the EpiPens are ready to be picked up.

- *Never be without an EpiPen when caring for an individual with a history of anaphylactic reaction!*

SUMMARY

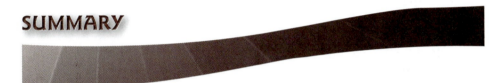

Anaphylaxis (anaphylactic reaction) is an emergency situation. The UAP must:

- Know an individual's history of allergies and reactions

- Know the emergency procedure to follow if a reaction occurs

- Be properly trained in the administration of epinephrine via EpiPen Auto-Injector

- React accordingly in an emergency situation

An individual's life is in the hands of the UAP. Her actions and inactions will determine the outcome for an individual who is experiencing anaphylaxis.

WORKBOOK REVIEW

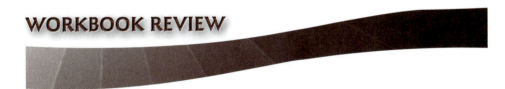

Go to the workbook and complete the exercises for Chapter 11.

REVIEW QUESTIONS

1. Anaphylaxis is:
   a. a rapid, severe allergic reaction
   b. an allergen
   c. a form of penicillin
   d. a chemical found in latex
2. The most common cause of anaphylaxis is:
   a. insect stings
   b. foods such as peanuts and milk
   c. latex
   d. penicillin
3. The medication of choice for the treatment of anaphylaxis is:
   a. penicillin
   b. epinephrine
   c. ibuprofen
   d. estradiol
4. Epinephrine is a/an:
   a. bronchoconstrictor
   b. bronchospasmodic
   c. bronchodilator
   d. antibiotic
5. Anaphylaxis requires treatment:
   a. within five (5) to ten (10) minutes
   b. immediately
   c. within thirty (30) minutes
   d. within two (2) hours
6. Immediately after administering an EpiPen, the UAP must:
   a. call emergency medical services (911) and the individual's licensed HCP
   b. monitor the individual for twenty-four (24) hours
   c. call the supervisor and the individual's licensed HCP
   d. call the individual's closest family member
7. An EpiPen is only injected into the:
   a. outer arm
   b. outer thigh
   c. chest
   d. buttock
8. Injection of an EpiPen into the hand or foot may cause:
   a. numbness in that area
   b. increased blood flow to that area
   c. loss of blood flow to that area
   d. swelling and pain in that area

9. After receiving an EpiPen injection, the individual needs to be:
   a. taken to the nearest emergency medical care center for evaluation
   b. put to bed so she can rest
   c. observed by the UAP for twenty-four (24) hours
   d. seen by her licensed HCP within twenty-four (24) hours for an evaluation
10. One of the best ways that a UAP may keep those in her care safe is by:
    a. asking other staff members for help in an emergency
    b. immediately contacting the licensed HCP and the supervisor in an emergency
    c. monitoring those who are the most ill
    d. knowing each individual's history of allergies and reactions

CLINICAL SCENARIOS

1. You are going on an outing to the state park with a group from a day program. Your assignment today includes monitoring James, who is allergic to bee stings. James is not able to self-administer an EpiPen injection.
   a. What should you do to prepare for this outing?
2. While at the park, you are assisting another group member when James approaches you. His face and arms are red and blotchy. His lips are swollen. He is wheezing.
   a. What is happening to James?
   b. What must you do immediately?
   c. What do you do next?

MODULE IV
Medications and Their Effects on the Body

Chapter 12
Body Organization and Systems

Learning Objectives

After reading this chapter and completing the review questions, you should be able to:

1. Spell and define terms.
2. Understand the organization of the body, from cell level to cavities and organs.
3. Understand each body system as it pertains to medication administration.
4. Describe three common disorders of each body system.

Key Terms

abrasion	cholecystitis	friction	musculoskeletal system
amputation	cholelithiasis	gastrointestinal system	nephritis
amyotropic lateral sclerosis	chronic bronchitis	glaucoma	nervous system
aphasia	cystitis	gout	organs
arthritis	cystocele	hernia	osteoarthritis
bursitis	decubitus ulcers	hydronephrosis	osteoporosis
cardiovascular system	diabetes mellitus	hypoxemia	otitis media
cataract	ecchymosis	integumentary system	otosclerosis
cavities	endocrine system	laceration	papules
cell	epilepsy	larynx	paralysis
cerebrovascular accident (CVA)	excoriation	lesions	Parkinson's disease
	fibromyalgia	membranes	pharynx
	fracture	multiple sclerosis	pressure ulcers

rectocele	rheumatoid arthritis	tracheostomy	vesicles
renal calculi	shearing	transient ischemic attack (TIA)	vulvovaginitis
reproductive system	systems		wheals
respiratory system	tissues	ulcers	
retinal or macular degeneration	total joint replacement	urinary incontinence	
	trachea	urinary system	

INTRODUCTION

The human body is made up of many systems that all work together. These systems help our bodies do all of the things they need to do in order to stay healthy—from breathing normally, to eating and digesting food, to moving and thinking. If one system is damaged or hurt, it may affect the way that other body systems work.

Medication is something that changes the way our body systems work and may affect more than one system. Not all of these effects are desired. For example, an antibiotic may be given to stop an infection but may upset the stomach or cause a skin rash at the same time.

In addition, over time, aging gradually causes changes to our body systems. These changes play an important role in medication administration.

This chapter reviews the organization of the body, its systems, and the common changes each system undergoes with aging.

ORGANIZATION OF THE BODY

All parts of the body are interdependent (work together). The basic unit of the body is the cell. Groups of similar cells are organized into tissues. Different tissues form organs. The organs are organized into systems that perform the body functions.

Cells

The **cell** is the basic unit of the body. Each cell performs basic activities that are important to the human body. These are breathing or respiration, nutrition, excretion (removal of body waste), and reproduction. Some cells are specialized, which means they perform a specific job that helps the body work well. Specialized cells include the following:

cell
The basic unit of the body.

- Epithelial cells: these cells form protective coverings; sometimes they make body fluids.

- Nerve cells: these cells carry electrical impulses that help us move, breathe, and use our senses.

- Muscle cells: these cells can shorten or lengthen; by changing their shape, they help move parts of the body.

- Connective tissue cells: these cells are present throughout the body; they support and connect body parts.

Tissues

tissue
A collection of specialized cells that perform a particular activity in the body.

As there are four types of specialized cells, there are also four types of **tissue** in the body. They are:

- Epithelial tissue: this tissue can absorb and produce fluids, eliminate waste, and protect structures in the body.

- Nervous tissue: this tissue forms the brain, spinal cord, and nerves throughout the body; it is also found in sensory organs like eyes, ears, and taste buds.

- Muscle tissue:

  - Skeletal, or voluntary, muscles are attached to bone for movement.

  - Cardiac muscle forms the walls of the heart.

  - Smooth, or involuntary, muscles form the walls of body organs such as the lungs or the bladder.

  - Connective tissue: this tissue forms blood, bone, and tissues that support and form connections for other tissue types such as ligaments and tendons.

Organs

organs
Perform specific activities that help the body to work as a whole.

Organs perform specific activities that help the body to work as a whole. They include structures like the heart and lungs, stomach, liver, and kidneys. However, blood vessels, glands, eyes, and ears are also organs.

Membranes

membranes
Sheets of tissue that line the body cavities.

Membranes have three jobs. They cover the body, line body cavities, and produce some body fluids. Important membranes include the following:

- Mucous membranes: these membranes produce a fluid called mucus; they line body cavities that open to the outside, such as the nose and throat.

- Synovial membranes: these membranes produce synovial fluid, which reduces friction in joint movement; they line joint cavities.

Cavities

cavities
Spaces in the body that contain the organs.

Although the body seems like a solid structure, almost half of it is made up of **cavities** or spaces that contain the organs. The two main cavities, the dorsal and ventral cavities, are divided into other cavities (Figure 12-1). A list of these follows:

1. Dorsal cavity

   - Cranial cavity: this cavity contains the brain and related structures.

   - Spinal cavity: this cavity contains the nerves and spinal cord.

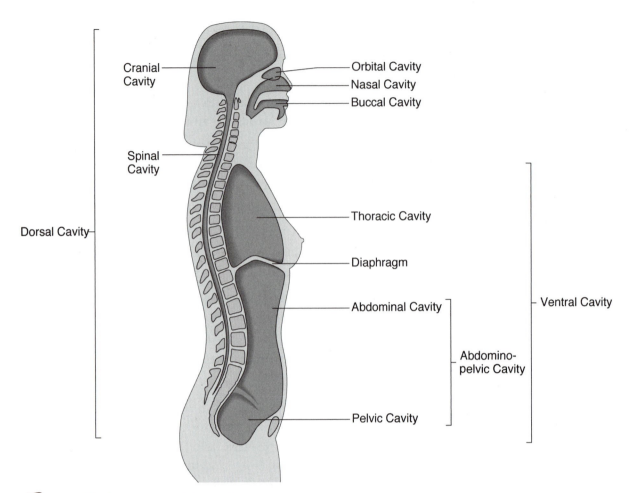

Figure 12-1 Side view of the body cavities. *(Delmar/Cengage Learning)*

2. Ventral cavity

* Thoracic cavity: this cavity contains the heart, lungs, major blood vessels, and thymus gland.

* Abdominal cavity: this cavity contains the stomach, small intestine, most of the large intestine, liver, gallbladder, pancreas, and the spleen.

* Pelvic cavity: this cavity contains reproductive organs and glands, along with the bladder, urethra, and rectum.

* Retroperitoneal space: this space contains the kidneys and ureters as well as the adrenal glands.

Systems

The body has ten (10) major **systems** that perform all of the functions of the body. Refer to Table 12-1 for a list of the systems and their basic functions.

systems
Groups of organs organized to work together, for example, the respiratory system.

Table 12-1 Systems of the Body: A List of the Body's Systems and Their Functions

SYSTEM	FUNCTION
Cardiovascular	Transports materials through the body; carries oxygen and nutrients (food) to the cells, carries waste away; as part of the immune system fights infections and protects against future infections
Endocrine	Produces hormones that regulate body processes
Gastrointestinal	Digests food, transports food, absorbs nutrients, and removes waste
Integumentary	Protects the body from injury and against infection, regulates body temperature, and removes some wastes
Muscular	Protects organs by forming body walls; forms walls of some organs, assists in movement by changing positions of bones at the joints
Nervous	Coordinates body functions
Reproductive	Reproduces the species, fulfills sexual needs, develops sexual identity
Respiratory	Brings in oxygen and removes carbon dioxide
Skeletal	Supports and protects body movement, produces blood cells, acts as a lever in movement
Urinary	Manages fluids and electrolytes, removes liquid wastes

Based on Hegner, B.R., Acello, B., and Caldwell, E. (2008). *Nursing assistant: a nursing process approach* (10th ed.), Figure 5-5. Clifton Park, NY: Delmar, Cengage Learning.

REVIEW OF BODY SYSTEMS

A brief look at each of the body systems follows.

Cardiovascular System

cardiovascular system Circulatory system; brings oxygen and nourishment to the cells and removes waste products.

The **cardiovascular**, or circulatory, **system** is the transport system of the body. It brings oxygen and nourishment to the cells and removes waste products. It is driven by the heart. When the system is disrupted, it can easily affect all of the body's activities.

The organs of the cardiovascular system include the following:

- Heart
- Blood vessels:
  1. Arteries, which carry blood away from the heart and to the cells
  2. Veins, which carry blood away from the cells and to the heart
  3. Capillaries, which connect the arteries and veins
- Lymphatic vessels: tubes that carry lymph or tissue fluid to the bloodstream
- Lymph nodes: filter the lymph fluid

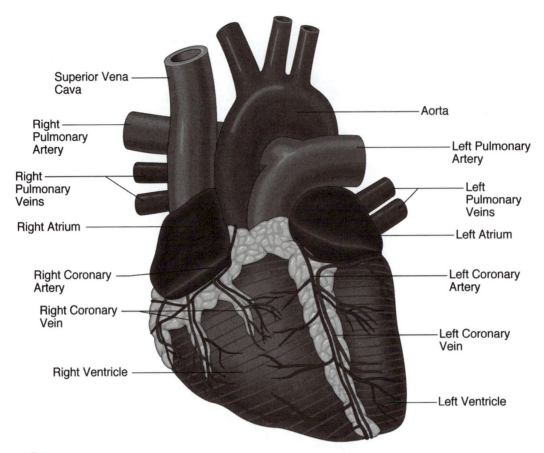

Figure 12-2 The heart and blood vessels. *(Delmar/Cengage Learning)*

- Spleen: produces some blood cells, helps destroy worn-out blood cells, and acts as a blood reservoir

- Blood

The heart is an organ made of muscle. It is about the size of a fist. It contains four chambers, separated by valves, that help to keep blood flowing in a constant forward motion (Figure 12-2). The four chambers are:

- The right atrium, which is on the upper right side of the heart

- The right ventricle, which is on the lower right side of the heart

- The left atrium, which is on the upper left side of the heart

- The left ventricle, which is on the lower left side of the heart

Nerve impulses cause the heart to contract in a regular rhythm depending on the needs of the body. When the body is at rest, the heart pumps more slowly. When the body is in motion, the heart pumps faster in order to provide more oxygen to the cells.

Common disorders of the cardiovascular system include:

- Diseases of the blood vessels, such as varicose veins or hypertension

- Diseases of the heart, such as congestive heart failure

- Blood abnormalities, or dyscrasias, such as anemia or leukemia

Common changes seen in the cardiovascular system with aging include the following:

- Longer period of time for the heart rate to increase to meet the demands placed on the heart and for the heart rate to return to a normal level

- Poor blood flow to the coronary arteries that provide blood to the heart

- Reduced cardiac output (amount of blood pumped from the heart to the body)

- Abnormal swelling of the lower legs due to weakness of the walls of the blood vessels

- Heart valves thicken and stiffen

- Stiffening of the arteries with loss of flexibility and elasticity (Ebersole & Hess, 2001)

Endocrine System

endocrine system
Made up of glands or distinct clusters of cells that release hormones.

The **endocrine system** is made up of glands or distinct clusters of cells. These glands release hormones or chemicals that control the body's activities and growth (Figure 12-3).

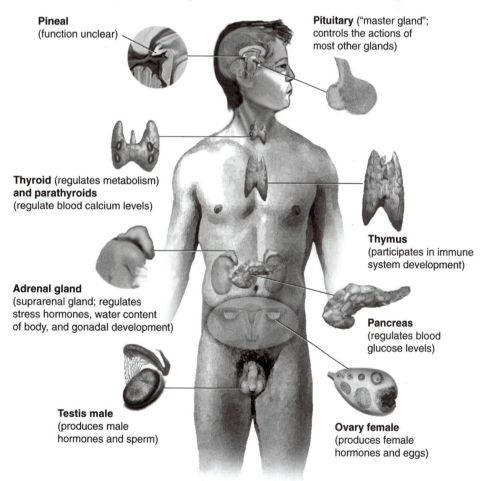

Pineal
(function unclear)

Pituitary ("master gland"; controls the actions of most other glands)

Thyroid (regulates metabolism) **and parathyroids** (regulate blood calcium levels)

Thymus (participates in immune system development)

Adrenal gland (suprarenal gland; regulates stress hormones, water content of body, and gonadal development)

Pancreas (regulates blood glucose levels)

Testis male (produces male hormones and sperm)

Ovary female (produces female hormones and eggs)

Figure 12-3 Endocrine system. *(Delmar/Cengage Learning)*

The endocrine glands and their functions are:

- Pituitary gland: also called the "master gland" because it controls most of the other glands. It affects growth, reproduction, and adrenalin production; it stimulates uterine contractions during childbirth and milk production; and it acts on the kidneys to prevent excess water loss.

- Pineal body: it is thought to be related to sexual growth, though not much is known about it.

- Adrenal glands: these produce adrenalin and noradrenalin, which help the body react quickly in an emergency. They also elevate blood sugar levels, control sodium and potassium levels, produce cortisone for emergency and healing responses, and influence sex hormones.

- Gonads: these are the male or female sex glands.

  - Ovaries: these produce estrogen and progesterone as well as special cells called ova (singular, ovum).

  - Testes: these produce testosterone as well as special cells called sperm.

- Thyroid gland: this releases thyroxine, which controls metabolism, and thyrocalcitonin, which controls calcium and phosphorus levels.

- Parathyroid glands: these produce parathormone, which helps control the body's use of calcium and phosphorus. Low calcium levels can cause severe muscle spasms.

- Islets of Langerhans: these produce insulin and glucagon, which control blood sugar.

Common disorders of the endocrine system include:

- Hyperthyroidism and hypothyroidism

- High or low blood sugar levels

- Mineral or electrolyte imbalances in the blood

- **Diabetes mellitus**

Common changes seen in the endocrine system with aging include the following:

diabetes mellitus
An imbalance in the body of carbohydrates.

- Tissue sensitivity to insulin decreases

- A significant decline in triiodothyronine (T_3)

- Production of epinephrine, norepinephrine, and dopamine decreases

- Pituitary gland decreases in size

- Decrease in estrogen, progesterone, and testosterone leading to atrophy (shrinkage) of the ovaries, uterus, and vaginal tissue in women and firmer testes and an enlarged prostate in men.

- Sexual capacity may be reduced even though libido (sex drive) remains the same in both men and women; intercourse may be less frequent and take longer but is not necessarily less satisfying (Ebersole & Hess, 2001)

Gastrointestinal System

gastrointestinal system
The digestive tract; helps the body to break down, transport, and absorb nutrients (food) as well as remove waste.

The **gastrointestinal system** is also called the digestive tract or the GI tract. This body system begins at the mouth and travels throughout the body all the way to the anus (Figure 12-4).

The gastrointestinal system includes the following structures:

- Mouth—including the teeth, tongue, and salivary glands
- Pharynx (throat)
- Esophagus
- Stomach
- Small intestine
- Liver, gallbladder, and pancreas
- Large intestine
- Rectum
- Anus

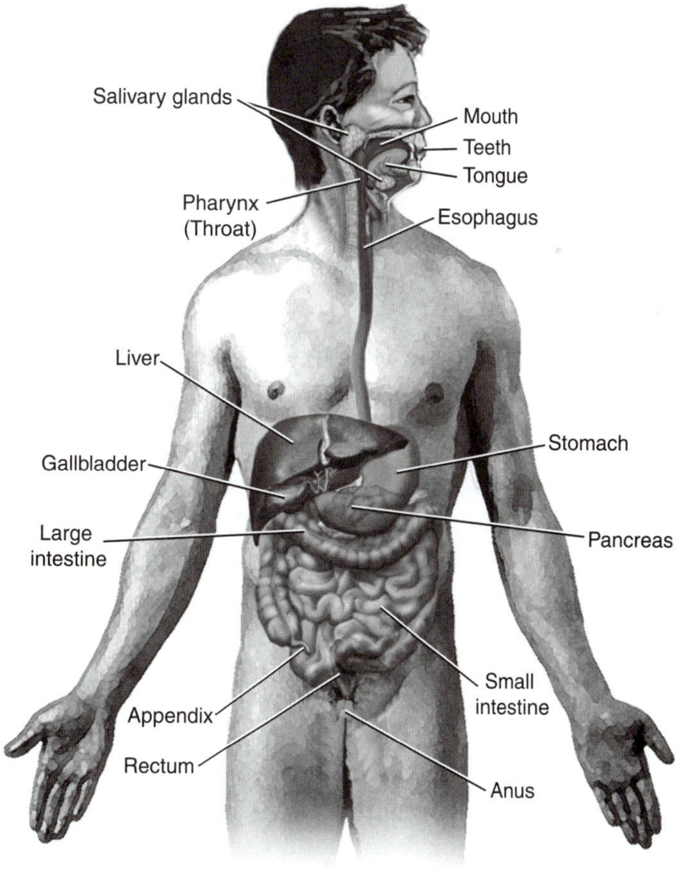

Figure 12-4 Gastrointestinal system. *(Delmar/Cengage Learning)*

These structures help the body to break down, transport, and absorb nutrients (food), as well as to remove waste.

Common disorders of the gastrointestinal tract include the following:

- Malignancies—cancers of the GI tract

- **Ulcers**—sores, which are most common in the stomach, duodenum (part of the small intestine), and colon (part of the large intestine)

- **Hernia**—this occurs when a structure pushes through a weakened area in a body wall that usually holds it in place; these are most common in the groin (inguinal hernia); near the umbilicus, or belly button (umbilical hernia); through a poorly healed incision (incisional hernia); or through the diaphragm (hiatal hernia)

- **Cholecystitis**—inflammation of the gallbladder

- **Cholelithiasis**—gallstones

- Diarrhea, constipation, or fecal impaction

Common changes seen in the gastrointestinal system with aging include the following:

- A decrease in saliva production causes dry mouth

- Esophagus becomes less effective in moving food into the stomach

- Hiatal hernias become more common

- Hydrochloric acid (HCL) is reduced along with a decrease in pepsin in the stomach

- Loss of smooth muscle in the stomach slows emptying time into the small bowel

- The absorption of nutrients and medications may be increased or delayed

- Secretions from the liver, gall bladder, and pancreas are changed

- Liver decreases in volume, weight, and liver blood flow decreases

- Smooth muscle and lymphatic changes in small bowel occur affecting absorption of fats, proteins, glucose, calcium, and iron.

- Changes in the large bowel may result in problems with removal of feces (stool), constipation, or fecal incontinence (Ebersole & Hess, 2001)

Integumentary System

The **integumentary system** includes the skin and most of the structures that are contained in it other than blood vessels. The skin is the largest organ in the body. It protects the other systems from infection, helps to regulate temperature, and eliminates some waste products.

integumentary system
Includes the skin; protects the other systems from infection; helps to regulate temperature and eliminate some waste.

The structures of the integumentary system include:

- Skin
- Hair
- Nails
- Sweat glands
- Nerves
- Oil glands

The skin does many things that keep the body healthy. First, it protects the inner structures and organs by forming a closed covering. This also helps to control our body temperature. Second, it stores fat and vitamins. Third, it passes some water, salts, and heat during perspiration or sweating. Fourth, it holds the nerve endings that alert us to changes in the environment around us.

The skin contains two layers: (1) the epidermis, which contains nerve endings but not blood vessels, and (2) the dermis, which contains blood vessels, nerve fibers, sweat and oil glands, and hair follicles.

The skin can tell us a lot about the body's general condition. An individual with a fever may have hot, dry skin. Flushing, or redness, usually indicates strenuous activity. Pallor, or paleness, can indicate many different ills. When oxygen content of the blood is low, the skin appears bluish or cyanotic.

Common disorders of the skin include many different types of lesions. **Lesions** are changes in the skin caused by injury or disease or as part of the aging process. Some examples of common skin lesions are:

- **Papules**—from chickenpox
- **Vesicles**—blisters
- **Wheals**—usually associated with itching as in hives
- **Excoriation**—a part of the skin has been scratched or scraped away

Lesions can be caused by allergic reactions, by parasites such as the scabies mite, or by an injury that can leave an **abrasion** (scrape), an **ecchymosis** (bruise), or a **laceration** (break in the skin).

The elderly population is susceptible to specific lesions, including senile purpura, which are dark purple bruises on the forearms and the back of the hands, and skin tears, in which only the epidermis is torn.

Pressure ulcers, or **decubitus ulcers**, may occur in people of any age. These ulcers are open areas of the skin that are over a bony area. They occur because of constant pressure on the skin. They can result from **shearing**, where the skin moves in one direction and the structures underneath move in the opposite direction, or from **friction**, where the skin rubs against another surface, even another area of skin.

Common changes seen in the integumentary system with aging include the following:

- Skin loses moisture and becomes dry and itchy
- Skin loses elasticity, becomes wrinkled, and tears easily

papules
A solid, raised, red area on the skin.

wheals
Hives.

abrasion
A scrape on the skin.

ecchymosis
A bruise.

laceration
A cut, a break in the skin.

shearing
An action where the skin moves in one direction and the structures underneath move in the opposite direction.

friction
Skin rubbing against another surface, even another area of skin.

- Wound healing slows

- The second layer of skin, the dermis becomes thinner

- Pigment spots (freckles and nevi) develop and/or enlarge

- Decrease in subcutaneous (fatty) tissue, which serves as our insulator changes; it is not uncommon to hear of older individuals complaining of being cold

- Hair on scalp grays and thins, hair loss is common in men, hair on arms and legs decreases, and women may develop hair on upper lip and chin

- Fingernails and toenails grow at a slower rate, the nail plate thickens, and the nail may have a yellow appearance

- Facial changes occur as fat deposits shift to less fat on face and extremities and more fat on the trunk; the size of the upper mouth, nose, and forehead are emphasized; eyelids appear swollen, and the eyes may appear sunken (Ebersole & Hess, 2001)

Musculoskeletal System

Because the skeletal and muscular systems work together to form the frame of the body and to move that frame, they are discussed together. The **musculoskeletal system** is made up of the skeleton, or the bony frame of the body, and of the muscles, or fibers and cells, that produce movement.

The musculoskeletal system contains the following structures:

musculoskeletal system
Made up of the skeleton, or the bony frame of the body, and of the muscles, or fibers and cells that produce movement.

- Skeletal muscles

- Bones

- Joints

- Tendons

- Ligaments

There are a total of 206 bones in the human body (Figure 12-5). Bones are solid structures made of calcium, minerals, and collagen fiber. They have a dense outer layer and a spongy inner layer. Bones are filled with marrow, which helps to produce red blood cells.

Joints are simply the places where bones meet and where there might be movement (Figure 12-6). For example, the lower and upper bones of the leg meet to form the knee joint. The bones in the skull meet but do not form a joint. Different joints make different types of movement. The shoulder joint moves in a variety of motions, while the elbow joint moves in only one direction.

Ligaments are bands of fibers, like rubber bands, that help to support the joints and hold the bones together at those joints. A bursa is a small sac, like a plastic baggie, that holds fluid that surrounds the joint, keeping it moving smoothly.

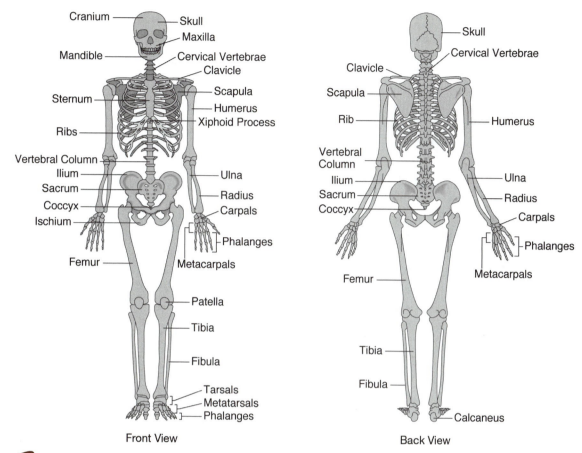

Figure 12-5 Major bones of the body. *(Delmar/Cengage Learning)*

Muscles in the body work in groups. There are over 500 muscles in the body, separated into three kinds:

1. Cardiac muscle, which forms the walls of the heart

2. Involuntary, or visceral muscles, which make up organ walls

3. Voluntary, or skeletal, muscles (Figure 12-7)

Muscles can only contract (shorten) and relax (lengthen). They are attached to bones by strong fibers called tendons. As muscles contract, they bend or straighten a joint. For example, when the hamstring muscles in the leg contract at the back of the thigh, they cause the knee to bend. To straighten the knee, the quadriceps muscles at the front of the thigh must contract. As muscles are used, they maintain or gain strength. If muscles are not used, they lose strength.

Common disorders of the musculoskeletal system include:

- **Bursitis**—inflammation of the bursa sacs around a joint

- **Arthritis**—inflammation of the joints; common forms of chronic arthritis are:

  - **Rheumatoid arthritis**—which affects the joint tissue and lining

  - **Osteoarthritis**—which affects cartilage in between the bones that form the joint

rheumatoid arthritis
A type of arthritis that affects the joint tissue and lining.

osteoarthritis
A type of arthritis that affects the cartilage in between the bones that form the joint.

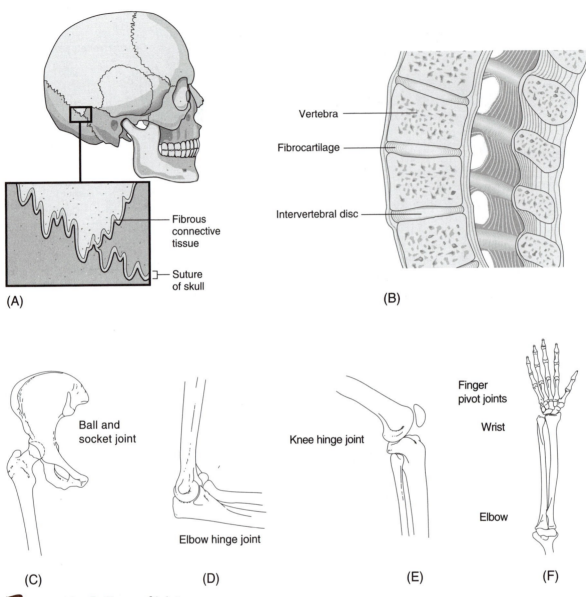

Figure 12-6 Types of joints. *(Delmar/Cengage Learning)*

- **Osteoporosis**—a metabolic disease that causes bones to lose their mass and become very spongy with very high risk for fracture

- **Gout**—a metabolic disease most common in the feet and legs

- **Fibromyalgia**—a chronic pain syndrome

- **Fracture**—any break in any bone

- **Total joint replacement**—such as at the hip or knee, where a joint is surgically removed and an artificial one is inserted

- Ruptured or slipped disc—places pressure on the spinal nerves and can cause pain, tingling, numbness, and/or weakness

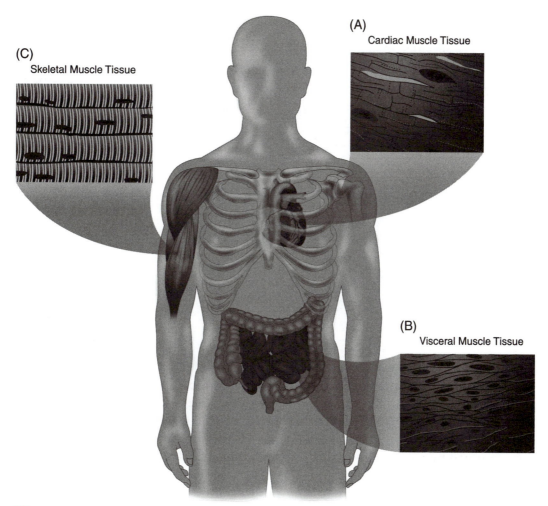

Figure 12-7 Types of muscle. A) cardiac muscle; B) visceral muscle; C) skeletal muscle.
(Delmar/Cengage Learning)

amputation
The surgical removal of a limb, for example, an arm or a leg.

- **Amputation**—of a limb, either an arm or a leg, or of fingers or toes, due to disease or trauma

Common changes seen in the musculoskeletal system with aging include the following:

- Height decreases by one and a half (1½) to two (2) inches, and the trunk of the body shortens
- Vetebral discs thin causing the trunk to shorten; many older adults may develop a stooped (forward bent) posture
- Skeletal muscles atrophy (shrink) especially in the legs
- Strength and stamina decrease to 65% to 85% of the maximum strength an individual had at twenty-five (25) years of age
- Bones become brittle
- Ligaments, tendons, and joints become hardened, stiff, and less flexible, leading to slower, painful movement (Ebersole & Hess, 2001)

Nervous System

The **nervous system** is the "driver" of the human body. The nervous system controls and coordinates all body activities, from movement to breathing to producing hormones. Some parts of this system control daily functions, while others are used only in a dangerous situation (Figures 12-8A and 12-8B, 12-9, and 12-10).

Structures of the nervous system include:

- Neurons
- Neurotransmitters
- Nerves
- Brain
- Spinal cord
- Nose, tongue, and skin
- Eyes
- Ears

Neurons are the cells of the nervous system. They conduct electrical impulses through extensions called axons and dendrites. An axon carries the impulse from the neuron and passes it on to the dendrites of the next neuron. Chemicals called neurotransmitters allow the impulses to pass from one neuron to the next. Axons and dendrites are usually found in bundles, wrapped by connective tissue and resembling cables. These cables are the nerves of the body (Figure 12-8A and B).

The nervous system is made up of two major components: the central nervous system and the peripheral nervous system. The central nervous system contains only the brain and spinal cord, while the peripheral nervous system connects them to various parts of the body (Figure 12-9).

The brain is like the powerhouse of the nervous system. It controls all mental activities—thoughts, movement, and emotions—as well as involuntary movements of the vital organs and also coordinates muscle activity and balance (Figure 12-10).

The spinal cord carries almost all of the nerves, except for the cranial nerves, that go directly from the brain to different areas in the head and face. It acts as the major cable that connects all of the body systems through the nerves, sending signals from the brain to the body and from the body to the brain (Figures 12-9 and 12-11).

Sensory receptors send information to the brain from the outside environment. The sensory dendrites in the nose carry the sense of smell, those in the tongue carry taste, and those in the skin carry temperature, pain, pressure, and body position.

Two other sensory receptors, the eye and the ear, are more highly developed end organs. The eye 1) controls the amount of light that enters and 2) changes the range of our vision from near to far through small muscles that change the shape of the lens within the eye. The ear 1) picks up sounds in the environment and 2) helps us to keep our balance by sending information about the position of the head from the inner ear to the brain.

nervous system
Controls and coordinates all body activities.

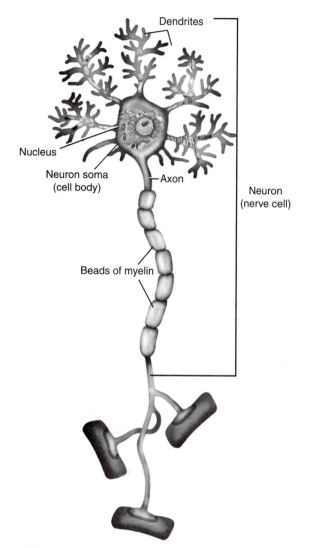

Figure 12-8a **The neuron.** *(Delmar/Cengage Learning)*

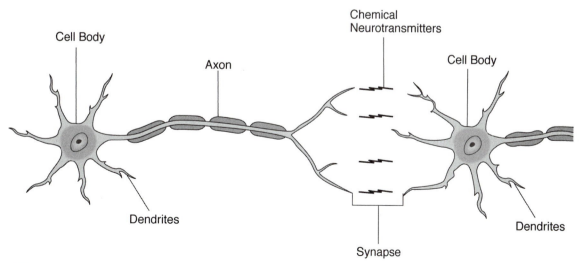

Figure 12-8b Chemicals called neurotransmitters help pass the messages across the synapse from one neuron to another. *(Delmar/Cengage Learning)*

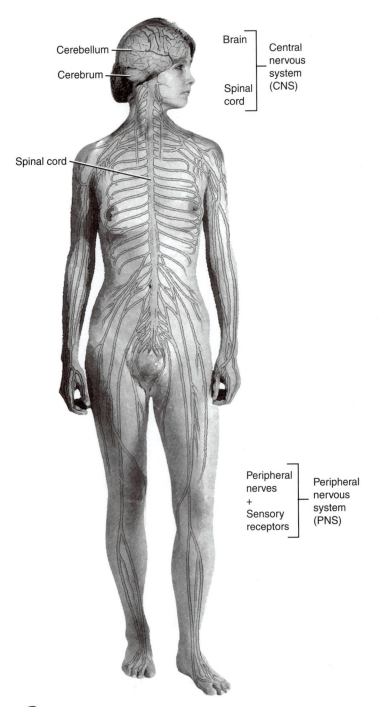

Cerebellum

Cerebrum

Brain

Central nervous system (CNS)

Spinal cord

Spinal cord

Peripheral nerves + Sensory receptors

Peripheral nervous system (PNS)

Figure 12-9 The peripheral nervous system connects the central nervous system to the different structures of the body. Messages are sent from these structures back to the brain through the spinal cord. *(Delmar/Cengage Learning)*

Common disorders of the nervous system include:

- Increased intracranial pressure—causes damage to the brain; can result from head injury, cerebrovascular accident (stroke), toxins, excessively high fever, or tumors

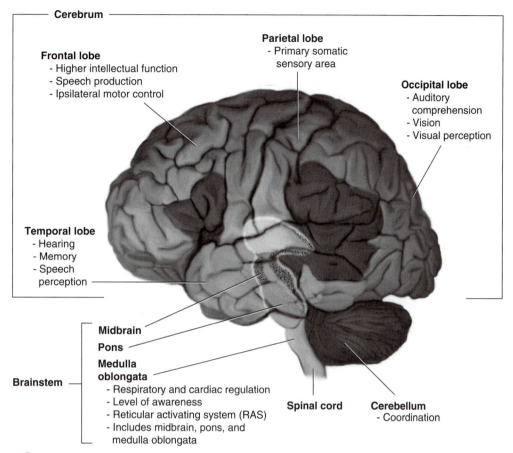

Figure 12-10 Each lobe of the brain is responsible for a different function (activity).
(Delmar/Cengage Learning)

- **Transient ischemic attack (TIA)**—a temporary decrease in blood flow to the brain; causes symptoms that are similar to a stroke but are temporary and reversible

- Stroke—**cerebrovascular accident (CVA)**, caused by complete or partial loss of blood flow to the brain

- **Aphasia**—difficulty expressing or understanding communication or language

- **Parkinson's disease**—causes tremors, muscle rigidity, and difficulty with voluntary movement

- **Multiple sclerosis**—caused by a loss of myelin around central nervous system fibers, which interferes with the workings of the nerve fibers

- **Amyotropic lateral sclerosis**—Lou Gehrig's disease; a progressive disease that causes muscle weakness and paralysis and is almost always fatal

- **Epilepsy**—a seizure disorder that involves recurring and temporary episodes of disrupted brain function resulting in seizures; seizures may involve movement and muscle rigidity (tonic-clonic or grand mal) or momentary loss of muscle tone (absence or petit mal)

Parkinson's disease
A nervous disorder that causes tremors, muscle rigidity, and difficulty with voluntary movement.

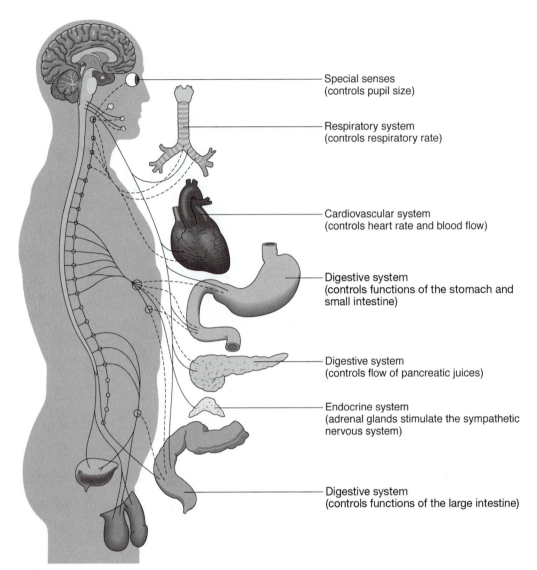

Special senses
(controls pupil size)

Respiratory system
(controls respiratory rate)

Cardiovascular system
(controls heart rate and blood flow)

Digestive system
(controls functions of the stomach and
small intestine)

Digestive system
(controls flow of pancreatic juices)

Endocrine system
(adrenal glands stimulate the sympathetic
nervous system)

Digestive system
(controls functions of the large intestine)

Figure 12-11 Autonomic nervous system. *(Delmar/Cengage Learning)*

- Spinal cord injury—results in **paralysis** (the loss of the ability to move or feel) below the level of the injury

- **Cataract**—the lens of the eye becomes cloudy and no light can pass through

- **Glaucoma**—increased pressure within the eye that causes gradual vision loss, leading to blindness

- **Retinal or macular degeneration**—breakdown of the retina inside the eye, which causes loss of central vision (directly in front of the pupil)

- **Otitis media**—infection of the middle ear, which is common in children

- **Otosclerosis**—a progressive form of deafness

- Partial or complete hearing loss

Common changes seen in the nervous system with aging include the following:

- Development of senile plaque and (less frequently) neurofibrillary tangles in the brain

- Changes in the neurotransmitter system

- Enlargement of the cerebral ventricles

- Decrease conduction time of the peripheral nerves

- Performance of tasks may take longer even though the intellectual performance of elders without brain dysfunction remains unchanged into and beyond eighty (80) years of age

- Learning is slower

- Forgetfulness

- Decrease in taste and smell

- A decline in vision due to physical changes in the eyes; older individuals require three times as much light to see things as they did when they were in their 20s; cataracts begin to develop; inability to see colors clearly

- Lack of tears

- Loss of hearing due to physical changes in the ears; loss of high frequencies

- Loss of feeling especially in the fingertips, palms of the hands, lower legs, and feet

- Increase difficulty with moving about their environment; with the ability of sensing changes about them; slower reaction times; leaving them at risk for falls (Ebersole & Hess, 2001)

Reproductive System

reproductive system
Produces reproductive cells and hormones that control sex characteristics.

The **reproductive system** is present in males and females. Both systems do two things: (1) they produce reproductive cells—sperm in the male and ovum in the female—and (2) they produce hormones that control sex characteristics—testosterone in the male and estrogen and progesterone in the female.

Structures in the male reproductive system (Figure 12-12) include:

- Testes

- Epididymis

- Vas deferens

- Seminal vesicles

- Ejaculatory duct

- Prostate gland

- Cowper's glands

- Penis

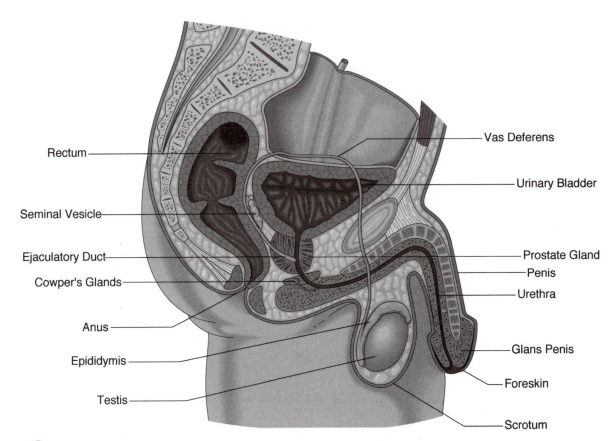

Figure 12-12 Cross section of the male reproductive system. *(Delmar/Cengage Learning)*

Structures in the female reproductive system (Figures 12-13 and 12-14) include:

- Vulva
- Clitoris
- Urinary meatus, or opening
- Vaginal meatus
- Ovaries
- Fallopian tubes
- Uterus
- Vagina

The male reproductive system produces sperm and the hormone testosterone. This allows the male to develop male sexual characteristics and reproduce.

Common disorders of the male reproductive system include:

- Prostate conditions such as enlargement or cancer
- Cancer of the testes

The female reproductive system triggers the process of menstruation and ovulation, beginning at puberty, in girls between the ages of nine (9) and seventeen (17). This is a monthly cycle in which the ovum, or egg, is

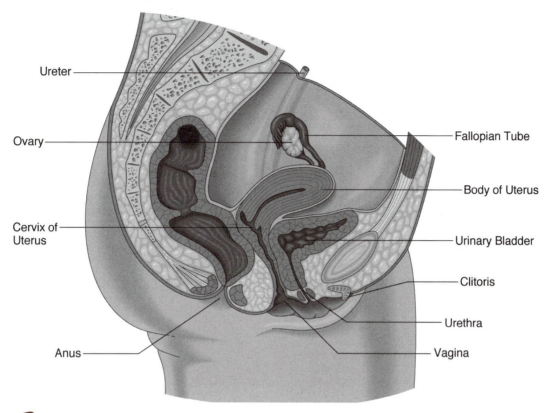

Figure 12-13 Cross section of the female reproductive system. *(Delmar/Cengage Learning)*

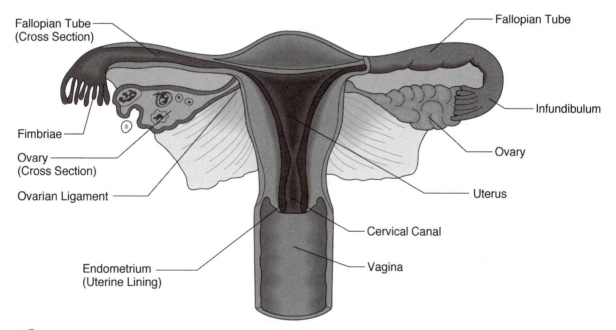

Figure 12-14 Front view of the internal female reproductive organs. *(Delmar/Cengage Learning)*

released from the ovary into the uterus for possible fertilization. This is called ovulation.

   If fertilization does not occur, the egg is flushed from the uterus with the lining of the uterus. This is called menstruation. Menopause is triggered when the last ova are released from the ovaries, usually in the mid-50s. Changes occur over time that stop the menstrual cycle. This can also be triggered by surgical removal of the ovaries.

Common disorders of the female reproductive system include:

- **Rectocele**—a hernia at the wall between the vagina and the rectum

- **Cystocele**—a hernia at the wall between the bladder and the vagina

- **Vulvovaginitis**—caused by a fungal infection

- Tumors of the uterus and ovaries

- Malignancies of the cervix

- Tumors of the breast

vulvovaginitis
A type of vaginal infection caused by a fungus.

Sexually transmitted diseases can affect men and women. They can be passed between mucous membranes, from a mucous membrane to the skin, or from the skin to a mucous membrane. They include:

- *Trichomonas vaginalis*—caused by a parasite

- Gonorrhea—caused by a bacterium

- Syphilis—caused by a microorganism

- Herpes—caused by a virus

- Venereal warts—caused by a virus

- Chlamydia—caused by infectious organisms

- Human immunodeficiency virus (HIV)—caused by a virus

Common changes seen in the reproductive system with aging include the following:

- For men: decrease in sperm count; smaller testes; less firm erections; erections take longer to occur

- For females: decrease estrogen production; ovaries deteriorate; vagina, uterus, and breast atrophy (shrink); intercourse may be uncomfortable; unable to become pregnant (Ebersole & Hess, 2001)

Respiratory System

If the nervous system is the body's "driver," then the **respiratory system** is its lifeline. This system brings in oxygen for the blood and removes the waste product, carbon dioxide. Without this extremely important exchange of gases, life cannot continue. The respiratory system goes from the nose to the alveoli (tiny air sacs deep in the lungs) (Figures 12-15 and 12-16).

respiratory system
Brings in oxygen for the blood and removes a waste product, carbon dioxide, from it.

Structures include:

- Nose

- Pharynx (throat)

- Larynx (voice box)

- Trachea (windpipe)

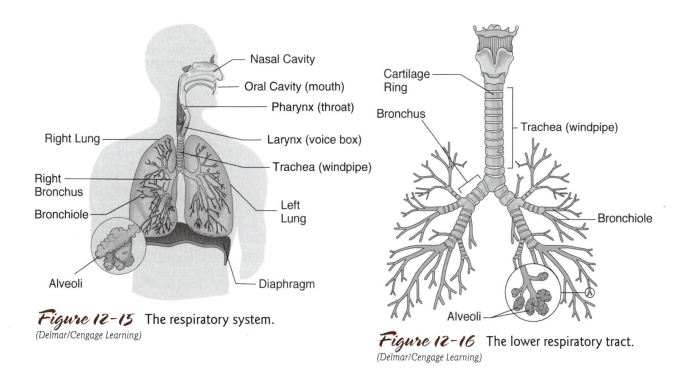

Figure 12-15 The respiratory system.
(Delmar/Cengage Learning)

Figure 12-16 The lower respiratory tract.
(Delmar/Cengage Learning)

- Bronchi (singular, bronchus)

- Lungs

The sinuses, diaphragm, and intercostal muscles between the ribs are called auxiliary structures. These help an individual to breathe.

Air enters the nose, where it is warmed, filtered, and moistened. It passes through the **pharynx** (throat), the **larynx** (voice box), and the **trachea** (windpipe) to the bronchi. Each bronchus travels to one of the lungs, right or left.

Once inside the lungs, the bronchus continues to branch into smaller divisions called bronchioles. Alveoli are at the end of each of the tiniest bronchioles. This is where the exchange of oxygen and carbon dioxide happens, between the alveoli and capillaries that pass by, carrying blood. The alveolus delivers oxygen into the blood, and the blood passes carbon dioxide back into the alveolus so it can be expelled from the body.

The respiratory system also plays a large part in voice production. As air leaves the lungs, it passes through the larynx, or voice box. Vocal cords, inside the larynx, can change shape and size to control airflow into the mouth, nasal cavities, and sinuses. Here, sounds can be formed by the tongue, teeth, and lips.

Common disorders of the respiratory system include:

- **Hypoxemia**—insufficient oxygen in the blood

- Upper respiratory infection—an infection in the nose, sinuses, and throat, for example, the common cold

- Pneumonia—inflammation of the lungs

- Chronic obstructive pulmonary disease (COPD)—a chronic and irreversible blockage of the respiratory system

- Asthma

- **Chronic bronchitis**—prolonged inflammation in the bronchi
- Emphysema—the alveoli become nonfunctional and cannot exchange gases

Surgical conditions include:

- **Tracheostomy**—a surgical opening in the trachea; it may be done as an emergency measure or for an individual who has used a ventilator for a long time
- Lung cancer
- Cancer of the larynx—may require removal of the larynx

Common changes seen in the respiratory system with aging include the following:

- Exercise tolerance decreases
- Trachea and larynx become stiff
- Respiratory muscle weaken
- Loss of elasticity of the chest wall
- Accessory structures become "floppy" because of muscle weakness
- Lungs become "flabbier"
- Alveoli enlarge
- Less effective cough response (Ebersole & Hess, 2001)

Urinary System

The **urinary system** has three functions. First, it removes liquid wastes. Second, it manages blood chemistry. Third, it manages fluid balance in the body. Without these functions, the body would quickly become bloated and unhealthy.

urinary system
Excretes liquid wastes, manages blood chemistry, and manages fluid balance in the body.

Structures of this system include (Figure 12-17):

- Kidneys
- Ureters
- Urinary bladder
- Urethra

The kidneys are the main organs in this system. They filter the blood, removing acids and salts, and flush them out of the body in urine. Urine is liquid waste containing these dissolved waste products mixed with water. After the urine is produced, it is passed through the ureters, one from each kidney, and into the urinary bladder. Once the bladder becomes partially full, with 150 to 300 mL of urine, it signals the brain to release urine through the urethra and out of the body through the urethral meatus, or opening. In males, the prostate gland sits between the bladder and the urethra.

Common disorders of the urinary system include:

- **Cystitis**—inflammation of the urinary bladder
- **Nephritis**—inflammation of the kidney

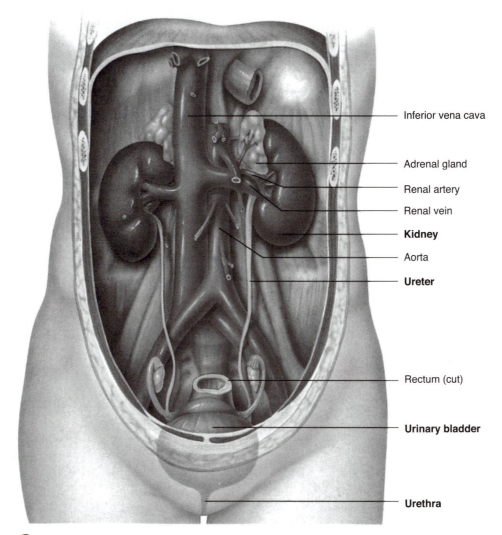

Figure 12-17 The urinary system. *(Delmar/Cengage Learning)*

Inferior vena cava

Adrenal gland

Renal artery

Renal vein

Kidney

Aorta

Ureter

Rectum (cut)

Urinary bladder

Urethra

- **Renal calculi**—kidney stones
- **Hydronephrosis**—a buildup of fluid in the kidney because of a blocked ureter or distended bladder, which causes damage to kidney cells
- **Urinary incontinence**—the involuntary release of urine caused by the lack of cerebral control or awareness, illness, or infection

Common changes seen in the urinary system with aging include the following:

- Decrease in size and function of the kidneys
- Decrease in the blood flow to the kidneys
- Decrease urinary bladder capacity; need to urinate more often; may have urinary incontinence; may have less bladder tone; men may have an enlarged prostate, which may cause urinary retention (Ebersole & Hess, 2001)

SUMMARY

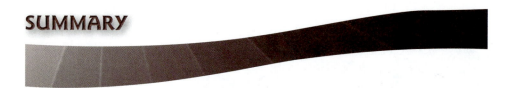

Our bodies are made up of many complex, integrated systems. Each system has its own set of structures that work together. The body uses all of these structures together in order to continue its own daily functioning. Damage to any system, or to part of any system, will affect the body's ability to work in an efficient manner.

WORKBOOK REVIEW

Go to the workbook and complete the exercises for Chapter 12.

REVIEW QUESTIONS

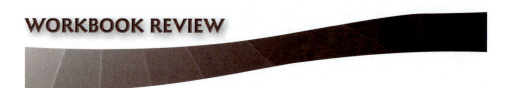

1. The four levels of organization in the body are:
   a. cells, tissue, organs, and systems
   b. epithelial, nervous, muscle, and connective
   c. heart, lungs, stomach, and kidneys
   d. tissue, organs, membranes, and cavities
2. The cardiovascular system:
   a. is made up of glands that release hormones
   b. helps the body to break down and transport nutrients
   c. brings oxygen and nourishment to cells and removes waste
   d. protects the body from infection
3. The endocrine system:
   a. includes glands such as the pituitary, adrenal, and thyroid glands
   b. is made up of the stomach, pancreas, and gallbladder
   c. is considered the control center of the body
   d. is responsible for the production of urine
4. Common disorders of the GI system include:
   a. varicose veins and anemia
   b. ulcers and hernias
   c. abrasions and lacerations
   d. bursitis and gout

5. The skin:
   a. can tell us whether an individual has a fever or illness or is low on oxygen
   b. is made up of muscle cells
   c. requires little attention—it cares for itself
   d. all of the above
6. Pressure ulcers:
   a. only occur in the elderly
   b. occur because of constant pressure on the skin over a bony area
   c. occur in the GI tract as the result of a stressful job
   d. are the result of an ecchymosis
7. The structures of the musculoskeletal system include:
   a. nerves and oil glands
   b. bones and joints
   c. bladder and kidneys
   d. ovary and uterus
8. The nervous system:
   a. is made up of glands that release hormones
   b. protects other systems from infection
   c. controls and coordinates all body activities
   d. brings in oxygen and removes carbon dioxide
9. Common disorders of the respiratory system include:
   a. hernias
   b. emphysema
   c. kidney stones
   d. myocardial infarction
10. The changes that occur to our bodies due to aging:
    a. affect all systems of the body except the nervous system
    b. occur gradually over time
    c. begin abruptly when we are in our 60s
    d. can easily be altered with diet, exercise, and medication
11. The main organs in the urinary system are the:
    a. lungs
    b. kidneys
    c. ureters
    d. bladder and urethra

CLINICAL SCENARIOS

1. Describe how muscles work to move the body.
2. Describe the specialized functions of the eye and ear.

Chapter 13
Vitamins, Minerals, and Dietary Supplements

Learning Objectives

After reading this chapter and completing the review questions, you should be able to:

1. Spell and define terms.
2. Discuss the role of good nutrition in an individual's general health.
3. Give five examples of when an individual may need additional dietary supplements.
4. Describe antioxidants and phytochemicals.
5. Discuss the role of vitamin and mineral supplements in an individual's daily diet.
6. List two guidelines for the administration of herbal medication.

Key Terms

antioxidants	free radicals	minerals	vitamins
avitaminosis	homeostasis	nutrients	water-soluble vitamins
electrolytes	hypervitaminosis	obesity	
fat-soluble vitamins	hypovitaminosis	phytochemicals	

INTRODUCTION

In the food we eat and the liquids we drink, there are vital **nutrients** that our bodies need to function. These include:

- Proteins
- Fats
- Carbohydrates
- Water
- Electrolytes
- Vitamins
- Minerals

Our bodies use these nutrients for heat and energy, to build and repair body tissues, to maintain the body's chemical balances, and to regulate body processes.

Poor nutrition can compromise an individual's health. One effect of poor nutrition is **obesity**. According to the Centers for Disease Control and Prevention (CDC), in the past six (6) years, the rate of obesity has risen significantly in the United States. Currently, approximately 67% of adults in the United States are overweight. Approximately 31% of adults are obese. Out of the 60 million adults who are obese, 9 million are morbidly (extremely) obese. In addition, 16.3% of children and adolescents aged 2 to 19 years are obese (Centers for Disease Control and Prevention, 2009).

Obesity has been linked to an increased risk of many health problems, including:

- Type 2 diabetes
- Coronary heart disease
- Cancers—endometrial, breast, and colon
- Stroke
- High blood pressure
- High cholesterol and high trigylcerides (dyslipidemia)
- Liver and gallbladder disease
- Osteoarthritis
- Complications in pregnancy or in the ability to conceive
- Sleep apnea and respiratory problems
- Early death (Centers for Disease Control and Prevention, 2009)

Good nutrition is a key to an individual's health. It may be achieved through moderation, variety, and balance in the diet.

obesity
An excess of fat in relation to lean body mass, with a body weight of 20% or more over ideal weight for height.

ADDING NUTRIENTS TO THE DIET

There are times and circumstances when an individual may need additional nutrients, such as a vitamin and/or mineral supplement. These times and circumstances include the following:

- During pregnancy and breast feeding
- During stages of growth and development throughout life
- When involved in a disease process
- Before and after surgery
- An individual with irregular eating habits
- An individual who diets
- An individual who is a vegetarian or who avoids entire food groups
- An individual with a deficiency disease or absorption disorder
- An individual who takes medications that interfere with nutrients
- An individual who abuses drugs or alcohol
- A woman at risk for osteoporosis
- A woman who bleeds excessively during menstruation
- During our elder years

An individual may be given a prescription for a vitamin and/or mineral supplement by her licensed health care provider. Vitamins may also be purchased as an over-the-counter medication. These are medications, just like any other medication, and should be treated as such. They are documented on the medication sheet and given on a schedule just as are other medications. These supplements may include **vitamins**, **minerals**, **antioxidants**, and **phytochemicals**.

VITAMINS

Vitamins are organic substances. This means that they are formed by an organism and can be retrieved from plant and animal sources, like vegetables, fruits, milk, and meats, or from the sunshine, as in vitamin D. Vitamins are either **fat soluble** or **water soluble**.

Table 13-1 has a complete list of both types of vitamins along with signs of deficiency and toxicity. Conditions that may occur related to a lack of a vitamin or too much of a vitamin include the following:

- **Avitaminosis**, an illness caused by a lack of vitamins in the diet
- **Hypervitaminosis**, a condition caused by an excessive amount of a vitamin in the body, which can lead to illness
- **Hypovitaminosis**, a condition caused by a lack of vitamins in the body, especially as related to poor nutrition; it can lead to avitaminosis

vitamins
Substances found in a variety of foods that are basic to good health.

minerals
Inorganic substances that are essential to the function of all body cells.

antioxidants
Chemical substances that neutralize free radicals.

phytochemicals
Any one of a hundred natural chemical substances found in plants.

fat-soluble vitamins
Vitamins that are stored in fat tissue and in the liver.

water-soluble vitamins
Vitamins that are not stored in the body and that need to be replenished daily.

Table 13-1 Vitamins

NAME	FOOD SOURCES	FUNCTIONS	DEFICIENCY/TOXICITY
Vitamin A	Oily saltwater fish Dairy products Eggs Dark-green leafy vegetables Deep yellow or orange fruit and vegetables	Vision in dim light Growth and development of bones Healing of wounds Resistance to infection Maintains healthy skin and mucus membranes	**Deficiency** Slow growth Bone and tooth deformities Itching Night blindness Dry skin Dry eyes Weight loss **Toxicity** Anorexia Irritability, lethargy, headache Joint pain, myalgia Stunted growth Loss of hair Jaundice, nausea, diarrhea Dry skin and hair

Vitamin D	Fish oils
	Fortified milk
	Fortified cereals
		Healthy bones and teeth
		Muscle function
		Absorption of calcium
			Deficiency
			Softening bones:
			   Rickets (in children)
			    Osteomalacia (in adults)
			Poorly developed teeth
			Muscle spasms
			Toxicity
			Convulsions
			Kidney stones, kidney damage
			Muscle/bone pain
			Nausea, anorexia, weight loss

Vitamin E	Meat, poultry eggs Vegetable oils Seeds, nuts Wheat germ, cereals	Decreases platelet clumping Normal metabolism Tissue protection of eyes, skin, liver, breasts, muscles, lungs	**Deficiency** Destruction of RCBs, muscle weakness **Toxicity** Prolonged bleeding time
Vitamin K	Egg yolk, cheese Liver Vegetable oil Green leafy vegetables Cabbage, broccoli	Blood clotting	**Deficiency** Prolonged blood clotting time Blood in urine and stool **Toxicity** None

(continues)

Table 13-1 Vitamins—*continued*

NAME	FOOD SOURCES	FUNCTIONS	DEFICIENCY/TOXICITY
Vitamin B_1	Pork, beef, liver Oysters Yeast Whole and enriched grains, wheat germ Beans, peas, collard greens, nuts, asparagus Oranges	Normal nervous and cardiovascular systems	**Deficiency** GI upset, constipation Neuritis, mental disturbance Cardiovascular problems Muscle weakness, fatigue **Toxicity** None known
Vitamin B_2	Milk, eggs Meat, liver Green vegetables Cereals Enriched bread Yeast, nuts	Aids metabolism of glucose, fats, and amino acids	**Deficiency** Skin & lip lesions Sore tongue Sensitivity to light, vision problems, itching eyes Dermatitis, rough skin **Toxicity** None
Vitamin B_6	Pork, beef, chicken, tuna, salmon Whole-grain cereals, wheat germ Legumes, peanuts, soybeans Bananas	Synthesis of amino acids Antibody production Maintenance of blood glucose level	**Deficiency** Anorexia, nausea, vomiting Dermatitis Neuritis, depression **Toxicity** None
Vitamin B_{12}	Seafood/shellfish Meat, poultry, liver Eggs Milk, cheese	Synthesis of RBCs Maintenance of nervous system	**Deficiency** Nerve, muscle, mental problems Pernicious anemia **Toxicity** None
Niacin	Milk Eggs Fish Poultry, meat Soy beans Nuts, peas, beans Green vegetables Peanut butter Enriched cereals	Lipid metabolism Nerve functioning	**Deficiency** Pellagra **Toxicity** Headache, flushing Increased blood glucose and uric acid

Table 13-1 Vitamins—*continued*

NAME	FOOD SOURCES	FUNCTIONS	DEFICIENCY/TOXICITY
Folic Acid	Organ meats Green leafy vegetables Avocado, beets Broccoli, kidney beans Orange juice	Synthesis of RBCs, leukocytes, DNA and RNA Needed for normal growth and reproduction	**Deficiency** Macrocytic anemia Irritability, behavior disorders **Toxicity** None
Vitamin C	All citrus fruits, cantaloupe Broccoli Tomatoes Brussel sprouts Cabbage Green peppers	Normal teeth, gums, and bone Prevention of scurvy Formation of collagen Healing of wounds Absorption of iron	**Deficiency** Scurvy Poor healing Muscle cramps/weakness Sore & bleeding gums/mouth, loose teeth Dry, scaly skin Bruising **Toxicity** Raise uric acid level, gout GI distress Kidney stones

Based on Woodrow, R. (2007). *Essentials of pharmacology for health occupations* (5th ed.), Table 11-1. Clifton Park, NY: Delmar, Cengage Learning.

MINERALS

Minerals are inorganic substances. That means that minerals are not made by an organism. Instead, minerals are found in many foods as well as in the earth's crust. Minerals may be isolated to form dietary supplements. Minerals do many things to keep the body healthy such as:

- Support the body's enzymes in their work activities
- Keep blood and body fluids chemically balanced
- Make up the major parts of skeletal bones
- Help regulate blood pressure and the contraction of the heart muscle
- Help heal wounds
- Help conduct nerve impulses

electrolytes
Acid, base, and salt particles formed by the breakdown of mineral compounds in body fluids.

Electrolytes are particles formed from the breakdown of mineral compounds in body fluids. The particles formed include acids, bases, and salts. They are found in body fluids that carry nourishment to the cells and remove wastes from the cells. Electrolytes support metabolism. Electrolytes are vital to normal cell functions. **Homeostasis** is a state of normal balance of electrolytes in body fluids.

Table 13-2 has a list of minerals along with signs of deficiency and toxicity.

Table 13-2 Minerals

NAME	FOOD SOURCES	FUNCTIONS	DEFICIENCY/TOXICITY
Calcium (Ca)	Milk, cheese, yogurt Sardines Salmon Green vegetables except spinach	Development of bones and teeth Contraction of cardiac, smooth and skeletal muscles Nerve conduction Blood clotting	**Deficiency** Osteoporosis, osteomalacia Rickets (in children) Muscle pathology Heart disease Increased clotting time **Toxicity** None known
Potassium (K)	Oranges, bananas Dried fruits Tomatoes Potato skins Cantaloupe Avocadoes Cooked dried beans Peas	Contraction of muscles Heartbeat regulation Transmission of nerve impulses Maintaining fluid balance	**Deficiency** (Hypokalemia) Muscle weakness Cardiac arrhythmias Lethargy, mental confusion **Toxicity** (Hyperkalemia) Confusion Weakness Cardiac arrhythmias
Sodium (Na)	Table salt Beef, eggs Milk, cheese	Maintaining fluid balance in blood Transmission of nerve impulses	**Deficiency** (Hyponatremia) Loss of weight, weakness, cramps **Toxicity** Increase in blood pressure
Chloride (Cl)	Table salt	Gastric acidity Regulation of osmotic pressure Activation of salivary amylase	**Deficiency** Imbalance in gastric acidity Imbalance in blood pH **Toxicity** Diarrhea
Magnesium (Mg)	Green vegetables Whole grains	Synthesis of ATP (adenosine triphosphate) Transmission of nerve impulses Relaxation of skeletal muscles	**Deficiency** (seldom) Imbalance Weakness, tremor Confusion **Toxicity** Diarrhea

Table 13-2 Minerals—*continued*

NAME	FOOD SOURCES	FUNCTIONS	DEFICIENCY/TOXICITY
Iron (Fe)	Meat Liver Eggs Poultry Spinach Dried fruits Dried beans Prune juice Enriched cereals	Hemoglobin formation	**Deficiency** (anemia) Pale Weakness Lethargy Vertigo Air hunger Irregular heartbeat **Toxicity** Lethargy, shock Vomiting, diarrhea Erosion of GI tract Liver or kidney damage
Iodine (I)	Freshwater shellfish and seafood Iodized salt	Major component of thyroid hormones Regulating rate of metabolism Growth, reproduction Nerve and muscle function Skin and hair growth	**Deficiency** Goiter Hypothyroidism **Toxicity** "Iodine goiter" Hyperactive, enlarged goiter
Zinc (Zn)	Meat Liver Oysters Poultry Fish Whole-grain bread and cereal	Wound healing Mineralization of bone Insulin glucose regulation Normal taste	**Deficiency** Poor wound healing Reduced taste perception Alcohol/glucose intolerance Anemia Slow growth Sterility Hair loss **Toxicity** GI distress, nausea, vomiting Copper deficiency with extended use of high levels of zinc

Based on Woodrow, R. (2007). *Essentials of pharmacology for health occupations* (5th ed.), Table 11-2. Clifton Park, NY: Delmar, Cengage Learning.

ANTIOXIDANTS

free radicals
Unstable and highly reactive molecules that can cause significant cell damage.

Antioxidants are substances that cancel the effects of **free radicals**. Free radicals are the elements that may cause cellular damage, including genetic changes. Free radicals are formed in the body as a product of metabolism. Free radicals are also found in the environment from substances such as cigarette smoke, pollution, and UV rays.

Antioxidants help to protect the body's cells from damage. It is felt that the damage caused by free radicals may lead to early aging. This damage may also contribute to the development of chronic diseases such as cataracts, cancer, and heart disease. Antioxidant vitamins include vitamins C and E and beta-carotene. These can be found in fruits and vegetables, nuts, and leafy greens. Tea leaves also contain antioxidants called polyphenols, which can prevent damage to DNA, an important structure in body cells.

PHYTOCHEMICALS

Phytochemicals provide nutritional value in the form of vitamins and minerals. Some also act as antioxidants, while others can form free radicals. Phytochemicals may help to prevent cancer and other diseases. Phytochemicals may also help to reduce damage caused by toxins such as pollution and cigarette smoke.

DIETARY SUPPLEMENTS

The use of dietary supplements has gained popularity in our society. To provide a layer of protection for the public, the U.S. Congress passed the Dietary Supplement Health and Education Act (DSHEA) in 1994. This act amended the Food, Drug, and Cosmetic Act. The act required:

- The wording "dietary supplements" on all product labels

- A "Supplement Facts" panel on the labels of most dietary supplements

- Supplement manufacturers to document substantiation of their claims

- A disclaimer on labels that the dietary supplements are not drugs and receive no FDA premarket approval

- Supplement labels *may not, without prior FDA review, bear a claim that they can prevent, treat, cure, mitigate, or diagnose disease*

The act recognized dietary supplements as distinct from food additives and drugs. By doing so, the act placed the responsibility for checking the safety of dietary supplements and for determining the truthfulness of its labels on the public. *The FDA does not authorize or test dietary supplements as it does for other medications.* Once a dietary supplement is marketed, the FDA does have the responsibility, however, to show that the supplement is unsafe. If the supplement is unsafe, the FDA can then take action to restrict the supplement's use.

To aid the public in its use of herbal medications and other dietary supplements, the FDA published a report titled *A FDA Guide to Dietary Supplements* in 2000. The guide provides basic information and guidelines on dietary supplements.

Herbal medications and other dietary supplements are easily purchased in health food stores, gyms, grocery stores, drugstores, discount department stores, pharmacies and on the Internet and at other locations throughout the United States. These items are used for a variety of reasons and sometimes in very large doses.

Herbal Medications

There are numerous types of herbal medications on the market. Some are more popular than others. Table 13-3 lists some of the more common herbs with their possible uses, cautions, and interactions.

It is important for the UAP to remember that herbal medications are *not* regulated by the FDA. They do *not* have to meet federal or state

Table 13-3 Herbs

HERBS	POSSIBLE USES	POSSIBLE SIDE EFFECTS, CAUTIONS, INTERACTIONS
Aloe vera	Topical use for minor burns, shallow wound healing	Do not use on deep, surgical wounds
Black cohosh	Phytoestrogen for menopausal symptoms and premenstrual syndrome (PMS)	Can cause bradycardia Do not take with estrogen or with history of breast cancer
Capsaicin	Topical pain reliever anti-inflammatory for arthritis For post-herpetic neuralgia and neuropathy	May cause local burning sensation that may fade with time
Chamomile	Sedative tea, insomnia, nausea	Individuals allergic to pollens such as ragweed, may be allergic to this herb
Chondroitin Sulfate	Anti-inflammatory for arthritis	Occasional mild GI effects such as nausea Reliability of content varies Shark cartilage or cattle cartilage may be contaminated
Echinacea	Proven *ineffective* in 2005 studies for prevention and treatment of colds	Can cause allergies and rashes Do not use in those with autoimmune disease such as HIV, MS, or lupus, and chronic use, longer than eight weeks
Ephedra	Banned by the FDA in 2004 due to danger of heart problems and stroke	
Flaxseed oil	For constipation Source of omega-3 fatty acids Possibly anti-inflammatory	May interact with anticoagulants to cause bleeding Diarrhea possible
Feverfew	Migraine headaches, prevention and treatment	No toxic reactions known Sensitive individuals may develop dermatitis from contact with skin

(continues)

Table 13-3 Herbs—*continued*

HERBS	POSSIBLE USES	POSSIBLE SIDE EFFECTS, CAUTIONS, INTERACTIONS
Garlic	To lower blood pressure and cholesterol Anti-infective, immune enhancing	There is a risk of bleeding with anticoagulants Nausea, vomiting, diarrhea, heartburn, flatulence (gas)
Ginger	Nausea, motion sickness	Doses higher than 6 grams may cause gastric irritation
Gingko (GBE)	Improve mental function and memory in elderly and Alzheimer's patients Antidepressant, anxiolytic, antioxidant	May interact with anticoagulants to cause bleeding and strokes Rare GI upset, headache
Ginseng	Antistress, antifatigue	Do not use long-term May cause hypertension, nausea, vomiting, diarrhea, nervousness, mental changes Do not take if pregnant
Glucosamine	Anti-inflammatory for arthritis	Elevated cholesterol Resistance to insulin Increase in blood sugar
Kava	FDA warning March 2002 Banned in Canada, Germany, S. Africa and Switzerland	Possible liver damage, often irreversible; deaths reported
Licorice	Anti-infective, for cough, anti-inflammatory, menopausal symptoms, PMS, peptic ulcer—deglycyrrhizinated licorice (DGL)	Hypertension, fluid retention Do not take with diuretics
Melatonin	For insomnia, improves sleep cycle, especially with older adults and for jet lag Boosts immune system Antioxidant protection	Side effects rare, nightmares Do not take if pregnant
SAM-e	Anti-inflammatory for osteoarthritis and fibromyalgia Antidepressant	Do not take with other antidepressants Not used to treat severe depression or bipolar disorder Package must be kept airtight and in a dark container; not stable herb
Saw palmetto	For benign prostatic hypertrophy (BPH) Antiandrogen	Rare GI upset See a licensed HCP for diagnosis and treatment
Soy	Menopause symptoms Phytoestrogen Cancer-preventing qualities	No known side effects Do not take with thyroid medicine.

Table 13-3 Herbs—*continued*

HERBS	POSSIBLE USES	POSSIBLE SIDE EFFECTS, CAUTIONS, INTERACTIONS
St. John's wort	Mild to moderate depression Not for severe depression or bipolar disorder	Photosensitivity—may cause hives Insomnia, irritability, headache Do not use with other antidepressants or alcohol Interacts with warfarin, oral contraceptives, anticonvulsants, digoxin, theophylline, and other drugs
Valerian	For anxiety, insomnia	Morning-after drowsiness Do not take if pregnant Use only short term

Based on Woodrow, R. (2007). *Essentials of pharmacology for health occupations* (5th ed.), Table 11-3. Clifton Park, NY: Delmar, Cengage Learning.

Note: There are many herbs on the market today. This is only a representative list of some of the more popular herbs and those that could cause problems. Always check current, reliable references before administering to an individual. Although some of the herbs listed here have been tested for use with the medical conditions mentioned, *these herbs are not approved by the FDA. There is no guarantee that these herbs will help the condition. There is always the possibility of adverse reactions.* **Do not administer without a licensed health care provider's order.**

standards for approval. As with OTC and prescription medications, herbal medications may interact with other medications an individual is taking. Herbal medications may cause side effects, allergic reactions, or other problems. The UAP needs to report an individual's use of herbal medications to her licensed health care provider.

It is recommended that the UAP have a written licensed health care provider's order to administer herbal medications. In some states, a licensed health care provider's order is required for administration. The container of herbal medication may need to be labeled by the pharmacist or licensed health care provider who is dispensing the medication. It is the UAP's responsibility to know her state regulations and workplace policies as they apply to the administration of herbal medications.

As for all medications, the UAP should never administer a medication that she is unfamiliar with. The UAP should, therefore, find a reference on herbal medications that is best for her. The most important thing to remember is that whatever reference is used, the reference must always be available. It must also be quickly and easily understood. It is the UAP's responsibility to *never* administer a medication of which she does not have basic knowledge.

Several references which the UAP may choose to use are as follows:

- PDR for Herbal Medicines
- The Pill Book: Guide to Natural Medicines (Kindle Edition)
- The Encyclopedia of Popular Herbs
- FDA Consumer: http://www.cfsan.fda.gov/dms/supplmnt
- Herbmed: http://www.herbmed.org

SUMMARY

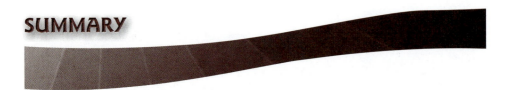

Good nutrition is a key to an individual's general health along with exercise and a healthy lifestyle. However, there are times when good nutrition is not enough to keep the body healthy. Nutritional supplements may be used to provide the additional nutrients an individual needs in her diet. The UAP can help to identify any signs of deficiency and to alert the appropriate clinicians. She can also administer dietary supplements as she would any other medication. Understanding the benefits and risks of dietary supplements will help the UAP in her daily care of individuals and in her communication with nursing staff and licensed health care providers.

WORKBOOK REVIEW

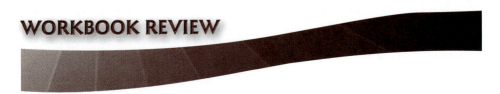

Go to the workbook and complete the exercises for Chapter 13.

REVIEW QUESTIONS

1. The vital nutrients our bodies need to function include:
   a. lipids, transfats and triglycerides
   b. electrolytes, vitamins, and minerals
   c. coffee and tea
   d. all of the above
2. Obesity:
   a. is the direct result of a disease process
   b. is on the decline in the United States
   c. is defined as a body weight of 20% or more over ideal weight for height
   d. is uncommon in children and adolescents
3. The following group of individuals would not need a vitamin and/or mineral supplement:
   a. individuals who diet
   b. healthy adults who eat a wide variety of foods
   c. women who are pregnant or breast feeding
   d. individuals with absorption disorders or deficiency diseases

4. Vitamin and mineral supplements:
   a. may be taken whenever an individual wants them
   b. can be shared with other individuals
   c. should be treated as any other prescribed medication
   d. do not have to be documented on a medication sheet

5. Vitamins are:
   a. organic substances found in plant and animal sources
   b. inorganic substances found in foods and in the earth's crust
   c. particles formed from the break down of mineral compounds in body fluids
   d. not made by an organism

6. Minerals are:
   a. organic substances found in plant and animal sources
   b. inorganic substances found in foods and in the earth's crust
   c. particles formed from the break down of mineral compounds in body fluids
   d. made by an organism

7. Electrolytes are:
   a. organic substances found in plant and animal sources
   b. inorganic substances found in foods and in the earth's crust
   c. particles formed from the break down of mineral compounds in body fluids
   d. made by an organism

8. Hypervitaminosis is:
   a. an excess of energy from taking vitamins
   b. an excess amount of vitamins in a bottle
   c. an excessive amount of a vitamin in the body that may lead to illness
   d. a lack of vitamins in the diet that may lead to illness

9. Antioxidants work to:
   a. help protect the body's cells from damage
   b. balance electrolytes in body fluids
   c. contribute to the development of chronic diseases
   d. filter oxygen from the body's cells

10. Phytochemicals:
    a. are artificial substances found in foods
    b. may act as antioxidants or form free radicals
    c. increase the damaging effects caused by toxins
    d. combine with antioxidants to form minerals

11. All of the following herbs may interact with anticoagulants to cause bleeding except:
    a. ginseng
    b. gingko
    c. flaxseed oil
    d. garlic

12. Soy:

    a. should only be used for a short time

    b. may cause high blood pressure

    c. may counteract thyroid medication

    d. may cause nightmares

CLINICAL SCENARIO

1. Mrs. Westerly's sister arrives at your workplace and gives you a bottle of OTC herbal supplements. She says that Mrs. Westerly has been taking these for the past few years and would like to keep taking them. As a UAP, what can you do with this bottle of medication?

Chapter 14
Topical Medications

Learning Objectives

After reading this chapter and completing the review questions, you should be able to:

1. Spell and define key terms.
2. List the seven main categories of topical medications.
3. Identify the action of each main category.
4. Explain the factors that affect the absorption of topical medication.
5. Compare and contrast scabicides and pediculicides.
6. Explain the importance of paying attention to detail when applying topical medication.
7. Describe antiseptics and disinfectants and their uses.

Key Terms

acne	corticosteroids	herpes zoster	photosensitivity
antifungals	Cushing's syndrome	hyperglycemia	rosacea
anti-infectives	demulcents	keratolytics	scabicides
antipruritics	disinfectants	malaise	varicella zoster
antiseptics	emollients	mucous membranes	
antivirals	glycosuria	pediculicides	
conjunctivitis	herpes simplex	perioral dermatitis	

INTRODUCTION

The skin is the largest organ of the body. Since it covers such a large area, many conditions may affect the skin. These conditions may cause discomfort, itching, and general **malaise**. Skin conditions may be mild, such as itching, or may be major, such as severe burns. The treatment of choice for most skin conditions involves the use of topical medications. This involves applying medications to a specific, local area of the body. However, there are times when oral medications or injections may be used to allow for internal treatment of the conditions. This chapter discusses topical medications.

malaise
A feeling of illness.

TOPICAL MEDICATIONS

Topical medications may be grouped into seven main categories. The medications are grouped according to the type of action they perform. These categories are:

- **Antipruritics** relieve itching.
- **Emollients** and **demulcents** soothe irritation.
- **Keratolytics** control conditions of abnormal scaling or peeling of the skin.
- **Scabicides** and **pediculicides** treat scabies or lice.
- **Antifungals** control conditions caused by fungi.
- Local **anti-infectives** prevent and treat infections.
- Medications to treat **acne**.

scabicides
Medications that treat scabies.

pediculicides
Medications that treat scabies or lice.

acne
A condition of the skin most common in adolescence and early adulthood that is usually on the face, neck, chest, back, and shoulders.

Several factors affect how fast a topical medication will be absorbed into the body. These factors include the following:

- The condition of the skin
- The area of the body where the medication is being applied
- Temperature of the skin
- The amount of moisture in the skin
- Thickness of the skin

For instance, if the skin is thick and calloused, absorption will be slower. If the skin is moist, raw, or open and warm, absorption will be faster.

To help increase the absorption of the medication, licensed health care providers may order the skin to be moistened before a medication is applied. Other times, to increase the absorption, the licensed health care provider might order plastic wrap to be placed over the ointment after it has been applied on the individual.

On occasion there may be times when the absorption needs to be slowed. During these times, the skin may be left open to the air to slow the absorption of the medication. The length of time the medication is left on the skin is very important. It is the UAP's responsibility to have a complete understanding of the directions for each topical medication *before applying it.*

Antipruritics

Antipruritics are used as a short-term treatment to relieve itching and discomfort. Antipruritics would be used to treat conditions such as:

- Dermatitis (rashes) caused by allergies or poison ivy
- Hives
- Insect bites

Adverse reactions:

- Skin irritation
- Rash
- Stinging and burning sensation
- Allergic reactions
- Sedation from antihistamines

Contraindications include the following:

- Prolonged use
- Allergies to medications belonging to the family of "caines"

Special considerations for antipruritics are as follows:

- Clean the area thoroughly before applying the medication.
- Rub the medication in gently until the medication is gone.
- Use caution if the individual has other known medication allergies.
- Do not get any of the medication near the individual's eyes or **mucous membranes**.
- Do not cover the area after applying the medication unless ordered to do so by the licensed health care provider.
- Do not use the medication any longer than what is ordered by the licensed health care provider.
- Notify the licensed health care provider immediately if the condition should worsen or irritation develops.

Refer to Table 14-1 for a further description of these medications.

mucous membranes The linings of the body cavities that open to the outside of the body.

Corticosteroids

Corticosteroids are used both topically and systemically to treat conditions of the skin. Topical medications come as ointments and creams. Corticosteroids would be used to treat conditions such as:

- Skin conditions caused by allergic reactions
- Psoriasis
- Seborrhea dermatitis

Table 14-1 Topical Medications for the Skin: Antipruritics, Corticosteroids, Emollients, Demulcents, and Keratolytics

GENERIC NAME	BRAND NAME	AVAILABLE	COMMENTS
Antipruritics			
benzocaine	Americaine, Solarcaine, Orajel	Ointment, spray, gel, lotion	Can cause hypersensitivity reaction
diphenhydramine	Benadryl, Caladryl	Lotion, cream, gel, spray	Antihistamine
dibucaine	Nupercainal	Ointment, cream	Potential for hypersensitivity
Corticosteroids			
corticosteroid	Cortaid, Topicort, Valisone, Aristocort, Synalar, others	Ointment, cream, lotion, solution	Used 1) as antipruitic to relieve itching and 2) for psoriasis and seborrhea
Emollients and Demulcents			
vitamins A and D	A & D	Ointment	
	Desitin (with zinc oxide)	Ointment	
Keratolytic			
coal tar	Zetar, Tegrin, Neutrogena	Shampoo, lotion	For dandruff, seborrheic dermatitis, or psoriasis
podophyllum	Podophyllin	Liquid	For anogenital warts; systemic toxicity possible
salicylic acid	Clearasil, Neutrogena	Cream, liquid, gel	For dandruff, psoriasis, acne, warts, corns, calluses (stains clothing)
sulfur	Many combinations with other kerolytics	Cream, lotion, shampoo	For acne, scabies, seborrheic dermatitis

Based on Woodrow, R. (2007). *Essentials of pharmacology for health occupations* (5th ed.), Table 26-1. Clifton Park, NY: Delmar, Cengage Learning.

Note: This table lists only typical medications and does not include all of those that are currently available.

Adverse reactions:

The following effects are seen especially with long term use of the medications:

- Thinning of the skin, with frequent skin tears and increased risk of infection
- Irritation of the skin
- Burning, stinging
- Ulceration
- Slow healing
- **Hyperglycemia**
- **Glycosuria**
- **Cushing's syndrome**

hyperglycemia
High level of blood sugar.

glycosuria
Sugar in the urine.

Cushing's syndrome
A condition caused by an excess amount of adrenal cortex hormones.

Contraindications include the following:

* Skin infections, bacterial or fungal infections, and cutaneous or systemic viral infections

* Open wounds

* Individuals with HIV, those on chemotherapy, or those who are otherwise immunosuppressed

* Pregnancy

* Breast feeding

* Acne, **rosacea**, or **perioral dermatitis**

rosacea
A chronic form of acne seen in adults of all ages usually on the nose, forehead, and cheeks.

perioral dermatitis
Inflammation of the skin in and/or around the mouth.

Special considerations for corticosteroids are as follows:

* Clean the area thoroughly before applying the medication.

* Rub the medication in gently until the medication is gone.

* Use caution if the individual has other known medication allergies.

* Do not get any of the medication near the individual's eyes or mucous membranes.

* Do not cover the area after applying the medication unless ordered to do so by the licensed health care provider.

* Do not use the medication any longer than what is ordered by the licensed health care provider.

* Notify the licensed health care provider immediately if the condition should worsen or irritation develops.

Refer to Table 14-1 for a further description of these medications.

Emollients and Demulcents

Emollients and demulcents are used topically to prevent or soothe minor skin conditions such as:

* Diaper rash

* Abrasions (cuts and scrapes)

* Minor burns

There are no specific adverse reactions.

Special considerations for emollients and demulcents are as follows:

* Clean the area well before applying the medication.

* Notify the licensed health care provider immediately if the area shows no sign of improvement or if the area worsens.

Refer to Table 14-1 for a further description of these medications.

Keratolytics

Keratolytic medications are used to control conditions of abnormal scaling or peeling of the skin. Keratolytic medications would be used to treat conditions such as:

- Dandruff
- Seborrhea
- Psoriasis
- Acne
- Hard corns
- Calluses
- Warts

Adverse reactions:

- Severe skin irritation
- Itching
- Stinging
- Irritation to the eyes or mucous membranes
- **Photosensitivity**
- Systemic effects in allergic individuals, such as headache, diarrhea, nausea, and vomiting

photosensitivity Sensitivity to the sun.

Contraindications include the following:

- Pregnancy
- Breast feeding
- Prolonged use
- Open wounds

Special considerations for keratolytic medications include the following:

- Use only as directed.
- Use the medication for the entire period of time that it is ordered even if the area has improved.
- Do not get any of the medication near the individual's eyes or mucous membranes.
- Do not get medication on the surrounding tissue when applying.
- If irritation occurs, notify the licensed health care provider immediately.

Refer to Table 14-1 for a further description of these medications.

Scabicides and Pediculicides

Scabies is caused by an itch mite that buries itself under the skin. Pediculosis is caused by an infestation of lice on the hairs of the scalp, pubic area, and trunk of the body. Both scabies and pediculosis are easily transmitted from individual to individual by direct and indirect contact. Indirect contact occurs through clothing or bed linens. In addition to treating these conditions with medications, all clothing and bedding must be laundered or washed in hot water or dry-cleaned.

Directions for Use:

Scabicides: Two medications are used to treat scabies. These are permethrin and lindane. The medication must be applied according to the directions on the package insert, left in place for the required amount of time, and then rinsed off thoroughly.

Pediculicides: There are also two forms of medication to treat this condition. The medications are Rid and lindane. Another name for lindane is Kwell.

Adverse reactions:

These effects rarely occur when applied topically according to the directions but may include:

conjunctivitis
The inflammation of the mucous membrane that lines the eyelids and covers the eye.

- Slight local skin irritation

- Rash

- **Conjunctivitis**

- Dermatitis with frequent application of the medication

Note: **With frequent overuse of these medications, with oral intake of them, and with inhalation of the vapors of the medication, central nervous system symptoms, hepatic toxicity, and renal toxicity may occur. Anemia and seizures have been reported with the use of lindane (Kwell). Because of the toxic effects of lindane, the individual's licensed HCP may order Stromectol to be given orally as a single dose with a repeat dose in ten (10) to fourteen(14) days. Stromectol is an oral antiparasitic medication used in an off-label fashion as an alternate medication. Stromectol is used (1) to treat large numbers of individuals infected with scabies in institutional settings and (2) to treat head lice that are resistive to standard therapy.**

Contraindications include the following:

- Do not use lindane (Kwell) if the individual is pregnant or is breast feeding.

- Do not use lindane (Kwell) in older adults and in those weighing less than 110 pounds.

- Do not use lindane (Kwell) on acutely, inflamed, raw, or draining areas

Special considerations for the scabicides and pediculicides include the following:

- Follow the directions for use carefully.

- Thoroughly launder or wash all clothing and bedding.

- Instruct the individual to inform his sexual partner(s) that he is receiving this treatment.

- Notify schools or work and day programs if head lice infestation should occur.

Refer to Table 14-2 for a further description of these medications.

Antifungals

Antifungal medications are used to treat monilial infections such as:

- Thrush

- Diaper rash

- Vaginitis

- Athlete's foot

- Jock itch

Table 14-2 Topical Medications for the Skin: Scabicides, Pediculicides, Antifungals, Antivirals, Burn Medications, and Acne Medications

GENERIC NAME	BRAND NAME	AVAILABLE	COMMENTS
Scabicides and Pediculicides			
permethrin	Acticin, Elimite	Cream	Apply from head to feet, wash off after 8–14 hours
	Nix	Liquid	Apply to hair, to remain on hair for 10 min
lindane	Kwell	Lotion, shampoo	Treat all hairy areas Toxic potential
pyrethrins	RID, RTC	Gel, shampoo	For lice only
Antifungals			
terbinafine	Lamisil	Cream, gel, spray, solution, tabs	Very effective for onychomycosis
clotrimazole	Mycelex, Lotrimin	Lozenges, cream, lotion, solution, vaginal cream, tabs	For oral, topical, or vaginal application
ketoconazole	Nizoral	Cream, shampoo	Topical antifungal, shampoo for dandruff
nystatin	Mycostatin	Oral suspension, lozenges, cream, lotion, ointment, vaginal tab, powder	Administer oral suspension or lozenges after meals, then nothing by mouth for 1 hour
tolnaftate	Tinactin	Aerosol spray, cream, powder, solution	Avoid inhaling spray or powder
Zinc undecylenate	Cruex, Desenex	Powder, soap, cream	Avoid inhaling powder

Table 14-2 Topical Medications for the Skin: Scabicides, Pediculicides, Antifungals, Antivirals, Burn Medications, and Acne Medications—*continued*

GENERIC NAME	BRAND NAME	AVAILABLE	COMMENTS
Antiviral			
acyclovir	Zovirax	Ointment, oral	Ointment is only effective for the first episode
			Oral treatment needs to begin within 72 hours of rash onset; most effective if begun within 48 hours of rash onset
valacyclovir	Valtrex	Oral	
Burn Medications			
nitrofurazone	Furacin	Cream, powder for solution	Watch for allergies
silver sulfadiazine	Silvadene	Cream	Watch for allergies
mafenide	Sulfamylon	Cream, 5% topical solution	Watch for allergies
Acne Medications			
benzoyl peroxide	Benzac, Oxy-10, Panoxyl-5 and 10	Bar, cream, gel, liquid, lotion	Antibacterial activity Drying actions, for type 1
isotretinoin	Accutane, Sotret	10, 20, 30, 40 mg caps	Absolutely contraindicated in pregnancy, for type 4 acne
salicylic acid	Clearasil,	Cream, liquid, gel	For type 1 acne
	Neutrogena	Cream, lotion	For type 1 acne

Based on Woodrow, R. (2007). *Essentials of pharmacology for health occupations* (5th ed.), Table 12-2. Clifton Park, NY: Delmar, Cengage Learning.

Note: This is a representative list. Other medications are available.

For effective treatment, the UAP must follow the licensed health care provider's order. If the order states "as directed," then the UAP must follow directions on the package insert. Good hygiene practice, including washing, drying, and exposure of the body part to air when possible, are very important to the healing process.

Note: In some states, a licensed health care provider's order that reads "as directed" is not permitted. Under this circumstance, the UAP should contact the individual's licensed HCP to obtain a HCP order that specifies the instruction(s) for use.

If the infection does not respond to treatment, the UAP needs to notify the licensed health care provider. The licensed HCP may order cultures to be done to determine the exact diagnosis and help in the selection of the appropriate medication.

Adverse reactions:

Although rare, these may include:

- Contact dermatitis
- Itching

- Burning
- Irritation

Contraindications include the following:

- Use of vaginal medications during pregnancy

Special considerations include the following:

- Carefully wash and dry the affected area.
- Expose the affected area to air whenever possible.
- With vaginitis and jock itch, do not wear tight clothing, panty-hose, or wet bathing suits.
- With athlete's foot, wear open-toed sandals instead of sneakers.
- Follow the directions carefully for application of the medication.
- Remove any stains on clothing and bedding with soap and water.
- Continue prescribed vaginal treatment even during menstruation.
- Continue treatment even if symptoms are gone. Follow the entire prescribed cycle of medication.
- Consult the licensed health care provider before using these medications during pregnancy.
- For oral medications (suspensions or lozenges), take after meals and after thorough rinsing of the mouth with water. No food or liquids for at least one (1) hour after taking the medication.
- For vaginal infections, no intercourse until the treatment is completed.
- The individual's sexual partner(s) may need to be treated if reinfection occurs.

Refer to Table 14-2 for a further description of these medications.

Anti-Infectives

Antivirals

Antiviral medications are used to treat viral infections such as:

- Cold sores or genital herpes (**herpes simplex**)
- Shingles (**herpes zoster**)
- Chickenpox (**varicella zoster**)

The medication is available in two forms: oral and ointment form.

Topical treatment is less effective than oral treatment. The ointment is not a cure and does not reduce the frequency of the outbreaks or delay the appearance of new lesions. However, the application of the ointment does decrease the duration of viral shedding, decrease pain and itching, and decrease the time it takes for crusting and healing of the lesions to occur.

It is effective in the first episode of genital herpes but shows little effect for recurrent episodes of genital herpes. The ointment needs to be applied as soon as possible, once the signs and symptoms of the infections are present.

Adverse reactions:

- Rash

- Hives

- Stinging

- Burning

- Itching

- Vulvitis

Special considerations for antiviral medications include the following:

- Do not get ointment in the eyes.

- Not effective in preventing infections.

Refer to Table 14-2 for a further description of these medications.

Antiseptics and Disinfectants

Antiseptics

antiseptics
Substances that are used to prevent or slow the growth of microorganisms.

disinfectants
Substances that can quickly kill microorganisms on any surface.

Antiseptics are substances that are used to prevent or slow the growth of microorganisms.

Although **disinfectants** are frequently too strong to be applied to the body, they are included in this group of substances. Following is a brief description of both antiseptics and disinfectants.

Antiseptics, with the exception of disinfectants, are generally applied directly to living tissue such as the skin or mucous membranes. Antiseptics can be used for:

- Cleaning and preparing the skin before injections or surgery

- Cleaning superficial skin wounds

- Irrigating the eye or body cavities

- Hand wash or surgical scrub

- Wet dressings

- Washing thermometers

Two major antiseptics in use today are chlorhexidene (Hibiclens) and povidone-iodine (Betadine). Other antiseptics include ethyl alcohol, hydrogen peroxide, and silver nitrate.

Adverse reactions of chlorhexidene (Hibiclens):

- Dermatitis and skin irritation

- Photosensitivity

- Allergic reactions, especially in the genital area

Contraindications for chlorhexidene (Hibiclens) include the following:

- Pregnancy

- Breast feeding

Special considerations for chlorhexidene (Hibiclens) include the following:

- Do not use for total body bathing.

- Do not get in the eyes and ears. If chlorhexidene accidentally enters the eyes or ears, flush immediately and call 911.

- Rinse thoroughly after use.

- Do not use on open skin lesions, mucous membranes, and genital areas.

Note: Chlorhexidene (Hibiclens) should be used on wounds involving only the superficial layer of skin. If the UAP is unsure of the depth of a wound or believes the wound is deeper than the superficial layer of skin, he is to check with his supervisor and/or the individual's licensed HCP before using Chlorhexidene (Hibiclens) on a wound.

Adverse reactions of povidone-iodine (Betadine):

- Skin irritation

- Burns

- Allergic reactions

Contraindications for povidone-iodine (Betadine) include the following:

- Known allergy to iodine

- Open wounds

Special considerations for povidone-iodine (Betadine) include the following:

- Use with caution in an individual with allergies.

- Do not get in the eyes and ears. If povidone-iodine accidentally enters the eyes or ears, flush immediately and call 911.

Disinfectants

Disinfectants can quickly kill microorganisms on any surface; however, they are typically strong enough to damage living tissue. Disinfectants are, therefore, only used directly on inanimate objects such as floors, walls, furniture, bathroom fixtures, medical and surgical instruments, and bed linens. Fungicides and germicides are types of disinfectants.

Examples of disinfectants include:

- Isopropyl alcohol, also called rubbing alcohol, used at full strength

- Lysol

- Staphene

- Household bleach

Refer to Table 14-3 for a list of common antiseptics and disinfectants.

Table 14-3 Antiseptics and Disinfectants

SUBSTANCE	BRAND NAME	USUAL CONCENTRATION	COMMON USES	COMMENTS
Ethyl alcohol		50%–70% solution	Skin antiseptic, disinfection of instruments	Not for use on open wounds; used to prepare the skin for injections; may dry skin Flammable
Isopropyl alcohol	Rubbing alcohol*	70%–95% solution	Skin antiseptic, disinfection of instruments	Not for use on open wounds; used to prepare the skin for injections; may dry skin and may prolong bleeding from injection sites Flammable
Benzalkonium chloride	Zephiran Benza	0.0025%–0.2% solution	Skin antiseptic, disinfection of instruments	Use on intact skin only
Chlorhexidine gluconate	Hibiclens Hibistat	0.5%–4% solution, liquid, foam	Antiseptic	Skin cleanser, surgical scrub, skin wound cleanser Rinse skin thoroughly
Cresol	Lysol	0.02%–50% solution, spray	Disinfectant	Use on inanimate objects only, such as contaminated linens, basins, and bedpans
Glutaraldehyde	Cidex Cidex-7	2%–3.2% solution	Disinfectant	Use on inanimate objects only
Hexachlorophene	pHisoHex Septisol	0.25%–3% topical emulsion, liquid soap, lotions, ointments, shampoos	Antiseptic	Skin scrub; rinse skin after use; may cause rash, dryness, and scaling on sensitive skin
Hydrogen peroxide		3%–6% solution	Antiseptic	Cleansing of wounds, mouthwash; store in a cool, dark place in a tightly closed container
Povidine-iodine	Betadine Operand	2%–10% aqueous solution ointment liquid scrub	Antiseptic	Topical antiseptic, surgical scrub; *check for allergies*

*Note: Common name for isopropyl alcohol.

Based on Broyles, B.E., Reiss, B.S., & Evans, M.E. (2007). *Pharmacological aspects of nursing care* (7th ed.). Table 9-1. Clifton Park, NY: Delmar, Cengage Learning.

Burn Medications

Burn treatment includes medications to prevent or treat infections. The two most commonly used medications for this purpose are silver sulfadiazine (Silvadene) and mafenide (Sulfamylon). Nitrofurazone (Furacin) is used for individuals that are allergic to sulfa. All burn medications must be applied with sterile gloved hand(s).

Adverse reactions:

- Pain
- Burning
- Itching
- Allergic reactions
- Staining of the skin (temporary)

Contraindications include the following:

- Impaired renal (kidney) or liver function
- History of allergy especially to sulfa drugs

Special considerations for burn medications include the following:

- Use sterile technique to prevent infection.
- Watch for allergic reactions.
- Keep careful intake and output records.
- Keep the burn area covered at all times with the medication and a sterile dressing.

Refer to Table 14-2 for a further description of burn medications.

Antibacterial Medications

There are many prescription and OTC antibacterial medications on the market, including ointments, creams, and solutions. In fact, there are too many to mention in this chapter. These medications have the potential to cause adverse effects, including local reactions, allergic reactions, and systemic reactions.

Adverse reactions:
Refer to the specific package insert or pharmacy information sheet that accompanies the medication.

Special considerations for antibacterial medications include the following:

- Follow the licensed health care provider's orders for application of the medication.
- If there is no improvement in the condition, the condition worsens, or there is an adverse effect that is noted, contact the licensed health care provider immediately.

Medications to Treat Acne

Acne is a condition of the skin most common in adolescence and early adulthood. Acne is usually seen on the face, neck, chest, back, and shoulders. There are four grades of acne depending on its severity. Type 1 is the least severe. Type 4 is the most severe. A brief description of the type of treatment for each grade of acne follows:

- Type 1—treated with mild OTC topical medications
- Type 2—treated with prescription topical antibiotics such as tetracycline or erythromycin
- Type 3—treated with a course of oral antibiotics such as tetracycline or erythromycin in addition to topical medications
- Type 4—treated with systemic hormones ("birth control pills") or Accutane

Two commonly used medications for acne are benzoyl peroxide and Accutane.

Adverse reactions for benzoyl peroxide:

- Skin irritation
- Mild stinging
- Redness
- Dry skin

Contraindications for benzoyl peroxide include the following:

- Pregnancy
- Breast feeding
- Skin disease, dermatitis, eczema, sunburn, and so on
- Sensitivity to benzoic acid or paraben

Special considerations for benzoyl peroxide include the following:

- Use medication every day as prescribed. Acne may actually worsen before it improves as it takes several weeks before the medication begins to work.
- Do not use with other topical acne products or retinoids.
- Avoid prolonged exposure to sunlight. Use sunscreen. Wear protective clothing. Avoid medications such as sulfa medications that make you more sensitive to the sun.
- Do not use near the eyes or mucus membranes.

Adverse reactions for Accutane:

- Inflammation of lips
- Dry skin
- Dry mouth
- Nosebleed
- Peeling
- Itching
- Photosensitivity
- Musculoskeletal pain

- Back pain
- Anorexia
- Colitis
- Increased appetite
- Nausea
- Vomiting
- Thirst
- Dizziness
- Drowsiness
- Fatigue
- Headache
- Lethargy
- Malaise
- Weakness
- Depression
- Emotional upset
- Psychosis
- Aggression
- Violent behavior
- Suicidal thought (rare)
- Decreased tolerance to contact lenses

Contraindications for Accutane include the following:

- Pregnancy
- Breast feeding
- Hypersensitivity to retinoid or paraben
- Use cautiously in individuals with psychiatric disorders
- Osteoporosis and other bone disorders
- Prolonged exposure to sunlight
- Do not drive or operate machinery at night due to decreased night vision and other visual disturbances

Special considerations for Accutane include the following:

- Use medication every day as prescribed. Acne may actually worsen before it improves, as it takes several weeks before the medication begins to work.
- Avoid cosmetic procedures to smooth the skin, including waxing, dermabrasion, or laser therapy during and for at least

six (6) months after Accutane therapy. These procedures may cause scarring while on Accutane.

- Do not take multivitamins or nutritional supplements that contain vitamin A, tetracycline antibiotics, certain antacids (those with aluminum hydroxide), and certain birth control pills (progestin-only pills).

- Use sunscreen. Wear protective clothing. Avoid medications such as sulfa medications that make you more sensitive to the sun.

- Make sure the UAP (and, if possible, the individual) receives, reads, and understands the pamphlet titled *Isotretinoin Medication Guide* every time he gets a prescription or refill for Accutane.

Note: **Accutane is absolutely contraindicated in pregnancy! There is an extremely high risk of birth defects. Prescribers, pharmacists, and individuals must agree to certain terms in a program known as the SMART program before this medication may be prescribed. The program requires women of childbearing age to (1) sign a consent form about Accutane and birth defects, (2) submit to periodic pregnancy tests, and (3) use two forms of birth control for a specified period of time.**

Refer to Table 14-2 for a further description of acne medications.

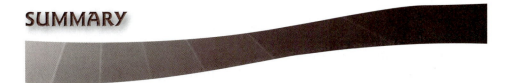

SUMMARY

Topical medications require close attention to detail. The UAP needs to know and understand not only the basic information about the medication but also the details about the application of the medication to the body. Applying the medication in an incorrect manner may result in an ineffective treatment. It may also result in harm to the individual. Remember, the first responsibility of the UAP is to keep the individual safe.

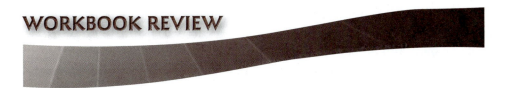

WORKBOOK REVIEW

Go to the workbook and complete the exercises for Chapter 14.

REVIEW QUESTIONS

1. Of the seven main categories of topical skin medications, which is used to treat infections caused by fungi?
   a. antipruritics
   b. scabicides and pediculicides
   c. antifungals
   d. anti-infectives

2. When determining how fast a medication will be absorbed by the skin, the following is *not* a factor:
   a. the temperature of the skin
   b. the weight of the individual
   c. the amount of moisture in the skin
   d. the thickness of the skin

3. A medication's absorption into the skin will be slower if:
   a. the skin is moist
   b. the skin is thick and calloused
   c. the skin is left open to the air
   d. the skin is warm

4. Antipruritics are used to:
   a. relieve itching and discomfort
   b. treat psoriasis
   c. soothe minor skin irritations
   d. treat fungal infections

5. Corticosteroids are prescribed for:
   a. treating hives and insect bites
   b. treating skin conditions caused by allergies or seborrhea
   c. treating scabies and lice
   d. treating infections

6. Emollients and demulcents are applied to:
   a. athlete's foot and jock itch
   b. dandruff and warts
   c. psoriasis and dermatitis
   d. abrasions, minor burns, and minor skin conditions

7. Keratolytics are used:
   a. for abnormal scaling or peeling of the skin
   b. to relieve itching
   c. to control conditions caused by fungi
   d. for treating lice

8. Scabies and pediculosis are different because:
   a. pediculosis is caused by mites buried in the skin, while scabies is an infestation of lice in the hair
   b. pediculosis is primarily on the feet, while scabies is on the trunk of the body

     c. scabies are mites buried in the skin, while pediculosis is an infestation of lice in the hair

     d. scabies cause an itch, but pediculosis causes a rash

9. When treating an infection with an antifungal medication:

     a. the area is to be washed, dried, and wrapped with a sterile dressing

     b. the area is to be rubbed vigorously to increase circulation

     c. the entire cycle of medication must be completed for treatment to be effective

     d. the individual with athlete's foot should wear closed-toe shoes

10. If the licensed health care provider's order for a topical medication states "as directed," the UAP should:

     a. apply the medication according to the directions of her coworker

     b. apply the medication according to the directions on the package insert accompanying the medication to be administered

     c. apply the medication according to the directions of his supervisor

     d. not apply the medication at all

11. Which statement is true about chlorhexidene (Hibiclens)?

     a. may be used to cleanse deep wounds

     b. does not cause photosensitivity

     c. must be rinsed off thoroughly

     d. is used as an alcohol hand sanitizer

12. Accutane may be used to treat acne in the following group of individuals:

     a. healthy adolescents

     b. pregnant women

     c. individuals with a major psychiatric disorder

     d. women with osteoporosis

CLINICAL SCENARIOS

1. Mrs. Salino has complained of itching and discomfort on her legs. Her licensed health care provider has seen her and diagnosed her with poison ivy. What type of topical medication do you think the licensed health care provider will prescribe? List the special considerations for this type of topical medication.

2. Mr. Foley has been diagnosed with a case of athlete's foot. What type of topical medication will the licensed health care provider prescribe? List five special considerations for topical medications used to treat athlete's foot.

Chapter 15
Eye and Ear Medications

Learning Objectives

After reading this chapter and completing the review questions, you should be able to:

1. Spell and define terms.

2. Discuss the uses, adverse reactions, and special considerations for various medications used to treat disorders of the eye.

3. Discuss the uses, adverse reactions, and special considerations for various medications used to treat disorders of the ear.

Key Terms

analgesics	aqueous humor	mydriatics	otitis media
anesthetics	blood dyscrasias	myopia	ototoxicity
antibacterials	glaucoma	nonsteroidal	phytophobia
anti-inflammatory medications	intraocular pressure	anti-inflammatory medications (NSAIDs)	wax emulsifiers
	miotics		

INTRODUCTION

The eyes can be susceptible to many different disorders caused by both internal and external factors. This chapter discusses five categories of medications used to treat disorders of the eye:

- Anti-infectants
- Anti-inflammatory medications
- Antiglaucoma medications

- Mydriatics
- Local anesthetics

otitis media
An infection of the middle ear.

The most common disorder of the ear is **otitis media**. Otitis media is a middle-ear infection that occurs mainly in children; however, otitis media also occurs in adults. Causes of otitis media include:

- Dental caries
- Water sports
- Infection due to foreign objects in the ear
- Injury to the tympanic membrane in the ear

This chapter discusses six categories of medications used to treat disorders of the ear:

- Antibacterials
- Antifungals
- Anti-inflammatory medications
- Local anesthetics
- Local analgesics
- Wax emulsifiers

EYE MEDICATIONS
Anti-Infectives

Anti-infective medications are used to treat bacterial infections in the eye. To make sure that the right medication is used, it is important for the licensed health care provider to first find out the cause of the infection. Once this is done, the licensed health care provider will order the specific medication and treatment for the individual.

Adverse reactions:

- Blurred vision
- Conjunctivitis
- Hives in an individual with an allergy to the medication
- Local burning
- Rash
- Stinging

Contraindications include the following:

- Individuals allergic to the medication
- Viral and fungal disease of the eye

Special considerations for these medications include the following:

- If there is no improvement in two (2) to three (3) days of treatment, the UAP should notify the individual's licensed health care provider.

- Administer the medication into the lower pocket of the eye. Do so carefully. Do not contaminate the tip of the eyedropper. Refer to Procedure 7-2 in Chapter 7 for a review of administration of eye medications.

- Hold the medication and notify the individual's licensed HCP immediately if the individual complains of burning and itching in the eye. If the licensed HCP does not respond to the call within a short period of time, send the individual to the urgent care center or emergency medical center for care.

- Frequently remind the individual to follow good handwashing practice. Good handwashing will help to prevent the spread of infection.

- Instruct the individual to not use makeup or wear contact lenses while being treated for infections.

- When administering more than one ophthalmic medication at the same time, administer the thickest medication last. In other words, administer liquid eyedrops before administering an eye ointment.

Table 15-1 gives a list of anti-infectives by generic and brand names with usual concentration.

Table 15-1 Anti-Infective Ophthalmic Medications by Generic and Brand Names with Usual Concentration

GENERIC NAME	BRAND NAME	USUAL CONCENTRATIONS
Ciproflaxin	Cipro	Ointment 3.5 g tube Solution 2.5 mL and 5 mL per dispenser
Erythromycin	Ilosone EES	Ointment 2%
Gentamycin	Garamycin	Ointment 0.1% Solution 0.3%
Polymixin B	Neosporin Opthalmic AK-Spore	Solution
Sulfacetamide sodium	AK-Sulf Bleph-10 Klaron Ocul-Sul	Ointment 10% Solution 10%, 15%, 30% in dropper bottles
Tobramycin	Tobrex	Ointment 0.3% Solution 0.3%

Note: This is a representative list of anti-infective ophthalmic medications.

Source: Based on Woodrow, R. (2007). *Essentials of pharmacology for health occupations* (5th ed.), Table 18-1. Clifton Park, NY: Delmar, Cengage Learning.

Anti-Inflammatory Medications

Anti-inflammatory medications are used to relieve inflammation of the eye from allergic reactions, burns, or irritation from a foreign substance.

Corticosteroids

Corticosteroids are used both as an anti-inflammatory medication and for an acute eye injury to prevent scarring.

Adverse reactions:

- Corneal ulcerations
- Decreased resistance to other bacterial, viral, or fungal infections
- Delayed healing of corneal wounds
- Increased **intraocular pressure**
- Stinging, burning, or eye pain
- Thinning of the cornea

intraocular pressure
The pressure within the eyeball.

Contraindications include the following:

- Acute bacterial, viral, or fungal infections
- Breast feeding
- Pregnancy
- Primary open-angle glaucoma
- Prolonged use

Special considerations for the use of corticosteroids include the following:

- When administering the medication, gently press on the inner corner of the eye after applying the medication. This decreases the systemic absorption of this medication. Refer to Chapter 7 for a review of administration of eye medications.
- Discard medication when treatment is completed. Do not use left-over medication for a new eye inflammation. For new inflammation, contact the individual's licensed health care provider for a new prescription.

Table 15-2 gives a list of corticosteroids by generic and brand names with dosage information.

Nonsteroidal Anti-inflammatory Medications (NSAIDs)

Nonsteroidal anti-inflammatory medications (NSAIDs) are used to treat inflammation of the eye after cataract surgery. NSAIDs are not usually used to treat other eye disorders. NSAIDs are used, however, as an alternate to corticosteroids when needed.

Contraindications include the following:

- Individuals with an allergy to aspirin and/or NSAIDs

Table 15-2 Anti-inflammatory Ophthalmic Medications by Generic and Brand Names with Dosage Information

GENERIC NAME	BRAND NAME	DOSAGE INFORMATION
Corticosteroids		
fluorometholone	FML	Ointment, suspension; varies with condition
prednisolone	Econopred, Pred Forte	Ointment, solution, suspension; varies with condition
	Many combinations with antibiotics	Ointment, solution, suspension; varies with condition
dexamethasone	Many combinations with antibiotics	Ointment, solution, suspension; varies with condition
Nonsteroidal Anti-inflammatory Drugs		
flubiprofen	Ocufen	Solution; varies with condition
ketorolac	Acular	Solution; varies with condition

Follow directions carefully! Do not use for longer than prescribed.

This table does not include all anti-inflammatory ophthalmic medications on the market.

Based on Woodrow, R. (2007). *Essentials of pharmacology for health occupations* (5th ed.), Table 18-1. Clifton Park, NY: Delmar, Cengage Learning.

Refer to Table 15-2 for a list of nonsteroidal anti-inflammatory medications by generic and brand names with dosage information.

Antiglaucoma Medications

Glaucoma is a condition of the eye in which there is increased intraocular pressure due to a blockage of the outflow of the fluid in the eye known as **aqueous humor**. Antiglaucoma medications are given to lower intraocular pressure.

aqueous humor
A clear, watery fluid that fills the eye.

Carbonic Anhydrase Inhibitors (CAIs)

Carbonic anhydrase inhibitors (CAIs) (1) decrease the amount of aqueous humor that is made by the body and (2) have a diuretic effect. This medication is administered orally.

Adverse reactions:

- **Blood dyscrasias**
- Confusion
- Constipation
- Diarrhea
- Drowsiness
- Fatigue
- Hepatic (liver) and renal (kidney) disorders
- Muscular weakness
- Nausea
- Numbness
- Photosensitivity

blood dyscrasias
An abnormal condition of the elements (parts) of the blood or of parts needed for clotting of the blood.

- Seizures
- Taste alteration
- Thirst
- Tingling
- Vomiting

Contraindications include the following:

- Breast feeding
- COPD
- Diabetes
- Liver or kidney disorders
- Pregnancy

Special considerations include the following:

- Report side effects to the individual's licensed HCP.
- Check with the individual's licensed HCP before the individual begins any new medication including OTCs and herbal medications.

Refer to Table 15-3 for a list of carbonic anhydrase inhibitors (CAIs) by generic and brand names with dosage information.

Miotics

Miotics work by contracting the pupil. Miotics reduce intraocular pressure by increasing the outflow of aqueous humor.

Adverse reactions:

- Blurred vision
- Bradycardia (pulse below 60)
- Bronchospasm
- Diarrhea
- Eye pain
- Headache
- Hypotension
- Increased sweating and salivation
- Increased tearing
- Local reactions
- **Myopia**
- Nausea
- **Photophobia**
- Poor vision in dim light
- Systemic reactions
- Twitching, stinging, and burning of the eye
- Vomiting

myopia
Nearsightedness.

photophobia
Sensitivity to light.

Table 15-3 Antiglaucoma Medications by Generic and Brand Names with Dosage Information

GENERIC NAME	BRAND NAME	DOSAGE INFORMATION
Carbonic Anhydrase Inhibitors		
acetazolamide	Diamox	Capsule, tablet 250–500 mg 4×/day (max 1 g/day)
dorzolamide	Trusopt	Ophthalmic solution, 1 gtt three times a day
Miotics		
*pilocarpine HCl	Isopto Carpine, Pilocar	Ophthalmic solution 0.25–8%, dose varies
pilocarpine gel	Pilopine HS	Ophthalmic gel 4% at bedtime
Beta-Adrenergic Blockers		
timolol	Timoptic, Timoptic-XE	Ophthalmic solution gel 0.25–0.5%, 1 gtt twice a day
timolol w/dorzolamide	Cosopt	Ophthalmic solution 1 gtt twice a day
betaxolol	Betoptic, Betoptic-S	Ophthalmic solution 0.5%, suspension 0.25% 1–2 gtt twice a day
Sympathomimetic		
dipivefrin	Propine	Ophthalmic solution 0.1%, 1 gtt q12h
Alpha Agonist		
brimonidine	Alphagan-P	Ophthalmic solution 0.15%, 1 gtt three times a day (8 hours apart)
Prostaglandin Analogs		
latanoprost	Xalatan	Ophthalmic solution 0.005%, 1 gtt at bedtime
travoprost	Travatan	Ophthalmic solution 0.004%, 1 gtt at bedtime

*Wide variation in strengths available. Check carefully for correct percentage.

Other antiglaucoma agents and combination drugs are available. This is a representative list.

Based on Woodrow, R. (2007). *Essentials of pharmacology for health occupations* (5th ed.), Table 18-2. Clifton Park, NY: Delmar, Cengage Learning.

Contraindications include the following:

- Acute inflammatory process
- Angle-closure glaucoma
- Corneal abrasion
- History of retinal detachment or retinal degeneration
- Use of soft contact lenses

Special considerations for miotics include the following:

- When administering the medication, apply gentle pressure to the inner corner of the eye after applying the medication. This decreases the systemic absorption of this medication. Refer to Procedure 7-2 in Chapter 7 for a review of administration of eye medications.
- Medication may cause temporary blurring of vision.
- Report any reactions to the licensed HCP for possible dosage adjustment.

- Give this medication before bedtime to reduce side effects.
- Do not drive at night.

Refer to Table 15-3 for a list of miotics by generic and brand names with dosage information.

Beta-Adrenergic Blockers

Timolol (Timoptic) is used to lower intraocular pressure in open-angle glaucoma by decreasing the production of aqueous humor.

Adverse reactions:

- Aggravation of preexisting cardiovascular or pulmonary disorders
- Changes to blood pressure and pulse
- Conjunctivitis
- Double vision
- Irritation of the eye

Contraindications include the following:

- Asthma and COPD
- Breast feeding
- Closed-angle glaucoma
- Diabetes
- Hyperthyroidism
- Individuals taking oral beta-blocker medications
- Individuals with sulfonamide allergy
- Pregnancy
- Pulse less than 60 beats per minute

Special considerations include the following:

- Check with the individual's licensed HCP before the individual begins any new medications including OTCs and herbal medications.
- Report any reactions to the licensed HCP for possible dosage adjustment.

Refer to Table 15-3 for a list of beta-adrenergic blockers by generic and brand names with dosage information.

Sympathomimetics

Sympathomimetics work to dilate the pupils. These medications (1) decrease the amount of aqueous humor made by the body and (2) increase the flow of aqueous humor from the eye. Sympathomimetics mimic the actions of the sympathetic nervous system.

Adverse reactions:

- Allergic reactions such as dermatitis and edema
- Blurred vision

- Burning

- Headache

- Pain

- Photophobia

- Stinging

- Systemic effects, including palpitations, tachycardia, and tremors

Contraindications include the following:

- Cardiac disorders

- Cerebral arteriosclerosis

- Diabetes

- Hypertension

- Narrow-angle glaucoma

- Thyroid disorders

Special considerations include:

- Do not drive after administration of medication.

- Do not use the solution if the solution becomes cloudy, changes color, or is different in any other way.

- Medication may cause temporary blurring of vision.

- Report any reactions to the licensed HCP for possible dosage adjustment.

- Store medication in a tightly closed container.

- Wear sunglasses to decrease sensitivity to light.

Refer to Table 15-3 for a list of sympathomimetics by generic and brand names.

Alpha Agonists

A medication called Brimonidine (Alphagan-P) decreases the amount of aqueous humor made by the body while having minimal effect on the cardiovascular and pulmonary systems. Brimonidine (Alphagan-P) is an alternate medication for individuals who are unable to use beta-blocker topical medications.

Adverse reactions:

- Dizziness

- Headache

The only special consideration for the use of Brimonidine (Alphagan-P) is the following:

- Report any reactions to the licensed HCP for possible dosage adjustment.

Refer to Table 15-3 for a list of alpha agonists by generic and brand names with dosage information.

Prostaglandin Analogs

A medication called latanoprost (Xalatan) causes the greatest reduction in intraocular pressure by increasing the outflow of aqueous humor.

Adverse reactions:

- Blurred vision

- Burning and stinging in the eye

- Change in length, thickness, and pigmentation of eyelashes

- Slow, gradual change in the color of the iris (may be permanent)

- Systemic effects, including upper respiratory tract infection and muscle and joint pain

Contraindications include the following:

- Breast feeding

- Contact lens wearers

- Hepatic (liver) and renal (kidney) disease

- Pregnancy

Special considerations for the use of Xalatan include the following:

- Refrigerate the unopened bottle. Once the bottle is opened, it can be stored at room temperature for up to six (6) weeks.

- Report any reactions, including changes in iris color, to the licensed HCP.

- Remove contact lenses before administration of the medication. Wait at least fifteen (15) minutes before reinserting contact lenses.

Refer to Table 15-3 for a list of prostaglandin analogs by generic and brand names with dosage information.

Mydriatics

Mydriatics are used to dilate the pupil prior to an ophthalmic exam.

Adverse reactions:

- Blurred vision (common)

- Confusion (caution in older adults)

- Dryness of skin

- Fever

- Flushing

- Increased intraocular pressure

- Local irritation, with short-lived burning sensation

Contraindications include glaucoma.

Special considerations for the use of mydriatics include the following:

- Use a sterile technique when giving this medication to avoid contamination of the medication.

- When administering the medication, apply gentle pressure to the inside corner of the eye. This will decrease the chance for systemic absorption of the medication. Refer to Procedure 7-2 in Chapter 7 for a review of administration of eye medications.

- Store medication in a tightly closed container.

- Do not use the solution if the solution becomes cloudy, changes color, or is different in any other way.

- Expect blurred vision and sensitivity to light with this medication. Wear dark glasses or stay out of the light.

- Do not drive while under the effect of the medication.

Refer to Table 15-4 for a list of mydriatics by generic and brand names, along with comments for use.

Local Anesthetics

Local **anesthetics** are applied to the eye topically before a minor surgical procedure. These medications are also used when removing foreign bodies from the eye or to decrease pain from a painful injury.

Adverse reactions are rare but may include anaphylaxis in an individual who is allergic to local anesthetics.

Contraindications include prolonged use.

Special considerations for the use of local anesthetics are as follows:

- Apply an eye patch after application of these medications to protect the eye. These medications cause the eye to lose its blink reflex.

- Remind the individual not to touch or rub her eye until the anesthetic has worn off.

Table 15-4 Mydriatics and Local Anesthetics for the Eye by Generic and Brand Names with Dosage Information

GENERIC NAME	BRAND NAME	DOSAGE INFORMATION	COMMENTS
Mydriatics			
*atropine	Atropine	Ointment, solution 0.5–2%	Administered 40–60 min before exam
*cyclopentolate	Cyclogyl	Ophthalmic solution 0.5–2%	
*phenylephrine	Neo-Synephrine	Ophthalmic solution 0.12%, 2.5%, 10%	Check carefully for percent
Local Anesthetics			
tetracaine	Pontocaine	Solution 0.5%	Apply eye patch
proparacaine	Ophthetic	Solution 0.5%	Apply eye patch

Wide variations in strengths available. Check carefully for correct percentage!

Based on Woodrow, R. (2007). *Essentials of pharmacology for health occupations* (5th ed.), Table 18-3. Clifton Park, NY: Delmar, Cengage Learning.

Refer to Table 15-4 for a list of local anesthetics by generic and brand names, along with comments for use.

Miscellaneous

At times, individuals who are comatosed, have allergies, or have a neurological disorder produce fewer tears. Fewer tears results in dry eyes and eye irritation, leading to itching and discomfort. To relieve these symptoms, a licensed HCP may order a lubricating solution (artificial tears) to be administered in the eyes. Artificial tears are also used for individuals wearing contact lenses or who have artificial eyes.

Names of several common brands of artificial tears include the following:

- Isopto Tears
- Lacril
- Tearisol
- Tears Naturale
- Visine (OTC)

Artificial tears are considered medications. These are administered and documented in the same manner and fashion as are all medications, OTCs, and herbal medications.

EAR MEDICATIONS
Antibacterials

Although otic **antibacterials** are available, the first-line treatment for ear infections is systemic antimicrobials taken preferably by mouth. This is due to the risk for **ototoxicity** from otic antibacterials administered into the ear. There are also topical forms of many antibiotics that may be applied to the outer ear.

Refer to Table 15-5 for a list of otic antibacterials by generic and brand names with adverse reactions.

ototoxicity
Damage to the eight cranial nerve and the organs of hearing and balance.

Antifungals

Otic antifungal medications are used to treat fungal infections and some bacterial infections of the ear.

Refer to Table 15-5 for a list of otic antifungals by generic and brand names with adverse reactions.

Anti-Inflammatory Medications

Otic anti-inflammatory medications are used to decrease redness, swelling, and pain caused by the body's reaction to infection. This provides the individual with comfort as the antimicrobial medication fights off the infection.

Table 15-5 Otic Medications with Generic and Brand Names with Adverse Reactions

OTIC MEDICATIONS	GENERIC NAME	BRAND NAME	ADVERSE REACTIONS
Antibacterials	Ciprofloxacin/hydrocortisone	Cipro-HC	Headache (rare)
	Polymyxin B	Neomycin	
		Cortisporin	Ototoxicity
	Ofloxacin	Floxin Otic	Itching on application
Antifungals	Acetic acid/hydrocortisone	VoSol HC	Burning and stinging on administration
Anti-inflammatory medications	1% hydrocortisone		
Local anesthetics and Local analgesics	Pramoxine and benzocaine (a combination medication)	Allergen	Allergic reaction to the local anesthetic
		Auralgan	
		Aurodex	
Wax Emulsifiers	Carbamide peroxide 6.5%	Debrox	Allergic reaction
		Murine Ear Wax Removal System	
		Bausch & Lomb Wax Removal System	

Note: This is a representative list of otic medications.

Source: Based on Broyles, B. E., Reiss, B. S., & Evans, M. E. (2007), *Pharmacological aspects of nursing care* (7th ed.). Table 18-4. Clifton Park, NY: Delmar Cengage Learning.

Refer to Table 15-5 for a list of otic anti-inflammatory medications by generic and brand names with adverse reactions.

Local Anesthetics and Local Analgesics

Otic local anesthetics and local **analgesics** are used in combination to treat congestion, pain, and swelling. These medications do not rid the body of infection; therefore, an antimicrobial medication is usually ordered along with these medications. It is best to warm these drops before administering them.

Refer to Table 15-5 for a list of otic local anesthetics and local analgesics by generic and brand names with adverse reactions.

Wax Emulsifiers

Wax emulsifiers are commonly used to remove a buildup of wax from an individual's ear(s). Drops of medication are administered into the ear(s) as per the licensed HCP order. The medication loosens the wax, permitting the wax to drain from the ear canal by gravity. The ear(s) then can be washed out in the bath or shower. The individual's licensed HCP may order the procedure to be repeated every one (1) to two (2) weeks.

Special considerations include the following:

- Warm the otic solution in a bowl of warm water to body temperature before administering the medication.
- Never use a cotton-tipped applicator (Qtip) in the ear.

Refer to Table 15-5 for a list of wax emulsifiers by generic and brand names with adverse reactions.

SUMMARY

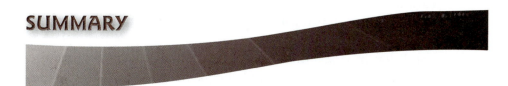

There are many different types of eye and ear medications available to treat various disorders. It is the UAP's responsibility to have a basic understanding of these disorders and medications. Doing so will help the UAP to give eye and ear medications safely and effectively.

WORKBOOK REVIEW

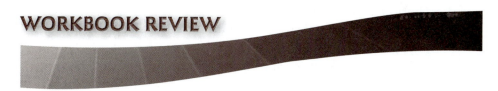

Go to the workbook and complete the exercises for Chapter 15.

REVIEW QUESTIONS

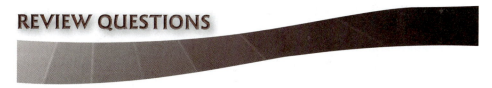

1. When giving eye medications using a tube or a dropper, it is important to:
   a. get it all over the surface of the eye
   b. squeeze the medication carefully into the lower pocket of the eye to prevent contaminating the tip of the eyedropper or tube of medication
   c. let the medication run into the other eye
   d. let the individual rub off the excess medication with her hand
2. When treating eye infections, improvement should be seen within:
   a. two (2) to three (3) days
   b. three (3) to five (5) days
   c. five (5) to seven (7) days
   d. seven (7) to ten (10) days

3. NSAIDs are used in eye disorders to:
   a. treat bacterial infections
   b. treat inflammation after cataract surgery
   c. reduce increased intraocular pressure
   d. prevent scarring in an acute eye injury

4. To reduce systemic absorption of eye medications, the UAP should instruct the individual to:
   a. apply gentle pressure to the inside corner of the eye
   b. rub her eyes after the medication is applied
   c. wear an eye patch
   d. let the medication run from one eye into the other

5. Glaucoma is:
   a. a condition in which there is increased intraocular pressure due to obstruction of the outflow of aqueous humor
   b. a condition of double vision
   c. another name for a bacterial infection of the eye
   d. another name for inflammation of the eye

6. A miotic medication will cause:
   a. dilation of the pupil
   b. contraction of the pupil
   c. swelling of the conjunctiva
   d. irritation of the eyelid

7. The antiglaucoma medication Xalatan, if unopened, must be stored:
   a. in the locked storage area
   b. at room temperature for six (6) weeks
   c. in the refrigerator
   d. in the freezer

8. A mydriatic medication will cause:
   a. dilation of the pupil
   b. contraction of the pupil
   c. swelling of the conjunctiva
   d. irritation of the eyelid

9. Local anesthetics are applied to the eye for:
   a. treatment of glaucoma
   b. treatment of infections
   c. contraction of the pupils
   d. removal of foreign bodies

10. An individual who has been given a local anesthetic on her eye should:
    a. wear an eye patch because of loss of the blink reflex
    b. hold her hand over her eye to protect it
    c. rub her eyes until the anesthetic wears off
    d. all of the above

11. Before administering a wax emulsifier, the UAP should:
    a. cool the medication by placing it in the refrigerator for ten (10) minutes
    b. have the individual lie flat on her back

c. warm the medication in a bowl of warm water to body temperature

d. set up a sterile field

12. An individual has a severe earache. What type of medication will the individual's licensed HCP order?

a. otic antifungal

b. otic antibacterial

c. otic local anesthetic with a local analgesic

d. antiviral

CLINICAL SCENARIOS

1. Robert Bern, a 35-year-old gentleman with Down syndrome, has been pulling at his right ear. When you speak to him, he appears to be ignoring you. Lately Robert has been watching TV with the volume turned up louder than usual. Today when you entered Robert's bedroom, you noticed that he was attempting to clean his ears with the tip of a pen. The tip of the pen is full of earwax.

a. What steps should you take to care for Robert?
Robert's licensed HCP orders a wax emulsifier, two drops of Debrox in each ear, to be administered every morning and every evening for two (2) days. On the third day, Robert is to have his ears irrigated (flushed).

b. What is your role as a UAP in the administration of Robert's Debrox and ear irrigation?

Chapter 16
Psychotropic Medications

Learning Objectives

After reading this chapter and completing the review questions, you should be able to:

1. Spell and define terms.
2. Describe the five classes of psychotropic medications.
3. Discuss the uses, adverse reactions, and special considerations for selected psychotropic medications.
4. Describe extrapyramidal symptoms, psuedoparkinsonism, and tardive dyskinesia.

Key Terms

agoraphobia

akathisia

anorexia

antianxiety medications

antidepressant medications

antimanic medications

antipsychotic medications

anxiety

ataxia

bipolar disorder

bradykinesia

carpopedal spasm

central nervous system (CNS) stimulants

diaphoresis

dyspepsia

dystonia

dysuria

edema

extrapyramidal symptoms

hypertensive crisis

hysteroid dysphoria

mental health

mydriasis

narcolepsy

neuroleptics

nystagmus

oculogyric crisis

orthostatic hypotension

paralytic ileus

polyuria

protrusion

pseudoparkinsonism

psychotic behavior

psychotropic medications

purpura

tardive dyskinesia

torticollis

trismus

INTRODUCTION

When defining the term **mental health**, it can be said that this is the overall health or well-being of the mind. An individual's mental health can affect his physical and emotional well-being. If there is a problem with the well-being of the mind, an individual may experience a physical, mental, or emotional disorder or illness. While the exact cause of mental illness is not known, it may be inherited genetically from parents or grandparents or brought on by biochemical changes in the brain. The environment and certain medications or drugs may also be factors.

PSYCHOTROPIC MEDICATIONS

psychotropic medications
Medications that affect the function, behavior, or experience of the mind.

Psychotropic medications affect the function, behavior, or experience of the mind. These medications are ordered by the licensed health care provider to reduce and control symptoms of mental or emotional illness. Psychotropic medications are not a cure that will make the illness go away. These medications do, however, help to manage the effects of mental or emotional illness in an individual's life. Psychotropic medications are usually used in combination with other treatments, including counseling or psychotherapy.

There are five classes of psychotropic medications:

* Medications for the treatment of ADHD, ADD, and narcolepsy

* **Antianxiety medications**, medications that counteract or relieve anxiety

* **Antidepressant medications**, medications that improve an individual's mood

* **Antimanic medications**, medications that treat the manic phase of bipolar disorder

* **Antipsychotic medications**, also called **neuroleptics**, that modify **psychotic behavior**

psychotic behavior
A significant distortion of reality that affects an individual's ability to function in daily life.

Medications for the Treatment of ADHD, ADD, and Narcolepsy

Central Nervous System (CNS) Stimulants
Central nervous system (CNS) stimulants are medications that improve the function of the central nervous system. These medications are used to treat (1) attention-deficit/hyperactivity disorder (ADHD) and attention deficit disorder without hyperactivity (ADD) and (2) **narcolepsy**.

Adverse reactions:

narcolepsy
Uncontrolled attacks of drowsiness or sleep during the daytime.

* Abdominal pain

* Anorexia

* Blurred vision

* Cardiac arrythmias

- Dizziness
- Dry mouth
- Headache
- Hypertension
- Nausea
- Nervousness
- Insomnia
- Irritability
- Seizures
- Psychosis from overdose
- Palpitations
- Tachycardia
- Tolerance and physical dependence with prolonged use
- Vomiting

Contraindications include the following:

- Treatment for obesity
- Individuals with anxiety or agitation
- History of drug dependence, alcoholism, or eating disorders
- Hyperthyroidism
- Cardiovascular disorders
- Closed-angle glaucoma
- Pregnancy
- Breast feeding
- Abrupt withdrawal (depression may result)
- Use with MAOIs

Special considerations for CNS stimulants are as follows:

- Individuals using CNS stimulants should be warned about the potential for abuse.
- Medication should be taken only as prescribed by an individual's licensed HCP.
- Medication should be taken early in the day to decrease insomnia.
- Do not stop abruptly. Doing so may cause depression, irritability, fatigue, agitation, and disturbed sleep.
- Observe older adults for possible dangerous cardiovascular side effects.
- Sustained-release medication are not to be chewed or crushed.
- Individuals need to get regular sleep in sufficient amounts.

Modafinil (Provigil)

Modafinil (provigil) is a new psychostimulant medication used for the treatment of (1) narcolepsy, (2) sleep apnea, and (3) shift-work sleep disorder in adults and adolescence over sixteen (16) years of age. The medication does not appear to be effective in treating adults with ADHD or in aiding in weight loss.

Adverse reactions are infrequent:

- Headache
- Nausea

Contraindication is allergy to the medication.
Special considerations for Modafinil (provigil) are as follows:

- Administer without food.
- Report the individual's response to the medication to his licensed HCP.

Strattera (Atomoxetine)

Strattera (atomoxetine) is the first nonstimulant medication to treat ADHD. Strattera is a selective norepinephrine reuptake inhibitor (SNRI). This medication has been shown to be effetive in adolescents and adults with ADHD and does not have a potential for abuse.

Adverse reactions:

- Constipation
- Decrease appetite
- Dry mouth
- **Dyspepsia** (upset stomach)
- Fatigue
- Nausea
- Possible suicidal tendencies (black box warning)
- Urinary hesitation
- Urinary retention
- Vomiting

Contraindications include the following:

- Allergy to medication
- Closed-angle glaucoma
- Cerebrovascular disease
- Heart disease
- Hepatic (liver) disease
- MAOI use within the past fourteen (14) days

Special considerations for Strattera (atomoxetine) are as follows:

- Medication should be taken in single morning dose or in divided doses in early morning and late afternoon to decrease insomnia.

Table 16-1 Selected Medications for the Treatment of ADHD, ADD, and Narcolepsy by Generic and Brand Names with Dosage Information

GENERIC NAME	BRAND NAME	DOSAGE INFORMATION	COMMENTS
amphetamines	Adderall	Oral 5–30 mg daily-twice a day	For narcolepsy, ADHD, ADD
	Adderall XR	Oral 5–30 mg daily	
methylphenidate	Ritalin	Oral 5–20 mg two-three times a day	For narcolepsy, ADHD, ADD, senile apathy, major depression
	Ritalin SR	Oral 10–20 mg two-three times a day	
	Metadate ER	(Note 8-hour duration of action)	For once-daily treatment of ADHD or ADD
	Medadate CD	Oral 20–60 mg every morning	
	Ritalin LA	Oral 18–54 mg every morning	Extended release tablet for once-daily treatment of ADD, ADHD, extended release tablet
	Concerta	Oral 18–54 mg every morning	
modafinil	Provigil	Oral 100–400 mg daily	For narcolepsy, sleep apnea, and shift-work sleep disorder
SNRI			
atomoxetine	Strattera	Oral 20–50 mg twice a day	For ADHD (black box warning: suicidal tendencies)

Based on Woodrow, R. (2007). *Essentials of pharmacology for health occupations* (5th ed.), Table 20-1. Clifton Park, NY: Delmar, Cengage Learning.

- Individuals need to establish an effective bedtime routine.
- Tell the individual taking Strattera that he should not drive or operate machinery while taking this medication.
- To decrease GI upset, encourage the individual to eat small, frequent meals and drink plenty of fluids.

Table 16-1 gives a list of selected medications for the treatment of ADHD, ADD, and narcolepsy by generic and brand names with dosage information.

Antianxiety Medications

Anxiety is a general feeling of worry or dread. Signs of anxiety include:

- Heart palpitations
- Chest pain
- Nausea
- Loss of appetite
- Upset stomach
- Tightness in the throat and skeletal muscles

- Hands that are shaking, sweating, or cold
- Feelings of tension
- Nervousness
- Indecisiveness
- Inability to sleep

If the feeling of anxiety affects an individual's ability to function, then the licensed health care provider may prescribe an antianxiety medication. Antianxiety medication is useful for short-term treatment of the following:

- Anxiety disorders
- Psychosomatic disorders
- Insomnia
- Nausea and vomiting
- Short-term relief of symptoms of anxiety
- Withdrawal symptoms of acute alcoholism
- Anxiety prior to surgery

Benzodiazepines

Benzodiazepines are commonly prescribed to treat anxiety.
Adverse reactions:

- Agitation
- Amnesia
- **Ataxia** (impaired coordination)
- Bizarre behavior
- Blood dyscrasias
- Confusion
- Daytime sedation
- Depression
- Dizziness
- Dryness of the mouth
- Drowsiness
- Fatigue
- Hallucinations
- Headache
- Hyperactivity
- Insomnia
- Itching
- Lethargy

- Muscle weakness

- Nausea

- Photophobia

- Rash

- Tremor

- Vomiting

Note: Benzodiazepines should not be taken for prolonged periods of time. These medications may result in tolerance and physical and psychological dependence. Sudden withdrawal after prolonged use may result in seizures, agitation, psychosis, insomnia, and gastric distress.

Contraindications include the following:

- Mental depression

- Individuals at risk for suicide

- Depressed vital signs

- Pregnancy

- Breast feeding

- Liver and kidney disorders

- Older adults

- Fragile and disabled individuals

- Individuals operating machinery

Special considerations for benzodiazepines are as follows:

- Be aware of the symptoms of blood dyscrasias—sore throat, fever, jaundice, unusual and progressive weakness, and **purpura** (bleeding into the skin).

- In the elderly or individuals who are generally weak, be especially aware of confusion, drowsiness, and ataxia. These may result in physical injury to the individual, such as a fall.

- Tell the individual taking benzodiazepines that he should not drive or operate machinery while taking these medications.

- Alcohol and other central nervous system depressants have an additive effect and should be avoided while taking these medications.

- Smoking may enhance absorption of the medication, and, as a result, larger doses may be needed to provide effective treatment.

- Physical dependence may occur and withdrawal symptoms may result. If the ordered dosage does not relieve anxiety, notify the licensed health care provider.

- *Do not* suddenly stop this medication.

Table 16-2 Selected Antianxiety Medications by Generic and Brand Names with Dosage Information

GENERIC NAME	BRAND NAME	DOSAGE INFORMATION	COMMENTS
Benzodiazepines (short-term use only)			
alprazolam	Xanax	Oral 0.125–0.5 mg 2–3 × day	Abrupt withdrawal may cause severe side effects
	Xanax XR	Oral 0.5–6 mg every morning	For panic disorder
chlordiazepoxide	Librium	Oral 5–25 mg 3 or 4 × day	
chlorazepate	Tranxene	Oral 15–60 mg daily in divided doses	For older adult patients no more than 15 mg daily
		7.5–15 mg daily in divided doses	
diazepam	Valium	Oral 2–10 mg three times a day	Also used as muscle relaxant
lorazepam	Ativan	Oral 2–3 mg daily in divided doses	For older adults who are agitated
oxazepam	Serax	Oral 10–15 mg 3–4 × day	For older adults who are agitated
Other Anxiolytics			
buspirone	Buspar	Oral 15–60 mg daily in divided doses	Slow onset of action, may be used long term
hydroxyzine	Atarax, Vistaril	Oral 25–100 mg 4 × day	Antiemetic, antipruritic, or preoperative medication

Based on Woodrow, R. (2007). *Essentials of pharmacology for health occupations* (5th ed.), Table 20-3. Clifton Park, NY: Delmar, Cengage Learning.

Table 16-2 gives a list of selected antianxiety medications by generic and brand names with dosage information.

Other Antianxiety Medications

Busipirone (BuSpar). Busipirone (BuSpar) is another type of antianxiety medication. Unlike the benzodiazepines, it does not impair psychomotor function and has little sedative effect. It appears to be more effective for cognitive and interpersonal problems, including anger and hostility related to anxiety. BuSpar works slower, taking two (2) to four (4) weeks to take full effect. BuSpar, however, has little potential for tolerance or dependence. The medication has been used without unusual adverse effects for as long as one (1) year.

Adverse reactions:

- Dizziness
- Drowsiness
- Headache
- Nausea

Contraindication include the following:

- Kidney impairment
- Liver impairment
- MAOI use within the past fourteen (14) days
- Allergy to the medication

Special considerations with BuSpar include the following:

- Take with food.
- Tell the individual taking BuSpar that he should not drive or operate machinery while taking this medication.
- Alcohol has an additive effect and should be avoided while taking this medication.

Hydroxyzine (Atarax)

Adverse reactions:

- Ataxia
- Dizziness
- Drowsiness
- **Mydriasis** (dilation of the pupils)
- Urinary retention

Contraindications include the following:

- Allergy to medications
- GI, liver, and respiratory disorders
- Closed-angle glaucoma

Special considerations for hydroxyine include the following:

- Tell the individual taking hydroxyine that he should not drive or operate machinery while taking this medication.
- Alcohol has an additive effect and should be avoided while taking this medication.

Table 16-2 gives a list of selected antianxiety medications by generic and brand names with dosage information.

Antidepressants

Depression is often described as a chemical imbalance in the brain. The neurotransmitters known as dopamine, serotonin, and norepinephrine are reabsorbed too quickly by nerve endings in the brain. A shortage results, causing an imbalance.

Depression is demonstrated differently in every individual who has it based on the cause and the individual. Depression may happen at the same time as an individual grows older. Depression, however, is not a normal part of the aging process. Even though depression may occur at the same time one is ill, depression is not a normal part of illness. The depression should be treated as a separate medical problem.

Symptoms of clinical depression include the following:

- Unusually deep sadness

- Major changes in eating patterns—an individual may stop eating or may eat constantly

- Major changes in sleep patterns—an individual may sleep whenever possible or may get very little sleep with episodes of insomnia at night

- Loss of interest in hobbies, work, friends and family, sex, food, and pleasurable activities

- Constant fatigue or loss of energy

- Feelings of worthlessness, helplessness, and guilt

- Thoughts of death or suicide

Antidepressants are prescribed to treat symptoms of depression. There are five categories of antidepressants:

- Selective serotonin reuptake inhibitors (SSRIs)

- Selective nonselective reuptake inhibitors (SNRIs)

- Tricyclic antidepressants

- MAO inhibitors (MAOIs)

- Heterocyclic antidepressants

Note: **It may take fourteen (14) to thirty (30) days before antidepressants become fully effective and make a noticeable difference.**

Selective Serotonin Reuptake Inhibitors (SSRIs)

Selective serotonin reuptake inhibitors (SSRIs) are considered to be the first-line treatment for depression. SSRIs block the reuptake (reabsorption) of serotonin in the brain. These medications have fewer side effects and are safer. Individuals are more likely to take their medications as prescribed. In addition, the cognition of older adults is not significantly impaired by SSRIs.

This group of antidepressants includes:

- Prozac

- Luvox

- Paxil

- Zoloft

These medications are used to treat:

- Depression

- Social anxiety disorder

- Obsessive-compulsive disorder (OCD)
- Panic disorder

Adverse reactions:

- Anxiety
- Agitation
- Amnesia
- Anorexia
- Chills
- Confusion
- Constipation
- Decreased libido (sex drive)
- Diarrhea
- Dizziness
- Drowsiness
- Dry mouth
- Fatigue
- Fever
- Headache
- Insomnia
- Nausea
- Nervousness
- Sexual dysfunction
- Sweating
- Tremor
- Weakness
- Weight gain or loss

Contraindications include the following:

- Use cautiously with individuals with bipolar disorders (may lead to manic attacks)
- Use cautiously with individuals at risk for suicide
- Pregnancy
- Breast feeding
- Underweight
- Eating disorders
- Diabetes
- Liver or kidney disease

Special considerations for SSRIs include the following:

- Monitor for the possibility of misuse or abuse.

- Monitor for the possibility of suicide.

- Monitor appetite and intake.

- Weigh weekly. Report weight gain or loss.

- Tell the individual taking SSRIs that he should not drive or operate machinery while taking this medication.

- Notify the licensed health care provider if the individual takes or plans to take any prescription or OTC medication or if he plans to drink alcohol.

- Notify the licensed health care provider if the individual is pregnant or planning to become pregnant or is breast-feeding.

- Report any adverse reactions to the licensed health care provider, especially a rash or hives.

Table 16-3 gives a selected list of SSRIs by generic and brand names with dosage information.

Table 16-3 Selected Antidepressants and Antimanic Medications by Generic and Brand Names with Dosage Information

GENERIC NAME	BRAND NAME	DOSAGE INFORMATION	COMMENTS
Tricyclics			
amitriptyline	Elavil	Oral 50–300 mg daily	All of these drugs interact with CNS drugs. Give at bedtime
desipramine	Norpramin	Oral 50–300 mg daily	Less sedation, orthostatic hypotension
doxepin	Sinequan, Adapin	Oral 50–300 mg daily	Also used topically for eczema
imipramine	Tofranil	Oral 50–300 mg daily	Also effective for bed wetting
nortriptyline	Aventyl, Pamelor	Oral 25–150 mg daily	Older adults and adolescent patients need lower dose
MAOIs			
isocarboxazid	Marplan	Oral 10–60 mg daily in divided doses	All of these drugs interact with many foods and other drugs, resulting in serious reactions
phenelzine	Nardil	Oral 45–90 mg daily in divided doses	
tranylcypromine	Parnate	Oral 20–60 mg daily in divided doses	

(continues)

Table 16-3 Selected Antidepressants and Antimanic Medications by Generic and Brand Names with Dosage Information—*continued*

GENERIC NAME	BRAND NAME	DOSAGE INFORMATION	COMMENTS
SSRIs			
citalopram	Celexa	Oral 20–60 mg daily	Take in morning or evening with or without food
escitalopram	Lexapro	Oral 10–20 mg daily	May be better tolerated than Celexa
fluoxetine	Prozac	Oral 10–80 mg daily	Delayed response, long half-life; take in morning
paroxetine	Paxil	Oral 10–60 mg daily	Older adults ½ dose; take in morning
	Paxil CR	Oral 12.5–62.5 mg daily	Do not give with antacids
sertraline	Zoloft	Oral 25–200 mg daily	Take in morning
SNRIs			
venlafaxine	Effexor	Oral 75–375 mg in divided doses	Take after meals to lessen nausea
	Effexor-XR	Oral 37.5–225 mg daily	Do not chew or crush, swallow whole
Heterocyclics			
buproprion	Wellbutrin	Oral 100–150 mg 2–3 × day	Take early in the day; space doses at least 6 hours apart to decrease seizure risk
	Wellbutrin SR	Oral 150–200 mg daily–2 × day	
	Wellbutrin XL	Oral 150–400 mg	8 a.m.
mirtazapine	Remeron	Oral 15–45 mg daily	Take at bedtime, sedation common
trazodone	Desyrel	Oral 25–100 mg at bedtime for insomnia	Take after meals to decrease dizziness and nausea; if drowsiness occurs, may give large portion of dose at bedtime
		Oral 150–600 mg in divided doses for depression	
Antimanic Agents			
lithium	Lithobid, Eskalith	900–1,800 mg in divided doses	0.8–1.5 mEq/ml (desired serum level)
carbamazepine	Tegretol	Oral 600–1,600 mg in divided doses	4–12 mcg/ml (desired serum level)
valproate	Depakote, Depakene	Oral 15–60 mg/kg/day in divided doses	50–100 mcg/ml (desired serum level)
	Depakote ER	Oral 250–1,000 mg/day	To prevent migraines
olanzapine/fluoxetine	Symbyax	Oral every night (various strengths)	For bipolar depression

Note: All tricyclics have a delayed response and mild tranquilizing effect. SSRIs also have delayed response.

Based on Woodrow, R. (2007). *Essentials of pharmacology for health occupations* (5th ed.), Table 20-3, Clifton Park, NY: Delmar, Cengage Learning.

Serotonin Nonselective Reuptake Inhibitors (SNRIs)

Effexor is a medication that is chemically different from other available antidepressants. Effexor inhibits the reuptake of norepinephrine and serotonin and slightly inhibits the uptake of dopamine. This medication is used for the treatment of depression.

Adverse reactions:

- Abnormal ejaculation or orgasm in men
- Anorexia
- Anxiety
- Blurred vision
- Constipation
- Dizziness
- Dry mouth
- General weakness
- Impotence
- Nausea
- Nervousness
- Sleepiness
- Sweating
- Vomiting

Contraindications include the following:

- Allergy to the medication
- MAOI use within the past fourteen (14) days

Special considerations for Effexor include the following:

- Regularly monitor the individual's blood pressure. Notify the licensed health care provider if the individual has high blood pressure. Effexor may cause an increase in blood pressure.
- Monitor for the possibility of misuse or abuse.
- Monitor for the possibility of suicide.
- Tell the individual taking SNRIs that he should not drive or operate machinery while taking this medication.
- Notify the licensed health care provider if the individual takes or plans to take any prescription or OTC medication or if he plans to drink alcohol.
- Notify the licensed health care provider if the individual is pregnant or planning to become pregnant or is breast-feeding.
- Notify the licensed health care provider if the individual has liver or kidney disease or a history of seizures.
- Report any adverse reactions to the licensed health care provider, especially a rash or hives.

Table 16-3 gives a selected list of SNRIs by generic and brand names with dosage information.

Tricyclic Antidepressants

Tricyclic antidepressants are prescribed for the treatment of depression. Tricyclic antidepressants block the reuptake (reabsorption) of norepinephrine and serotonin. They usually work best in instances of depression where the cause is felt to be inherited or biochemical rather than environmental. Tricyclic antidepressants are often admininstered at bedtime because of their mild sedative effect.

The most common adverse reactions for tricyclic antidepressants are related to their effect on the parasympathetic nervous system. They can include:

- Blurred vision
- Constipation
- **Diaphoresis** (perspiration, sweating)
- Dilation of the urinary tract
- Disturbance of accommodation (the inability to adapt to changes in the environment, which may result in a secondary physical injury)
- Dry mouth
- Flushing
- Increased intraocular pressure
- **Paralytic ileus** (bowel obstruction due to paralysis of the bowel wall)
- Urinary retention

Other adverse reactions that are more generalized include:

- Anxiety
- **Anorexia** (loss of appetite)
- Ataxia
- Blurred vision
- Cardiac arrythmias
- Confusion, especially in older adults
- Constipation
- Dizziness
- Drowsiness
- Excitement
- Fatigue
- Headache
- Hypertension
- Hypotension, particularly orthostatic hypotension

- Insomnia
- Nausea
- Numbness and tingling in the extremities
- Palpitations
- Postural hypotension
- Seizures
- Skin rash
- Tachycardia
- Tremors
- Urinary retention
- Vomiting
- Weight gain or loss

Contraindications include the following:

- Cardiac disorders
- Renal (kidney) disorders
- GI disorders
- Liver disorders
- Use in older adults
- Glaucoma
- Obesity
- Seizure disorder
- Pregnancy
- Breast feeding
- Use with MAOIs
- Use with SSRIs (may increase trigylceride blood levels)

Special considerations for tricyclic antidepressants include the following:

- Be alert to the possibility of suicide.
- Tell the individual taking tricyclic antidepressants that he should not drive or operate machinery while taking this medication.
- Alcohol and other central nervous system depressants have an additive effect and should be avoided while taking these medications.
- Tell the individual to change positions slowly when sitting up from lying down or when standing from sitting to decrease the risk of **orthostatic hypotension**.

orthostatic hypotension
A drop in blood pressure after an individual sits up from lying down or stands up from a sitting position too quickly.

Table 16-3 gives a list of selected tricyclic antidepressants by generic and brand names with dosage information.

Monoamine Oxidase Inhibitors (MAOIs)

MAOIs are indicated for use in treating atypical depressions or depressions associated with panic disorders or phobias. Examples follow:

- **Agoraphobia**—an irrational fear of leaving the house and of open spaces

- **Hysteroid dysphoria**—a general dissatisfaction, restlessness, depression, and anxiety that can escalate to hysteria

- Depression in individuals who have not responded to tricyclic antidepressants

MAOIs increase the amount of serotonin, norepinephrine, and dopamine at the nerve endings in the brain by inhibiting an enzyme known as the MAO enzyme. Because of (1) the potential serious side effects from MAOIs and (2) the medication interaction with food and other medications, these medications are rarely used today.

Note: As a safety precaution, be aware that MAOIs should not be taken with or within fourteen (14) days of Effexor, tricyclic antidepressants, or SSRIs.

Adverse reactions:

- Abdominal pain

- Agitation

- Anorexia

- Blurred vision

- Chest pain

- Chills

- Constipation

- Diarrhea

- Dizziness

- Drowsiness

- Dryness of the mouth

- **Dysuria** (difficulty or pain during urination)

- **Edema** (swelling)

- Headache

- Hypertension or **hypertensive crisis**, which may be fatal

- Impotence

- Insomnia

- Muscle twitching

- Nausea

- Nervousness

- Orthostatic hypotension

hypertensive crisis
A life-threatening situation requiring immediate emergency care. Symptoms include severe headache, palpitations, sweating, chest pain, possible intracranial hemorrhage, and death.

- Palpitations

- Photosensitivity

- Restlessness

- Stiff neck

- Tachycardia

- Tremors

- Vertigo

- Vomiting

- Weakness

Contraindications include the following:

- Cerebrovascular disease

- Heart disease

- Liver disease

- Renal (kidney) disease

- Pregnancy

- Breast feeding

- Abrupt discontinuance

Special considerations for MAOIs are specified below.

MAOIs should not be given in the following situations:

- In combination with sympathomimetics (medications that mimic the sympathetic nervous system)

- In combination with Demerol

- In individuals undergoing elective surgery

- In combination with alcohol, hypotensive medications, or narcotics

- An individual taking MAOIs must avoid the foods and beverages listed in Table 16-4. *These foods and beverages must be avoided while the individual is taking the MAOI and for two (2) weeks after the medication is discontinued.* These foods and beverages contain tyramine, which can cause fatal hypertension when taken in combination with MAOIs.

- Notify the licensed health care provider immediately if the individual complains of headache, stiff neck, pounding heartbeat, nausea, or vomiting.

- Tell the individual to rise slowly from a lying position to minimize risk of orthostatic hypotension.

- Tell the individual not to drink alcohol or caffeinated beverages.

- Tell the individual not to take OTC or herbal medications while taking MAOIs.

- If the individual has more than one licensed HCP, make sure that each licensed HCP knows the individual's medication list.

Table 16-4 Foods and Beverage to Be Avoided When Taking MAOIs

TYPE OF FOOD	TYRAMINE-CONTAINING FOODS
alcohol	beer, wines (especially red wines and Chianti)
dairy products	cheese (except for cottage cheese), sour cream, yogurt
fruits	avocados, bananas, canned figs, papaya products (including meat tenderizers), raisins
meats	beef or chicken liver, bologna/hot dogs, meat extracts, pate, pepperoni, pickled or kippered herring, salami, sausage
other	chocolate
sauces	soy sauce
vegetables	pods of broad beans (fava beans)
yeast	all yeast or yeast extracts

Source: Moini, J. (2009). *Fundamental pharmacology for pharmacy technicians*, Table 4-3. Clifton Park, NY: Delmar, Cengage Learning.

Table 16-3 gives a list of selected MAOIs by generic and brand names with dosage information.

Heterocyclic Antidepressants

Heterocyclic antidepressants are considered the second generation of antidepressants. These medications have a different effect on dopamine, norepinephrine, and serotonin. Examples of medications in this group are as follows:

- Wellbutrin (buproprion)
  - Useful in treating individuals with severe depression along with extreme fatigue, lethargy, and psychomotor retardation
  - Helps to decrease relapse rates in individuals who quit smoking
  - Useful in treating individuals who experienced sexual dysfunction with other antidepressants
- Desyrel (trazodone)
  - Highly sedating
  - Used in low dose as a sleep medication
  - Used in higher dose for older adults experiencing agitation secondary to dementia
  - Useful in treating side effects caused by SSRIs
- Remeron (mirtazaoine)
  - Useful in treating agitated depression
  - Mixed anxiety and depression
  - Fibromyalgia
  - Treating individuals with a poor appetite

Adverse reactions:

- Agitation (with Wellbutrin)
- Anxiety (with Wellbutrin)
- Confusion (Desyrel)
- Dizziness (Desyrel)
- Dry mouth (Desyrel)
- Drowsiness (common except Wellbutrin)
- Impotence (Desyrel)
- Insomnia (with Wellbutrin)
- Nausea(Desyrel)
- Restlessness (with Wellbutrin)
- Weight gain (Desyrel and Remeron)

Contraindications include the following:

- Those at risk for suicide
- Seizure disorder
- Cardiac disorders
- Liver disorders

Special considerations for Heterocyclic antidepressants are as follows:

- Do not crush or chew sustained release medications.
- Do not abruptly stop the medication.
- Do not administer medication at bedtime. May cause insomnia.
- Tell the individual to rise slowly from a lying position to minimize risk of orthostatic hypotension.
- Tell the individual not to drink alcohol.
- Tell the individual not to take OTC or herbal medications.
- Be alert to the possibility of suicide.
- Tell the individual that he should not drive or operate machinery while taking this medication.
- Monitor vital signs, especially for orthostatic hypotension.

Table 16-3 gives a list of selected heterocyclic antidepressants by generic and brand names with dosage information.

Antimanic Medications

Lithium is the primary medication used to treat the manic phase of **bipolar disorder**. Bipolar disorder was previously called manic depression or manic-depressive psychosis. Lithium treats and prevents the symptoms in the manic phase, including:

- Boisterousness
- Decreased need for sleep

- Delusions of grandeur
- Euphoria
- Exalted feelings
- Excitement
- Hyperactivity
- Impaired ability to concentrate
- Overproduction of ideas

Treatment of bipolar disorder is long term. Once a maintenance dose is established, blood levels to check the amount of lithium in the body will need to be drawn every few months.

Adverse reactions to lithium can *initially* include:

- Cardiac arrythmias
- Fine tremors in the hands
- General discomfort
- GI upset (take medication with meals to decrease upset)
- Hypotension
- Thirst
- **Polyuria** (frequent urination)
- Transient, mild nausea
- Thyroid problems

Lithium intoxication may occur if lithium levels are too high in the body. Early signs of lithium intoxication are:

- Ataxia (impaired coordination)
- Confusion
- Diarrhea
- Dizziness
- Drowsiness
- Dry mouth
- Giddiness
- Lethargy
- Muscle weakness
- **Nystagmus** (involuntary jerking movement of the eyes)
- Photophobia
- Polyuria
- Slurred speech
- Swallowing difficulty

- Tremors

- Vomiting

As lithium intoxication progresses, symptoms may also include:

- Blurred vision

- Cardiovascular collapse

- Coma

- Seizures

- Tinnitus

If the UAP observes any of these symptoms in an individual taking lithium, the UAP should hold the individual's dose of lithium and notify the individual's licensed HCP *immediately*.

Contraindications include the following:

- Seizure disorders

- Parkinsonism

- Cardiovascular disorders

- Kidney disorders

- Older adults

- Fragile, disabled individuals

- Thyroid disease

Special considerations for lithium include the following:

- Administer medication with meals to decrease GI upset.

- Tell the individual to drink ten (10) to twelve (12) 8-ounce glasses of water daily.

- Tell the individual to avoid alcohol and caffeinated drinks.

- Tell the individual that he may experience a metallic taste. The metallic taste is usually temporary. Report the individual's complaints of a metallic taste to the individual's licensed HCP. Since a lower dose of lithium may decrease or eliminate the metallic taste, the individual's licensed HCP may adjust the individual's dose of lithium.

- Advise women taking lithium to avoid pregnancy while they are taking the medication.

- Educate the individual and her family about the signs of lithium intoxication. Advise them to notify the individual's licensed HCP immediately if they notice signs of intoxication.

Table 16-3 gives a list of selected antimanic medications by generic and brand names with dosage information.

Antipsychotic Medications

Psychotic behavior comes from a significant distortion of reality that affects an individual's ability to function in daily life. An example of psychotic behavior would be someone believing that he is a major hero figure, like Batman, and going through daily life as though that were actually true. Psychotic behavior may involve hallucinations as well as altered thought processes.

Neuroleptics are used to treat:

- Acute and chronic schizophrenia
- Organic psychoses (caused by biochemical changes in the brain)
- The manic phase of bipolar disorder
- Psychotic disorders

Antipsychotic medications, also called **neuroleptics**, are used to modify psychotic behavior. There are two types of antipsychotic medications: (1) typical antipsychotics, such as Thorazine, and (2) atypical antipsychotics, such as respiridone. Typical antipsychotics block dopamine receptors in the brain. Atypical antipsychotics block both serotonin and dopamine receptors in the brain.

General adverse reactions:

- Agitation
- Allergic reactions
- Anorexia
- Blurred vision
- Bradycardia
- Confusion
- Constipation
- Depression
- Dizziness
- Drowsiness
- Dryness of the mouth
- **Dystonia**
- Elevated blood sugars (with atypical antipsychotics)
- Fainting
- Fever
- Insomnia
- Headache
- Jaundice
- Motor restlessness
- Nasal congestion
- Ocular changes

dystonia
Literally, difficult, or bad tone; symptoms include spasms and rigidity in various muscle groups.

- Orthostatic hypotension
- Photosensitivity
- Postural hypotension
- Rash
- Restlessness
- Seizures
- Skin pigmentation changes
- Tachycardia
- Toxic psychosis
- Urinary retention
- Vertigo
- Weakness
- Weight gain (clozapine and olanzapine)

Other adverse reactions:

- **Extrapyramidal symptoms**, or EPS—These are abnormalities of movement that mimic movements that would be brought on after an injury to the brain. These symptoms may be very frightening to the individual experiencing them. Extrapyramidal symptoms (EPS) include dystonia. Dystonia may be demonstrated by:
  - Spasm in the neck muscles
  - **Torticollis**—a muscle spasm of the neck in which the head is pulled to one side and turned so the chin is pointing to the other side of the body
  - Rigidity of back muscles
  - **Carpopedal spasm**—spasm and rigidity in the hands and feet
  - **Trismus**—spasms in the jaw muscles
  - Difficulty in swallowing
  - **Oculogyric crisis**—severe and repeated upward rolling of the eyeballs
  - **Protrusion**—sticking out of the tongue
  - **Akathisia**—an inability to sit down; the individual experiences severe restlessness and an urgent need to move. Symptoms include agitation, fidgeting, and pacing repeatedly.
- **Pseudoparkinsonism**—This is a collection of symptoms that mimic those of parkinsonism. These are more common in older adults. Symptoms include:
  - **Bradykinesia** (a decrease in spontaneous movement)
  - Drooling
  - Hypersalivation
  - A rigid or masklike facial expression

- Rigidity
- Tremors
- Postural abnormalities
- Shuffling gait

- **Tardive dyskinesia**—This causes involuntary rhythmic movements of the face, mouth, jaw, tongue, trunk, and extremities.

Note: Parkinsonism symptoms and tardive dyskinesia may become permanent and irreversible. The UAP should observe individuals on these medications closely and report any symptoms to his supervisor and the individual's licensed HCP immediately. Individuals need to be assessed by their licensed HCP often.

Contraindications include the following:

- Seizure disorders
- Parkinsonian syndrome
- Cerebral vascular disease
- Severe depression
- Pregnancy
- Breast feeding
- Blood dyscrasias

Special considerations for antipsychotic medications include the following:

- Tell the individual taking neuroleptics that he should not drive or operate machinery while taking this medication.

- Alcohol and other central nervous system depressants have an additive effect and should be avoided while taking these medications.

- Tell the individual to change positions slowly when sitting up from lying down or when standing from sitting to minimize the risk of orthostatic hypotension.

- In some states, the use of these medications requires approval by the court. The UAP should consult with his workplace to determine if such is required in his state.

- Instruct the individual to avoid exposure to sunlight or to artificial UV rays, use sunscreen, and wear protective clothing when outdoors.

- Encourage the individual to eat a balanced diet and to drink plenty of fluids.

- Notify the licensed health care provider if the individual has constipation. The licensed health care provider may prescribe a laxative or stool softener.

tardive dyskinesia
Involuntary movements of the face, trunk, and extremities that develop as a side effect of long term use of neuroleptics.

Table 16-5 gives a list of selected antipsychotic medications by generic and brand names with dosage information.

Table 16-5 Selected Antipsychotic Medications by Generic and Brand Names with Dosage Information

GENERIC NAME	BRAND NAME	DOSAGE INFORMATION	COMMENTS
Typical*			
chlorpromazine	Thorazine	Oral 200–800 mg daily	Primarily for agitation: also for nausea and vomiting and severe behavior problems
haloperidol	Haldol	Oral 1–20 mg daily	For agitation, especially with schizophrenia and delusions in older adults
prochlorperazine	Compazine	Oral supp, 5–10 mg Per rectum 25 mg 2 × day	For agitation; primarily for nausea and vomiting in adults
thioridazine	Mellaril	Oral 10–200 mg 4 × day	For psychoneurosis, agitation, or combativeness
trifluoperazine	Stelazine	Oral 2–40 mg 2 × day	Tranquilizer for psychotic disorders
thiothixene	Navane	Oral 2–40 mg 2 × day	For chronic schizophrenic or behavioral management of withdrawn patients
fluphenzine HCl	Prolixin	Oral 2.5–20 mg daily in divided doses	For older adults, reduce dose to ½ or ¼
perphenazine	Trilafon	Oral 8–64 mg daily in divided doses	For psychosis, nausea, and vomiting in adults
Atypical			
aripiprazole	Abilify	Oral 5–30 mg daily	For schizophrenia
clozapine	Clozaril	Oral 12.5–900 mg in divided doses	
olanzapine	Zyprexa	Oral 5–20 mg daily	Reduce dose by ½ for older adults For acute agitation
quetiapine	Seroquel	Oral 50–750 mg daily in divided doses	Monitor for orthostatic hypotension
risperidone	Risperdal Risperdal Consta	Oral 1–4 mg 2 × day	Reduce dose by ½ for older adults For schizophrenia
ziprasidone	Geodon	Oral 20–80 mg 2 × day	Greater risk of cardiac disorders For acute psychosis/agitation

*These drugs frequently cause EPS with long-term use. Monitor closely.

Based on Woodrow, R. (2007). *Essentials of pharmacology for health occupations* (5th ed.), Table 20-4. Clifton Park, NY: Delmar, Cengage Learning.

SUMMARY

Psychotropic medications are a complex group of medications with a number of unique characteristics. It is the UAP's responsibility to be aware of the many reactions and considerations to be used with these medications. This does not mean that the UAP is expected to memorize all of the possible reactions from the medications.

The UAP needs to:

- Be observant for any and all changes in an individual

- Recognize any unusual reaction and report it to the licensed health care provider in a timely fashion

- Use available references to recall the considerations for each type of medication

- Remember, "when in doubt, ask"—ask the licensed health care provider, the pharmacist, or licensed clinicians

- Use reference materials to resolve a question *before* giving a medication.

WORKBOOK REVIEW

Go to the workbook and complete the exercises for Chapter 16.

REVIEW QUESTIONS

1. Mental illness:
   a. is not important to an individual's overall well-being
   b. occurs only when one has a break in reality with hallucinations
   c. may be due to drinking beverages from aluminum cans
   d. may be inherited from one's parents or grandparents
2. Psychotropic medications:
   a. distort perception of reality
   b. affect the function, behavior, or experience of the mind
   c. are medications that cure mental illness
   d. do not require an order from a licensed health care provider

3. Benzodiazepines are commonly used to treat:
   a. anxiety
   b. depression
   c. the manic phase of bipolar disorder
   d. psychotic behavior
4. An individual taking benzodiazepines:
   a. may use moderate amounts of alcohol
   b. may use OTC medications without the approval of his licensed HCP
   c. may experience physical dependence that results in withdrawal symptoms
   d. should have no problem driving or using machinery
5. Depression:
   a. does not occur normally with aging or illness and should be treated as a separate issue
   b. causes an individual to have increased energy
   c. is treated with antimanic agents
   d. causes euphoria
6. Whenever an individual is taking an antidepressant, the UAP should:
   a. try to cheer the individual up
   b. be alert to the possibility of suicide
   c. minimize contact to avoid upsetting the individual
   d. tell the individual that he should try to get over it
7. An individual taking MAOIs should:
   a. avoid foods and beverages containing tyramine, like cheese and bananas
   b. feel free to drink alcohol and caffeinated beverages
   c. stay in bed to avoid leaving the house
   d. all of the above
8. Early signs of lithium intoxication include:
   a. ataxia, nystagmus, slurred speech
   b. torticollis
   c. oculogyric crisis
   d. toxic psychosis
9. Psychotic behavior:
   a. is similar to anxiety
   b. is a response to a distorted perception of reality
   c. triggers the manic phase in bipolar disorder
   d. causes dizziness and photosensitivity
10. Extrapyramidal symptoms as an adverse reaction to neuroleptics include:
    a. dystonia and akathisia
    b. drowsiness and jaundice
    c. blurred vision and nasal congestion
    d. all of the above

Chapter 17
Analgesics, Anesthetics, Hypnotics, and Sedatives

Learning Objectives

After reading this chapter and completing the review questions, you should be able to:

1. Spell and define terms.
2. Discuss the uses, adverse reactions, and special considerations for analgesics, anesthetics, hypnotics, and sedatives.
3. Lists three ways pain affects an individual's quality of life.
4. Describe a pain assessment scale.
5. List six signs of pain the UAP should look for in an individual with dementia or who is in a coma.

Key Terms

acute pain	euphoria	pain	somnolence
addiction	hypnotic	paresthesias	Stevens-Johnson
analgesic-antipyretics	migraines	phantom pain	Syndrome
analgesics	myocardial	psychological	tinnitus
anesthetics	infarction (MI)	dependence	tolerance
asthenia	opiates	radiating pain	
chronic pain	opioids	sedative	

INTRODUCTION

As discussed in Chapter 12, the nervous system controls and coordinates all body activities. The nervous system is made up of the central nervous system, peripheral nervous system, and sensory receptors that send information to the brain. Disorders to the nervous system may result in minor or major changes to the body that may be temporary or permanent.

For instance, throughout an individual's lifetime, she may experience (1) acute or chronic discomfort or pain due to injury, illness, surgery, or other circumstance(s) and (2) insomnia.

This chapter will discuss various types of medications available to manage or control pain, and insomnia.

PAIN

pain
An abnormal sensation that causes suffering or distress.

Pain is defined as an abnormal sensation that causes suffering or distress. Because of the effects pain has on the quality of an individual's life, it is considered the "fifth" vital sign. An individual experiencing pain may restrict her daily activities and mobility; may experience depression, hopelessness, and anxiety; may withdraw from others; and may develop behaviors that are unusual for the individual, such as crying all of the time, being combative, and being uncooperative.

There are four types of pain: (1) **acute pain**, (2) **chronic pain**, (3) **phantom pain**, and (4) **radiating pain**. All types of pain are serious and need to be treated. Pain is personal, different from individual to individual. Pain is what the specific individual describes it as.

UAPs have an important role of observing the individuals in their care for pain and for medicating the individuals as ordered. Pain assessment scales may be used to help the UAP to determine the amount of pain an individual is experiencing. Figure 17-1 is an example of a pain assessment scale. This scale may be used with children, adults, and individuals who do not speak or understand English.

For an individual who is unable to use a pain assessment scale, such as an individual with dementia or who is in a coma, to communicate the amount of pain she is experiencing, the UAP needs to observe for signs of pain. Signs of pain the UAP should look for include the following:

acute pain
Occurs suddenly and without warning. Usually is the result of injury or surgery. Decreases over time as healing takes place.

chronic pain
Lasts longer than six (6) months. May be caused from multiple medical conditions.

phantom pain
Is the result of an amputation. Pain is real, not imaginary.

radiating pain
Moves from place of origin to other places, for instance, chest pain moving to the arm or jaw.

- Changes in facial expression, crying, moaning, rigid posture, or protecting their body (guarding) upon movement

- Withdrawing or moving away from the UAP when touched

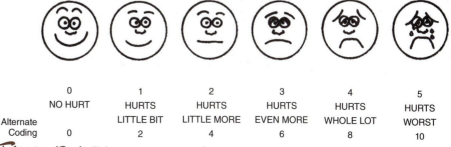

0 NO HURT	1 HURTS LITTLE BIT	2 HURTS LITTLE MORE	3 HURTS EVEN MORE	4 HURTS WHOLE LOT	5 HURTS WORST
Alternate Coding 0	2	4	6	8	10

Figure 17-1 Pain assessment scale *(FACES Pain Rating Scale from Hockenberry, M. J., Wilson, D: Wong's essentials of pediatric nursing, ed.8 St. Louis 2009, Mosby. Used with permission. Copyright Mosby.)*

- Being combative or resistive to care
- Restlessness
- Irregular breathing
- Sweating
- Irritability
- Agitation
- Refusal to eat or drink
- Withdrawal from activities
- Refusal to get out of bed

For an individual experiencing pain, it is best to medicate her "around the clock" with additional doses when needed. Medicating an individual around the clock will provide the best control of her pain by preventing pain from developing or worsening. If an individual is experiencing pain and she does not have an order for pain medication, the UAP should contact the individual's licensed HCP.

Approximately thirty (30) to sixty (60) minutes after medicating an individual for pain, the UAP needs to observe the individual:

- To see if the pain medication has been effective
- To see if the individual is having adverse effects from the medication

If the medication is not effective or if the individual is experiencing adverse effects, the UAP must contact the individual's licensed HCP.

ANALGESICS

Analgesics are medications used to relieve pain caused by many different conditions. There are three classes of analgesics:

- Narcotic analgesics
- **Analgesic-antipyretics** (nonnarcotic)
- Adjuvant

Narcotic Analgesics

Narcotic analgesics, also called **opiates** or **opioids**, are used in the relief of moderate to severe pain. There are natural opioids, such as morphine and codeine. There are also synthetic opioids, such as meperidine (Demerol) and propoxyphene (Darvon).

Chronic use of opioids are known to cause **tolerance** and **psychological dependence**. These medications are, therefore, not used for extended periods of time except to manage chronic pain for individuals with such issues as cancer pain or terminal illness or with nonmalignant pain who do not benefit from other pain relief. However, individuals who require opioids for pain management rarely experience **addiction** or psychological dependence. Even then, for an individual who is dying,

tolerance
A condition in which the individual's body adjusts to the dose of a medication and a larger amount of the medication is needed to achieve the desired or wanted effect.

psychological dependence
A mental or emotional craving for the effects produced by a substance; without it, there are no physical withdrawal symptoms.

addiction
The compulsive, uncontrollable use of a substance.

dependence should not be a consideration; rather, adequate control of pain should be the primary concern.

Adverse effects:

- Agitation
- Blurred vision
- Bradycardia
- Confusion
- Constipation
- Dependence—physical and/or psychological
- Dizziness
- Flushing of the face
- Hallucinations
- **Euphoria** (excitement)
- Flushing
- Headache
- Hypotension
- Hives
- Itching
- Light-headedness
- Nausea
- Respiratory depression
- Restlessness
- Sedation
- Seizures (with large doses)
- Slowed pulse, heartbeat, and respirations
- Sweating
- Rash
- Urinary retention
- Vomiting

Contraindications include the following:

- Head injury
- Cardiac disease
- Hypotension
- CNS depression
- Liver disease
- Kidney disease
- Thyroid disease

- COPD
- Asthma
- Pregnancy
- Breast feeding
- Older adults
- Fragile, disabled adults
- Individuals prone to addiction
- Individuals at risk for suicide
- Alcoholism
- Allergy to opiates

Special considerations when giving narcotic analgesics include the following:

- Always count respirations before giving these medications. If the respiratory rate is twelve (12) or lower, hold the medication. Call the individual's licensed HCP immediately.
- Be aware that physical dependency may occur with long-term use.

Table 17-1 gives a list of selected narcotic analgesics by generic and brand names with dosage information and uses.

The medication naloxone hydrochloride (Narcan) works to reverse the effects of opioids, including slowed respiration, hypotension, and sedation.

Adverse reactions:

- Cardiac arrest
- Increased blood pressure
- Nausea
- Seizures
- Sweating
- Tachycardia
- Vomiting

Analgesic-Antipyretics

Analgesic-antipyretics, also known as nonnarcotic and nonopioid analgesics, work to (1) relieve mild to moderate pain, (2) reduce fever, and (3) provide an anti-inflammatory effect. Many analgesic-antipyretics are available over-the-counter. These medications may also be used along with narcotic analgesics to control severe pain.

Salicylates and Other NSAIDs

Salicylates have been in use for a very long time. Salicylates reduce pain, relieve inflammation, and relieve fever. Individuals on long-term

Table 17-1 Selected Narcotic Analgesics by Generic and Brand Names with Dosage Information

GENERIC NAME	BRAND NAME	DOSAGE INFORMATION	USES
butorphanol	Stadol Stadol NS	1 mg (one spray) nasal spray q3–4h as needed	Moderate to severe acute pain (e.g., migraine)
codeine	Codeine	15–60 mg oral q4h as needed Oral 10–20 mg q4–6h as needed	Mild to moderate acute, chronic, or cancer pain
fentanyl citrate	Sublimaze	Oral 200–400 mcg q4–6h as needed	Moderate to severe acute, chronic, or cancer pain
	Duragesic	Transdermal q72h	Not for acute pain
hydrocodone	Lorcet	Oral 5–10 mg q4–6h as needed	Moderate acute, chronic, cancer pain
with acetaminophen	Lortab Vicodin	Max 4 grams acetaminophen per day	
hydromorphone	Dilaudid	Oral 1–4 mg q3–4h as needed Rectal 3 mg q6–8h as needed	Moderate to severe acute, chronic, or cancer pain
meperidine	Demerol	50–150 mg oral q3–4h as needed	Moderate to severe acute pain, not for chronic pain, not for older adults
methadone	Dolophine	2.5–10 mg oral initially q3–4h as needed; maintenance 5–20 mg oral q6–8h as needed	Severe acute, chronic, and cancer pain; also for narcotic withdrawal
morphine sulfate	Morphine	Oral 10–30 mg or rectal 10–20 mg q4h as needed	Moderate to severe acute, chronic, or cancer pain
	MS Contin SR Avinza SR cap	Oral, Rectal 15–100 mg q8–12h Oral 30–120 mg q24h	Don't crush! overdose can be fatal
oxycodone	Oxycontin	Oral 10–80 mg SR q8–12h Oral 5–10 mg q6h as needed	Serious abuse potential, overdose can be fatal; Do not crush.
	Roxicodone	Oral 1–2 tab or 5–10 ml 6 h as needed	Moderate to severe acute, chronic, or cancer pain
with aspirin	Percodan	Oral 1–2 tab q4–6h as needed	
with acetaminophen	Tylox, Percocet	Oral Max 4 grams acetaminophen/day	
pentazocine	Talwin-NX	Oral 50–100 mg q3–4h as needed	Moderate to severe pain; not for older adults
propoxyphene HCL	Darvon	Oral 65–100 mg q4h as needed	Mild to moderate acute, chronic, or cancer pain
with acetaminophen	Darvocet	Oral Max 4 grams acetaminophen/day	Not for older adults

Combination Opioid Products (Check for allergies, especially for aspirin combinations.)

Based on Woodrow, R. (2007). *Essentials of pharmacology for health occupations* (5th ed.), Table 19-1. Clifton Park, NY: Delmar, Cengage Learning.

salicylate treatment need to be monitored for side effects, especially older adults who are at risk for ulceration and bleeding, which may be "silent."

Adverse reactions:

- Anaphylaxis
- Bleeding
- Coma
- Depression
- Dizziness
- Drowsiness
- Euphoria
- Frequent bruising
- GI upset
- Headache
- Hearing loss with overdose
- Kidney insufficiency and failure
- Liver dysfunction
- Prolonged bleeding time
- Rash
- Respiratory failure
- Sweating
- **Tinnitus** (ringing in the ears)
- Ulceration

Contraindications include the following:

- GI ulcer and bleeding
- Bleeding disorders
- Anticoagulant use
- Asthma
- Pregnancy
- Breast feeding
- Vitamin K deficiency
- Allergy to aspirin

Special considerations for salicylates and NSAIDs are as follows:

- Take with food or milk to decrease GI upset or use enteric-coated tablets or buffered aspirin.
- Keep out of reach of children especially flavored aspirin.

Table 17-2 gives a list of selected analgesic-antipyretics by generic and brand names with dosage information.

Table 17-2 Selected Analgesics-Antipyretics by Generic and Brand Names with Dosage Information

GENERIC NAME	BRAND NAME	DOSAGE INFORMATION	COMMENTS
acetylsalicylic acid	Aspirin, ASA, Ecotrin, Ascriptin, Bufferin	5–10 gr oral or rectal supp q4h as needed; large doses for arthritis	Give with milk or food
acetaminophen	Tylenol, Panadol, Tempra	325–650 mg oral or rectal supp q4h as needed (max 4 grams/day)	No anti-inflammatory action
combinations			
ASA and caffeine	Anacin	2 tabs oral q6h as needed, max 8/day	
ASA and meprobamate	Equagesic	1–2 tabs oral 3–4×/day	Used to treat pain accompanied by anxiety and/or tension
ASA, acetaminophen, and caffeine	Excedrin	2 tabs/caps oral q6h as needed, max 8/day	Also for pain of migraine headaches
butalbital, caffeine, and acetaminophen	Esgic, Fioricet	1–2 tabs/caps oral q4h as needed, max 6/day	See Equagesic
tramadol	Ultram	50–100 mg oral q4–6h as needed, max 400 mg daily	Strong analgesic, not controlled
with acetaminophen	Ultracet	Oral 2 tabs q4–6h, max 8 tabs/24h	

This is only a representative list.

Based on Woodrow, R. (2007). *Essentials of pharmacology for health occupations* (5th ed.), Table 19-2. Clifton Park, NY: Delmar, Cengage Learning.

Acetominophen. Acetominophen is used to treat mild to moderate pain and to relieve fever. Acetominophen has fewer side effects than salicylates.

Adverse reactions:

- Blood dyscrasias
- Hives
- Kidney insufficiency
- Rash
- Severe liver toxicity

Contraindications include the following:

- Repeated administration with anemia
- Cardiac conditions
- Asthma
- Kidney disease
- Liver disease

Special considerations with acetaminophen include the following:

- Be aware that toxicity may occur with a single dose.

- Use caution with frequent use of acetaminophen and alcohol. There is a potential for severe liver damage.

- Do not use acetaminophen with other acetaminophen-containing medications. If an individual has orders for multiple medications containing acetaminophen, the UAP should hold the medications and contact her supervisor and the individual's licensed HCP immediately.

Table 17-2 gives a list of selected analgesic-antipyretics by generic and brand names with dosage information.

Tramadol. Tramadol (Ultram) is a nonnarcotic analgesic that is similar in effect to opioids. Tramadol inhibits the reuptake of norepinephrine and serotonin in the brain.

Adverse reactions:

- Allergic reactions

- Anxiety

- Confusion

- Constipation

- Dizziness

- Headache

- Itching

- Malaise

- Nausea

- Orthostatic hypotension

- Rash

- **Somnolence** (drowsiness)

- Sweating

Contraindications include the following:

- Increased intracranial pressure

- Head injury

- Kidney disease

- Liver disease

- Seizure disorders

- Pregnancy

- Breast feeding

- Abrupt discontinuance

- Allergy to opiates

Special considerations for Tramadol (Ultram) are as follows:

- Always count respirations before giving these medications. If the respiratory rate is twelve (12) or lower, hold the medication. Call the individual's licensed HCP immediately.

- Do not administer OTC or herbal medications without first talking with the individual's licensed HCP.

- Tell the individual that she should not drive or operate machinery while taking this medication.

Table 17-2 gives a list of selected analgesic-antipyretics by generic and brand names with dosage information.

Adjuvant Analgesics

Adjuvant analgesics are medications that are used to treat conditions other than pain. When combined with narcotic analgesics and analgesic-antipyretics, however, these medications increase the analgesic effect of the medications. In addition, adjuvant analgesics reduce pain on their own and decrease the side effects of analgesics.

Two classes of medications commonly used for analgesia are tricyclic antidepressants and anticonvulsants. In addition, Lidocaine (Lidoderm), a local anesthetic, is available topically as a patch.

Tricyclic Antidepressants

Tricyclic antidepressants are used to treat (1) nerve pain due to herpes, arthritis, diabetes, and cancer; (2) migraine or tension headaches; (3) insomnia; and (4) depression. The pain is often described as "burning." Medications often used are as follows:

- Elavil

- Pamelor

- Tofranil

Adverse reactions:

- Constipation

- Delirium

- Dry mouth

- Heart block in individuals with cardiac disease

- Orthostatic hypotension

- Sedation

- Tachyarrythmias

- Urinary retention

Note: Adverse effects may be additive with narcotic analgesics.

Table 17-3 Selected Adjuvant Analgesics by Generic and Brand Names with Dosage Information

GENERIC NAME	BRAND NAME	DOSAGE INFORMATION	COMMENTS
Tricyclic Antidepressants			
amitripytyline	Elavil	Oral 10–100 mg at bedtime	Caution combining with opioids
nortriptyline	Pamelor	Oral 10–150 mg at bedtime	
imipramine	Tofranil	Oral 10–150 mg at bedtime	
Anticonvulsants			
carbamazepine	Tegretol	Oral 200 mg 2 × /day	Especially for trigeminal neuralgia Monitor serum levels periodically
gabapentin	Neurontin	Oral 600–3600 mg/day in divided doses 3–4×/day	For nerve pain, especially postherpetic neuralgia
lamotrigine	Lamictal	Oral 25–200 mg twice a day	Use when unresponsive to others
Local Anesthetic			
Lidocaine	Lidoderm	1–3 Patches 5% daily	For postherpetic neuralgia (12 hrs off and 12 hrs on)

Note: All adjuvants should be started at the lower end of the dosage range and increased in small amounts weekly.

Based on Woodrow, R. (2007). *Essentials of pharmacology for health occupations* (5th ed.), Table 19-3. Clifton Park, NY: Delmar, Cengage Learning.

Contraindications include the following:

- Allergy to the medication
- Being in the recovery phase of **myocardial infarction (MI)** (heart attack)

For special considerations for tricyclic antidepressants, see Chapter 16.

Table 17-3 gives a list of selected adjuvant analgesics by generic and brand names with dosage information.

Anticonvulsants

Anticonvulsants are also used for nerve pain due to neuralgia, herpes zoster (shingles), and cancer. Pain is described as "sharp," "shooting," "shocklike," or "lightninglike." Medications commonly used are as follows:

- Neurontin
- Tegretol
- Lamictal

Adverse reactions:

- Anorexia
- Blurred vision
- Bone marrow suppression
- Confusion
- Constipation

- Diplopia
- Dizziness
- Gingivitis
- Hepatitis
- Hypotension
- Nausea
- Nystagmus
- Rash
- Sedation
- **Stevens-Johnson syndrome**
- Unsteadiness
- Vomiting

Stevens-Johnson syndrome
A serious, sometimes fatal, inflammatory disease. Signs and symptoms include the sudden onset of fever, blisters on the skin, and ulcers on the mucous membranes of the lips, eyes, mouth, nose, and genitals.

Contraindications include the following:

- Allergy to the medications
- Psychiatric conditions
- Pregnancy
- Sinoatrial and atrioventricular block
- Blood disorders
- Abrupt discontinuation

For special considerations, refer to Chapter 18.

Table 17-3 gives a list of selected adjuvant analgesics by generic and brand names with dosage information.

Lidocaine

Lidocaine (Lidoderm) is a local anesthetic used for the treatment of postherpetic neuralgia, including diabetic neuropathy and musculoskeletal pain, such as osteoarthritis and low back pain.

Adverse reactions are usually mild:

- Allergic reactions to the medication
- Edema (swelling)
- Hives
- Redness

Contraindications include the following:

- Sensitivity to local anesthetics
- Liver disease
- Nonintact skin
- Pregnancy
- Breast feeding

Special considerations are as follows:

- *The lidocaine patch must be applied to intact skin.*

- Patches may be cut into smaller pieces with scissors before removal of the release liner to fit the specific area that it is being applied to.

- Patches work for only twelve (12) hours within a twenty-four (24)-hour period, then are removed.

Table 17-3 gives a list of selected adjuvant analgesics by generic and brand names with dosage information.

ANTIMIGRAINE MEDICATIONS

Migraine headaches are thought to be due to an imbalance of chemicals in the brain and altered nerve activity that cause the blood vessels of the brain to dilate. Studies have shown that serotonin levels drop during a migraine headache when the blood vessels are dilated.

Migraines are the most common type of vascular headache. A migraine usually begins on one side of the head, spreads to the other side of the head, and becomes generalized. It may last for several hours or for days. The severity of the headache varies.

In addition to headache, individuals may experience the following symptoms:

- Constipation

- Diarrhea

- Nausea

- Photophobia

- Sensitivity to noise

- Visual changes

- Vomiting

Migraine headaches may be triggered by the following:

- Changes in weather

- Stress or emotional upset

- High altitude

- Polluted air

- Smoking

- Certain foods, chocolate, aged cheese, food additives, and alcohol, especially red wine and beer

- Hormonal changes

Migraines may be effectively treated with analgesics, NSAIDs, and narcotic analgesics. Early treatment is the key, beginning, hopefully, in the very early stages of the migraine.

Serotonin Receptor Agonists (SRAs)

When other medications fail to relieve an individual's migraine headache, serotonin receptor agonists (SRAs) are an effective treatment. In addition to relieving pain, SRAs also relieve nausea and vomiting related to the migraine. SRAs work by causing constriction in the arteries in the brain.

Three SRAs available today are as follows:

- Imitrex (sumatriptan)—first SRAs to receive approval
- Maxalt (rizatriptan)
- Relpax (eletriptan)

Adverse reactions:

- Angina
- Arrythmias
- **Asthenia** (absence or loss of strength, weakness)
- Cardiac arrest
- Diarrhea
- Dizziness
- Drowsiness
- Fatigue
- Flushing
- Malaise
- MI (heart attack)
- Nausea
- Pain or pressure in the chest, neck, or jaw
- Palpitations
- **Paresthesias** (an abnormal sensation of crawling or burning of the skin)
- Tingling
- Vomiting

Contraindications include the following:

- Cerebrovascular or cardiovascular disease
- Liver disease
- Kidney disease
- Use in older adults
- Pregnancy
- Breast feeding

Table 17-4 Selected Antimigraine Medications by Generic and Brand Names with Dosage Information

GENERIC NAME	BRAND NAME	DOSAGE FORMS	INITIAL DOSE ADULT	REPEAT TIME (HOURS)	DAILY MAXIMUM DOSE (MG)
eletriptan	Relpax	Tablet	20–40 mg	2	80
rizatriptan	Maxalt	Tablet	5–10 mg	2	30
	Maxalt-MLT	OD tablet*	5–10 mg	2	30
sumatriptan	Imitrex	Nasal	20 mg	2	40
		Tablet	25–100 mg	2	200

*OD, orally disintegrating tablet.

Based on Woodrow, R. (2007). *Essentials of pharmacology for health occupations* (5th ed.), Table 19-4. Clifton Park, NY: Delmar, Cengage Learning.

Special considerations are as follows:

- Do not administer within fourteen (14) days of an MAOI.
- Monitor blood pressure and pulse closely. Notify individual's licensed HCP if changes in blood pressure and/or pulse occur.
- Report individual's response to medication to her licensed HCP.

Table 17-4 gives a list of selected antimigraine medications by generic and brand names with dosage information.

ANESTHETICS

Anesthetics are medications used to (1) prevent pain, (2) relax muscles, and (3) induce lack of sensation during surgery and other procedures. There are three main types of anesthetics. They are as follows:

- General anesthetic
- Regional anesthetic
- Local anesthetic

General Anesthetics

General anesthetics are used to block pain in the brain. General anesthetics cause loss of consciousness. These anesthetics are administered in two ways:

- Inhalation
- Intravenous

Regional Anesthetics

Regional anesthetics block nerve impulses to a specific area of the body to produce a loss of feeling without loss of consciousness. Regional anesthetics may be mdministered with or without sedation. An anesthetic medication is injected along a specific nerve pathway.

Table 17-5 Local Anesthetics by Generic and Brand Names with Routes and Adverse Reactions

GENERIC NAME	BRAND NAME	ROUTE(S)	ADVERSE REACTIONS
bupivacaine HCl	Marcaine HCl	injection	Usually dose related: apnea, hypotension, heart block
dyclonine HCl	Dyclone	topical	Hives, edema, burning, hypotension, blurred vision
lidocaine HCl	Xylocaine HCl	topical, injection	Drowsiness, lightheadedness, euphoria, tinnitus, blurred vision, numbness of lips
procaine HCl	Novocain	injection	Nervousness, dizziness, hypotension, postspinal headache
tetracaine HCl	Pontocaine	topical, injection	Nervousness, blurred vision, drowsiness, nausea, vomiting, chills, hypotension, edema

Based on Moini, J. (2009). *Fundamental Pharmacology for Pharmacy Technicians*, Table 9-3. Clifton Park, NY: Delmar, Cengage Learning.

Local Anesthetics

With the use of local anesthetics, the individual remains awake during the surgery or procedure but remains free of pain. Local anesthetics may be applied in the following two ways:

- Topical—direct application of the local anesthetic to the tissues in the form of ointment, lotions, solutions, or sprays as previously discussed with the Lidoderm patch.

- Injections—anesthetic is injected into a local area to create a local nerve block such as is done when stitching a laceration or extracting (pulling) teeth.

Table 17-5 gives a list of selected local anesthetic medications by generic and brand names with routes and adverse reactions.

SEDATIVES AND HYPNOTICS

Sedatives and hypnotics are used to treat disorders that cause anxiety and insomnia. Whether a medication acts as a sedative or a hypnotic depends on the dose given. A **sedative** calms, soothes, or quiets without causing sleep, while a **hypnotic** is a dose high enough to cause sleep. The two classes of sedatives and hypnotics are as follows:

- Barbiturates
- Nonbarbiturates

sedative
A medication that calms, soothes, or quiets without causing sleep.

hypnotic
A medication that causes sleep.

Barbiturates

Barbiturates are seldom used today as a sedative or hypnotic. They have been found to be involved in many suicides and fatalities due to accidental overdoses, especially when combined with alcohol or other

CNS depressants. Use of barbiturates is restricted to those instances in which an individual can be closely monitored.

Adverse reactions:

- Agitation
- Anxiety
- Ataxia
- Bradycardia
- Confusion
- Constipation
- Dizziness
- Drowsiness
- Excessive movement of the body
- Fever
- Headache
- Hypotension
- Nausea
- Nightmares
- Rash
- Vomiting

Special considerations when giving barbiturates include the following:

- Warning: Barbiturates may cause physical dependency and addiction.

- Observe the individual for signs of respiratory dysfunction, including dilated pupils and a respiratory rate of less than twelve (12) breaths a minute. If these signs are noted, immediately call the individual's licensed HCP. If no response from the licensed HCP within a short period of time, call 911 or your local emergency medical services and one's supervisor.

- Observe the individual for signs of toxicity, including bluish lips, cold and clammy skin, delirium, hallucinations, insomnia, nausea, and vomiting. If these signs are noted, immediately call the individual's licensed HCP. If no response from the licensed HCP within a short period of time, call 911 or your local emergency medical services and one's supervisor.

- Instruct the individual to avoid the use of alcohol.

- Individuals should not drive or operate machinery while taking this medication.

- Do not suddenly stop the medication.

Nonbarbiturates

For the most part, nonbarbiturates have replaced the use of barbiturates. However, because withdrawal may occur with long-term use of nonbarbiturates and respiratory distress may occur when taken with alcohol, only short-term use of nonbarbiturates is recommended. Before beginning treatment with nonbarbiturates, the cause(s) for the insomnia and/or anxiety should be determined.

Nonbarbiturates include the following medications:

- Chloral hydrate (Aquachloral)
- Temazepam (Restoril)
- Zaleplon (Sonata)
- Zolpidem tartrate (Ambien)

Adverse reactions of chloral hydrate (Aquachloral):

- Ataxia
- Dependence with withdrawal symptoms
- Diarrhea
- Dizziness
- Nausea
- Rash
- Vomiting

Adverse reactions with benzodiazepines, temazepam (Restoril):

- Amnesia
- Bizarre behavior
- Confusion
- Daytime sedation
- Dependence with withdrawal symptoms
- Hangover effect
- Headache
- Hallucinations
- Increased risk of falls

Contraindications for all sedative and hypnotics include the following:

- Allergy to the medication
- Severe liver impairment
- Severe kidney impairment
- Abrupt discontinuation

- Individual prone to addiction

- Depression

- Individual who is mentally impaired

- Individual at risk for suicide

- Pregnancy

- Breast feeding

- COPD

- Sleep apnea

Special considerations are as follows:

- Take only limited doses for short periods of time.

- Always count respirations before giving these medications. If the respiratory rate is twelve (12) or lower, hold the medication. Call the individual's licensed HCP immediately.

- Instruct the individual to avoid the use of alcohol.

- Do not administer OTC or herbal medications without first contacting the individual's licensed HCP.

- Individuals should not drive or operate machinery while taking this medication.

- Do not suddenly stop the medication.

Table 17-6 gives a selective list of sedatives and hypnotics by generic and brand names with dosing information.

Table 17-6 Selected Sedatives and Hypnotics by Generic and Brand Names with Dosage Information

GENERIC NAME	BRAND NAME	DOSAGE INFORMATION	COMMENTS
Nonbarbituarates			
chloral hydrate		Oral 500 mg–1 g or rectal ½ h before bedtime	Short-term treatment of insomnia only (loses effectiveness within 2 weeks)
			Preop sedation
estazolam	Prosom	0.5–2 mg oral at bedtime	Rapid onset, intermediate duration
flurazepam	Dalmane	15–30 mg oral at bedtime	Rapid onset, long half-life
temazepam	Restoril	7.5–30 mg oral at bedtime	Intermediate onset and duration
triazolam	Halcion	0.125–0.25 mg oral at bedtime	Can cause amnesia, hallucinations, bizarre behavior, rapid onset, short duration
zolpidem	Ambien	5–10 mg oral	Rapid onset 30 min
			Short half-life (less than 3 hrs)
zaleplon	Sonata	Oral 5–10 mg at bedtime	Rapid onset, very short half-life

Based on Woodrow, R. (2007). *Essentials of pharmacology for health occupations* (5th ed.), Table 19-5. Clifton Park, NY: Delmar, Cengage Learning.

SUMMARY

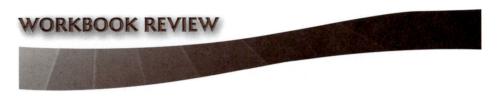

Pain and insomnia significantly impact an individual's quality of life. It is, therefore, the UAP's responsibility to have a basic understanding of these disorders and the medications used to manage and control them. This understanding will help the UAP to (1) observe the individuals in her care for pain; (2) administer analgesics, hypnotics, and sedatives safely and effectively; and (3) observe individuals in her care who have received anesthetics for various procedures and surgery.

WORKBOOK REVIEW

Go to the workbook and complete the exercises for Chapter 17.

REVIEW QUESTIONS

1. The four types of pain are:
   a. sudden pain, chronic pain, ghost pain, radiating pain
   b. acute pain, chronic pain, phantom pain, radiating pain
   c. acute pain, chronic pain, ghost pain, rotating pain
   d. sudden pain, chronic pain, phantom pain, rotating pain
2. Analgesics are used to relieve:
   a. hypotension
   b. pain
   c. nausea
   d. constipation
3. Analgesics are most effective when administered:
   a. before meals
   b. when needed
   c. during waking hours
   d. around the clock
4. Migraine headaches:
   a. begin in the center of the forehead then spread to the back of the head
   b. are the same for all individuals
   c. are due to a chemical imbalance in the brain and altered nerve activity
   d. last one (1) to two (2) hours

5. Anesthetics are used to:
   a. stop seizures
   b. treat Alzheimer's disease
   c. prevent pain and promote muscle relaxation
   d. treat insomnia

6. General anesthetics are administered by:
   a. inhalation
   b. patch
   c. spray
   d. lotion

7. A sedative is:
   a. a medication that causes increased energy
   b. a medication that causes sleep
   c. a medication that causes a calming effect without sleep
   d. a medication that causes tremors

8. A hypnotic is:
   a. a medication that causes increased energy
   b. a medication that causes sleep
   c. a medication that causes a calming effect without sleep
   d. a medication that causes tremors

9. Barbiturates are:
   a. the most frequently used sedative today
   b. preferred over nonbarbiturates
   c. used only in restricted circumstances
   d. used to treat severe pain

10. Nonbarbiturates are:
   a. used for long-term treatment of insomnia
   b. connected to many suicides and fatalities due to accidental overdoses
   c. completely safe
   d. recommended for short-term use only

Chapter 18
Anticonvulsants, Antiparkinsonian Medications, and Medications for the Treatment of Alzheimer's Disease

Learning Objectives

After reading this chapter and completing the review questions, you should be able to:

1. Spell and define terms.
2. Discuss the uses, adverse reactions, and special considerations for various medications used to treat seizure disorders, Parkinson's disease, and Alzheimer's disease.
3. State the mood changes that occur in an individual with Alzheimer's disease.

Key Terms

Alzheimer's disease	antiparkinsonian medications	epilepsy	status epilepticus
anticonvulsants		Parkinson's disease	syncope

INTRODUCTION

Alzheimer's disease, Parkinson's disease, and seizure disorders affect millions of individuals in the United States today. These diseases significantly impact an individual's quality of life as well as his family and friends. At times an individual may not even be able to perform his own daily activities. Medications, along with other treatments, provide an individual with the opportunity to live his life to the fullest.

ANTICONVULSANTS

Anticonvulsants are medications used to treat seizures in individuals with **epilepsy**. Epilepsy is a not a mental illness. It is a disorder of the nervous system. Epilepsy is caused by recurring and temporary periods of disrupted brain activity. It may be caused by anything that affects the brain. About 70% of the time, the cause is unknown (Epilepsy Foundation, 2009 J).

According to the Epilepsy Foundation, more than three (3) million Americans of all ages have epilepsy. Approximately 200,000 additional new cases of seizure disorders and epilepsy are diagnosed each year. Over their lifetime, 1 in 10 adults in the United States will have a seizure (Epilepsy Foundation, 2009 J).

The goal of anticonvulsant therapy is to prevent seizures (1) without oversedating the individual and (2) while minimizing adverse side effects. An individual's daily dose is adjusted based on his response to the medication. (Epilepsy Foundation, 2009 f)

Refer to Chapter 34 for detailed information on epilepsy, including the care of an individual having a seizure.

Adverse reactions:

- Ataxia
- Coarsening of facial features
- Confusion
- Constipation
- Dizziness
- Enlargement of the lips
- Fever
- Headache
- Insomnia
- Jerking of the eyeballs
- Muscle twitching
- Nausea
- Nervousness
- Rash similar to measles
- Slurred speech
- Vomiting
- Weight gain

Contraindications include the following:

- Pregnancy
- Breast feeding
- Liver disease
- Kidney disease

anticonvulsants
Medications used to treat seizures in individuals with epilepsy.

epilepsy
A seizure disorder caused by recurring and temporary episodes of disrupted brain function.

- Pancreatitis (inflammation of the pancreas)
- Diabetes
- Congestive heart failure
- Bradycardia
- Heart block
- Hypotension
- Blood disorders
- Abrupt sudden discontinuation

Special considerations for these medications include the following:

- Be aware that some of these medications can discolor urine pink.
- Do not stop these medications suddenly. Doing so may cause seizures. If there is an order to suddenly stop an anticonvulsant medication, contact the individual's licensed HCP to clarify the order before discontinuing the medication.
- Do not administer Tegretol with grapefruit juice.
- Give medications with food or milk to decrease GI upset.
- Instruct the individual to not drive or operate machinery while taking this medication.
- Instruct the individual to use good oral hygiene while taking this medication to prevent complications.
- Individual should wear a Medic-Alert tag or bracelet at all times in case of accident or injury.
- Always administer medication on time. *Never* omit (skip) doses of medication. Doing so may lead to **status epilepticus**.

status epilepticus
A condition of non-stop seizure activity.

Table 18-1 gives a list of selected anticonvulsants by generic and brand names, along with adverse reactions and dosage information.

ANTIPARKINSONIAN MEDICATIONS

antiparkinsonian medications
Medications used to give relief of the symptoms of Parkinson's disease.

Antiparkinsonian medications are used to give relief of the symptoms of **Parkinson's disease**. Parkinson's disease is a slowly progressing, chronic disease of the brain. The nerve centers in the brain responsible for the control of certain involuntary body movements degenerate gradually over a period of time. There is a decrease in the production in the neurotransmitter dopamine.

Parkinson's disease
A nervous disorder that causes tremors, muscle rigidity, and difficulty with voluntary movement.

There are approximately one (1) million individuals in the United States with Parkinson's disease. Two-thirds (2/3) of these individuals develop the disease between the ages of 45 and 69. An individual has about a 2% chance of developing Parkinson's disease in his lifetime (Broyles, Reiss, & Evans, 2007).

Symptoms of Parkinson's disease include the following:

- Slow movement
- Rigidity

Table 18-1 Anticonvulsant Medications by Generic and Brand Names with Adverse Reactions and Dosage Information

GENERIC NAME	BRAND NAME	DOSAGE INFORMATION	ADVERSE REACTIONS	COMMENTS
carbamazepine	Tegretol	Oral 400 mg–1.2 g daily in divided doses, suspension, tablets	Dizziness, vertigo, drowsiness, edema, arrhythmias, skin rashes, nausea, vomiting, abdominal pain, aplastic anemia, blurred vision	Psychomotor (partial or mixed seizures)
	Tegretol XR	Oral 200–600 mg twice a day		Extended release, do not crush or chew
clonazepam	Klonopin	Oral, dose varies	Palpitations, bradycardia, hair loss, hirsutism, skin rash, sore gums, drowsiness, ataxia, dysuria	Absence seizures
ethosuximide	Zarontin	Oral 250 mg–1.5 g daily in divided doses	Hiccups, ataxia, dizziness, hyperactivity, anxiety, epigastric distress, nausea, leukopenia	Absence seizures
felbamate	Felbatol	Oral 3600 mg daily in divided doses	Vomiting, constipation, insomnia, headache, fatigue, nausea, dizziness, anorexia, fever	Partial seizures
levetiracetam	Keppra	Oral, 1000–3000 mg daily in divided doses	Somnolence, dizziness, ataxia, depression, nervousness, vertigo, amnesia, anxiety, hostility, paresthesia, psychotic symptoms, pharyngitis, rhinitis, sinusitis, increased cough, abdominal pain, constipation, diarrhea, dyspepsia, gastoenteritis, gingivitis, nausea, vomiting, headache, anorexia, diplopia, coordination difficulties	Partial seizures
phenobarbital sodium	Luminal	Oral, 60–100 mg as a single dose or in divided doses	Nightmares, insomnia, hangover, dizziness, bradycardia, nausea, coughing, hiccups, liver damage	Grand mal and partial seizures
phenytoin, phenytoin sodium	Dilantin	Oral 300–600 mg daily in divided doses	Nystagmus, diplopia, blurred or dimmed vision, drowsiness, ataxia, slurred speech, hypotension, nausea, epigastric pain, pruritus, acute renal failure, hyperglycemia, gingival hyperplasia, hirsutism	Grand mal, psychomotor, or focal seizures, frequently combined with phenobarbitol
primidone	Mysoline	Oral, 250 mg three to four times a day	Drowsiness, sedation, vertigo, nausea, anorexia, nystagmus, swelling of eyelids, alopecia	Grand mal, psychomotor, or focal seizures
topiramate	Topamax	Oral 50–200 mg daily twice a day	Dizziness, drowsiness, fatigue, malaise, poor memory and concentration, nervousness, psychomotor slowing, speed and language problems, agitation, anxiety, confusion, depression, ataxia, tremor, paresthesia, hyperesthesia	Partial seizures, may affect cognitive function at higher doses

Table 18-1 Anticonvulsant Medications by Generic and Brand Names with Dosage Information—*continued*

GENERIC NAME	BRAND NAME	DOSAGE INFORMATION	ADVERSE REACTIONS	COMMENTS
valproic acid	Depakene Depokote	Oral 15–60 mg/kg daily in divided doses	Breakthrough seizures, sedation, drowsiness, dizziness, ataxia, nausea, hypersalivation, hepatic failure, depression, skin rash	Absence, partial, and grand mal seizures
	Depokote ER	8%–20% higher than daily dose		One dose/day. Do not crush or chew
fosphenytoin	Cerebyx	Administered by injection only	Ataxia, agitation, dizziness, drowsiness, speech disorder, EPS, headache, nervousness, weakness, confusion, paresthesia, hypotension, tachycardia, double vision, nystagmus, tinnitus, nausea, vomiting, constipation, dry mouth, anorexia, pink urine, hepatitis, high blood sugar, rash, itching, altered taste, weight loss, Stevens-Johnson syndrome, coma	*Do not confuse with Celexa or Celebrex*
gabapentin	Neurontin	Oral 300–600 mg three times a day	Drowsiness, anxiety, dizziness, malaise, vertigo, weakness, ataxia, altered reflexes, paresthesia, tremor, amnesia, abnormal thinking, difficulty concentrating, hostility, hypertension, abnormal vision, nystagmus, double vision, dry throat, nausea, vomiting, constipation, upset stomach, anorexia, dry mouth, erectile dysfunction, joint pain, fractures, cough, itching, dental abnormalities, inflammation of the gums, increased appetite, weight gain	Partial seizures, minimal interactions with other medications
lamotrigine	Lamictal	Oral 100–300 mg twice a day	Dizziness, vertigo, headache, drowsiness, ataxia, incoordination, sleep disorders, insomnia, tremors, depression, anxiety, irritability, impaired memory, poor concentration, malaise, seizures, palpitations, nausea, vomiting, diarrhea, constipation, upset stomach, dry mouth, anorexia, liver toxicity, muscle spasm, neck pain, cough, shortness of breath, loss of hair, rash, Stevens-Johnson syndrome, hives, allergic reaction with anaphylaxis	Partial seizures, watch liver function. *Do not confuse with Lamisil (an antifungal)*

Based on Broyles, B. E., Reiss, B. S., & Evans, M. E. (2007). *Pharmacological aspects of nursing care* (7th ed.), Table 32-2. Clifton Park, NY: Delmar, Cengage Learning and Woodrow, R. (2007). *Essentials of pharmacology for health occupations* (5th ed.), Table 22-1. Clifton Park, NY: Delmar, Cengage Learning.

- Tremors
- Balance and postural problems

Four classes of medication used to treat Parkinson's are as follows:

- Dopamine replacement
- Dopamine agonists
- COMT inhibitor
- Other medications

Dopamine Replacements

Sinemet (a combination of carbidopa and levodopa) is used most often for the long-term treatment of Parkinson's disease. Sinemet is recommended as the initial treatment for individuals over seventy (70) years of age and individuals with dementia. Sinemet crosses over into the brain and is converted into dopamine.

Adverse reactions:

- Agitation
- Anxiety
- Anorexia
- Behavioral changes
- Confusion
- Depression
- Dizziness
- Dyskinesias (involuntary movements of many parts of the body)
- Hypotension
- Nausea
- Psychosis
- **Syncope** (fainting)
- Vomiting

syncope
Fainting.

Note: Adverse reactions may be severe. A decrease in dose or gradual discontinuation of the medication may be necessary.

Contraindications include the following:

- Abrupt sudden discontinuation
- Bronchial asthma
- Emphysema
- Cardiac disease
- Hypotension
- Active peptic ulcer

- Diabetes

- Liver disorder

- Kidney disorder

- Glaucoma

- Pregnancy

- Breast feeding

- Psychosis

Special considerations for Sinemet include the following:

- Do not stop these medications suddenly. These medications should be tapered off for one (1) to two (2) weeks rather than being stopped quickly. Stopping the medication quickly may cause an exacerbation of parkinsonian symptoms. If these medications are being stopped suddenly, call the individual's licensed HCP for further instructions before discontinuing the medications.

- Give the medication with or after a meal to decrease GI upset.

- Administer medication on a regular schedule.

- Maintain the individual's physical activity, self-care, and social interaction.

- Instruct the individual to rise slowly.

- Instruct the individual to not drive or operate machinery while taking this medication.

Table 18-2 gives a list of selected antiparkinsonian medications by generic and brand names with dosage information.

Dopamine Agonists

Dopamine agonists are used along with levodopa (Sinemet) to delay the beginning of the complications caused by the levodopa (Sinemet). This class of medications include the following medications:

- Bromocriptine (parlodel)

- Pramipexole (Mirapex)

- Ropinirole (Requip)

Because of the high rate of adverse reactions, bromocriptine (parlodel) is not usually used alone. Pramipexole (Mirapex) and ropinirole (Requip), however, are used for beginning therapy in individuals under seventy (70) years of age. These medications have a protective effect. They may delay the "wearing off effect" seen with Sinement. Using these medications may help postpone the need for treatment with Sinemet for several years.

Adverse reactions:

- Confusion

- Hallucinations

- Hypotension

Table 18-2 Antiparkinsonian Medications by Generic and Brand Names with Dosage Information

GENERIC NAME	BRAND NAME	DOSAGE INFORMATION	COMMENTS
Dopamine Replacement			
carbidopa and levodopa	Sinemet	Oral 10/100–200/2,000 mg in 3–6 divided doses after meals	
	Sinemet CR	Oral 25/100–400/2,000 mg in 2–4 divided doses after meals	Separate doses by at least 6 hours
Dopamine Agonists			
bromocriptine	Parlodel	Oral 1.25 mg twice a day with meals	Used with Sinemet; dosage gradually increased to optimum maintenance dose (up to 40 mg/day)
pramipexole	Mirapex	Oral 0.125 mg three times a day	Increase to a maximum daily dose of 4.5 mg for desired effect balanced against side effects
ropinirole	Requip	Oral 0.25 mg three times a day	Increase to a maximum daily dose of 24 mg for desired effect balanced against side effects
Anticholinergics			
benztropine	Cogentin	Oral 1–6 mg daily in single dose or divided doses	Not for the older adult For drug-induced parkinsonism and other forms of parkinsonian syndrome
trihexyphenidyl	Artane	Oral 1–15 mg daily in divided doses	For drug-induced parkinsonism and other forms of parkinsonian syndrome
COMT Inhibitor			
entacapone	Comtan	Oral 200 mg–1,600 mg with each Sinemet	Use only with Sinemet
Other Drugs			
amantadine	Symmetrel	Oral 100–300 mg daily in divided doses	Also for drug-induced parkinsonism
selegiline	Eldepryl	Oral 5 mg twice a day (second dose no later than 2 P.M.)	Used when levodopa wears off, levodopa dosage can be decreased

Based on Woodrow, R. (2007). *Essentials of pharmacology for health occupations* (5th ed.), Table 22-2. Clifton Park, NY: Delmar, Cengage Learning.

- Nausea
- Psychosis
- Somnolence
- Syncope
- Vomiting

Contraindications include the use of sedatives and hypnotics. These medications may increase the risk for somnolence.

Special considerations are as follows:

- Do not stop these medications suddenly. These medications should be tapered off for one (1) to two (2) weeks rather than being stopped quickly. Stopping the medication quickly may cause an exacerbation of parkinsonian symptoms. If these medications are being stopped suddenly, call the individual's licensed HCP for further instructions before discontinuing the medications.

- Give the medication with food to decrease GI upset.

- Administer medication on a regular schedule.

- Maintain the individual's physical activity, self-care, and social interaction.

- Instruct the individual to rise slowly.

- Instruct the individual to not drive or operate machinery while taking this medication.

Table 18-2 gives a list of selected dopamine agonists by generic and brand names with dosage information.

COMT Inhibitors

COMT inhibitors block the enzyme that metabolizes levodopa (Sinemet). This allows the individual to take less Sinemet. Taking less medication means the individual will have fewer adverse reactions to the Sinemet (levodopa).

Adverse reactions:

- Diarrhea

- Dyskinesia

- Hallucinations

- Nausea

- Orange discoloration of urine

- Orthostatic hypotension

- Vomiting

Contraindications include the following:

- Use of nonselective MAOIs

- Use of CNS depressants

Special considerations are as follows:

- Do not stop these medications suddenly. These medications should be tapered off for one (1) to two (2) weeks rather than being stopped quickly. Stopping the medication quickly may cause an exacerbation of parkinsonian symptoms. If these medications are being stopped suddenly, call the individual's licensed HCP for further instructions before discontinuing the medications.

- Administer medication on a regular schedule.

- Maintain the individual's physical activity, self-care, and social interaction.
- Instruct the individual to rise slowly.
- Instruct the individual to not drive or operate machinery while taking this medication.

Other Medications

Selegine

After an individual has been on levodopa (Sinemet) for several years and this medication has begun to "wear off," an individual's licensed HCP may prescribe Selegine (Eldepryl). Selegine (Eldepryl) will be administered along with the individual's levodopa (Sinemet). Selegine is not administered alone.

Adverse reactions:

- Agitation
- Anxiety
- Arrhythmias
- Confusion
- Delusions
- Depression
- Diarrhea
- Dizziness
- Dry mouth
- Dyskinesias
- Hallucinations
- Headache
- Hypertension
- Insomnia
- Leg pain
- Lethargy
- Light-headedness
- Loss of balance
- Nausea
- Orthostatic hypotension
- Palpitations
- Syncope
- Urinary retention
- Vivid dreams
- Weight loss

Contraindications are as follows:

- Abrupt sudden discontinuation
- Do not use with the following medications:
  - Meperidine (Demerol)
  - Tricyclic antidepressants
  - Selective serotonin reuptake inhibitors (SSRIs)
  - Sympathomimetics

Special considerations are as follows:

- Do not stop these medications suddenly. These medications should be tapered off for one (1) to two (2) weeks rather than being stopped quickly. Stopping the medication quickly may cause an exacerbation of parkinsonian symptoms. If these medications are being stopped suddenly, call the individual's licensed HCP for further instructions before discontinuing the medications.
- Give the medication with food to decrease GI upset.
- Administer medication on a regular schedule.
- Maintain the individual's physical activity, self-care, and social interaction.
- Instruct the individual to rise slowly.
- Instruct the individual to not drive or operate machinery while taking this medication.

Anticholinergic Medications

Anticholinergic medications were the first medications used to treat Parkinson's disease. Today they are still useful in treating mild forms of Parkinson's disease.

Adverse reactions:

- Blurred vision
- Confusion
- Constipation
- Depression
- Dizziness
- Drowsiness
- Dry mouth
- Nausea
- Tachycardia
- Urinary retention

Contraindications are as follows:

- Older individuals due to the risk for mental dysfunction.
- Individuals with benign prostatic hypertrophy (BPH) due to the risk for urinary retention.

- Do not stop these medications suddenly. These medications should be tapered off for one (1) to two (2) weeks rather than being stopped quickly. Stopping the medication quickly may cause an exacerbation of parkinsonian symptoms. If these medications are being stopped suddenly, call the individual's HCP for further instructions before discontinuing the medications.

- Give the medication with food to decrease GI upset.

- Administer medication on a regular schedule.

- Maintain the individual's physical activity, self-care, and social interaction.

- Instruct the individual to rise slowly.

- Instruct the individual to not drive or operate machinery while taking this medication.

Amantadine

Amantadine (Symmetrel) is used to treat parkinsonian symptoms in an individual with prolonged use of phenothiazines, carbon monoxide poisoning, or cerebral arteriosclerosis in older adults.

Adverse reactions:

- Anxiety

- Confusion

- Congestive heart failure

- Constipation

- Depression

- Dizziness

- Edema

- GI distress

- Hallucinations

- Headache

- Hypotension

- Insomnia

- Irritability

- Nervousness

- Urinary retention

- Weakness

Contraindications include the following:

- Liver disease

- Kidney disease

- Cardiac disorders

- Psychosis

- Neurosis

- Depression

- Epilepsy

- Individuals taking CNS medications

Special considerations include the following:

- Do not stop these medications suddenly. These medications should be tapered off for one (1) to two (2) weeks rather than being stopped quickly. Stopping the medication quickly may cause an exacerbation of parkinsonian symptoms. If these medications are being stopped suddenly, call the individual's licensed HCP for further instructions before discontinuing the medications.

- Give the medication with food to decrease GI upset.

- Administer medication on a regular schedule.

- Maintain the individual's physical activity, self-care, and social interaction.

- Instruct the individual to rise slowly.

- Instruct the individual to not drive or operate machinery while taking this medication.

Table 18-2 provides additional information on selegiline, amantadine, and anticholinergics.

ALZHEIMER'S DISEASE

Alzheimer's disease is the most common form of dementia. Four (4) million Americans are currently affected by Alzheimer's disease. It is estimated that by 2030, as many as fourteen (14) million Americans will have the disease (Broyles et al., 2007).

The cause of Alzheimer's disease is unknown. There is some family tendency to develop the disease. Women are more likely to develop the disease than men. Individuals usually develop the disease in their mid-60s or older. Younger individuals, however, do develop the disease, but this is much less common.

The disease causes a progressive decline in cognitive ability that eventually affects all aspects of an individual's life. There is no known prevention or cure at this time.

Behavioral problems commonly seen with Alzheimer's disease include the following:

- Agitation

- Anxiety

- Childish behavior

- Confusion

- Disorientation

- Dizziness

- Inability to remember recent events or to retain new information
- Inattention
- Increased tendency to misplace or lose things
- Impaired balance
- Mood changes with depression
- Paranoia

Two classes of medication are being used for the treatment of Alzheimer's disease. They are as follows:

- Cholinesterase inhibitors
- NMDA receptor antagonists

These medications (1) help with the symptoms of the disease and (2) slow the progress of the disease. They do not, however, cure the disease.

Cholinesterase Inhibitors

Cholinesterase inhibitors prevent the breakdown of acetylcholine in the brain. Doing this improves cognitive function such as memory.
Medications in this class include the following:

- Tacrine (Cognex)
- Donepezil (Aricept)
- Rivastigmine (Exelon)

Adverse reactions:

- Anxiety
- Anorexia
- Confusion
- Diarrhea
- Dizziness
- Drowsiness
- Dry mouth
- Hallucinations
- Hypertension
- Insomnia
- Headache
- Nausea
- Psychosis
- Rash
- Significant liver toxicity—Tacrine (Cognex)
- Sweating

- Syncope
- Tremors
- Urinary incontinence
- Vomiting
- Weight loss

Contraindications include the following:

- GI bleeding
- Jaundice
- Kidney disease
- Pregnancy
- Breast feeding

Special considerations are as follows:

- Closely monitor cognitive status. Report improvement or decline to the individual's licensed HCP.
- Observe for signs and symptoms of infection. If noted, contact the individual's licensed HCP.
- Give medication with food to decrease GI upset.
- Weigh weekly. Report weight loss to the individual's licensed HCP.
- Report to the individual's licensed HCP if the individual is smoking.
- Do not administer OTC's or herbal medications before talking with the individual's licensed HCP.

NMDA Receptor Antagonist

The first NMDA has been approved for the treatment of moderate to severe Alzheimer's disease. The medication is memantine (Namenda). Namenda may be used alone or along with donepezil (Aricept).

Adverse reactions:

- Agitation
- Cerebrovascular disorder
- Confusion
- Constipation
- Dizziness
- Falls
- Headache

Contraindications include the following:

- Pregnancy
- Breast feeding
- Kidney disease

Table 18-3 Medications for Alzheimer's Disease by Generic and Brand Names with Dosage Information

GENERIC NAME	BRAND NAME	DOSAGE INFORMATION	COMMENTS
Cholinesterase Inhibitors			
donepezil	Aricept	Oral 5–10 mg at bedtime	May be taken with or without food
rivastigmine	Exelon	Oral 1.5 mg twice a day with food	Increase to 3–6 mg twice a day (higher doses may be more beneficial)
tacrine	Cognex	Oral 10–40 mg four times a day on empty stomach	
galantamine	Reminyl	Oral 4–12 mg twice a day with food	Caution with liver/kidney disease
NMDA Receptor Antagonist			
memantine	Namenda	Oral 5 mg/day initially then increase to 10 mg twice a day	Can be used alone or in combination with donepezil CNS side effects, especially agitation

Based on Woodrow, R. (2007). *Essentials of pharmacology for health occupations* (5th ed.), Table 22-3. Clifton Park, NY: Delmar, Cengage Learning.

Special circumstances are as follows:

• Administer with or without food. Ask the individual his preference.

Table 18-3 gives a list of selected medications for the treatment of Alzheimer's disease by generic and brand names, along with adverse reactions.

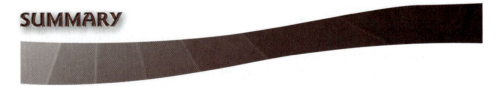

SUMMARY

The UAP plays an important role in the care of an individual with a seizure disorder, Parkinson's disease, or Alzheimer's disease. By administering medications as ordered, observing the individual for responses to the medication(s) and/or adverse reactions, and communicating effectively with the individual's licensed HCP, the UAP helps to ensure that the individual has the best quality of life possible.

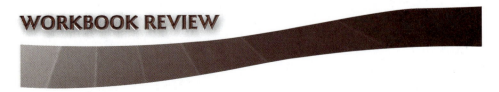

WORKBOOK REVIEW

Go to the workbook and complete the exercises for Chapter 18.

REVIEW QUESTIONS

1. The goal of anticonvulsant therapy is to:
   a. prevent seizures
   b. control tremors and shuffling gait
   c. decrease depression
   d. control bladder spasms

2. Anticonvulsants:
   a. may be stopped suddenly without problems
   b. may be taken while pregnant
   c. should be taken without food
   d. should always be administered on time

3. Status epilepticus is:
   a. due to administering medications too close together
   b. an emergency situation requiring immediate medical attention
   c. a status report on an individual's epilepsy
   d. a minor seizure condition that requires periodic monitoring

4. Parkinson's:
   a. is a sudden-onset neurological disorder caused by trauma
   b. involves all of the major organs of the body
   c. is a slowly progressing, chronic disease of the brain
   d. is cured with radiation treatment and medications

5. Symptoms of Parkinson's disease include:
   a. abdominal pain
   b. hematuria
   c. balance and postural problems
   d. rash and itching

6. If an individual suddenly stops taking his antiparkinsonian medications, he may experience:
   a. increased heart rate
   b. worsening of his parkinsonian symptoms
   c. light-headedness
   d. all of the above

7. The medication Sinemet (levodopa):
   a. is used for the treatment of individuals under the age of seventy (70)
   b. crosses over into the brain and is changed into norepinephrine
   c. "wears off" after a period of time
   d. must always be administered without other medication

8. Alzheimer's disease is:
   a. a disease only of the elderly
   b. a progressive disorder with devastating mental decline
   c. a curable disease
   d. all of the above

9. Behavioral problems seen with Alzheimer's disease include:
   a. lethargy and fatigue
   b. confusion, disorientation, and agitation
   c. increase attention to small details
   d. all of the above

10. When administering medications to individuals with epilepsy, Parkinson's disease, and/or Alzheimer's disease, it is important for the UAP to:
   a. allow the individual to self-medicate at all times
   b. permit the individual to have access to his medications as he wishes
   c. administer an individual's medication on time and as ordered, observe an individual for response or side effects to the medication, and communicate effectively with his licensed HCP.
   d. administer medications when the individual asks for them and allow the individual to make his own appointments with his licensed HCP

Chapter 19
Medications for Treating Infections

Learning Objectives

After reading this chapter and completing the review questions, you should be able to:

1. Spell and define terms.
2. Describe how infection occurs.
3. Name at least three infectious diseases.
4. List the signs of a serious infection.
5. List the emergency supplies and medications that should be available when administering medication to a individual.
6. Describe the various types of antimicrobials used to treat infection along with adverse reactions and special considerations for these medications.
7. Describe the various types of antifungal medications along with adverse reactions and special considerations for these medications.
8. Describe the various types of antiviral and antiretroviral medications along with adverse reactions and special considerations for these medications.
9. Discuss the symptoms and treatment of tuberculosis.
10. State the general recommendations for immunization.

Key Terms

acquired
  immunodeficiency
  virus (AIDS)
active immunization

allergic reaction
anaphylactic reaction
antibiotics

antifungal
  medications
antimicrobials

culture
cyanosis
drug-resistant organism

electrolyte imbalance	hypesthesia	opportunistic	toxicity
fungus	immunity	pancytopenia	tuberculosis (TB)
helminthiasis	immunization	passive immunization	urticaria
herpes zoster	infection	pruritis	varicella zoster
human immunodeficiency virus (HIV)	local anesthesia	stomatitis	virus
	microorganisms		

INTRODUCTION

There are many different types of **antimicrobials** (medications) that are used to treat infections. This chapter provides the UAP with a few examples of the most frequently used antimicrobials. These antimicrobials include antibiotics, antifungals, antivirals, anthelmintics, and antiprotozoas.

antimicrobials
Medications that kill or prevent the growth of microorganisms. (Myers, 2006)

INFECTIONS

We are all constantly surrounded by **microorganisms**. These are organisms so small that they cannot be seen without a microscope. Many are not harmful to us, but some can cause infectious disease.

Infectious diseases may be caused by a virus, bacteria, fungus, protozoa, or other microorganisms. An **infection** happens when microorganisms enter the body or a body part, multiply, and produce injury or illness. Bacteria and viruses multiply very quickly. Because of this, they can often become resistant to medications. This is called a **drug-resistant organism** (Hegner et al., 2008).

microorganism
A living thing, whether plant or animal, too small to be seen with the naked eye. (Hegner, Acello, & Caldwell, 2008)

drug-resistant organism
A microorganism that is not killed by medication and which can potentially cause death. (National Institute of Allergies and Infectious Diseases, 2008)

Drug Resistance

According to the National Institute of Allergies and Infectious Diseases, bacteria and viruses become resistant to medications for several reasons:

1. Overuse of antimicrobials (medications). Licensed health care providers may prescribe inappropriate antimicrobials for an individual who has a viral infection or an undiagnosed condition.

2. An antimicrobial (medication) is stopped before an infection is fully treated. An individual is told to take the medication for ten (10) days but stops taking it after only five (5) days because she feels better.

3. The practice of adding antibiotics to agricultural feed to encourage growth in farm animals. More than half of the antibiotics produced in the United States are used for agricultural purposes (National Institute of Allergies and Infectious Diseases, 2008).

Two examples of organisms resistant to most antimicrobials are:

1. MRSA (methicillin-resistant Staphylococcus aureus)

2. VRE (vancomycin-resistant enterococci)

Treatment options are limited for individuals with MRSA or VRE. Death rates are high for individuals with these infections.

Danger Signs of a Serious Infection

Below is a list of symptoms that must *not* be ignored. If the UAP observes any of these symptoms in an individual for whom she is caring, she *must* get medical attention for that individual *immediately*:

- Burning or pain with urination
- Cough or shortness of breath
- Increase pain at the site of an injury, surgery, or IV
- Pain in the muscles
- Redness, swelling, or warmth at the site of an injury, surgery, or IV
- Shaking chills
- Sudden onset of confusion, especially in the elderly
- Sudden onset of fever (in adults, a fever of 101°F or higher)

Protect Yourself

Because the UAP works in various settings, she will often come into contact with sick individuals. In order to keep herself healthy and prevent the spread of infection, there are steps a UAP can take to minimize her risk of developing an infection. These steps include:

- *Wash one's hands frequently*—handwashing is the single most important way to prevent the spread of infection!
- Stay home if you are ill—do not go to work with a fever, flu symptoms, and so on.
- Do not smoke—if one does, trying to quit is one of the best gifts one can give oneself.
- Reduce stress whenever possible.
- Exercise regularly—one does not have to join a gym; even a walk around the block every day is good exercise.
- Get a good amount of sleep—try to get six (6) to eight (8) hours of sleep in a twenty-four (24)-hour period.
- Keep one's immunizations (vaccinations) up to date.
- Unless your licensed health care provider advises you otherwise, get a flu shot every year.
- Stay well hydrated—drink at least eight (8) glasses of water every day.
- Eat at least five (5) servings of fruits and vegetables daily.
- Do not share food or drink with another individual or anything else that touches one's mouth, such as lip balm, lipstick, or a toothbrush.
- Keep fingers away from one's eyes, nose, and mouth—if one must touch one of these areas for any reason, *wash hands* immediately afterward.

GENERAL INFORMATION ON ANTIBIOTICS

Antibiotics are a type of medication used to treat bacterial infections. Antibiotics do this by slowing the growth of bacteria or by destroying bacteria. Antibiotics are among the most commonly used medications. A licensed health care provider will often perform a **culture** to find out what type of bacteria is causing an illness. This helps to guarantee that an appropriate antibiotic is prescribed for the individual who needs it.

Some antibiotics may interfere with birth control medications. It is important for the UAP to inform the licensed health care provider if an individual is taking birth control medication. If the individual is independent with this form of medication or with her birth control method, the UAP needs to refer the individual to her licensed HCP or pharmacist for advice. Pregnancy may occur if an alternate method of birth control is not used.

Adverse Reactions

As with most medication, an antibiotic may cause an adverse reaction in an individual who takes it. These may include the following:

- **allergic reaction**—can be seen as hives or a rash, fever, headache, nausea, vomiting, and/or diarrhea

- **anaphylactic reaction**—a severe allergic reaction *that may cause death* if not treated immediately; symptoms include swelling in the face or inside the throat, difficulty breathing, **cyanosis**, collapse of the circulatory system, and convulsions

There are certain emergency supplies and medications that should be readily available whenever the UAP gives a medication, especially an antibiotic such as a penicillin or a cephalosporin. The UAP may need to use them if an individual goes into anaphylactic shock. It is strongly recommended that the UAP know the following:

- The location of emergency supplies in her workplace

- How to administer or use them, if needed

- How to call for assistance in an emergency situation

- Her workplace policy for emergencies.

Emergency supplies should include:

- Epinephrine (Adrenalin)

- Diphenhydramine (Benadryl)

- Corticosteroids

- Blood pressure equipment

- Oxygen

- Oral airways

- Cardiac support system

antibiotics
A type of medication used to treat bacterial infections.

culture
A laboratory test done to determine the type of invading organism causing an infection.

allergic reaction
Hypersensitivity, many times noted by a rash or hives.

anaphylactic reaction
A severe allergic reaction *that may cause death* if not treated immediately; anaphylactic shock.

cyanosis
A blue or purplish coloration of the skin because of decreased oxygen intake.

It is very important to find out if an individual is allergic to any medications and to report these to the licensed health care provider. Medication allergies can cause a severe adverse reaction in an individual who is mistakenly given a medicine to which she is allergic. Even if an individual does not have any known allergies, an individual can develop a medication allergy at any time.

After giving an antibiotic, *always* observe the individual for at least thirty (30) minutes to check for any unusual reactions.

Major Antibiotic Groups

Antibiotics are divided into these major groups:

- Aminoglycosides
- Cephalosporins
- Macrolides
- Penicillins
- Quinolones
- Tetracyclines

Aminoglycosides

Aminoglycosides work by killing bacteria (Table 19-1). They are used to treat:

- Active tuberculosis
- Plague
- Subacute bacterial endocarditis (inflammation of the inner lining of the heart)
- *Haemophilus influenzae*; causes sinusitis and chronic bronchitis in adults
- Pneumonia
- Peritonitis
- Respiratory tract infections
- Urinary tract infections
- Infections caused by *E. coli*

Adverse reactions:

- Ataxia (lack of coordination)
- Can cause reversible renal (kidney) damage if noted early
- Can cause irreversible hearing loss
- Headache
- Muscular weakness
- Nausea
- **Pruritus** (itching)

- Skin rashes
- **Stomatitis** (inflammation inside the mouth)
- Tinnitus (ringing in the ears)
- Vertigo (a sensation of spinning)
- Vomiting

Contraindications for aminoglycosides are as follows:

- Tinnitus
- Vertigo
- High-frequency hearing loss
- Dehydration
- Pregnancy
- Breast feeding
- Elderly individuals

Special considerations for aminoglycosides include the following:

- Observe the individual taking an aminoglycoside closely for as long as she is taking the medication. The individual can develop **toxicity**. Signs of toxicity include nausea, vomiting, tinnitus, vertigo, sudden onset of hearing loss, and decreased urine output.

- Encourage the individual to drink at least eight (8) glasses of water daily to reduce the chance of toxicity.

toxicity
A condition that results from exposure to a poison or to poisonous amounts of a substance.

Refer to Table 19-1 for a list of selected aminoglycosides by generic and brand names with dosage information.

Cephalosporins

Like penicillins, cephalosporins kill bacteria (Table 19-2). They are used to treat:

- Mild to severe respiratory infections
- Otitis media (middle ear infection)
- Skin and soft tissue infections
- Septicemia
- Gastrointestinal infections
- Genitourinary tract infections

Table 19-1 Selected Aminoglycosides

GENERIC NAME	BRAND NAME	ROUTE	ADULT DOSE RANGE
Kanamycin Sulfate	Kantrex	Oral	8 to 12 g/day in divided doses depending on use
Neomycin Sulfate	Mycifradin	Oral	4–12 g/day in divided doses

Based on Broyles, B. E., Reiss, B. S., & Evans, M. E. (2007). *Pharmacological aspects of nursing care* (7th ed.), Table 7-5. Clifton Park, NY: Delmar, Cengage Learning.

- Meningitis
- Bone and joint infections

Adverse reactions:

- Abdominal pain
- Diarrhea
- Dizziness
- Dyspepsia (upset stomach)
- Headache
- Itching
- Mild to severe allergic reaction
- Rash

Contraindications include the following:

- Renal (kidney) problems
- Allergies to medications, especially to penicillin
- Long-term use
- Pregnancy
- Breast feeding

Special considerations for cephalosporins include the following:

- Oral doses may be taken on a full or empty stomach, taken with food, or crushed and mixed with food.

Note: **Remember that the UAP needs a written licensed HCP order to crush medication or to mix medication in food.**

- Tell the individual to avoid drinking alcohol when taking some cephalosporins, such as Mandol and Cefizox. Cephalosporins may cause a severe hypersensitivity to alcohol, with symptoms including flushing of the skin, chest pain, palpitations, tachycardia (rapid heartbeat), hypotension (low blood pressure), fainting, and arrhythmias (irregular heartbeat).

Refer to Table 19-2 for a list of selected cephalosporins by generic and brand names with dosage information.

Macrolides

Macrolides are another type of antibiotic. They include:

- Erythromycins
- Azithromycin
- Clarithromycin (Table 19-3)

Erythromycins. This type of antibiotic can slow the growth of bacterial cells or kill them. The type of action that occurs depends on the type of bacteria and on the concentration of the medication. Erythromycins are

Table 19-2 Selected Cephalosporins

GENERIC NAME	BRAND NAME	ROUTE	ADULT DOSE RANGE
Cefaclor	Ceclor	oral	250–500 mg every 8 hrs
Cefadroxil	Duricef	oral	1 or 2 g per day given in a single dose or in a divided dose (twice a day)
Cefixime	Suprax	oral	400 mg daily
Cefpodoxime	Vantin	oral	100–400 mg every 12 hrs
Cefuroxime	Ceftin	oral	125–500 mg every 12 hrs
Cephalexin	Keflex	oral	250–500 mg every 6 hrs
Cefdinir	Omnicef	oral	300 mg every 12 hrs or 600 mg every 24 hrs

Based on Broyles, B. E., Reiss, B. S., & Evans, M. E. (2007). *Pharmacological aspects of nursing care* (7th ed.), Table 7-2. Clifton Park, NY: Delmar, Cengage Learning and Woodrow, R. (2007). *Essentials of pharmacology for health occupations* (5th ed.), Table 17-1. Clifton Park, NY: Delmar, Cengage Learning.

often used for individuals who are allergic to penicillin. They are also used to treat penicillin-resistant microorganisms.

Erythromycins are prescribed for:

- Pneumococcal and diplococcal pneumonia
- Pelvic inflammatory disease
- *Neisseria gonorrhoeae*
- Legionnaires' disease
- Upper and lower respiratory tract infections
- Skin and soft tissue infections

Adverse reactions:

- Abdominal discomfort
- Diarrhea
- Fever
- Skin rashes
- Nausea
- **Urticaria** (hives)
- Vomiting

Contraindications include the following:

- Liver problems
- Alcoholism
- Individuals with hypertension who are taking calcium channel blockers
- Individuals who are taking Diflucan (an antifungal medication)

Special considerations include the following:

- Administer on an empty stomach one (1) hour before or two (2) hours after a meal—enteric-coated tablets may be given regardless of meals.

- Do not administer these medications with fruit juices.

Azithromycin. Azithromycin works by inhibiting the growth of bacterial cells. It is used to treat:

- Lower respiratory infections caused by *H. influenzae, Moraxella catarrhalis,* or *Streptococcus pneumoniae*

- Upper respiratory infections, such as streptococcal pharyngitis or tonsillitis

- *Streptococcus pyogenes* infection in the nasopharynx (part of the throat behind the nasal cavity)

- Uncomplicated skin infections from staph or strep bacteria

- Nongonococcal urethritis and cervicitis from *Chlamydia trachomatis*

Adverse reactions:

- Abdominal pain

- Diarrhea

- Dizziness

- Fatigue

- Headache

- Nausea

- Somnolence (drowsiness)

- Vertigo

- Vomiting

Contraindications include the following:

- Liver problems

- Alcoholism

- Individuals with hypertension who are taking calcium channel blockers

Special considerations include the following:

- Administer the medication at least one (1) hour before or at least two (2) hours after a meal.

- Avoid antacids containing aluminum or magnesium.

Clarithromycin. Clarithromycin also slows the growth of bacteria. It is prescribed for:

- Upper respiratory infections, including streptococcal pharyngitis and sinusitis

- Lower respiratory infections, including bronchitis and pneumonia

- Prevention of bacterial infection in the inner lining of the heart during certain cardiac, dental, respiratory, gastrointestinal, and genitourinary tract procedures when taken one (1) hour prior to the procedure

Adverse reactions:

- Abdominal pain or discomfort
- Abnormal taste sensations
- Certain types of colitis
- Diarrhea
- Dyspepsia (upset stomach)
- Headache
- Nausea

Contraindications include the following:

- Liver problems
- Alcoholism
- Individuals with hypertension who are taking calcium channel blockers

Special considerations for an individual taking clarithromycin are minimal and include the following:

- Administer the medication at any time regardless of meals.
- Report diarrhea with a fever to the individual's licensed health care provider. If the individual's symptoms do not improve in forty-eight (48) to seventy-two (72) hours, inform the licensed HCP.

Refer to Table 19-3 for a list of selected macrolides by generic and brand names with dosage information.

Penicillins

Penicillins are a type of antibiotic that kill bacterial cells (Table 19-4). They are used to treat diseases such as:

- Pneumonia
- Gonorrhea

Table 19-3 Selected Macrolides

GENERIC NAME	BRAND NAME	ROUTE	DOSAGE INFORMATION
erythromycin	E-mycin, Ery-Tab, EES	Oral	250 mg every 6 hrs, 500 mg every 12 hrs 400–800 mg every 6–12 hrs
clarithromycin	Biaxin Biaxin XL	Oral	250–500 mg every 12 hrs 1000 mg daily
azithromycin	Zithromax	Oral	500 mg × 1, then 250 mg daily

Based on Woodrow, R. (2007). *Essentials of pharmacology for health occupations* (5th ed.). Table17-1. Clifton Park, NY: Delmar, Cengage Learning.

- Syphilis
- Meningitis
- Diptheria
- Sinusitis
- Bronchitis
- Acute osteomyelitis
- Otitis media
- Infections caused by *Staphylococci*, *Streptococci*, *E. coli*, and *Salmonella* bacteria

Adverse reactions:

- Allergic reaction or anaphylactic shock (most common reactions)
- Diarrhea
- Chills
- Fever
- Itching
- Nausea
- Rash
- Vomiting

Contraindications include the following:

- History of allergy
- Renal (kidney) problems
- **Electrolyte** (fluid) **imbalance**

electrolyte imbalance
An imbalance of the basic minerals and salts important to our body functions. These are soduim, potassium, calcium, chloride, bicarbonate, and sulfate. (Potter et al., 2009)

Special considerations for penicillins include the following:

- Administer the medication either one (1) hour before or two (2) hours after a meal.
- Administer the medication with 8 ounces of water.
- Do not administer the medication with soft drinks, fruit juices, or wine. The acid in these liquids may destroy the medication.

Refer to Table 19-4 for a list of selected penicillins by generic and brand names with dosage information.

Quinolones
Quinolones work by killing bacterial cells. Specific examples of quinolones include:

- Ciprofloxacin (Cipro)
- Enoxacin (Penetrex)
- Gatifloxacin (Tequin)
- Levofloxacin (Levaquin)

Table 19-4 Selected Penicillins

GENERIC NAME	BRAND NAME	ROUTE	DOSAGE INFORMATION
penicillin VK	Veetids	Oral	250–500 mg every 6 hrs
amoxicillin	Amoxil, Trimox	Oral	250 mg–1 g every 8 hours; 875 mg every 12 hrs
ampicillin	Principen	Oral	250–500 mg every 6 hours
Extended-spectrum amoxicillin-clavulanate	Augmentin Augmentin XR	Oral	250 mg every 8 hours, 500–875 mg every 12 hours 2000 mg every 12 hours
carbenicillin	Geocillin	Oral	382–764 mg 4 ×/day

Based on Woodrow, R. (2007). *Essentials of pharmacology for health occupations* (5th ed.), Table17-1. Clifton Park, NY: Delmar, Cengage Learning.

- Lomefloxacin (Maxaquin)
- Moxifloxacin (Avelox)
- Norfloxacin (Noroxin)
- Ofloxacin (Floxin) (Table 19-5)

Quinolones are used to treat:

- Mild to moderate genitourinary tract infections, such as cystitis, urinary tract infection, prostatitis, and the sexually transmitted diseases gonorrhea and chlamydia
- Upper respiratory infections
- Infectious diarrhea
- Ophthalmic infections
- Bone and joint infections
- Dental work, gum, and tooth infections

Adverse reactions:

Refer to Table 19-5 for the adverse reactions to quinolones. Some are common to quinolones as a group, and some are specific to each medication.

Contraindications include the following:

- Elderly individuals, especially those with gastrointestinal diseases or arteriosclerosis
- Pregnancy
- Breast feeding
- Severe renal (kidney) problems/disease
- Seizure disorders
- Cardiac (heart) disease

Special considerations:

There are no special considerations to be listed here. Consult with the individual's licensed health care provider or pharmacist for specific instructions.

Refer to Table 19-5 for a list of selected quinolones by generic and brand names with dosage information.

Table 19-5 Selected Quinolones with Adverse Reactions

GENERIC NAME	BRAND NAMES	ROUTE	ADULT DOSE RANGE	ADVERSE REACTIONS
ciprofloxacin	Cipro	oral	250–750 mg every 12 hrs	Nausea, diarrhea, vomiting, rash, headache, tremors, abdominal pain, dry painful mouth, cartilage and tendon damage possible, phototoxicity, Stevens-Johnson syndrome*
	Cipro XR	oral	500–1000 mg daily (UTIs only)	
enoxacin	Penetrex	oral	200 to 400 mg every twelve hours	Anorexia, bloody stools, gastritis, stomatitis, anxiety, tremors, cartilage and tendon damage possible, Stevens-Johnson syndrome*
levofloxacin	Levaquin	oral	250–500 mg every 24 hrs	Nausea, vomiting, diarrhea, dry or painful mouth, headache, dizziness, cartilage and tendon damage possible, phototoxicity, photosensitivity, cardiovascular collapse
lomefloxacin	Maxaquin	oral	400 mg daily	Confusion, tremor, vertigo, anxiety, anorexia, coma, bad taste in the mouth, dysphagia, tongue discoloration, cartilage and tendon damage possible, cardiovascular collapse
moxifloxacin	Avelox	oral	400 mg daily	Anaphylaxis after the first dose, cardiovascular collapse, loss of consciousness, vertigo, dysphagia, cartilage and tendon damage possible
norfloxacin	Noroxin	oral	400 mg every twelve hours	Nausea, vomiting, diarrhea, dry or painful mouth, headache, dizziness, photosensitivity, cartilage and tendon damage possible, cardiovascular collapse
ofloxacin	Floxin	oral	200 to 400 mg every twelve hours	Nausea, vomiting, diarrhea, abdominal pain, headache, dizziness, anxiety, hypertension, cartilage and tendon damage possible, photosensitivity, rash

*Note: Stevens-Johnson syndrome is a serious, sometimes fatal inflammatory disease. Symptoms include sudden onset of fever, blister-like lesions on the skin, and ulcers on the lips, eyes, mouth, nasal passages, and genitals (Myers, 2006).

Based on Woodrow, R. (2007). *Essentials of pharmacology for health occupations* (5th ed.), Table 17-2. Clifton Park, NY: Delmar, Cengage Learning.

Tetracyclines

Tetracyclines are a type of antibiotic that slow or inhibit the growth of bacterial cells (Table 19-6).

Tetracyclines are prescribed for:

- Rickettsial disease, from bacteria carried by lice, fleas, ticks, and mites; causes typhus, Rocky Mountain spotted fever, rickettsial pox, and some other less common diseases
- Respiratory infections

- Venereal diseases

- Acne

- Amebiasis

Adverse reactions:

- Anorexia

- Colitis

- Diarrhea

- Nausea

- Photosensitivity

- Secondary fungal infection

- Vomiting

Contraindications include the following:

- Pregnancy

- Breast feeding

- Individuals exposed to direct sunlight

- Individuals with liver disease

- Individuals with renal (kidney) disease

- Individuals with an esophageal blockage or problem

Special considerations when taking tetracyclines include the following:

- Administer medication on an empty stomach one (1) hour before or two (2) hours after a meal.

- Administer the medication with eight (8) ounces of water.

- Do not administer this medication with milk or any dairy products because these can make tetracycline less effective.

- Store the medication away from light, heat, humidity, and cold.

- Tell the individual taking the tetracycline to avoid direct or artificial sunlight because the medication causes increased sensitivity to sunlight, which may result in sunburn.

- Do not administer antacids, laxatives, or iron supplements within one (1) to two (2) hours of administering the tetracycline. These may reduce absorption of the medication.

Refer to Table 19-6 for a list of selected tetracyclines by generic and brand names with dosage information.

Monobactams

Monobactams, like quinolones, work by killing bacteria. The most widely known monobactam is aztreonam (Azactam). This medication is administered only by the parenteral route (injection) directly into the muscle (intramuscular) or into the vein (intravenous).

Table 19-6 Selected Tetracyclines

GENERIC NAME	BRAND NAME	ROUTE	ADULT DOSE RANGE
demeclocycline hydrochloride	Declomycin	oral	150 mg every 6 hrs; or 300 mg every 12 hrs. For gonorrhea initial 600 mg first day, then 300 mg every 12 hours
doxycycline	Doryx, Doxy Caps Vibramycin, Vibra-Tabs	oral	100 mg every 12 hours first day, then 100 mg daily or 50–100 mg every 12 hrs 100–200 mg daily in divided doses
minocycline hydrochloride	Minocin	oral	200 mg at first, then 100 mg every 12 hrs; or 100–200 mg at first, then 50 mg every 6 hrs
tetracycline hydrochloride	Achromycin, Sumycin, Panmycin	oral	250–500 mg every 6 hrs; or 500 mg–1 g every 12 hrs. For gonorrhea 1.5 grams first dose, then 500 mg every 6hrs

Based on Woodrow, R. (2007). *Essentials of pharmacology for health occupations* (5th ed.), Table 17-2. Clifton Park, NY: Delmar, Cengage Learning.

Note: A UAP may or may not be permitted to administer medications by the parenteral route. State regulations and workplace policy will vary. It is the UAP's responsibility to work within her scope of function and to administer parenteral medications only if she has been trained to do so and only if her state regulations and workplace policy permit her to do so. However, administration of medications by the intravenous (IV) route is performed ONLY by licensed health care providers.

Azactam is used for:

- Urinary tract infections
- Lower respiratory tract infections
- Skin and skin structure infections
- Intra-abdominal infections
- Gynecologic infections
- Septicemia

Adverse reactions:

- Abdominal cramps
- Anaphylaxis
- Diarrhea
- Fever
- Headache
- Hypotension
- Malaise (general discomfort)

- Nausea

- **Pancytopenia** (a decrease in the number of white blood cells, platelets, and mature red blood cells in the bloodstream)

- Purpura (hemorrhage into the skin)

- Seizures

- Skin rash

- Vomiting

- Weakness

The only known contraindication is a sensitivity to Azactam or any of its ingredients.

There are no special considerations to be listed here. Consult with the individual's licensed health care provider or pharmacist for specific instructions (Schull, 2007).

Oxazolidinones

These are a new class of antibiotics. Linezolid (Zyvox) is the first of this type to be developed and the first entirely new type in thirty-five (35) years. It kills bacteria by stopping protein production, which keeps them from multiplying. Zyvox is mainly for use in hospitals or other institutional care settings. It is currently prescribed for:

- Vancomycin-resistant *Enterococcus faecium* infections (vancomycin is a type of antibiotic)

- Nosocomial pneumonia

- Complicated and uncomplicated skin and skin structure infections

- Community-acquired pneumonia

Adverse reactions:

- Anemia

- Colitis

- Diarrhea

- Headache

- Nausea

- Vomiting

Contraindications include the following:

- Blood disorders

- Cardiac (heart) disease

- Hypertension

- Gastrointestinal disease

- Hyperthyroidism

- Pregnancy

- Breast feeding

Special considerations include the following:

- Do not administer Zyvox if the individual is taking OTC cold medications that contain pseudoephedrine, such as Sudafed, or phenylpropanolamine, such as Neo-Synephrine. The interaction causes a risk of increased blood pressure. Notify the licensed health care provider if the individual has orders for Zyvox and OTC cold medications.

- Tell the individual to avoid eating foods or drinking beverages high in tyramine content. These foods will interact with Zyvox. These foods include the following:

  - Yogurt
  - Sour cream
  - All cheeses
  - Liver, especially chicken liver
  - Pickled herring
  - Figs
  - Raisins
  - Bananas
  - Pineapple
  - Avocados
  - Broad beans (Chinese pea pods)
  - Meat tenderizers
  - Alcoholic beverages, especially red wine and beer
  - All fermented or aged foods, such as corned beef, bologna, and pepperoni

Miscellaneous Antibiotics

These are antibiotics that do not fall into any other class of antibiotics previously discussed. They include:

- Chloramphenicol (AK-Chlor)
- Clindamycin HCl (Cleocin)
- Imipenem and cilastatin (Primaxin)
- Lincomycin HCl (Lincocin)
- Metronidazole HCl (Flagyl)
- Polymyxin B, bacitracin, and neomycin (Neosporin)
- Spectinomycin HCl (Trobicin)
- Vancomycin HCl (Vancocin HCl)

Refer to Table 19-7 for a list of miscellaneous antibiotics by generic and brand names with dosage information and adverse reactions.

Table 19-7 Miscellaneous Antibiotics with Adverse Reactions

GENERIC NAME	BRAND NAMES	ROUTE	ADULT DOSE RANGE	ADVERSE REACTIONS
chloramphenicol	AK-Chlor	oral	Dose is based on body weight— usual dose 12.5 mg per kg (5.7 mg per pound) every 6 hrs	Bone marrow depression, blood cell abnormalities, headache, confusion, nausea, vomiting, diarrhea, stomatitis
Clindamycin HCl	Cleocin	oral	150–450 mg every 6 hrs	Diarrhea, rash, GI upset, jaundice, anaphylaxis, kidney dysfunction
lincomycin HCl	Lincocin	oral	500 mg every 6 to 8 hrs	Nausea, vomiting, diarrhea, changes in blood cell formation
metronidazole HCl	Flagyl	oral	250–500 mg every 6 hrs to every 8 hrs	Nausea, vomiting, diarrhea, skin rash, seizures, peripheral neuropathy
	Flagyl ER	oral	750 mg daily	
polymyxin B, bacitracin, neomycin	Neosporin	eyedrops, ointment	1 to 3 times daily	Ear damage, damage to kidney cells
vancomycin HCl	Vancocin HCl	oral	125–500 mg every 6 hrs	Nausea, chills, fever, hives, rashes on the eyes

Based on Woodrow, R. (2007). *Essentials of pharmacology for health occupations* (5th ed.), Table 17-2. Clifton Park, NY: Delmar, Cengage Learning.

ANTIFUNGAL MEDICATIONS

A **fungus** is a plantlike organism that may be parasitic or may grow in dead and decaying organic matter. The classification of fungus includes mold and yeasts. Common fungal diseases include *Candida* infections such as thrush, athlete's foot, tinea (also known as ringworm), and aspergillosis, a fungus that infects mainly the lungs. Fungal infections are also commonly found in the folds of the skin under the breast, in the abdomen, and in the groin.

Antifungal medications work by killing fungal cells. They do not work against bacteria, rickettsiae, or viruses. They are used to treat fungal infections that are systemic or that are present on the skin or mucous membranes.

antifungal medication
Medications that control conditions caused by fungi.

Refer to Table 19-8 for the adverse reactions specific to each medication.

Contraindications vary for each of the antifungal medications. Consult with the individual's licensed health care provider or pharmacist for specific warnings.

Special considerations for antifungal medications include the following:

- If the individual being treated has a vaginal fungal infection, tell her that sexual intercourse should be avoided over the course of treatment. Her infection can be spread by intercourse. Her partner could become infected and then possibly reinfect her.

- If the individual being treated has a *Candida* infection, instruct her on proper hand washing procedure and individual hygiene including:

    - Drying the genital area after bathing, showering, or swimming

    - Wiping from front to back after a bowel movement

    - Avoiding heavily fragranced products such as soaps, bubble baths, toilet paper, and feminine hygiene sprays

Refer to Table 19-8 for a list of antifungal medications by generic and brand names with dosage information.

Table 19-8 Selected Antifungal Medications with Adverse Reactions

GENERIC NAME	BRAND NAME	ROUTE	ADULT DOSE RANGE	ADVERSE REACTIONS
amphotericin B	Fungizone	IV, *administered only by licensed HCP*	Dose varies with individual's condition and product formulation	Headache, chills, fever, hypotension, increased respiratory rate, malaise, muscle and joint pain, weakness, loss of appetite, nausea, vomiting, cramps, renal (kidney) toxicity, anemia, low potassium
clotrimazole	Lotrimin Mycelex	Cream, lotion, solution	2 times a day, morning and evening	Reddened areas, stinging, blistering, peeling, edema, itching, hives, burning, and general irritation of the skin
Fluconazole	Diflucan	oral	50–400 mg daily	Nausea, headache, skin rash, vomiting, abdominal pain, diarrhea, liver abnormalities, dizziness, headache, Steven-Johnson Syndrome
flucytosine	Ancobon	oral	Dose is based on body weight—usual dose 12.5–37.5 mg per kg (5.7 to 17 mg per pound) every 6 hrs	Nausea, vomiting, diarrhea, rash, anemia
Griseofulvin	Grifulvin V	oral	300–750 mg total per day given in 2–4 doses a day	Skin rashes, hives, oral thrush, nausea, vomiting, epigastric distress, diarrhea, headache, fatigue, dizziness, thirst, sensitivity to sun, liver toxicity
Itraconazole	Sporanox	oral	Capsule: 200–400 mg daily for weeks or months Oral solution: 100–200 mg daily for days or weeks	Nausea, vomiting, headache

(continues)

Table 19-8 Selected Antifungal Medications with Adverse Reactions—*continued*

GENERIC NAME	BRAND NAME	ROUTE	ADULT DOSE RANGE	ADVERSE REACTIONS
ketoconazole	Nizoral	oral	200–400 mg daily for days or weeks	Anaphylaxis (rare), nausea, vomiting, abdominal pain, itching, headache, fever, diarrhea, impotence
miconazole nitrate	Monistat	cream	as directed by licensed HCP	Vulvovaginal burning, itching or irritation, cramping, headache, hives, skin rash
nystatin	Mycostatin	oral	500,000–1 million units 3–4 times a day	Almost nontoxic—large oral doses occasionally cause diarrhea, nausea, and vomiting
		cream, ointment powder	Apply as directed by licensed HCP	
terbinafine	Lamisil	oral	250 mg daily	Diarrhea, dyspepsia, abdominal pain, rash, hives, itching, taste disturbances

Based on Woodrow, R. (2007). *Essentials of pharmacology for health occupations* (5th ed.), Table 17-2. Clifton Park, NY: Delmar, Cengage Learning.

ANTIVIRAL MEDICATIONS

A **virus** is a parasitic organism that may cause disease by invading normal cells. Common viruses include the common cold, smallpox, herpes, influenza, rabies, hepatitis B, hepatitis C, and AIDS.

Antiviral medications are used to treat specific viral diseases. Common antiviral medications include:

virus
A parasitic organism that may cause disease by invading normal cells.

- Acyclovir (Zovirax)
- Famiciclovir (Famvir)
- Penciclovir (Denavir)
- Trifluridine (Viroptic Ophthalmic Solution 1%)
- Amantadine (Symmetrel)
- Rimantadine (Flumadine)
- Oseltamivir (Tamiflu)
- Zanamivir (Relenza)

Refer to Table 19-9 for dosage information on these medications.

Acyclovir (Zovirax)

Acyclovir kills viral cells by keeping them from multiplying. Acyclovir is used to treat initial episodes and manage recurring episodes of genital herpes. It is not a cure for genital herpes but helps to manage outbreaks

Table 19-9 Selected Antiviral Medications

GENERIC NAME	BRAND NAME	ROUTE	ADULT DOSAGE RANGE
Acyclovir	Zovirax	oral	200–800 mg 5 times a day
Famiciclovir	Famvir	oral	500 mg every 8 hrs
Penciclovir	Denavir	cream	Apply to the affected area(s) of the skin every 2 hrs, while awake, for 4 days
Trifluridine	Viroptic Ophthalmic Solution 1%	eye drops	One drop every 2 hrs while awake
Amantadine	Symmetrel	oral	100–200 mg daily
Rimantadine	Flumadine	oral	Adults 100 mg two times a day Elderly—100 mg daily
Oseltamivir Phosphate	Tamiflu	oral	75 mg twice a day for 5 days
Zanamivir	Relenza	nasal spray	10 mg every 12 hrs for 5 days

Based on Woodrow, R. (2007). *Essentials of pharmacology for health occupations* (5th ed.), Table 17-3. Clifton Park, NY: Delmar, Cengage Learning and Dwyer Schull, P. (2007). *Premier 2008 edition nursing spectrum drug handbook.* USA: Nursing Spectrum.

of the virus. This medication is also used to treat **herpes zoster** (shingles) and **varicella zoster** (chickenpox).

Adverse reactions:

- Anorexia
- Confusion
- Diarrhea
- Dizziness
- Nausea
- Vomiting
- Fatigue
- Edema
- Leg pain
- Skin rash
- Swelling of the lymph nodes in the groin
- Headache

Contraindications include the following:

- Pregnancy
- Breast feeding
- Renal (kidney) disease
- Dehydration
- Neurological abnormalities with high doses

Special considerations for acyclovir include the following:

- Use gloves when applying acyclovir to lesions to prevent unintended application of acyclovir to other body sites and to avoid passing the virus to anyone else.

- Tell the individual being treated that sexual intercourse should be avoided when lesions are visible because of the risk of passing the virus on to others.

- Keep this medication in the container it came in, tightly closed, and out of reach of children. Store it at room temperature and away from excess heat and moisture (not in the bathroom).

Famciclovir (Famvir)

Famciclovir also kills viral cells by preventing multiplication of the cells. It is prescribed for treatment of acute herpes zoster (shingles) and for recurring genital herpes in individuals who have a healthy immune system.

Adverse reactions:

- Diarrhea

- Fatigue

- Headache

- Nausea

Contraindications are the same as for Acyclovir.
Special considerations when taking famciclovir include the following:

- Treatment is most effective when started within forty-eight (48) hours of the onset of the rash.

- May be administered without regard to mealtimes.

- Keep this medication in the container it came in, tightly closed, and out of reach of children. Store it at room temperature and away from excess heat and moisture (not in the bathroom).

Penciclovir (Denavir)

Penciclovir stops viral cells from multiplying. Penciclovir is prescribed for treatment of herpes virus types 1 and 2. Penciclovir cream is used to treat recurring cold sores.

Adverse reactions:

- Headache

- Itching

- Loss of feeling (**local anesthesia**) or decreased sensitivity (**hypesthesia**) at the application site

- Pain

- Rash

- Reaction at the application site

- Taste distortion

local anesthesia
Loss of sensation at the site of application of a topical medication or anesthetic.

hypesthesia
Diminished sensitivity to stimulation.

Contraindications include the following:

- History of allergy to penciclovir, acyclovir (Zovirax), or other antiviral medications
- Pregnancy
- Breast feeding

Special considerations for penciclovir include the following:

- Use penciclovir only on the lips and face. Do not use this medication on mucous membranes inside the mouth, nose, genitals, or rectal area.
- Use gloves for application. Wash hands thoroughly before and after applying. If the individual being treated is self-administering, tell her to wash her hands thoroughly before and after applying the cream.
- Keep this medication in the container it came in, tightly closed, and out of reach of children. Store it at room temperature and away from excess heat and moisture (not in the bathroom).

Amantadine Hydrochloride (Symmetrel)

It is not entirely clear how this medication works against influenza A, which is the main virus it is used to treat. Influenza A is a virus that causes respiratory tract illnesses. Amantadine hydrochloride is also used for treating Parkinson's disease and involuntary body movements caused by medications or drugs.

Adverse reactions:

- Anxiety
- Anorexia
- Blurred vision
- Confusion
- Constipation
- Depression
- Difficulty sleeping
- Difficulty urinating
- Dizziness
- Edema, especially of the hands, legs, or feet
- Episodes of low blood pressure after body position changes
- Headache
- Nausea
- Nervousness
- Shortness of breathe
- Weakness

Contraindications include the following:

- Individuals with mental disorders
- Seizure disorders
- Cardiovascular disorders
- Hypotension
- Renal (kidney) problems
- Liver disease
- Older adults—need a reduced dose
- Pregnancy
- Breast feeding

Special considerations for amantadine hydrochloride include the following:

- Give the medication after meals.
- Tell the individual being treated that she should not change position or stand up too quickly, as this could cause a sudden drop in blood pressure (orthostatic hypotension) that could result in fainting.

Rimantadine (Flumadine)

Rimantadine also works against influenza A. It is used to prevent and treat illnesses caused by various strains of the influenza A virus.

Adverse reactions:

- Dizziness
- Insomnia
- Nervousness
- Nausea
- Vomiting

For contraindications, consult with the individual's licensed health care provider or pharmacist for specific warnings.

Special considerations for rimantadine include the following:

- This can be given to prevent illnesses caused by the influenza A virus. The medication should be started as soon as possible after an outbreak of the virus in the community.
- Observe elderly individuals being given this medication. They may suffer from gastrointestinal problems, insomnia, and nervousness.

Oseltamivir Phosphate (Tamiflu)

Oseltamivir phosphate is used to treat viral infections caused by influenza A and B. Oseltamivir is typically prescribed for individuals who have been ill for two (2) days or less and who demonstrate an uncomplicated acute illness from the virus.

Adverse reactions:

- Diarrhea

- Nausea

- Vomiting

For contraindications, consult with the individual's licensed health care provider or pharmacist for specific warnings.

Special considerations for oseltamivir phosphate include the following:

- May be administered with or without food; however, some individuals may have a better reaction if they take it with food.

Zanamivir (Relenza)

Zanamivir is also prescribed for individuals who are acutely ill because of the influenza A and B viruses. Zanamivir is an inhalant rather than a tablet like oseltamivir phosphate.

Adverse reactions:

- Airway irritation

- Bronchspasm

- Diarrhea

- Headache

- Nausea

- Signs and symptoms that indicate nasal illness

For contraindications, consult with the individual's licensed health care provider or pharmacist for specific warnings.

Special considerations for zanamivir include the following:

- Because it is an inhalant, the individual being treated may need assistance with the inhaler. If she is self-administering, provide many opportunities for demonstration of proper inhaler use. Refer to Chapter 7 if a review of the technique is required.

ANTIRETROVIRAL MEDICATIONS

human immunodeficiency virus (HIV)
A retrovirus that causes acquired immunodeficiency syndrome, or AIDS.

Antiretroviral medications have been approved by the Food and Drug Administration since 1987 for treatment of HIV infection. The **human immunodeficiency virus (HIV)** is a retrovirus that causes acquired immunodeficiency syndrome, or AIDS. There are four classes of medications currently used to treat HIV infection:

1. Nucleoside reverse transcriptase inhibitors—these medications slow the spread of HIV infection in the body and delay the onset of opportunistic infections.

2. Nonnucleoside reverse transcriptase inhibitors—these medications stop some of the infected cells from changing and multiplying.

3. Protease inhibitors—these medications stop the virus from being duplicated by infected cells.

4. Fusion inhibitors—these medications prevent the virus and the cell from joining together. Therefore, HIV is unable to infect the cell and multiply.

These medications are also being used in combinations of three, a treatment called highly active antiretroviral therapy (HAART). It is important to remember that antiretroviral medications do not cure the HIV infection or AIDS.

The adverse reactions that individuals experience from these medications are serious and can be severe, especially since their immune systems are already compromised. Reactions, including anemia, pancreatitis, and peripheral neuropathy, should be reported to the individual's licensed health care provider immediately.

Consult with the individual's licensed health care provider or pharmacist for information on contraindications and special instructions.

Refer to Tables 19-10, 19-11, and 19-12 for specific information on the three classes of medication listed earlier.

Table 19-10 Nucleoside Reverse Transcriptase Inhibitors with Adverse Reactions

GENERIC NAME	BRAND NAME	ADVERSE REACTIONS
abacavir	Ziagen	Malaise, fever, rash, GI disturbances
didanosine, ddI	Videx	Peripheral neuropathy, pancreatitis
lamivudin, 3TC	Epivir	Nausea, headache, diarrhea, fatigue, anemia, neuropathy
stavudine	Zerit	Peripheral neuropathy, pancreatitis
zalcitabine, ddC	Hivid	Peripheral neuropathy, pancreatitis, oral ulcers
zidovudine, AZT	Retrovir	Anemia, fatigue, headache, nausea, myopathy
Zidovudine, lamivudine	Combivir	Anemia, diarrhea, fatigue, headache, nausea

Based on Woodrow, R. (2007). *Essentials of pharmacology for health occupations* (5th ed.), Table 17-3. Clifton Park, NY: Delmar, Cengage Learning and Dwyer Schull, P. (2007). *Premier 2008 edition nursing spectrum drug handbook*. USA: Nursing Spectrum.

Table 19-11 Nonnucleoside Reverse Transcriptase Inhibitors with Adverse Reactions

GENERIC NAME	BRAND NAME	ADVERSE REACTIONS
delavirdine	Rescriptor	Short-lived rash
efavirenz	Sustiva	Initial dizziness, short-lived rash, insomnia
nevirapine	Viramune	Hepatitis, short-lived rash

Based on Woodrow, R. (2007). *Essentials of pharmacology for health occupations* (5th ed.), Table 17-3. Clifton Park, NY: Delmar, Cengage Learning and Dwyer Schull, P. (2007). *Premier 2008 edition nursing spectrum drug handbook*. USA: Nursing Spectrum.

Table 19-12 Protease Inhibitors with Adverse Reactions

GENERIC NAME	BRAND NAME	ADVERSE REACTIONS
amprenavir	Agenerase	Depression, diarrhea, nausea, vomiting, itching, rash, taste disorders
indinavir	Crixivan	Kidney stones in <10% of people— good hydration is vital; occasional nausea and GI upset
nelfinavir	Viracept	Diarrhea, occasional nausea
ritonavir	Norvir	Nausea, diarrhea, numb lips for up to 5 weeks, occasional hepatitis
saquinavir hard gel cap	Invirase	Abdominal discomfort, diarrhea, nausea
saquinavir soft gel cap	Fortovase	Abdominal discomfort, diarrhea, nausea

Based on Woodrow, R. (2007). *Essentials of pharmacology for health occupations* (5th ed.), Table 17-3. Clifton Park, NY: Delmar, Cengage Learning and Dwyer Schull, P. (2007). *Premier 2008 edition nursing spectrum drug handbook*. USA: Nursing Spectrum.

ANTITUBERCULAR MEDICATIONS

Tuberculosis (TB) is a contagious respiratory disease that is spread through the air. It can be caught after an infected individual coughs, laughs, sings, sneezes, or talks. Tuberculosis is seen mostly among individuals with AIDS, drug abusers, homeless people, immigrants, and prison inmates. There are many drug-resistant strains of TB being seen at present.

Symptoms of Tuberculosis

Symptoms of TB include:

- Anorexia
- Fatigue
- Low-grade fever in the afternoon and evening
- Night sweats
- Productive cough
- Spitting of blood after coughing
- Weakness
- Weight loss

Treatment of Tuberculosis

Treatment of TB requires medication therapy with antitubercular medications for six (6) to twelve (12) months combined with proper diet and plenty of rest. Within two (2) to three (3) weeks of beginning treatment, the individual usually can no longer spread the disease as long as she remains on her medication. It is very important that an individual being treated for TB complete her entire course of medication to avoid relapse.

Adverse reactions to antitubercular medications:

- Decrease in vision
- Diarrhea
- Fever
- Hearing loss
- Hypoglycemia
- Kidney damage
- Kidney failure
- Liver damage
- Low potassium level
- Nausea
- Psychosis
- Rash
- Seizures
- Vomiting

Contraindications for antitubercular medications are as follows:

- Allergy to antitubercular medications, sulfates, or other aminoglycosides
- Renal impairment
- Liver impairment
- Diabetes
- Black or Hispanic women with isoniazid (INH)
- Chronic alcoholism
- Pregnancy
- Breast feeding
- Cataracts
- Eye inflammation
- Gout
- Diabetic retinopathy

Special considerations for antitubercular medications include the following:

- Monitor the individual for hearing loss, kidney damage and failure, changes in vision, jaundice, and rash. If noted, immediately contact the individual's licensed HCP.
- Administer medications exactly as prescribed. Do not skip doses.
- Administer medications with food except rifampin (Rimactane).

- Administer oral doses of rifampin (Rimactane) one (1) hour before or two (2) to three (3) hours after meals with a full glass of water. For individuals who are unable to swallow capsules, open capsule and mix medication with syrup. Shake well and administer.

- Inform the individual that rifampin (Rimactane) and rifapentine (Priftin) may turn body secretions (tears, urine, and so on) red-orange in color. This medication may also permanently discolor contact lenses.

- Inform individuals on isoniazid (INH) to avoid foods containing tyramine. Refer to Table 16-1 in Chapter 16 for a list of foods containing tyramine.

- Offer the individual small frequent meals and plenty of fluids to decrease GI upset.

- Instruct the individual to avoid the use of alcohol.

- Instruct the individual to not drive or use machinery while taking these medications.

Table 19-13 gives a list of selected antitubercular medications by generic and brand names with dosage information.

Table 19-13 Antitubercular Medications by Generic and Brand Names with Dosage Information

GENERIC NAME	BRAND NAME	DOSAGE INFORMATION
cycloserine	Seromycin	0.5–1 g daily in divided doses
ethambutol HCl	Myambutol	15–25 mg/kg as a single dose every 24 hours Administer with food.
isoniazid (INH)	Laniazid Nydrazid	5 mg/kg daily with a maximum dose of 300 mg daily
Pyrazinamide (PZA)	Tebrazid	15–35 mg/kg once daily
rifabutin	Mycobutin	300 mg once daily in a single dose or in two (2) divided doses
rifampin	Rimactane Rifadin	600 mg daily in one dose Administer one (1) hour before or two (2)–three (3) hours after meals
rifapentine	Priftin	600 mg twice a day Administer one (1) hour before or two (2)–three (3) hours after meals
streptomycin sulfate		15 mg/kg up to 1 g/day Elderly 10 mg/kg up to 750 mg/day

Based on Broyles, B. E., Reiss, B. S., & Evans, M. E. (2007). *Pharmacological aspects of nursing care* (7th ed.), Table 7-10. Clifton Park, NY: Delmar, Cengage Learning and Woodrow, R. (2007). *Essentials of pharmacology for health occupations* (5th ed.), Table 17-2. Clifton Park, NY: Delmar, Cengage Learning.

Precautions

The UAP may come into contact with people who are diagnosed with TB. If this happens, there are specific precautions that must be followed in addition to standard precautions (Figure 19-1). These precautions are taken to prevent the spread of highly contagious diseases such as TB. Figure 19-2 highlights airborne precautions while Figure 19-3 highlights droplet precautions.

ANTHELMINTICS

These are a class of medications used to treat **helminthiasis**, or an infestation of the intestine with parasitic worms.

There are four types of parasitic worms that infest humans:

1. *Platyhelminthes*, or flatworms

2. *Acanthocephala*, or spiny-headed worms

3. *Nemathelminthes*, or threadworms and roundworms

4. *Annelida*, or segmented worms

Helminthiasis may occur in any country or society, though it is most often related to unsanitary living conditions. *Nemathelminthes*, such as

helminthiasis
A condition in which there is an intestinal infestation with parasitic worms.

G U I D E L I N E S *for*

Standard Precautions

1. Wash hands.
2. Wear gloves for any contact with blood, body fluids, mucous membranes, or nonintact skin, such as when:
   – Hands are cut, scratched, chapped, or have a rash
   – Cleaning up body fluid spills
   – Cleaning potentially contaminated equipment
3. Carry gloves with you so they will always be with you when you need them.
4. If you are allergic to latex gloves, follow your licensed Health care provider's advice. Three possible options are:
   – Change to nonlatex gloves.
   – Apply a skin barrier cream to your hands before putting on latex gloves; the cream protects hands against most irritants, including latex.
   – Put on glove liners that prevent direct contact between the skin of the hands and the latex gloves.
5. Change gloves:
   – After contact with each individual
   – Before touching noncontaminated articles or environmental surfaces
   – Between tasks with the same individual if there is contact with infectious materials
6. Dispose of gloves according to workplace policy.
7. Wear a waterproof gown for procedures likely to produce splashes of blood or other body fluids.

– Remove a soiled gown as soon as possible and dispose of it properly according to workplace policy.
– Wash your hands.
8. Wear a mask and protective eyewear or face shield for procedures likely to produce splashes of blood or other moist body fluids. This is to prevent contact between pathogens and your mucous membranes.
The surgical mask covers both the nose and the mouth. The mask is used once and discarded. When a mask is required, a new one is put on for each individual receiving care. If the mask becomes wet, a new one must be put on because the mask loses its effectiveness when moist.
9. Goggles or a face shield help protect the mucous membranes of the eyes from splashes or sprays of blood and other body fluids. A surgical mask must be worn with goggles and with a face shield to protect the nose and mouth.
10. When using personal protective equipment (PPE), you should:
    – Know where to obtain these items in your work place.
    – Always remove the items before leaving the work area, whether the individual's room, an isolation room, or the utility room.
    – Place used PPE items in the proper container for laundering, decontamination, or disposal, according to your workplace policy.

Figure 19-1 Guidelines for Standard Precautions
(Reprinted with permission from Brevis Corporation (www.brevis.com))

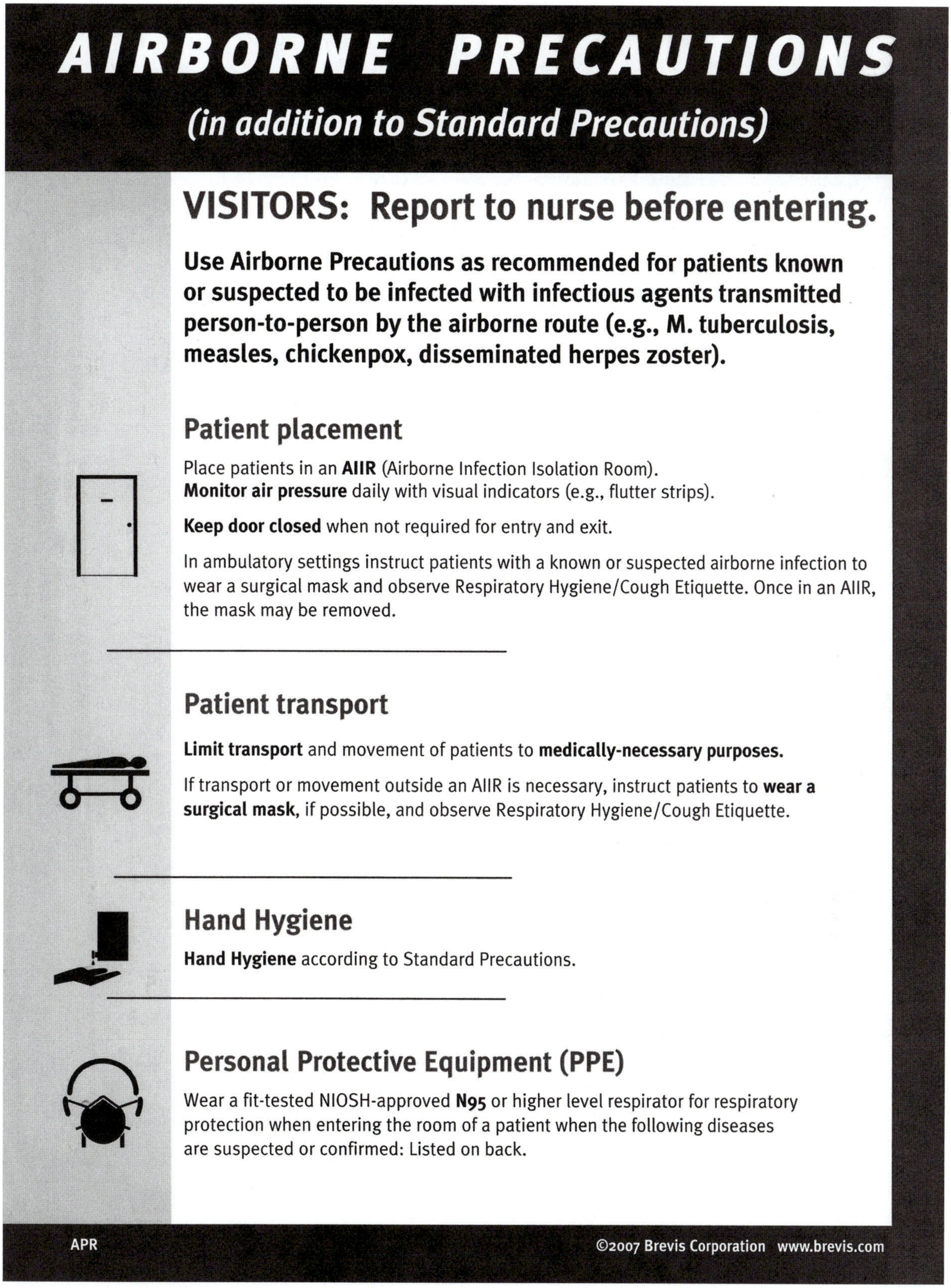

AIRBORNE PRECAUTIONS

(in addition to Standard Precautions)

VISITORS: Report to nurse before entering.

Use Airborne Precautions as recommended for patients known or suspected to be infected with infectious agents transmitted person-to-person by the airborne route (e.g., M. tuberculosis, measles, chickenpox, disseminated herpes zoster).

Patient placement

Place patients in an **AIIR** (Airborne Infection Isolation Room).
Monitor air pressure daily with visual indicators (e.g., flutter strips).

Keep door closed when not required for entry and exit.

In ambulatory settings instruct patients with a known or suspected airborne infection to wear a surgical mask and observe Respiratory Hygiene/Cough Etiquette. Once in an AIIR, the mask may be removed.

Patient transport

Limit transport and movement of patients to **medically-necessary purposes.**

If transport or movement outside an AIIR is necessary, instruct patients to **wear a surgical mask,** if possible, and observe Respiratory Hygiene/Cough Etiquette.

Hand Hygiene

Hand Hygiene according to Standard Precautions.

Personal Protective Equipment (PPE)

Wear a fit-tested NIOSH-approved **N95** or higher level respirator for respiratory protection when entering the room of a patient when the following diseases are suspected or confirmed: Listed on back.

APR

©2007 Brevis Corporation   www.brevis.com

Figure 19-2 Airborne Precautions
Source: Reprinted with permission from Brevis Corporation (www.brevis.com)

DROPLET PRECAUTIONS

(in addition to Standard Precautions)

STOP VISITORS: Report to nurse before entering.

Use Droplet Precautions as recommended for patients known or suspected to be infected with pathogens transmitted by respiratory droplets that are generated by a patient who is coughing, sneezing or talking.

Personal Protective Equipment (PPE)

Don a mask upon entry into the patient room or cubicle.

Hand Hygiene

Hand Hygiene according to Standard Precautions.

Patient Placement

Private room, if possible. Cohort or maintain spatial separation of 3 feet from other patients or visitors if private room is not available.

Patient transport

Limit transport and movement of patients to **medically-necessary purposes**.

If transport or movement in any healthcare setting is necessary, instruct patient to **wear a mask** and follow Respiratory Hygiene/Cough Etiquette.

No mask is required for persons transporting patients on Droplet Precautions.

DPR7 ©2007 Brevis Corporation www.brevis.com

Figure 19-3 Droplet Precautions

Source: Reprinted with permission from Brevis Corporation (www.brevis.com)

roundworms, pinworms, and hookworms, cause the most common infestations worldwide. *Platyhelminthes*, such as tapeworms and flukes, also cause disease in humans.

Anthelmintics include:

- Ivermectin (Stromectol)
- Mebendazole (Vermox)
- Praziquantel (Biltricide)
- Pyrantel pamoate (Antiminth)
- Thiabendazole (Mintezol)

Refer to Table 19-14 for adverse reactions specific to each medication.

Table 19-14 Antihelmintics with Adverse Reactions

GENERIC NAME	BRAND NAME	INFECTED BY	ADVERSE REACTIONS
ivermectin	Stromectol	Strongyloidaisis (roundworm)	Diarrhea, nausea, vomiting, anorexia, abdominal pain, dizziness, tremor, vertigo, itching, rash, fatigue
ivermectin	Stromectol	Onchocerciasis (filarial worm)	"Mazzotti reaction": itching, edema, rash; enlargement and tenderness of lymph nodes in the groin, armpits, and neck; joint pain and inflammation Abnormal sensations in the eyes Rapid heartbeat, low blood pressure on body position change, headache, muscle pain
mebendazole	Vermox	Roundworm, hookworm, whipworm	Diarrhea, fever, dizziness, abdominal pain that is short-lived
mebendazole	Vermox	Pinworm	Same
praziquantel	Biltricide	Blood fluke	Abdominal pain, nausea, anorexia, dizziness, headache, malaise, drowsiness, itching, hives, fever
praziquantel	Biltricide	Other flukes	Same
praziquantel		Tapeworms	Same
pyrantel pamoate	Antiminth	Pinworm, roundworm	Dizziness, drowsiness, headache, anorexia, nausea, abdominal bloating, rash
thiabendazole	Mintezol	Roundworm, pinworm, hookworm, threadworm	Low blood pressure, slow heartbeat, anorexia, nausea, vomiting, jaundice, a stop in the flow of bile, liver damage, headache, blurred vision, foul smelling urine, seizures

Based on Broyles, B. E., Reiss, B. S., & Evans, M. E. (2007). *Pharmacological aspects of nursing care* (7th ed.), Table 8-2. Clifton Park, NY: Delmar, Cengage Learning and Dwyer Schull, P. (2007). *Premier 2008 edition nursing spectrum drug handbook*. USA: Nursing Spectrum.

Special considerations must be given when treating an individual for worms because of the risk of reinfestation. For example, if an individual is being treated for an infection of pinworm or threadworm, all of her family members must also be treated. Her close contacts—friends and coworkers—must also be examined and, if necessary, treated. Body weight is measured before treatment begins. The medicines Antiminth and Vermox may be taken with food; however, Mintezol is typically taken after meals.

Education is an important part of the treatment as well, with focus on ways to avoid reinfestation, including:

- Cook beef and pork thoroughly to prevent the possibility of tapeworms.

- Avoid walking barefoot in areas where hookworms are known to cause infection.

- Wash fruits and vegetables thoroughly to prevent the possibility of roundworms.

- Teach proper hygiene, especially handwashing, before meals and after using the bathroom.

ANTIPROTOZOAL MEDICATIONS

Protozoa are another family of parasites that cause diseases including:

- Malaria, an infection of the blood

- Giardiasis, an infection of the small intestine

- Trichomoniasis, an infection of the vagina; also found in the male urethra and in the male or female rectum

- Amebiasis, an infection of the intestinal tract caused by ingesting microorganisms that live in the intestine; this usually happens by taking in food or water contaminated with feces; can also be sexually transmitted

- *Pneumocystis carinii* pneumonia, an **opportunistic** infection common in individuals with **AIDS**

Antiprotozoal medications include:

- Atovaquone (Mepron)

- Chloroquine (Aralen)

- Chloroquine phosphate (Aralen Phosphate)

- Hydroxychloroquine sulfate (Paquenil)

- Metronidazole (Flagyl)

- Paromomycin sulfate (Humatin)

- Pentamidine (Pentam 300)

- Primaquine phosphate

- Trimetrexate (NeuTrexin)

opportunistic
An organism that can cause disease only in a host whose resistance is already lowered by other diseases or medications.

AIDS
Acquired immune deficiency syndrome is a set of symptoms and infections resulting from damage to the immune system caused by the human immunodeficiency virus (HIV).

Table 19-15 Antiprotozoal Medications with Adverse Reactions

GENERIC NAME	BRAND NAME	DISEASE	ADVERSE REACTIONS
atovaquone	Mepron	Mild to moderate *Pneumocystis carinii* pneumonia (PCP)	Headache, insomnia, cough, diarrhea, nausea, vomiting, rash, fever
chloroquine phosphate		Malaria	Fatigue, irritability, psychoses, nightmares, heart block, low blood pressure, eczema, vomiting, abdominal cramps, visual disturbances
chloroquine phosphate	Aralen Phosphate	Amebiasis (hepatic)	Same
hydroxychloroquine sulfate	Plaquenil	Malaria	GI distress, visual disturbances, degeneration of the retina, vertigo, nerve deafness, tinnitus
metronidazole	Flagyl	Amebiasis, trichomoniasis, giardiasis	Rash, flushing of the skin, headache, vertigo, confusion, insomnia, depression, increased urine output, cystitis, nausea, vomiting, anorexia, abdominal cramps, dry mouth, bitter taste, low white blood cell count
paromomycin sulfate	Humatin	Amebiasis	Headache, vertigo, abdominal cramps, diarrhea, nausea, ear damage, kidney cell damage
primaquine phosphate		Malaria	Nausea

Based on Broyles, B. E., Reiss, B. S., & Evans, M. E. (2007). *Pharmacological aspects of nursing care* (7th ed.), Table 8-1. Clifton Park, NY: Delmar, Cengage Learning and Dwyer Schull, P. (2007). *Premier 2008 edition nursing spectrum drug handbook.* USA: Nursing Spectrum.

Refer to Table 19-15 for the adverse reactions specific to each medication. Special considerations are varied and are specific to the medication and to the protozoa:

- Observe a dark-skinned individual who is taking primaquine phosphate closely. This individual may have a hemolytic reaction. If this occurs, the individual may experience unusual bleeding, such as a nosebleed or blood in the urine. This should be reported to the individual's licensed health care provider immediately.

- Administer before or after meals to prevent GI distress.

- Educate the individual taking this medication about the nature of her disease and ways of becoming infected. Teach the individual about good hygiene habits, especially handwashing, after using the bathroom and before eating.

- When an individual is being treated for trichomoniasis, all sexual partners must also be treated to ensure the effectiveness of the medication.

- Instruct the individual who is taking Flagyl to not use alcohol while taking this medication. The combination may cause nausea, vomiting, headache, and abdominal cramps and may color the urine reddish brown.

IMMUNIZATION

Immunity is protection against or resistance to a disease from the development of antibodies.

Immunity is built up in the body through a mechanism called the *antigen–antibody response*. An antigen, some type of organism, enters the body and triggers a series of complex activities. Mechanical and chemical forces begin to defend and protect the cells and tissues in the body.

Antibodies are made by the body and then released into the body's fluids, where they can fight the antigens and prevent further illness.

Immunity helps the body to:

- Protect itself against specific infectious microorganisms
- Protect itself against cancer and immunodeficiency disease
- Defend body cells and tissues that are attacked by foreign substances or organisms
- Accept or reject blood or organs taken into the body through a blood transfusion or an organ transplant

Immunization is the process of either triggering the antigen–antibody response or of providing temporary immunity by administering an immunizing medication such as a vaccine.

Active immunization occurs when a vaccine is given, causing the body to form antibodies. **Passive immunization** occurs when a preformed antibody or antitoxin is given so that the body does not have to produce it.

immunity
The state of being protected from or resistant to a specific disease because of the development of antibodies.

immunization
The process of inducing or providing immunity artificially by administering an immunobiologic.

General Recommendations for Immunization

Recommendations for immunization are based on a number of factors. They are based on facts about immunizing medications, on scientific understanding of active and passive immunization, and on judgments by clinical specialists as well as public health officials. It is important to note that benefits and risks exist in the use of all products. Vaccines are not 100% safe or 100% effective. Individuals may still get the disease for which they took the vaccine. Adverse reactions are always a possibility as with any medication.

The benefits of immunization include partial to complete protection from specific illnesses. The risks of immunization can be anything from common and undesirable side effects to severe and life-threatening conditions. Recommendations on immunization have to balance the benefits and risks in order to provide the best protection from infections for the highest number of individuals. The recommendations may apply only in the United States since disease occurrence and vaccines may be different in other countries.

For the most up-to-date information about vaccines, immunization recommendations, and requirements, contact:

CDC Info Contact Center	800-232.-4636
National Immunization Hotline	800-232-2522 (English) 800.232.0233 (Spanish)
National Immunization Program at the Centers for Disease Control and Prevention	http://www.cdc.gov.nip

SUMMARY

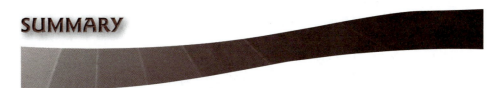

Infectious illnesses are the number one killer of human beings in the world. Around 13 million individuals die each year as a result of untreated or untreatable infection. Diseases including AIDS, the Ebola virus, Lyme disease, mad cow disease, and even drug-resistant tuberculosis are all of concern. It is important that the UAP have a good understanding of the causes and treatments of various infections. This will help the UAP give the best and safest care possible to the individuals with whom she works.

WORKBOOK REVIEW

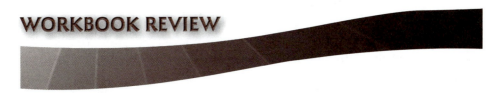

Go to the workbook and complete the exercises for Chapter 19.

REVIEW QUESTIONS

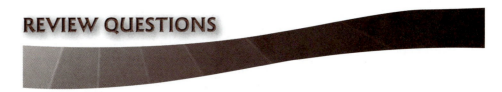

1. A microorganism:
   a. is found only on animals living in unsanitary conditions
   b. can enter the body through intact, healthy skin
   c. can be passed from one individual to another through water
   d. is a living thing too small to be seen with the naked eye
2. An infection happens when:
   a. a microorganism invades the body, multiplies, and causes injury or illness
   b. an individual takes the wrong medication
   c. an individual gets an injury from a fall
   d. an individual comes into contact with a sick individual

3. Drug-resistant organisms:
   a. are not a problem in the United States
   b. are increasing because of the overuse of antibiotics
   c. cause only minor illnesses
   d. all of the above

4. If one observes that an individual in her care has a sudden high fever with muscle pain and enlarged lymph nodes, she should:
   a. continue to observe her for twenty-four (24) hours
   b. get medical help for her immediately
   c. offer Tylenol for the fever and pain
   d. call the individual's family to tell them

5. What can the UAP do to keep herself from getting a serious infection?
   a. wash her hands frequently
   b. do not come in close contact with others
   c. limit her intake to no more than four (4) glasses of water a day
   d. avoid fresh fruits and vegetables—they may be contaminated

6. If the UAP gives an individual an antibiotic. The individual develops a rash, fever, and headache. This is:
   a. nothing to worry about
   b. a typical reaction to antibiotics
   c. an allergic reaction
   d. a reason to give a higher dose of the antibiotic

7. Anaphylactic shock:
   a. is a severe allergic reaction that may cause death
   b. is a minor allergic reaction that requires only close observation
   c. is a minor side effect to antibiotic medications
   d. all of the above

8. One example of an emergency medication for anaphylactic shock is:
   a. penicillin
   b. erythromycin
   c. epinephrine
   d. Flagyl

9. An adverse reaction to a medication is:
   a. an unwanted action or effect that is harmful to the body
   b. an expected side effect that is beneficial to the body
   c. the way an individual acts if she does not want to take her medication
   d. the way an individual acts if her medication makes her feel sick

10. Examples of a virus include:
    a. bursitis and arthritis
    b. herpes and influenza
    c. strep and salmonella
    d. hypertension and tachycardia

11. Common fungal infections include:
    a. pneumonia and bronchitis
    b. otitis media and meningitis
    c. athlete's foot and ringworm
    d. nausea and vomiting

12. In addition to following proper handwashing procedures, individual hygiene instruction for a woman being treated for a vaginal *Candida* infection includes:
    a. using tampons to prevent vaginal drainage
    b. wiping from front to back after having a bowel movement
    c. applying fragranced products after bathing to decrease body odor
    d. all of the above

13. When applying the antiviral Zovirax, gloves should be used:
    a. to prevent applying it to other body parts and to avoid passing the virus to anyone else
    b. if it is the policy of the workplace
    c. if one has a cold and does not want to infect the individual she is caring for
    d. if one has not washed her hands before applying the medication

14. Orthostatic hypotension is:
    a. a drop in blood pressure from changing position too slowly
    b. an increase in blood pressure from changing position too slowly
    c. a drop in blood pressure from changing position too quickly
    d. an increase in blood pressure from changing position too quickly

15. If an individual taking antiretroviral medications for HIV or AIDS demonstrates symptoms including sudden severe abdominal pain, fever, nausea, and tingling in the arms and legs:
    a. offer Tylenol for the pain and fever
    b. report symptoms to the individual's licensed health care provider and hold the medications until one hears from the individual's licensed HCP
    c. observe the individual for twenty-four (24) hours before contacting the licensed health care provider
    d. call emergency medical services and have the individual taken to the emergency room

16. Tuberculosis is:
    a. a contagious respiratory disease
    b. another name for the common cold
    c. a type of bronchitis
    d. easily treated with a ten (10)-day regime of a cephalosporin

17. If an individual is being treated for TB:
    a. it is okay to stop taking her medication once she feels better
    b. she needs to complete the medication course as ordered by her licensed HCP to avoid a relapse
    c. she can get better even if she is not eating a proper diet and getting rest
    d. she needs to be in total isolation the entire time

18. Antiprotozoal medications are ordered to treat:
    a. vaginal infections
    b. urinary infections
    c. ringworm
    d. malaria

19. Immunity is:

a. being especially vulnerable to viral infections

b. being protected from or resistant to a specific disease because of the development of antibodies

c. becoming ill after having a vaccination

d. having an allergic reaction to an antifungal medication

20. Immunity protects the body from specific microorganisms. It also helps the body to:

a. accept or reject blood or organs taken into the body through transfusion or transplant

b. prevent osteporosis

c. cure itself of cancer

d. heal after surgery

21. An immunization:

a. can kill a fungus

b. can kill a virus

c. can kill bacteria

d. can trigger a body to make antibodies

CLINICAL SCENARIOS

1. Name three infections for which the UAP would be asked to give an individual penicillin. What reactions should the UAP watch for? What are the special considerations for penicillin?

2. What is HAART therapy? What types of medications are used for HAART therapy?

3. Tom Blie was recently diagnosed with active tuberculosis (TB) and placed on medication. How long will Tom be on medication? Why? Will Tom be on precautions? If so,

a. for how long will Tom be on precautions?

b. What type of precautions will Tom be on?

4. Are immunizations always beneficial? If not, why not?

Chapter 20
Medications for Treating Cancer

Learning Objectives

After reading this chapter and completing the review questions, you should be able to:

1. Spell and define terms.
2. Discuss the uses of chemotherapy in treating cancer along with side effects and adverse reactions.
3. Explain the care of an individual being treated for cancer.
4. Briefly describe other methods of treatment for an individual who has cancer.

Key Terms

antiangiogenesis

antineoplastic
   medications

brachytherapy

chemotherapy

exacerbation

external radiation
   therapy

gene therapy

hyperthermia

immunotherapy

internal radiation
   therapy

local hyperthermia

malignant cells

metastasis

petechiae

photodynamic therapy
   (PDT)

radiation therapy

regional hyperthermia

remission

systemic radiation
   therapy

targeted therapy

thermal ablation

whole body
   hyperthermia

INTRODUCTION

Cancer is a word used to describe many different diseases. The American Cancer Society (ACS) describes cancer as "a group of cells that divide quickly and grow out of control." Many factors may be involved in these cells becoming damaged, abnormal, and growing out of control. These factors include biological, environmental, and hereditary factors (American Cancer Society, 2009a).

These damaged cells are called **malignant cells**. These malignant cells multiply quickly, creating a mass of cells that damage the cells around them. This is called **metastasis**. In metastasis, malignant cells destroy and take the place of normal cells. Metastasis is what causes cancer to spread so quickly. Malignant cells can be carried by the lymph and blood vessels or can pass easily across the body cavities.

According to the American Cancer Society, cancer of some type affects one out of four men and one out of five women in the United States. The key to the successful treatment of cancer is early detection (American Cancer Society, 2009b).

Over the past fifty (50) years, great strides have been made in the treatment of cancer. Today individuals with cancer have numerous options for treatment, including the following:

- Chemotherapy

- Radiation therapy

- Surgery

- Immunotherapy

- Hyperthermia

- Photodynamic therapy (PDT)

- Targeted therapy

- Antiangiogenesis

- Gene therapy (American Cancer Society, 2009b)

The type of treatment administered by an individual's licensed HCP depends upon the following:

- The specific type of cancer the individual has

- The location of the cancer

- How advanced the cancer is (its staging)

- How quickly the cancer will metastasis

- The individual's health (American Cancer Society, 2009b)

CHEMOTHERAPY

In **chemotherapy**, **antineoplastic medications** are used to the destroy the abnormal, damaged, "cancer" cells (malignant cells). The goal of chemotherapy is to "cure" the individual of his cancer. If a "cure" is not possible, then the goal is to put the body into a state of **remission**. Remission allows the individual to live as long as possible without an **exacerbation** of cancer symptoms.

Antineoplastic medications are also known as "chemo medications." These medications may be used as follows:

- Before or after surgery for cancer

- With radiation treatment

malignant cells
Cells or groups of cells that invade local tissue and destroy normal cells.

metastasis
The spread of malignant cells to other areas of the body through lymph or blood vessels or by passing through the body cavities.

chemotherapy
Treatment of disease by using anticancer medications that destroy cancer cells.

remission
The time when the symptoms of a disease are stable or absent.

exacerbation
The time when a disease process and its symptoms are most severe and debilitating.

- Alone as the primary treatment for cancer
- With other forms of cancer treatments (American Cancer Society, 2009b)

Antineoplastic medications may be administered in the following ways:

- Orally—an individual may be permitted to take this medication at home
- By injection like a flu shot—this is usually administered at the licensed HCP office, a clinic, or a hospital or at times at the individual's home
- Most often, the medication is administered intravenously (IV) by a licensed HCP through a needle or a catheter (American Cancer Society, 2009a)

Chemotherapy, also known as chemo, may be administered daily, weekly, or even once a month (American Cancer Society, 2009a).

There are eight classes of antineoplastic medications. They are as follows:

- Antimetabolites
- Alkylating medications
- Plant alkaloids
- Antibiotic antineoplastics
- Steriod hormones
- Antiestrogen
- Antiandrogen
- Biological response modifiers

Refer to Table 20-1 for a list of antineoplastic medications by generic and brand names.

Chemotherapy and the administration of antineoplastic medications are very complex. The UAP is not expected to know the names, dosages, and routes of all of these medications. However, the UAP needs to know the frequent possible side effects and adverse reactions an individual in his care may have. Knowing this information will help the UAP provide the care and comfort the individual will need as he undergoes the treatment for his cancer.

Side Effects/Adverse Reactions

According to the ACS, some individuals have no side effects from chemotherapy. At other times chemotherapy makes an individual feel ill. Antineoplastic medications are very strong. Because of this, these medications kill healthy cells along with cancer cells. The killing of healthy

Table 20-1 Antineoplastic Medications by Generic and Brand Names

GENERIC NAME	BRAND NAME	GENERIC NAME	BRAND NAME
Antimetabolites		**Antibiotic Antineoplastics**	
cytarabine	Cytosar-U	bleomycin	Blenoxane
fluorouracil	Adrucil	daunorubicin	Cerubidine
methotrexate	Rheumatrex	doxorubicin	Adriamycin
mercaptopurine	Purinethol	mitomycin	Mutamycin
Alkylating Agents		etoposide, VP-16	VePesid
busulfan	Myleran	**Steroid Hormones**	
carboplatin	Paraplatin	dexamethasone	Decadron
carmustine, BCNU	BiCNU, Gliadel	prednisone	Deltasone
chlorambucil	Leukeran	**Antiestrogen**	
cisplatin	Platinol	tamoxifen	Nolvadex
cyclophosphamide	Cytoxan	anastrozole	Arimidex
ifosfamide	IFEX	**Antiandrogen**	
thiotepa	Thioplex	leuprolide	Lupron Depot
Plant Alkaloids		bicalutamide	Casodex
vinblastine	Velban	**Biological Response Modifiers**	
vincristine	Oncovin	interferon	Roferon-A
paclitaxel	Taxol		Intron A
		bevacizumab	Avastin
		rituximab	Rituxan
		tositumomab	Bexxar
		trastuzumab	Herceptin

Note: This listing is not complete but is representative of the most used drugs.

Based on Woodrow, R. (2007). *Essentials of pharmacology for health occupations* (5th ed.), Table 14-1. Clifton Park, NY: Delmar, Cengage Learning.

cells causes side effects. Side effects from chemotherapy may include the following:

- Anemia, causing skin, mouth, and gums to look pale
- Diarrhea
- Dryness and sores in the mouth
- Dry skin
- Easy bruising and bleeding
- Fatigue
- Hair loss on the entire body
- High risk for infection due to a lower white blood cell count
- Infertility, which is usually permanent

- Loss of sexual desire, which is usually temporary

- Nausea

- Shortness of breath

- Vomiting

- Weakness (American Cancer Society, 2009a)

CARE OF INDIVIDUALS UNDERGOING CHEMOTHERAPY

When an individual is receiving chemotherapy treatment, he is going to need support and understanding. Remember, not only is he ill from the chemotherapy, but he also has a diagnosis of cancer. There are several things the UAP can do to make the individual's daily life more comfortable and also to keep the individual as healthy as possible.

Observe, Report, and Record

During daily care and tasks, observe the individual's general response to treatment. Be alert for any signs of side effects and adverse reactions. Report any changes in the individual's condition to his licensed health care provider. Record observations, changes, and licensed HCP recommendations and orders on the appropriate forms.

Risk for Infection

An individual having chemotherapy is at high risk for infection, including bacterial, fungal, and viral infections. The medications used in chemotherapy lower an individual's white blood cell count. White blood cells fight off infection. With a lower white blood cell count, the individual is at high risk for infection. To protect the individual from infections, the UAP may do the following:

- Wear a clean uniform with hair clean and either short or tied back.

- Keep her fingernails short and clean, free of nail polish.

- Keep the individual's living environment clean.

- Do not keep fresh flowers or plants in the individual's room or home.

- If the individual has a cat litter box, place the box away from kitchen and food areas; clean the box daily.

- Wash hands often, especially before providing care to the individual, with warm water and soap.

- Individual should avoid crowds; if he must be with crowds (in a public place), he should wear a surgical mask.

- Individual needs to stay away from others who are ill.

- Monitor vital signs.

- Observe the individual for signs and symptoms of infection; if symptoms are noted, they must be reported to the individual's licensed HCP as soon as possible and documented in the individual's progress notes. Signs and symptoms of infection include the following:

  - Fever greater than 100.5°F orally—*do not take a rectal temperature*

  - Change in level of consciousness

  - Cough or shortness of breath

  - Nasal congestion

  - Pain, heat, redness, and swelling at the site of an injury, surgical wound, catheter, or IV site

  - Pain or burning on urination

  - Pain, redness, or irritation inside the mouth

  - Change in vital signs (pulse, respirations, and/or blood pressure)

  - Shaking chills

  - Sore throat

  - Warm, flushed, dry skin (American Cancer Society, 2009b)

- Follow basic food safety guidelines, including the following:

  - Individual should not eat or drink raw milk or milk products or unpasteurized milk or milk products, including cheese and yogurt made from unpasteurized milk

  - Individual should not eat raw or undercooked meat, fish, chicken, eggs, or tofu

  - Individual should not eat raw honey

  - Individual should not eat outdated foods

  - Individual should not eat uncooked:

    - Hotdogs, deli meats, or processed meats (unless they have just been cooked before eating)

    - Vegetables and fruits

    - Grain products (American Cancer Society, 2009b)

- Administer antibiotics as ordered by the individual's licensed health care provider.

- Educate the individual, his family, and visitors about the spread of infectious diseases and how they can avoid passing on an infection:

  - Family and friends should not visit if they are ill.

  - Hands need to be washed often, including before eating and after touching face and mucous membranes.

  - Individual should not use hot tubs or play, wade, or swim in ponds, lakes, or rivers.

- Individual needs to use condoms to avoid sexually transmitted infections.

- Bath towels, drinking glasses, utensils, and so on are not to be shared.

- Individual should not change a child's diaper.

- All cuts, scrapes, and so on experienced by the individual should be cleaned with warm water and soap and a clean bandage applied. Staff should then be notified (American Cancer Society, 2009b).

Self-Care Needs

- Assist the individual as needed with daily bathing, making sure feet, groin, armpits, and other moist, sweaty areas are washed and dried well.

- Individual should not have manicures or pedicures or use false nails or nail tips.

- Individuals should wear shoes at all times to avoid injury and infections.

- Individuals should use an electric razor. Razors are not to be shared.

- Provide good mouth care. Teeth are to be brushed at least twice a day, preferably with a soft-bristled toothbrush. Check with the individual's licensed HCP to see (1) if it is okay to floss, (2) if a special toothbrush is needed, and (3) if a special mouthwash is needed. *Do not use OTC alcohol-based mouthwash or lemon glycerin swabs.*

- Prevent constipation and straining by encouraging the individual to drink 2 quarts of fluid each day. If permitted, encourage the individual to exercise. If unsure if the individual may exercise, check first with the individual's licensed HCP.

- Women are not to use tampons, vaginal suppositories, or douches without a written order from their licensed HCP.

- Individuals should use a water-based lubricant during intercourse to avoid injury or abrasion of the skin and mucous membranes.

- Advise the individual not to smoke.

- For individuals receiving radiation therapy, obtain specific instructions for care from his radiation oncologist (specialist) regarding care to the area of the body receiving treatment and any special precautions the UAP may need to follow.

- Provide emotional support. Encourage individuals to be honest about how they feel and to talk with their loved ones and with their licensed HCPs (American Cancer Society, 2009b).

Nutritional Needs

Chemotherapy treatment can induce anorexia, nausea and vomiting, and inflammation of the mouth and mucous membranes. The UAP can provide for the individual's nutritional needs by taking the following steps:

- Encourage him to eat small, frequent meals. If he is able to eat, offer six small meals a day.

- Check with the individual's licensed HCP to see if the individual may benefit from high-protein drinks like Ensure or Boost.

- Offer ice chips or sugarless hard candies to keep the individual's mouth moist.

- Offer the individual's favorite beverages frequently throughout the day.

- If needed, offer special mouth care frequently.

- Encourage the individual to eat whatever he wants, whenever he wants to eat.

- Assist him in choosing foods if he wants or needs help. Recommend moist foods. Advise him to avoid hot, spicy, and acidic foods and drinks to lessen the severity of nausea and vomiting.

- Record intake at every meal and output every time the individual urinates.

- If ordered, administer antiemetic medications to relieve nausea and vomiting. When an individual is taking these medications, the following considerations apply:

  - If the individual vomits within thirty (30) minutes of taking the medication, notify the licensed health care provider for instructions.

  - If vomiting continues after the second dose, contact the individual's licensed HCP for instructions.

Special Considerations

When caring for an individual who is undergoing chemotherapy, the UAP must be alert for early signs of bleeding. If these occur, the early signs of bleeding must be reported to the individual's licensed HCP as soon as possible and documented in the individual's progress notes.
Signs of bleeding include the following:

- Excessive or unusual bruising

- Nosebleeds

- Bleeding gums

- Rectal bleeding

- Abnormal vaginal bleeding

- Small, purplish, hemorrhagic spots on the skin called **petechiae** (American Cancer Society, 2009b)

petechiae
Tiny purple, or red spots appearing on the skin due to tiny hemorrhages under the skin.

OTHER TREATMENTS FOR CANCER
Radiation Therapy

radiation therapy
A treatment that uses high-energy particles or waves to destroy or damage cancer cells.

Radiation therapy uses high-energy particles or waves to destroy or damage cancer cells. Radiation therapy may be administered (1) alone or (2) along with other treatments, such as with surgery or with chemotherapy. Often it is used along with other treatments to treat cancers of the head, neck, bladder, and lung and Hodgkin's disease.

Radiation therapy uses special equipment to deliver high doses of radiation to cancer cells. The radiation kills or damages the cancer cells. The goal of radiation therapy is to damage as many cancer cells as possible with as little harm as possibile to the healthy cells nearby. At times, radiation therapy is administered as a substance by mouth or intravenously (IV).

Radiation therapy may be administered in the three following ways:

- **External radiation therapy**: a machine delivers high-energy waves of radiation from outside the body to the tumor and some nearby tissue.

- **Internal radiation therapy**, also called **brachytherapy**: a radioactive source in the form of a seed, wire, or pellet is implanted (placed into) in the body or near the tumor. This has very little effect on healthy tissue.

- **Systemic radiation therapy**: radioactive medications called radiopharmaceuticals are administered by mouth or by injection. The medication travels throughout the body to the cancer cells (American Cancer Society, 2009b).

Surgery

The oldest form of cancer treatment is surgery. Surgery plays an important role in diagnosing cancer and finding out how far cancer has spread. Surgery offers the best chance for cure for many types of cancer, especially for those that have not spread (metastasized).

The goal of surgery is to remove the cancer cells along with surrounding tissues in order to stop the cancer from spreading. Surgery is also used to lessen some complications of cancer, such as when a tumor is obstructing (blocking) a duct or an airway.

The more common types of surgery are as follows:

- Preventive surgery: done to remove body tissue likely to become cancerous (malignant) though there are no signs of cancer at the time of surgery, such as the removal of precancerous polyps.

- Diagnostic surgery: done to get a tissue sample to determine whether cancer is present in the sample or to tell what type of cancer is in the sample.

- Staging surgery: done to find out how much cancer there is and how far the cancer has metastisized (spread).

- Curative surgery: done when a tumor is in one specific area and all of the tumor can be removed.

- Debulking (cytoreductive) surgery: done to remove part but not all of a tumor. It is done when removing all of the tumor would cause too much damage. As much of the tumor is removed as possible. Chemotherapy or radiation therapy is then administered. This is commonly used for advanced cancers such as advanced ovarian caner.

- Palliative surgery: done (1) to treat complications of advanced surgery or (2) to correct a problem that is causing pain, discomfort, or disability. For instance, this surgery would be used to remove part of a tumor that is blocking an individual's airway, making it difficult for the individual to breath. This surgery is not done to cure the individual.

- Supportive surgery: done to help with other types of treatment. For instance, this surgery would be done to insert a catheter into a large vien. The catheter, known as a port-a-cath, would be used to draw blood and administer antineoplastic medications.

- Reconstructive (restorative) surgery: done (1) to restore the function of an organ or body part after surgery or (2) to change the way an individual looks after major surgery, such as breast reconstruction after a mastectomy (American Cancer Society, 2009b).

Immunotherapy

Immunotherapy uses an individual's immune system to fight cancer. In immunotherapy, the individual's immune system is able to recognize cancer cells and destroy them. At this time, monoclonal antibodies are the most widely used form of cancer immunotherapy. Immunotherapy is usually used in combination with other treatments. Immunotherapy is also called biologic therapy or biotherapy. Several immunotherapies for cancer have been approved by the FDA. Others have shown promise and are in clinical trials (American Cancer Society, 2009b).

immunotherapy
A treatment for cancer in which the individual's immune system is used to fight cancer.

Hyperthermia

Hyperthermia uses heat to treat cancer. There are two main ways in which hyperthermia may be used:

1. **Local hyperthermia**, also called **thermal ablation**: a small area of cancer cells is destroyed by very high temperatures.

2. **Regional hyperthermia**, also called **whole body hyperthermia**: used along with other cancer treatments such as radiation therapy, chemotherapy, or immunotherapy. The temperature of the entire body or a part of the body is raised to higher-than-normal level (American Cancer Society, 2009b).

Photodynamic Therapy (PDT)

Photodynamic therapy (PDT) uses medications, known as photosensitizing medications, along with light to kill cancer cells. To work, the photosensitizing medications must be "turned on" by certain types of light. The photosensitizing medications are injected into the individual's bloodstream or applied to the skin. Once the medications are absorbed by the cancer cells, the special light is applied only to the area to be treated. The light causes the medication to react with oxygen. The reaction of the medication with oxygen forms a chemical that kills the cancer cells (American Cancer Society, 2009b).

Targeted Therapy

Targeted therapy is a new type of cancer treatment that causes little damage to healthy cells. Targeted therapy uses medications or other substances to recognize and attack only cancer cells. Each type of targeted therapy works differently. All targeted therapies, however, change the way cancer cells grow, divide, repair themselves, and interact with other cells. Some of the cancers that may be treated with targeted therapy include cancers of the head, neck, lung, breast, pancreas, liver, colorectal, and kidney. A major focus of cancer research today is in the area of targeted therapies (American Cancer Society, 2009b).

Other Treatments

Two additional areas of interest to researchers for cancer treatment include (1) **antiangiogenesis** and (2) **gene therapy**.

Antiangiogenesis is a form of targeted therapy. To grow, a tumor needs nutrients. Just like the body, a tumor gets its nutrients through an individual's blood supply. As a tumor grows, it makes new blood vessels to meet its increased need for nutrients. Antiangiogenesis uses medications or substances to stop tumors from making new blood vessels. Tumors cannot grow without a new blood supply to feed itself (American Cancer Society, 2009b).

Gene therapy has not yet been approved by the FDA for use with the general public. It is still being researched. Treatment with gene therapy is available only in clinical trials. According to the ACS, "It will probably be several years before gene therapy is ready for use to the general public" (American Cancer Society, 2009b).

SUMMARY

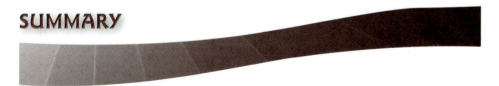

An individual being treated for cancer may be vulnerable physically as well as emotionally. By understanding the mechanism of cancer and cancer treatments, the UAP can provide the care needed to help the individual at every level of his daily life.

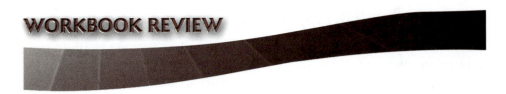

WORKBOOK REVIEW

Go to the workbook and complete the exercises for Chapter 20.

REVIEW QUESTIONS

1. According to the American Cancer Society, cancer will affect:
   a. one in every two men and two in every three women
   b. one in every four men and one in every five women
   c. one in every three men and one in every seven women
   d. almost all Americans
2. Malignant cells are:
   a. cells that have changed but can still function normally
   b. cells that multiply slowly
   c. locally invasive and destructive to normal cells
   d. cells that are not damaging to other cells
3. Metastasis occurs when:
   a. malignant cells are spread to other areas of the body
   b. malignant cells damage cells around them
   c. malignant cells can no longer function normally
   d. an individual receives chemotherapy treatment
4. It is important to minimize the risk of infection for an individual receiving chemotherapy because:
   a. it is a standard precaution
   b. the individual is more susceptible to many bacterial, fungal, and viral infections
   c. the licensed health care provider has ordered it
   d. all of the above
5. Early signs of bleeding:
   a. include nasal congestion, cough, and shortness of breath
   b. must be reported to the individual's licensed HCP as soon as possible
   c. may be observed closely for twenty-four (24) hours and then reported to the licensed HCP
   d. are not a concern to the UAP unless they worsen
6. The UAP may assist with nutritional needs for an individual receiving chemotherapy by:
   a. encouraging small, frequent meals and plenty of fluids
   b. offering spicy foods
   c. offering large meals three times a day
   d. recommending dry foods like crackers or plain bread

7. Signs of infection in an individual receiving chemotherapy include:
   a. a fever above 100.5°F orally
   b. increased appetite and thirst
   c. constipation
   d. all of the above

8. Immunotherapy treats cancer by:
   a. using medications that destroy cells
   b. using an individual's immune system to fight cancer
   c. using electromagnetic waves
   d. surgically removing cancer cells and surrounding tissues

9. Radiation therapy treats cancer by:
   a. using medications that destroy cells
   b. using an individual's immune system to fight cancer
   c. using electromagnetic waves
   d. surgically removing cancer cells and surrounding tissues

10. Surgery is used with individuals who have cancer to:
   a. remove localized malignant cells and lessen some complications of cancer
   b. using an individual's immune system to fight cancer
   c. kill malignant cells with chemical medications
   d. repair damage done by malignant cells

Chapter 21
Medications for Treating Cardiovascular Disorders

Learning Objectives

After reading this chapter and completing the review questions, you should be able to:

1. Spell and define terms.
2. List the warning signs of a heart attack.
3. State two primary causes of chest pain.
4. State the uses, adverse reactions, and special considerations of various medications used to treat cardiovascular disorders.

Key Terms

angina pectoris

angioedema

antiarrhythmic medications

anticoagulants

antihypertensive medications

antilipidemic medications

arrhythmia

arteriosclerosis

atrial fibrillation

atrial flutter

bradycardia

cardiac glycosides

cardiomyopathy

cardiovascular disease (CVD)

colony-stimulating factors (CSFs)

congestive heart failure

embolus

hypertension

hypoglycemia

hypotension

lipids

myalgia

myasthenia gravis

myopathy

platelet inhibitors

systemic lupus erythematosis

tachycardia

thrombolytic medications

thrombus

vasoconstrictors

vasodilators

INTRODUCTION

arteriosclerosis
Thickening, hardening, and loss of elasticity of the artery walls.

cardiovascular disease (CVD)
Diseases of the heart and blood vessels.

cardiomyopathy
Any disease that affects the structure and function of the heart.

angina pectoris
Chest pain caused by a lack of blood supply to the heart.

Cardiovascular disease (CVD) is currently the leading cause of death in the United States. Cardiovascular disease includes disorders such as **arteriosclerosis** and **cardiomyopathy** (Myers, 2006). Cardiomyopathy includes diseases that affect the structure and function of the heart.

Chest pain may be a warning sign that there is an underlying problem with the heart. The UAP should, therefore, take all complaints of chest pain seriously. When chest pain occurs, the individual should stop her activities and rest. The chest pain should be reported to the individual's licensed HCP. Once the individual having the symptoms is seen by a licensed health care provider, the licensed HCP can determine the cause of the chest pain and treat the individual appropriately.

Causes for chest pain may include the following:

- **Angina pectoris**
- Anxiety
- Gastrointestinal disorders, such as hiatal hernia or gastritis
- Medication side effects/adverse reactions
- Musculoskeletal, such as rib fractures
- Myocardial infarction (MI) (heart attack)
- Respiratory disease, such as pneumonia
- Stress (Myers, 2006)

The risk factors for chest pain and possible heart attack include:

- Diabetes mellitus
- High cholesterol levels
- Family history or heredity
- Ethnic background
- Gender—men tend to have more heart attacks than do premenopausal women
- History of stroke or vascular disease
- Hypertension
- Obesity
- Lack of physical activity
- Postmenopausal women are at greater risk than premenopausal women
- Smoking
- Stress (Myers, 2006)

The signs and symptoms of a heart attack include the following:

- Chest pain that lasts for two (2) minutes or longer; pain is described as crushing or as severe indigestion and spreads to the jaw or arm
- Cyanosis (blue or purplish discoloration of the skin)

- Fear that death is near
- Feelings of anxiety
- Irregular pulse and respiration
- Nausea
- Restlessness
- Shortness of breath
- Sweating
- Vomiting
- Weakness (Myers, 2006)

Individuals may try to ignore the symptoms of a heart attack. They may think they are having indigestion. If a UAP notices that an individual is having symptoms of a heart attack, the UAP should call 911 or the emergency medical services (EMS) number for her location immediately. An individual may die from a heart attack because she hesitates to get the medical help she needs.

CARDIOVASCULAR MEDICATIONS

Cardiovascular medications are used to treat disorders that affect the (1) heart, (2) blood vessels, and (3) blood. Types of cardiovascular medications discussed in this chapter are as follows:

- Cardiac glycosides
- Antiarrhythmic medications
- Vasodilators
- Vasoconstrictors
- Antihypertensive medications
- Antilipidemic medications
- Anticoagulants
- Platelet inhibitors
- Thrombolytic medications
- Colony-stimulating factors (CSFs)
- Medications used to treat anemias

Cardiac Glycosides

Cardiac glycosides (1) strengthen the heartbeat, (2) slow the heart rate (pulse), and (3) improve the contractions of the heart muscle as it pumps blood throughout the body. Cardiac glycosides are used to treat the following:

- **Congestive heart failure**
- **Tachycardia**, pulse (heart rate) of more than 100 beats per minute (bpm) but regular

- **Atrial fibrillation**, an irregular heart rate occurring in the atria of the heart
- **Atrial flutter**, a type of atrial fibrillation with a heart rate of 230 to 380 beats per minute (bpm)

The most commonly used cardiac glycosides are digitalis medications. Of these, lanoxin (Digoxin) is the most commonly used.

Adverse reactions:

- Anorexia
- Arrhythmias
- Asthenia
- Blurred or yellow vision
- Confusion
- Diarrhea
- Excessive slowing of the pulse (a sign of digitalis overdose)
- Fatigue
- Headache
- Nausea
- Tachycardia
- Vomiting
- Weakness

Digitalis toxicity is another adverse reaction. Table 21-1 highlights the signs and symptoms of digitalis toxicity.

Contraindications are as follows:

- Allergy to digitalis medications
- Severe respiratory disease
- Hypothyroidism
- Acute MI
- Acute myocarditis
- Severe heart failure
- Impaired renal function
- Arrhythmias not caused by heart failure
- Pregnancy
- Breast feeding
- High doses in elderly individuals

Special considerations in the use of digitalis medications include the following:

- Take the individual's apical pulse for one (1) full minute before giving the medication. If the individual's pulse is below 60 or if it

Table 21-1 Signs and Symptoms of Digitalis Toxicity

IMMEDIATELY REPORT THESE SIGNS AND SYMPTOMS TO THE INDIVIDUAL'S LICENSED HCP	
Signs and Symptoms of Digitalis Toxicity	**Comments**
anorexia, nausea, vomiting	**early signs of toxicity**
abdominal cramping	
abdominal distention	
cardiac arrhythmias of all kinds	especially a heart rate (pulse) of less than 60 beats per minute
confusion	
diarrhea	
electrolyte imbalance	
fatigue	
headache	
insomnia	
irritability	
lethargy	
mental disorders such as psychosis	especially with elderly individuals
muscle weakness	
restlessness	
seizures	
tremors	
vertigo	
visual disturbances including blurred vision, double vision, and yellow halos	

Based on Woodrow, R. (2007). *Essentials of pharmacology for health occupations* (5th ed.), pages 465–466. Clifton Park, NY: Delmar, Cengage Learning.

is below a specified rate, do not give the medication. Immediately notify the individual's licensed health care provider.

- Observe for signs of digitalis toxicity. If signs and symptoms of digitalis toxicity are noted, hold the medication. Notify the individual's licensed health care provider at once.

- Do not administer OTC and herbal medications unless they are ordered by the individual's licensed HCP.

- Do not suddenly stop administering this medication. To prevent complications for the individual, the medication should be gradually discontinued.

- There are differences between various generic and brand names and dosage forms of these medications. Do not change the brand or dosage form(s) of this medication without first checking with the individual's licensed HCP.

Table 21-2 Cardiac Glycosides and Antiarrhythmics by Generic and Brand Names with Dosage Information

GENERIC NAME	BRAND NAME	DOSAGE INFORMATION	COMMENTS
Cardiac Glycoside			
digoxin	Lanoxin, Lanoxicaps	Oral: tablets, liquid-filled capsules, elixir I.V. dose varies	Maximum dose 0.125 mg (long term in the elderly individual)
Antiarrhythmics			
atenolol	Tenormin	Oral 50 mg daily	Beta-blocker
propranolol	Inderal	Oral 10–30 mg 3–4 ×/day	Beta-blocker
verapamil	Isoptin, Calan	Oral 240–480 mg daily in divided doses	Calcium channel blocker
amiodarone	Cordarone	Oral, dose varies	Antiarrhythmic and vasodilator
procainamide	Pronestyl, Procanbid	Oral, dose varies	
propafenone	Rythmol Rythmol SR	Oral 150–300 mg every 8 hours Oral 225–425 mg every 12 hours	Antiarrhythmic for ventricular arrhythmias
quinidine		Oral tabs, extended release dose varies	Antiarrhythmic
disopyramide	Norpace, Norpace CR	Oral 150 mg every 6 hours or oral 300 mg every 12 hours, extended release	Ventricular antiarrhythmic Not for elderly individuals

Note: Other antiarrhythmics are available.

Based on Woodrow, R. (2007). *Essentials of pharmacology for health occupations* (5th ed.), Table 25-1. Clifton Park, NY: Delmar, Cengage Learning.

- Refer to a current edition of a reliable medication reference, as needed, for specific precautions and medication interactions associated with digitalis medications.

Table 21-2 gives a list of cardiac glycosides by generic and brand names with dosage information.

Antiarrhythmic Medications

arrhythmia
An irregular heartbeat caused by a disruption of the pacemaker (sinoatrial node) in the heart, which sets the rhythm of the heartbeat.

An **arrhythmia** is an irregular heartbeat caused by a disruption of the pacemaker (sinoatrial node) in the heart, which sets the rhythm of the heartbeat. **Antiarrhythmic medications** are used to treat an arrhythmia (irregular heartbeat). Antiarrhythmic medications include the following:

- Adrenergic blockers
- Calcium channel blockers
- Disopyramide (Norpace), a synthetic medication
- Procainamide (Pronestyl)

Adverse reactions of antiarrhythmic medications include **hypotension** (low blood pressure) and **bradycardia** (pulse less than 60 beats per minute).

Special considerations for antiarrhythmic medications are as follows:

- Avoid giving OTC and herbal medications unless they are ordered by the individual's licensed HCP.

- Advise the individual to move slowly when changing body positions in early treatment to minimize the risk of orthostatic hypotension.

- Make sure that emergency supplies are available when giving an individual an antiarrhythmic. The medication may cause a serious adverse reaction.

- Refer to a current edition of a reliable medication reference, as needed, for specific precautions and medication interactions associated with antiarrhythmic medications.

Table 21-2 gives a list of selected antiarrhythmic medications by their generic and brand names with dosage information.

Adrenergic Blockers

Adrenergic blockers have a complex action. These medications are used to treat arrhythmias, hypertension (high blood pressure), some types of chronic angina, and, with caution, some patients with lung disorders that cause bronchospasms. Examples of these medications include Tenormin and Inderal.

Adverse reactions:

- Bradycardia (pulse less than 60 beats per minute) with heart block and cardiac arrest

- Bronchospasm, especially if individual has history of asthma

- Constipation

- Diarrhea

- **Hypoglycemia** (low blood sugar)

- Hypotension with vertigo and syncope (fainting)

- Impotence (rare)

- Nausea

- Rash

- Vomiting

- With long-term treatment:
  - Confusion
  - Dizziness
  - Fatigue
  - Irritability
  - Insomnia
  - Nightmares
  - Sleepiness

- Visual disturbances
- Weakness

Contraindications for adrenergic blockers are as follows:

- Sudden withdrawal after prolonged use
- Major surgery
- Diabetes
- Liver impairment
- Kidney impairment
- Asthma
- Allergic rhinitis
- Bradycardia
- Heart block
- Congestive heart failure
- Pregnancy
- Breast feeding
- COPD

Special considerations for adrenergic blockers are as follows:

- Take the individual's apical pulse for one (1) full minute before giving the medication. If the individual's pulse is below 60 or if it is below a specified rate, do not give the medication. Immediately notify the individual's licensed HCP.
- Do not administer OTC and herbal medications unless they are ordered by the individual's licensed HCP.
- Administer with meals at the same time everyday to decrease GI upset.
- Do not suddenly stop administering this medication. To prevent complications for the individual, the medication should be gradually discontinued.
- Advise the individual to move slowly when changing body positions in early treatment to minimize the risk of orthostatic hypotension.

Observe the individual closely for signs and symptoms of hypoglycemia. Refer to Chapter 22 for a list of the signs and symptoms of hypoglycemia.

- Make sure that emergency supplies are available when giving an individual an adrenergic blocker. The medication may cause a serious adverse reaction.

Calcium Channel Blockers

Calcium channel blockers work to dilate the main coronary arteries increasing the flow of blood and oxygen to the body. These medications are used to treat arrhythmias, hypertension (high blood pressure), and angina. Verapamil (Isoptin) is a calcium channel blocker.

Adverse reactions:

- Abdominal discomfort

- Bradycardia (pulse below 60 beats per minute) with heart block

- Constipation

- Edema (swelling)

- Hypotension (low blood pressure) with vertigo and headache

- Nausea

Contraindications for calcium channel blockers are as follows:

- Heart block

- Heart failure

- Angina

- Liver failure

- Kidney failure

- Pregnancy

- Breast feeding

- Hypotension

- Heart block

- Certain arrhythmias

- Severe heart failure

- Use with caution in elderly individuals

Special considerations for calcium channel blockers are as follows:

- *Do not administer with grapefruit juice!*

- Observe closely for signs and symptoms of heart failure.

- Observe for signs and symptoms of hyperglycemia in individuals with diabetes. Refer to Chapter 22 for a list of signs and symptoms of hyperglycemia.

- Do not crush or break extended-release forms of the medication. Instruct individual not to chew extended-release forms of medication.

- Instruct individual to limit her intake of caffeine and alcohol.

- Do not administer OTC or herbal medications unless they are ordered by the individual's licensed HCP.

- Instruct the individual to avoid sun exposure and to wear sunscreen and protective clothing when outdoors.

Disopyramide (Norpace)

Disopyramide (Norpace) is used to treat ventricular arrhythmias (irregular heartbeats of the ventricles of the heart).

Adverse reactions:

- Bloating
- Blurred vision
- Chest pain
- Constipation
- Dizziness
- Dry mouth
- Edema (swelling)
- Flatulence (gas)
- Hypotension
- Nausea
- Urinary retention
- Vomiting
- Weight gain

Contraindications for disopyramide (Norpace) are as follows:

- Heart block
- Congestive heart failure
- Liver disorders
- Kidney disorders
- Pregnancy
- Breast feeding
- Use in elderly individuals

Special considerations for disopyramide (Norpace) are as follows:

- Take the individual's apical pulse for one (1) full minute before giving the medication. If the individual's pulse is below 60 or above 120 or if it is below or above a specified rate, do not give the medication. Immediately notify the individual's licensed health care provider.
- Observe closely for signs and symptoms of heart failure.
- Observe for signs and symptoms of fluid retention, for example, weight gain, and swelling of lower extremities.
- Advise the individual to move slowly when changing body positions in early treatment to minimize the risk of orthostatic hypotension.
- Do not administer OTC and herbal medications unless they are ordered by the individual's licensed HCP.

Procainamide (Pronestyl)

Once other treatments have established a regular heart rhythm in an individual, procainamide (Pronestyl) may be ordered by the individual's licensed HCP to keep an individual's heart rate regular.

Adverse reactions:

- Allergic reaction including fever, rash, and weakness
- Blood dyscrasias
- Diarrhea
- Hypotension
- Nausea
- Tachycardia (pulse over 100 beats per minute)
- Vomiting

Contraindications for procainamide (Pronestyl) are as follows:

- Heart block
- Congestive heart failure
- Allergic reactions to local anesthetics
- **Myasthenia gravis**
- Pregnancy
- Breast feeding
- Liver disorders
- Kidney disorders
- **Systemic lupus erythematosis**

Special considerations for procainamide (Pronestyl) are as follows:

- Do not crush or break tablets. Instruct the individual not to chew the tablets.
- Administer at prescribed times. Do not skip doses.
- Instruct individual to avoid alcohol.
- Do not administer OTC and herbal medications unless they are ordered by the individual's licensed HCP.

myasthenia gravis
An abnormal condition with fatigue and muscle weakness, especially in the face and throat.

systemic lupus erythematosis
A chronic inflammatory disease affecting many systems of the body.

Quinidine

Like procainamide (Pronestyl), Quinidine may be ordered by the individual's licensed HCP to keep an individual's heart rate regular after other treatments have established a regular heart rhythm in the individual. Brand names for quinidine are Quinaglute and Cardioquin.

Adverse reactions are many. Treatment may need to be discontinued because of the adverse reactions.

Common adverse reactions include the following:

- Anorexia
- Diarrhea
- Nausea
- Vomiting

Additional adverse reactions include the following:

- Apprehension
- Blood dyscrasias
- Confusion
- Fever
- Headache
- Hearing disturbances
- Hypoglycemia
- Liver disorders
- Respiratory arrest
- Severe hypotension
- Syncope
- Tachycardia
- Tinnitus (ringing in the ears)
- Tremor
- Vascular collapse
- Vertigo
- Vision disturbances

Contraindications for quinidine are as follows:

- Heart block
- Electrolyte imbalance
- Digoxin toxicity
- Congestive heart failure
- Hypotension
- Myasthenia gravis
- Asthma
- Other respiratory disorders
- Pregnancy
- Breast feeding
- Liver disorders
- Kidney disorders

Special considerations for quinidine are as follows:

- Administer with food to decrease GI upset.
- *Do not administer with grapefruit juice!*
- Do not crush or break extended-release tablets. Instruct individual not to chew the extended-release tablets.

- Administer at prescribed times. Do not skip doses.
- Instruct individual to avoid licorice and grapefruit juice.
- Do not administer OTC and herbal medications unless they are ordered by the individual's licensed HCP.

Vasodilators

Vasodilators are medications that (1) dilate (enlarge) blood vessels and (2) increase their ability to carry blood. Vasodilators make blood flow easier, lower blood pressure, and relieve chest pain due to a decrease of blood supply and oxygen to the heart muscle.

Nitrates

Nitrates are most commonly used to treat angina pectoris. Nitrates are also used to treat the following conditions:

- Congestive heart failure related to acute myocardial infarction
- For prevention of angina pain

Two nitrates used in the treatment and management of angina are nitroglycerin and isosorbide (Isordil, Sorbitrate).

Nitroglycerin is available in the following forms:

- Sublingual tablets
- Sublingual spray
- Timed-release capsules
- Transderm patch (Nitrodur, Transderm-Nitro)
- Nitro-Bid ointment (topical)
- IV administration

Isosorbide (Isordil, Sorbitrate) is available in the following forms:

- Sublingual tablets
- Regular-release tablets
- Timed-release capsules
- Tablets

General adverse reactions:

- Abdominal pain
- Apprehension
- Dizziness
- Contact dermatitis (rash)
- Flushing
- Headache
- Hypotension
- Nausea

- Syncope
- Tachycardia
- Vomiting

Contraindications for nitrates are as follows:

- Glaucoma
- Intracranial pressure
- Severe anemia
- Hypotension
- Allergy to nitrates
- Acute MI
- Use of Viagra (sildenafil citrate)

Special considerations for nitrate preparations include the following:

- If an individual taking a vasodilator complains of headache and light-headedness, take her blood pressure. If the blood pressure is low, notify her licensed health care provider.
- If chest pain is not relieved by a total dose of three tablets of nitroglycerin in fifteen (15) minutes, immediately call emergency medical services. Have the ambulance take the individual to the nearest emergency medical care center. Notify the individual's licensed HCP of her transfer to the emergency medical care center.

Note: **Nitroglycerin is commonly administered as one tablet every five (5) minutes for a total of three tablets in fifteen (15) minutes. An individual's licensed HCP, however, will provide specific orders to be followed for chest pain.**

- Advise the individual to move slowly when changing body positions to decrease the risk of orthostatic hypotension.
- With transdermal patch and topical application, apply to skin site with little hair and movement. Check area(s) of application for rash or skin irritation.
- With administration of sublingual tablets, instruct individual to hold tablets under her tongue or in her buccal pouch until dose dissolves. Individual is *not* to chew or swallow the medication.
- With sublingual spray, spray directly onto the oral mucosa. Do not allow individual to inhale the spray.
- Administer tablets and capsules with water. Do not crush or break tablets or capsules. Instruct the individual not to chew the medication.
- With Isosorbide (Isordil, Sorbitrate), administer medication thirty (30) minutes before or one (1) to two (2) hours after a meal.
- Instruct the individual to avoid the use of alcohol.

Table 21-3 gives a list of selected vasodilators by generic and brand names.

Table 21-3 Vasodilators by Generic and Brand Names with Dosage Information

GENERIC NAME	BRAND NAME	DOSAGE INFORMATION
Nitrates		
nitroglycerin	Nitrostat tabs sublingual	1–3 tabs every 5 min × 3 doses maximum in 15 min as needed
	Nitrolingual spray	1–2 sprays (0.4–0.8 mg) SL every 5 min × 3 doses maximum in 15 min as needed
	Caps E.R.	2.5–9 mg oral every 8–12 hours
	Nitro-Bid oint 2%	1–2 inches every 8 hours (while awake and at bedtime)
	Nitro-Dur, Transderm-Nitro	1 transdermal patch 2.5–19 mg daily, rotate site; on 12 hours/off 12 hours
isorbide dinitrate	Tabs sublingual	2.5–5 mg × 3 doses maximum in 30 min
	Tabs oral	Prophylactic 10–40 mg two times a day—three times a day before meals
	Caps, tabs extended release	Oral 20–40 mg every 6–12 hours
isosorbide mononitrate	Monoket, Ismo	10–20 mg oral, twice a day, 7 hours apart
	Imdur (SR)	30–60 mg oral once to twice a day

Based on Woodrow, R. (2007). *Essentials of pharmacology for health occupations* (5th ed.), Table 25-3. Clifton Park, NY: Delmar, Cengage Learning.

Vasoconstrictors

Vasoconstrictors are medications administered intravenously by licensed health care providers. Vasoconstrictors (1) constrict blood vessels and (2) increase blood pressure. Licensed HCPs use these medication mainly on a short-term basis to treat shock. Levophed is a vasoconstrictor.

Antihypertensive Medications

Hypertension is high blood pressure. Hypertension is defined as a systolic blood pressure equal to or greater than 140 or a diastolic blood pressure equal to or greater than 90. Hypertension is staged as mild, moderate, or severe. If left untreated, high blood pressure can increase an individual's risk for heart disease, stroke, and kidney disease.

Hypertension is treated with a category of medications known as **antihypertensive medications**. Classes of antihypertensive medications include the following:

- Thiazide diuretics
- Beta-adrenergic blockers
- Calcium channel blockers
- Angiotensin-converting enzyme (ACE) inhibitors (ACEIs)
- Angiotensin receptor blockers (ARBs)
- Other antihypertensives

Thiazide Diuretics

Thiazide diuretics are used as initial treatment of hypertension either alone or in combination with other antihypertensive medications. Thiazide diuretics are as effective as other treatments and are cost effective.

Adverse reactions:

- Anorexia

- Diarrhea

- Fatigue

- Headache

- Hyperglycemia (high blood sugar)

- Hypotension

- Low chloride level

- Low potassium level

- Muscle weakness or spasm

- Nausea

- Photosensitivity (rare)

- Rash (rare)

- Vertigo

- Vomiting

- Weakness

Contraindications are as follows:

- Diabetes

- History of gout

- Severe kidney disease

- Impaired liver function

- Prolonged use

- Elderly individuals because of a greater sensitivity to thiazides

- Individuals with an allergy to sulfa medications

Special considerations include the following:

- Administer with food to decrease GI upset.

- Administer in the morning to prevent disruption of sleep at night.

- Instruct individual to avoid the use of alcohol.

- Advise the individual to move slowly when changing body positions to decrease the risk of orthostatic hypotension.

- Explain to the individual that she must keep taking the medication even if she feels better. Antihypertensives control high blood pressure but do not cure it.

- Do not administer OTC and herbal medications, especially cough, cold, and allergy medications, unless ordered by the individual's licensed HCP.

- Notify the individual's primary licensed HCP and other licensed health care providers caring for the individual if the individual is self-administering OTC and herbal medications.

Beta-Adrenergic Blockers

Beta-adrenergic blockers may be used as an initial treatment for hypertension, especially for individuals with hypertension who also have angina, who have had an MI, or who have certain types of arrhythmias. Two beta-adrenergic blockers used as antihypertensive medications are propranolol (Inderol) and atenolol (Tenormin).

Adverse reactions, contraindications, and special considerations for beta-adrenergic blockers are discussed under the previous section for antiarrhythmic medications.

Table 21-4 gives a list of selected beta-adrenergic blockers by generic and brand names with dosage information.

Calcium Channel Blockers

Calcium channel blockers may also be used as an initial treatment for hypertension. In particular, diltiazem (Cardizem) and nifedipine (Procardia) are effective in treating individuals with hypertension who have diabetes or are at a high risk for coronary artery disease.

Adverse reactions, contraindications, and special considerations for calcium channel blockers are discussed under the previous section for antiarrhythmic medications.

Table 21-4 gives a list of selected calcium channel blockers by generic and brand names with dosage information.

Angiotensin-Converting Enzyme (ACE) Inhibitors (ACEIs)

Angiotensin-converting enzyme (ACE) inhibitors (ACEIs) work very well alone in treating hypertension. In addition, these medications work well with other antihypertensive medications.

ACEIs are the medication of choice for individuals with hypertension who also have heart failure, diabetes, kidney failure, and/or cerebrovascular disease. In fact, ACEIs are known to slow the progression of renal disease. Two ACEIs are captopril (Capoten) and enalapril (Vasotec).

Adverse reactions:

- Anorexia

- Arrhythmias

- Blood dyscrasias

- Cardiac arrest

- Chronic dry cough

Table 21-4 Antihypertensives by Generic and Brand Names with Dosage Information

GENERIC NAME	BRAND NAME	DOSAGE INFORMATION
Beta-Adrenergic Blockers		
atenolol	Tenormin	25–100 mg oral daily
carvedilol	Coreg	6.25–25 mg oral twice a day with food
metoprolol	Lopressor	100–450 mg oral daily in divided doses
	Toprol XI	50–100 mg oral daily (SR)
propranolol	Inderal	80–240 mg oral daily in 2–3 divided doses
	Inderal LA	80–160 mg oral daily (SR)
Calcium Channel Blockers		
amlodipine	Norvasc	2.5–10 mg oral daily
diltiazem	Cardizem CD	120–360 mg oral daily (SR)
	Cardizem LA	
	Diltiazem SR	120–180 mg oral twice a day (SR)
nifedipine	Procardia XL	30–90 mg oral daily (SR)
	Adalat CC	
verapamil	Calan SR, Isoptin SR	120–240 mg oral once to twice a day (SR)
ACE Inhibitors (ACEIs)		
benazepril	Lotensin	10–20 mg once to twice a day
captopril	Capoten	12.5–50 mg oral twice a day to three times a day
enalapril	Vasotec	5–20 mg oral twice a day
lisinopril	Zestril	2.5–40 mg oral daily
ramipril	Altace	2.5–20 mg oral once to twice a day
trandolapril	Mavik	1–4 mg oral daily
Angiotensin Receptor Blockers (ARBs)		
losartan	Cozaar	25–50 mg oral once to twice a day
telmisartan	Micardis	25–80 mg oral daily
valsartan	Diovan	80–320 mg oral daily
Other Antihypertensives		
clonidine	Catapres	0.1–1.2 mg oral daily in divided doses
	Catapres TTS	Weekly patch (delivers 0.1–0.3 mg per 24 h)
hydralazine	Apresoline	10–50 mg oral four times a day
methyldopa	Aldomet	200–500 mg oral two–four times a day
prazosin	Minipres	1–20 mg oral daily in 2–3 divided doses

Note: Extended release products (ER/SR) must not be crushed, cut, or chewed! Quick release of the medication can cause the blood pressure to drop suddenly, sending the individual into shock.

Note: Other antihypertensives are available.

Based on Woodrow, R. (2007). *Essentials of pharmacology for health occupations* (5th ed.), Table 25-2. Clifton Park, NY: Delmar, Cengage Learning.

- Diarrhea
- Dizziness
- Drowsiness
- Erectile dysfunction
- Fatigue
- Fever
- Headache
- Hepatitis
- High potassium level
- Hypotension
- Insomnia
- Kidney failure
- Loss of taste
- Nasal congestion
- Pancreatitis
- Photosensitivity
- Rash
- Severe hypotension
- Tachycardia
- Weakness

Contraindications for ACEIs are as follows:

- Systemic lupus
- Scleroderma
- Heart failure
- **Angioedema** (swelling of the face, neck, lips, larynx, hands, feet, genitalia, or internal organs)
- Pregnancy
- Breast feeding
- Use cautiously in elderly individuals and individuals of color with hypertension

Special considerations for ACEIs include the following:

- Do not suddenly stop administering the medication. Individuals may experience seizures.
- Do not crush or break extended-release capsules. Instruct the individual not to chew the capsules.
- Advise individual that the coating on the capsules may be visible on her stools. Coating on the capsules is not absorbed into the body.
- Administer medication with meals to decrease GI upset.

- Advise individual to avoid exposure to sun, use sunscreen, and wear protective clothing when outdoors.

- Inform female individuals that medication may interfere with birth control pills and other forms of hormonal contraception. An alternative birth-control method should be used to prevent pregnancy.

- Advise the individual to move slowly when changing body positions to decrease the risk of orthostatic hypotension.

Table 21-4 gives a list of selected ACEIs by generic and brand names with dosage information.

Angiotensin Receptor Blockers (ARBs)

Angiotensin receptor blockers (ARBs) work in a similar fashion as ACEIs. ARBs, however, have fewer adverse reactions than the ACEIs. These medications are, therefore, used in individuals who cannot tolerate ACEIs. ARBs are also used for individuals with hypertension who have other serious diseases such as heart failure and renal disease. Two ARBs are losartan (Cozaar) and valsartan (Diovan).

Adverse reactions are uncommon and include the following:

- Angioedema

- Diarrhea

- Dizziness

- Headache

- High potassium level

- Hypotension

- Insomnia

- Nausea

- Upper respiratory infections

- Vomiting

Contraindications for ARBs are as follows:

- Kidney impairment

- Heart failure

- Pregnancy

- Breast feeding

Special considerations for ARBs are as follows:

- Administer medication with or without food.

- Be aware that it may take three (3) to six (6) weeks for the medication to take maximum effect.

- Instruct individual to avoid potassium supplements and salt substitutes containing potassium unless approved by her licensed HCP.

- Instruct individual to avoid alcohol.

Table 21-4 gives a list of selected ARBs by generic and brand names with dosage information.

Other Antihypertensive Medications

Additional antihypertensive medications that may be used to treat individuals with hypertension include the following:

- Methyldopa (Aldomet)

- Hydralazine (Apresoline)

- Clonidine (Catapres)

- Prazosin (Minipres)

Methyldopa (Aldomet) and hydralazine (Apresoline) are used to treat moderate to severe hypertension. Both medications are usually used with a diuretic. Methyldopa (Aldomet) is contraindicated with elderly individuals.

Refer to a current edition of a reliable medication reference, as needed, for specific information on these medications, including adverse reactions, contraindications, and special considerations for use.

Table 21-4 gives a list of selected other antihypertensives by generic and brand names with dosage information.

Antilipidemic Medications

A buildup of **lipids** (fatty substances) in the body may:

- Block the flow of blood to the heart and other organs

- Increase the risk of coronary artery disease

- Be an underlying cause in hypertension

- Play a role in the development of dementia

For these reasons, licensed health care providers treat an individual with elevated lipid levels. Treatment usually includes the following:

- Diet with a restriction on foods high in saturated fats and cholesterol

- Exercise

- Weight control

- Smoking cessation

- Antilipidemic medications

Antilipidemic medications are used to lower high blood levels of lipids (fatty substances). The goal of therapy is to have an individual's LDL cholesterol below 100 mg/dl.

There are five categories of antilipidemic medications available to lower lipid levels. These are:

- HMG-CoA reductose inhibitors (Statins)

- Bile acid sequestrants

- Nicotinic acid (niacin)

- Fibric acid derivatives (Fibrates)
- Cholesterol absorption inhibitors

HMG-CoA Reductose Inhibitors (Statins)

HMG-CoA reductose inhibitors (statins) are (1) the strongest medications to lower lipids as a monotherapy, (2) considered the first choice of treatment for managing high cholesterol, and (3) moderately effective in decreasing triglyceride levels. Usually, these medications are very well tolerated by most individuals. Atorvastatin (Lipitor) and simvastatin (Zocor) are two statins.

Adverse reactions:

- Abdominal pain or cramps
- Arrhythmias
- Constipation
- Destruction of muscle tissue leading to renal failure (rare)
- Diarrhea
- Drowsiness
- Elevated liver enzymes
- Fatigue
- Flatulence (gas)
- Headache
- Hepatitis
- Hypoglycemia
- Liver failure
- Muscle weakness
- **Myalgia**
- Nausea
- Rash
- Rectal hemorrhage
- Syncope
- Upper respiratory infection
- Vomiting

myalgia
Muscle pain usually accompanied by a feeling of weakness, distress, or discomfort.

Contraindications for HMG-CoA reductose inhibitors (statins) are as follows:

- Liver disease
- Kidney disease
- Myalgia
- Muscle weakness
- Pregnancy
- Breast feeding

Special considerations for HMG-CoA reductose inhibitors (statins) include the following:

- If the individual complains of unexplained muscle pain, weakness, or tenderness, especially with fever or malaise, notify her licensed HCP immediately.
- Administer with food.
- *Do not administer with grapefruit juice or antacids!*
- Zocor may take up to four (4) weeks to have maximum effect.
- Instruct individual to avoid alcohol and red yeast rice.

Table 21-5 gives a list of selected HMG-CoA reductose inhibitors (statins) by generic and brand names with dosage information.

Table 21-5 Antilipemic Medications by Generic and Brand Names with Dosage Information

GENERIC NAME	BRAND NAME	DOSAGE INFORMATION
Statins		
atorvastatin	Lipitor	10–80 mg oral at bedtime
lovastatin	Mevacor	20–80 mg oral at bedtime
pravastatin	Pravachol	10–80 mg oral at bedtime
rosuvastatin	Crestor	5–40 mg oral at bedtime
simvastatin	Zocor	10–80 mg oral at bedtime
Bile Acid Sequestrants		
cholestyramine	Questran, Questran Light	4 g three times a day before meals; mix powder with water, milk, or juice
colestipol	Colestid granules	5–20 g in 2–4 divided doses; mix with above fluids
	Colestid tabs	2–16 g oral in 2 divided doses with a full glass of water
Nicotinic Acid		
niacin	Niaspan, Slo-Niacin	Dose varies with response; take after meals or a snack
Fibric Acid Derivatives		
fenofibrate	Tricor	54–160 mg oral daily with food
gemfibrozil	Lopid	600 mg oral twice a day before meals
Cholesterol Absorption Inhibitor		
ezetimibe	Zetia	10 mg oral daily
Combinations		
atorvastatin/amlodipine	Caduet	Oral daily dose varies with response
ezetimibe/simvastatin	Vytorin	Oral daily in evening, dose varies with response
lovastatin/niacin	Advicor	Oral daily at bedtime, dose varies with response

Note: Other antilipemic medications are available.

Based on Woodrow, R. (2007). *Essentials of pharmacology for health occupations* (5th ed.), Table 25-3. Clifton Park, NY: Delmar, Cengage Learning.

Bile Acid Sequestants

Bile acid sequestants work by decreasing the total amount of cholesterol in the body. Bile acid sequestants may be used alone or with statins. Cholestyramine (Questran) and colestipol (Colestid) are bile acid sequestants.

Adverse reactions:

- Anemia
- Anxiety
- Bloating
- Constipation
- Fecal impaction
- Headache
- Heartburn
- Liver dysfunction
- Nausea
- Vomiting

Contraindications for bile acid sequestants are as follows:

- Allergy to medication
- Biliary cirrhosis and obstruction
- GI obstruction
- Fecal impaction

Special considerations for bile acid sequestants include the following:

- With Questran, mix powder with soup, cereal, pulpy fruit, milk, or water.
- Observe individuals for jaundice (yellowing of skin or eyes), easy bruising, and bleeding. Report these observations to the individual's licensed HCP.
- With Colestid, mix granules with at least ninety (90) mL of water, fruit juice, soup, cereal, or crushed pulpy fruit. Stir until completely mixed then administer.
- With Colestid, give tablets with large amounts of water. Do not crush, cut, or break tablets. Instruct individual not to chew tablets.
- Administer these medications one (1) hour before or four (4) to six (6) hours after other medications.

Table 21-4 gives a list of selected bile acid sequestants by generic and brand names with dosage information.

Nicotinic Acid (Niacin)

Nicotinic acid (niacin) (1) lowers total cholesterol, (2) lowers LDL, (3) lowers triglycerides, and (4) raises HDL.

Adverse reactions:

- Arrhythmias
- Blurred vision

- Chills
- Diarrhea
- Dizziness
- Fatigue
- Flushing
- Glucose intolerance
- Headache
- Hives
- Insomnia
- Itching
- Irritation
- Liver toxicity, especially with higher doses
- Nausea
- Rash
- Syncope
- Tingling
- Vomiting

Contraindications for nicotinic acid (niacin) are as follows:

- Liver disease
- Peptic ulcer disease
- Diabetes
- Gout
- Pregnancy
- Breast feeding
- Severe hypotension

There are no special considerations for nicotinic acid (niacin). Table 21-5 gives information on nicotinic acid (Niacin).

Fibric Acid Derivatives (Fibrates)

Fibric acid derivatives (fibrates) are used to treat (1) individuals with very high triglyceride levels and (2) individuals with complex forms of hyperlipidemia. Fibric acid derivatives (fibrates) may be used alone or with other antilipidemic medications. Fenofibrate (TriCor) and gemfibrozil (Lopid) are fibric acid derivatives (fibrates).

Adverse reactions:

- Allergic reactions (rare)
- Arrhythmias
- Asthma

- Blood dyscrasias
- Diarrhea
- Dyspepsia (upset stomach)
- Gallstones
- Hypoglycemia
- Jaundice
- **Myopathy**
- Nausea
- Rectal hemorrhage
- Seizures
- Vomiting

myopathy
An abnormal condition of skeletal muscle with muscle weakness, wasting, and changes in the muscle tissue.

Contraindications for fibric acid derivatives (fibrates) are as follows:

- Allergy to medication
- Gallbladder disease
- Liver disease
- Renal disease
- Peptic ulcer disease
- Pregnancy
- Breast feeding

Special considerations for fibric acid derivatives (fibrates):

- Administer fenofibrate (TriCor) with meals.
- Administer Lopid thirty (30) minutes before meals.
- Administer bile acid sequestrants at least one (1) hour before or four (4) to six (6) hours after fenofibrate (TriCor).
- Be aware that it may take up to two (2) months for fenofibrate (TriCor) to have maximum effect.
- If the individual complains of unexplained muscle pain, weakness, or tenderness, especially with fever or malaise, notify her licensed HCP immediately.

Table 21-5 gives a list of selected fibric acid derivatives (fibrates) by generic and brand names with dosage information.

Cholesterol Absorption Inhibitor

Ezetimibe (Zetia) is a cholesterol absorption inhibitor. Zetia slows down the absorption of cholesterol in the intestines. Zetia may be taken along with statins to lower LDL. Ezetimibe (Zetia) is well tolerated.

Adverse reactions include:

- Anorexia
- Back pain

- Diarrhea
- Dizziness
- Dry mouth
- Fatigue
- Headache
- Joint pain
- Nausea
- Vomiting

Contraindications for Ezetimibe (Zetia) are as follows:

- Allergy to medication
- Liver disease
- Pregnancy
- Breast feeding

Special considerations for Ezetimibe (Zetia) include the following:

- Administer with or without food.
- Administer at least two (2) hours before or four (4) hours after bile acid sequestrants.
- Advise individual to use hard candy or gum to relieve dry mouth.
- Administer at least one (1) hour before or two (2) hours after administering antacids.

Table 21-5 gives information on Ezetimibe (Zetia).

Anticoagulants

Anticoagulants are medications that prevent or delay clotting of the blood. Anticoagulants are divided into two general groups: coumarin derivatives and heparins. Anticoagulants may be used as follows:

1. Before surgery
2. For an individual who is immobilized, such as an individual who is on prolonged bed rest
3. To treat clot formation (Myers, 2006)

Note: Anticoagulants do not dissolve blood clots. Anticoagulants do, however, prevent the blood clot from getting larger.

A formed blood clot is called a **thrombus**. When a thrombus breaks away from the place where it was formed, it becomes an **embolus** that travels in the bloodstream. An embolus may block a blood vessel, causing a stroke, a heart attack, or other significant damage to an organ (Myers, 2006).

thrombus
A blood clot that has formed inside a blood vessel.

embolus
A blood clot that has disconnected from the point where it was formed.

Coumarin Derivatives

Warfarin Sodium (Coumadin). Warfarin sodium (Coumadin) is an oral anticoagulant. It usually takes twelve (12) to twenty-four (24) hours for Coumadin to work. Coumadin is used for:

- Long-term therapy
- With various heart conditions, such as atrial fibrillation and MI
- Treating and preventing clots in blood vessels
- Treating embolism in the lungs (pulmonary embolism)
- Preventing clots with heart valve replacement

Adverse reactions:

- Allergic reaction
- Bleeding
- Abdominal cramps
- Alopecia
- Anorexia
- Dermatitis
- Diarrhea
- Fever
- Hematuria
- Hepatitis
- Itching
- Nausea
- Necrosis of the skin and other tissues
- "Purple toes" syndrome—painful, purple lesions on toes and sides of both feet
- Rash
- Stomatitis
- Vomiting

Contraindications are as follows:

- Allergy to medication
- Uncontrolled bleeding
- Open wounds
- Severe liver disease
- Bleeding tendency
- Blood dyscrasias
- Recent eye, brain, or spinal cord injury or surgery

- Unsupervised senile, alcoholic, or psychotic individuals
- Pregnancy
- Breast feeding
- Use with caution in elderly and fragile, disabled individuals

Special considerations for warfarin sodium (Coumadin) include the following:

- Explain to the individual that OTC and herbal medications may not be used without the approval of the individual's licensed HCP. As with all medications, OTC and herbal medications require the written approval of the individual's licensed HCP.
- Monitor the individual's stools and urine for blood.
- Be aware that Coumadin may cause a red-orange discoloration of urine.
- Instruct the individual to avoid the use of alcohol. Alcohol may decrease the individual's response to the medication.
- Instruct the individual to avoid sports and activities that may cause bleeding.
- Have the individual shave only with an electric razor. Do not use a razor with blades.
- Use special mouth care. Be careful when brushing and flossing teeth.
- Individual should wear an ID tag and carry an ID card identifying her as a user of an anticoagulant.
- Notify the individual's licensed HCP if the individual has diarrhea or a fever or if any unusual symptoms occur, such as pain or swelling or unusual bleeding, including:
  - Bleeding of gums when brushing the teeth
  - Blood in urine (red or dark brown urine)
  - Blood in stools (red or black stools)
  - Continued bleeding from cuts
  - Frequent bruising
  - Heavier menstrual bleeding
  - Nosebleeds

Refer to Table 21-6 for information on warfarin sodium (Coumadin).

Heparins

Heparins are administered only by licensed healthcare providers. Depending on the type of heparin being administered, licensed HCPs may administer heparins (1) intravenously or (2) subcutaneously. When administered intravenously, the action of heparin is immediate.

Table 21-6 Anticoagulants and Platelet Inhibitors by Generic and Brand Names with Dosage Information

GENERIC NAME	BRAND NAME	DOSAGE INFORMATION
Anticoagulants		
Coumarin Derivatives		
warfarin sodium	Coumadin	Oral dose varies, based on PT/INR (lab) results
Platelet Inhibitors		
aspirin	Ecotrin, Ascriptin, others	81–325 mg oral daily
clopidogrel	Plavix	75 mg oral daily with or without food
dipyridamole	Persantine	75–100 mg oral four times a day with warfarin
dipyridamole with aspirin	Aggrenox	I cap oral twice a day

Note: Many other products are available.

Based on Woodrow, R. (2007). *Essentials of pharmacology for health occupations* (5th ed.), Table 25-4. Clifton Park, NY: Delmar, Cengage Learning.

Platelet Inhibitors

Platelet inhibitors work by stopping platelets from sticking together to form clots. Platelet inhibitors are used for individuals with a history of a recent stroke, recent MI, or a diagnosis of peripheral vascular disease (PAD). Platelet inhibitors help to reduce the recurrence of heart attacks and strokes as well as to reduce the incidence of death from these disorders. Aspirin and clopidogrel (Plavix) are platelet inhibitors.

Clopidogrel (Plavix) may be used in individuals who do not tolerate aspirin or have not had good results with the use of aspirin.

Adverse reactions include:

- Anorexia
- Bruising
- Confusion
- Convulsions
- Coma
- Dizziness
- Drowsiness
- Flushing
- GI bleeding
- Hallucinations

- Heartburn
- Hearing loss
- Itching
- Nausea
- Rapid pulse
- Rash
- Tinnitus
- Vomiting
- Visual changes

Contraindications are as follows:

- Active bleeding
- Bleeding disorders
- Allergy to medication
- Kidney impairment
- Severe liver impairment
- Anticoagulant use
- Pregnancy
- Breast feeding

Special considerations for platelet inhibitors include the following:

- Do not administer OTC and herbal medications unless ordered by the individual's licensed HCP.
- Tell the individual to avoid alcohol, caffeine, and nicotine.
- Administer with food to decrease GI upset.

Table 21-6 gives a list of selected platelet inhibitors by generic and brand names with dosage information.

Thrombolytic Medications

Thrombolytic medications are administered only by licensed healthcare providers in an emergency room or the intensive care unit. Thrombolytic medications may be administered (1) intravenously or (2) subcutaneously. These medications work with an individual's body to dissolve clots. Licensed HCPs administer thrombolytic medications within the first few hours of a heart attack (MI) or stroke (CVA).

Colony-Stimulating Factors (CSFs)

Individuals with anemia from (1) chronic renal failure, (2) HIV, and (3) chemotherapy lack the ability to produce the red blood cells they desperately need. **Colony-stimulating factors (CSFs)**, such as epoetin alfa (Epogen, Procrit) and darbepoetin alfa (Aranesp), stimulate an individual's bone marrow to make more red blood cells. The CSF filgrastim (Neupogen) decreases the effects of chemotherapy on an individual's bone marrow, allowing for more intense chemotherapy treatments.

Colony-stimulating factors (CSFs) are administered only by licensed health care providers. Colony-stimulating factors (CSFs) may be administered (1) intravenously or (2) subcutaneously.

Medications for the Treatment of Anemia

This chapter discusses medications to treat two forms of anemia:

1. Iron-deficiency anemia
2. Megaloblastomic anemia

Iron-Deficiency Anemia

Iron-deficiency anemia is caused by an inadequate supply of iron. Signs and symptoms of iron deficiency anemia include the following:

- Pallor
- Fatigue
- Weakness

Causes of iron-deficiency anemia include:

- Poor dietary intake of iron
- Poor absorption of iron in the digestion system
- Chronic bleeding (Myers, 2006)

Treatment of iron-deficiency anemia includes oral iron preparations:

- Ferrous fumarate (Femiron, Feostat, Hemocyte, Ircon, Neo-Fer)
- Ferrous gluconate (Fergon)
- Ferrous sulfate (Feosol, Fer-in-Sol, Slow-Fe)

Adverse reactions:

- Constipation
- Diarrhea
- Epigastric pain
- Nausea
- Tarry stools
- Vomiting

Special considerations for iron preparations include the following:

- Dilute liquid preparations with water or fruit juice. Administer through a plastic straw to avoid discoloration of tooth enamel and mask the taste.
- Store medication in a tight, light-resistant container.

- Monitor the individual for signs of toxicity:
  - Cyanosis
  - Diarrhea
  - Pale color of skin
  - Nausea
  - Vomiting
- Administer the medication between meals with water. If GI upset occurs, administer after meals or with food.
- Do not administer with milk or antacids.
- Tell the individual that iron may cause dark green or black stools, constipation, or diarrhea.

Megaloblastic Anemia

Megaloblastic anemia is a disorder that causes problems with various types of blood cells. Megaloblastic anemia is usually related to severe pernicious anemia or folic acid deficiency anemia (Myers, 2006). Medications used to treat this disorder include folic acid and vitamin B12.

Folic Acid (Folvite). Adverse reactions:

- Allergic reaction, including rash, itching, redness
- Altered sleep pattern
- Anorexia
- Bitter taste
- Bronchospasm
- Flatulence (gas)
- Hyperactivity
- Impaired judgment
- Malaise
- Nausea
- Poor concentration

Contraindications for folic acid (Folvite) are as follows:

- Pernicious, aplastic, or normocytic anemia
- Use cautiously in individuals who are breast feeding

There are no special considerations for folic acid (Folvite).

Vitamin B12. Vitamin B12 is an injectable medication administered only by licensed HCPs.
Adverse reactions:

- Anaphylactic shock
- Anxiety

- Back pain
- Congestive heart failure
- Diarrhea
- Dizziness
- Dyspepsia (upset stomach)
- Flushing
- Headache
- Heart failure
- Itching
- Nausea
- Nervousness
- Pulmonary edema
- Rash
- Sore throat
- Thrombosis
- Vomiting

Contraindication for Vitamin B12 is an allergy to Vitamin B12, cobalt, or components of the medication.

There are no special considerations for Vitamin B12.

SUMMARY

The cardiovascular system is one of the vital systems in the body. Keeping this body system healthy will help to keep an individual healthy. Sometimes this has to be done with the use of medications. It is the UAP's responsibility to have a basic knowledge of these medications. In addition, the UAP must be able to observe and report any unusual circumstances that may arise while she is giving care.

WORKBOOK REVIEW

Go to the workbook and complete the exercises for Chapter 21.

REVIEW QUESTIONS

1. Early symptoms of a heart attack:
   a. include headache, nasal congestion, nausea, and chest pain
   b. must be reported to the individual's licensed HCP if the symptoms do not pass within thirty (30) minutes
   c. must be observed for twenty-four (24) hours before contacting the individual's licensed HCP
   d. require immediate emergency medical care

2. Risk factors for possible heart attack include:
   a. exercising on a regular basis
   b. eating a balanced diet
   c. obesity
   d. sleeping six (6) to eight (8) hours a night

3. Lanoxin (Digoxin):
   a. strengthens heart contractions and slows the heartbeat
   b. causes rapid, irregular heartbeat
   c. can be given if the individual's heartbeat is less than 60 beats per minute
   d. all of the above

4. An arrhythmia is:
   a. a slow but regular heartbeat
   b. a fast but regular heartbeat
   c. an irregular heart beat
   d. a lack of a heartbeat

5. Vasodilators work by:
   a. tightening and constricting blood vessels
   b. increasing blood pressure
   c. causing angina pectoris
   d. relaxing and dilating blood vessels

6. Orthostatic hypotension is:
   a. low blood pressure in the feet
   b. not something an individual taking vasodilators needs to worry about
   c. a drop in blood pressure after standing up or sitting up
   d. a warning sign of a heart attack

7. A buildup of lipids in the blood:
   a. may increase an individual's strength
   b. may increase the risk of coronary artery disease
   c. may increase an individual's life expectancy by approximately ten (10) years
   d. may decrease one's risk for cancer

8. A thrombus is:
   a. an irregular heartbeat
   b. a blood clot
   c. an increased respiratory rate
   d. an antiplatelet medication
9. Two common platelet inhibitors are:
   a. Coumadin and nitrates
   b. digitalis and iron
   c. folic acid and nicotine
   d. aspirin and Plavix
10. Iron-deficiency anemia is caused by:
    a. low levels of iron in the blood
    b. irregular heartbeat
    c. an embolism
    d. taking medications that contain iron

Chapter 22
Medications for Treating Endocrine Disorders

Learning Objectives

After reading this chapter and completing the review questions, you should be able to:

1. Spell and define terms.
2. Discuss the uses, adverse reactions, and special considerations for various medications used to treat endocrine system disorders.
3. Describe diabetes mellitus and give the warning signs.
4. State signs and symptoms of hypoglycemia and hyperglycemia.

Key Terms

diabetes mellitus	hyperglycemia	lactic acidosis	thrombophlebitis
hormones	hypoglycemia		

INTRODUCTION

The endocrine system contains glands that produce **hormones** to control growth and regulate body activities. If these glands make too much or too little of the hormones they produce, disorders result.

The endocrine system is made up of the following glands:

- Adrenal glands
- Gonads, testis (male) and ovaries (female)
- Pancreas
- Parathyroid
- Pineal gland

hormone
A substance made by the body that controls growth and regulates body activities.

- Pituitary
- Thymus
- Thyroid

Refer to Chapter 12 for additional information on the endocrine system and the glands listed above.

ADRENAL GLANDS

The adrenal glands make a hormone known as corticosteroids. Corticosteroids help the body to (1) control the body's response to fight infection or injury, (2) relieve inflammation, (3) decrease swelling, and (4) control symptoms of certain conditions.

When there is a deficiency (lack) of corticosteroids in the body, adrenal corticosteroids may be administered as replacement therapy. When inflammation and swelling are present, adrenal corticosteroids may also be administered as an anti-inflammatory.

Treatment with adrenal corticosteroids is supportive, not curative. Adrenal corticosteroids are administered along with other medications. Because of the potential for serious side effects, adrenal corticosteroids are used for only a short period of time. Cortisone acetate and prednisone are adrenal corticosteroids.

Adverse reactions with prolonged use (may be very serious):

- Adrenal suppression
- Anxiety
- Arrhythmias
- Bronchospasm
- Cataracts
- Delayed wound healing
- Easy bruising
- Facial edema
- Fat embolism (clot)
- Gastric ulcers
- Heart failure
- Hyperglycemia (high blood sugar)
- Increased appetite
- Increased intracranial pressure
- Increased intraocular (eye) pressure
- Increased risk of infection
- Muscle pain or weakness
- Osteoporosis
- Petechiae

- Psychosis
- Seizures
- Shock
- Skin thinning and tearing
- Spontaneous fractures
- Blood clotting disorders
- **Thrombophlebitis**
- Weight gain

Contraindications for adrenal corticosteroids are as follows:

- Allergy to corticosteroids
- Intolerance to alcohol
- An active untreated infection
- Systemic fungal infections
- Hypothyroidism
- Cirrhosis
- Hypertension
- Congestive heart failure
- Individuals with psychosis
- Diabetes
- Glaucoma
- History of gastric or esophageal irritation or ulcers
- Pregnancy
- Breast feeding
- History of blood clotting disorders
- History of seizures

Special considerations for adrenal corticosteroids include the following:

- Administer doses with meals or snack.
- If possible, administer single dose, alternate-day dose, and morning dose before 9 a.m. Evenly space multiple doses throughout the day. Do not administer the last dose of the day near bedtime.
- Monitor individual closely for signs and symptoms of infection. If noted, immediately contact the individual's licensed HCP.
- Watch for weight gain, swelling, and signs of low potassium level (weakness, confusion, depression). If noted, immediately contact the individual's licensed HCP.
- Do not suddenly stop the medication. Doing so may result in adrenal insufficiency, shock, and death.

thrombophlebitis
Inflammation of the vein along with the formation of a clot.

Table 22-1 Adrenal Corticosteroids by Generic and Brand Names with Dosage Information

GENERIC NAME	BRAND NAME	DOSAGE INFORMATION
Adrenal Corticosteroids		
cortisone	Cortone	Oral, for replacement
dexamethasone	Decadron	Oral, inhalation
fludrocortisone	Florinef	Oral, for orthostatic hypotension
hydrocortisone	Cortef	Oral
methylprednisolone	Medrol	Oral
prednisone	Deltasone, Sterapred	Oral, tablet or solution; do not confuse with prednisolone
triamcinolone	Aristocort, Kenalog	Oral, inhalation

Note: Many other products available. Topical products are discussed in Chapter 14.

Based on Woodrow, R. (2007). *Essentials of pharmacology for health occupations* (5th ed.), Table 23-1. Clifton Park, NY: Delmar, Cengage Learning.

- Do not administer OTC and herbal medications unless they are ordered by the individual's licensed HCP.
- Individual should carry identification stating that he is on long-term corticosteroid therapy.

Refer to Table 22-1 for a list of selected adrenal corticosteroids by generic and brand names with dosage information.

PANCREAS

Within the pancreas, the islets of Langerhans are the glands that produce insulin. There are three major conditions related to insulin:

- **Hyperglycemia**, a condition in which there is too much sugar in the blood
- **Hypoglycemia**, a condition in which there is too little sugar in the blood
- **Diabetes mellitus**, a metabolic disorder that causes an inability to use insulin

The warning signs and symptoms of diabetes are listed in Table 22-2. Signs and symptoms of hyperglycemia and hypoglycemia are listed in Table 22-3.

Insulin

Insulin is used for:

- Insulin-dependent diabetes mellitus (IDDM), or Type 1
- Non–insulin-dependent diabetes mellitus (NIDDM), or Type 2, when other treatments are not successful
- Non–insulin-dependent diabetes mellitus (NIDDM), or Type 2, at the time of surgery, fever, severe injury, infection, serious liver or kidney conditions, endocrine conditions, gangrene, or pregnancy.

Table 22-2 Warning Signs and Symptoms of Diabetes

TYPE I INSULIN DEPENDENT DIABETES (IDDM)	TYPE 2 NON-INSULIN DEPENDENT DIABETES (NIDDM)
• Frequent urination (polyuria)	• Easily fatigued
• Excessive thirst (polydipsia)	• Skin infections
• Extreme hunger (polyphagia)	• Slow-healing wounds
• Unexplained weight loss	• Itching
• **Hyperglycosuria**	• Itching of the vulva in women
	• Burning on urination
	• Vision changes
	• Obesity

Delmar/Cengage Learning

hyperglycosuria
Too much sugar in the urine.

Table 22-3 Signs and Symptoms of Hypoglycemia and Hyperglycemia

HYPOGLYCEMIA	HYPERGLYCEMIA
• Hunger	• Early signs: Headache, drowsiness, and/or confusion
• Weakness	• Breath has sweet, fruity odor
• Dizziness	• Thirsty
• Shakiness	• Weakness
• Cold, moist, clammy, pale skin	• Flushed, dry, hot skin
• Headache	• Nausea, vomiting
• Rapid, shallow respirations	• Rapid, deep respirations
• Irritability, nervousness	• Low blood pressure
• Rapid pulse	• Full, bounding pulse
• Confusion	
• Unconsciousness	• Unconsciousness
• Seizures	
• Blood sugar below normal: less than 50 mg/dL	• Blood sugar above normal: more than 300 mg/dL

Delmar/Cengage Learning

Adverse reactions:

- Allergic reaction, including anaphylaxis
- Fatigue
- Flushing
- Hunger
- Hypoglycemia (low blood sugar)
- Hives
- Itching
- Local reaction at injection site, including redness, stinging, and/ or warmth

- Lethargy
- Low potassium level
- Rash
- Weakness

Special considerations for using insulin include the following:

- Monitor individual for signs and symptoms of hypoglycemia and hyperglycemia. If noted, immediately follow the individual's licensed HCP orders for care and notify the individual's licensed HCP.
- Monitor blood sugar levels before administering insulin to prevent episodes of hypoglycemia and to make sure that the proper dose is given.
- An individual who has an infection or is under unusual stress may need a higher dose of insulin at that time. Notify the individual's licensed HCP if the individual is ill or under stress.
- Do not give OTC and herbal medications without permission from the individual's licensed HCP.
- Instruct the individual to wear a medical ID stating that he is a diabetic and is taking insulin.

Note: Insulin is given via subcutaneous injection. This method of medication administration is not taught in this manual. The UAP should administer insulin only if insulin administration is permitted by his state regulations and workplace policies and after he has been given appropriate training in that technique.

Oral Antidiabetic Medications

Oral antidiabetic medications are used to manage and treat non–insulin dependent diabetes mellitus (NIDDM), Type 2 diabetes. Oral antidiabetic medications may be administered alone, with other oral antidiabetic medications, or with insulin.

Oral antidiabetic medications may be ordered as a single daily dose or two divided doses. Single daily doses are administered before breakfast. Doses ordered twice a day are administered before breakfast and at the evening meal.

Sulfonylureas

Sulfonylureas are oral antidiabetic medications. These medications are used to (1) increase insulin production from the cells of the pancreas and (2) improve insulin activity in the body.

Adverse reactions:

- Abdominal pain
- Allergic reaction
- Anorexia
- Blood dyscrasias, including anemia
- Blurred vision

- Cardiovascular death possible (controversial at this time)
- Diarrhea
- Dizziness
- Drowsiness
- Eczema
- Fatigue
- Headache
- Heartburn
- Hypoglycemia
- Hives
- Increased appetite
- Itching
- Joint pain
- Liver impairment, including jaundice
- Nausea
- Photosensitivity
- Rash
- Tingling in the extremities
- Vertigo
- Vomiting
- Weakness
- Weight gain

Contraindications for sulfonylureas are as follows:

- Allergy to sulfonylureas
- Diabetic coma
- Ketoacidosis
- Sole therapy for Type 1 diabetes (IDDM)
- Unstable diabetes
- Severe kidney disease
- Liver disease
- Thyroid disease or other endocrine diseases
- Uncontrolled infection
- Serious burns
- Pregnancy
- Breast feeding
- Do not use Diabinese for elderly individuals.

Special considerations for using sulfonylureas include the following:

- Monitor blood sugar levels before giving the medication to prevent episodes of hypoglycemia and to make sure that the proper dose is given.

- Monitor individual for signs and symptoms of hypoglycemia and hyperglycemia. If noted, immediately follow the individual's licensed HCP orders for care and notify the individual's licensed HCP.

- Administer single daily doses before breakfast. Doses ordered twice a day are administered before breakfast and at the evening meal.

- Do not give OTC and herbal medications without written permission from the individual's licensed HCP.

Refer to Table 22-4 for a list of selected sulfonylureas by generic and brand names with dosage information.

Biguanides

The medication metformin hydrochloride (Glucophage) is used to manage Type 2 diabetes (NIDDM). Glucophage may be used alone or with sulfonylureas.

Adverse reactions:

- Bloating

- Decrease Vitamin B12 level

- Diarrhea

- Flatulence (gas)

- Hypoglycemia

- Nausea

- Unpleasant or metallic taste

- Vomiting

lactic acidosis
A buildup of an end product of metabolism in the bloodstream.

Lactic acidosis can also occur. This is a buildup of an end product of metabolism in the bloodstream. Lactic acidosis is indicated only by a blood test. Lactic acidosis is fatal in around 50% of all cases.

Contraindications for metformin hydrochloride (Glucophage) are as follows:

- Allergy to metformin hydrochloride (Glucophage)

- Kidney impairment

- Liver impairment

- Congestive heart failure

- Pregnancy

- Breast feeding

- Use in elderly individuals

Table 22-4 Oral Antidiabetic Medications by Generic and Brand Names with Dosage Information

GENERIC NAME	BRAND NAME	DOSAGE INFORMATION
First-Generation Sulfonylureas		
acetohexamide	Dymelor	Oral 250–1500 mg/day before meals or in divided doses
chlorpropamide	Diabinese	Oral 100–500 mg/day with meals (do not use for elderly individuals)
tolazamide	Tolinase	Oral 100–1000 mg/day or in divided doses before meals
tolbutamide	Orinase	Oral 250–3000 mg/day or in divided doses
Second-Generation Sulfonylureas		
glimepiride	Amaryl	Oral 1–8 mg/day with meals
glipizide	Glucotrol	Oral 2.5–40 mg/day before meals or in divided doses
	Glucotrol XL	Oral 5–20 mg/day with meals
glyburide	Diabeta, Micronase	Oral 1.25–20 mg/day or in divided doses with meals
	Glynase	Oral 1.5–12 mg/day with meals
Alpha-Glucosidase Inhibitors		
acarbose	Precose	Oral 25–100 mg three times a day with first bite of each meal
miglitol	Glyset	
Biguanides		
metformin	Glucophage	Oral 500–2,550 mg/day in divided doses with meals
	Glucophage XR	Oral 500–2,000 mg/day in divided doses with meals
Meglitinides		
nateglinide	Starlix	Oral 60–120 mg three times a day with meals
repaglinide	Prandin	Oral 0.5–4 mg before each meal
Thiazolidinediones		
pioglitazone	Actos	Oral 15–45 mg/day
rosiglitazone	Avandia	Oral 4 mg/day or twice a day in divided doses
Combinations		
glyburide/metformin	Glucovance	Oral 1.25/250–10/2,000 mg/day twice a day with meals
rosiglitazone/metformin	Avandamet	Oral 2/500–8/2,000/day in divided doses with meals

Note: In older adults, the licensed HCP should start with the lowest dose possible and increase slowly.

Based on Woodrow, R. (2007). *Essentials of pharmacology for health occupations* (5th ed.), Table 23-4. Clifton Park, NY: Delmar, Cengage Learning.

Note: Administration of metformin hydrochloride (Glucophage) with a radiocontrast dye is contraindicated. The combination of these two substances could lead to acute changes in kidney function. Before an individual undergoes testing that requires the administration of a radiocontrast dye, the UAP will need to contact the individual's licensed HCP to obtain instructions about the administration of the individual's metformin hydrochloride (Glucophage).

Special considerations for metformin hydrochloride (Glucophage) include the following:

- Administer with food to decrease GI upset.

- Do not crush or cut extended-release tablets. Instruct individual not to chew extended-release tables.

- Monitor individual for signs and symptoms of lactic acidosis. Signs and symptoms of lactic acidosis include the following:

  - Weakness

  - Fatigue

  - Muscle pain

  - Shortness of breath

  - Abdominal pain

  - Dizziness

  - Light-headedness

  - Slow or irregular heartbeat

Refer to Table 22-4 for dosage information on metformin hydrochloride (Glucophage).

Thiazolidinediones (TZDs)

Thiazolidinediones (TZDs) are used to treat Type 2 diabetes. Thiazolidinediones (TZDs) may be used alone or with sulfonylureas, metformin, or insulin.

Adverse reactions:

- Anemia

- Back pain

- Diarrhea

- Edema

- Fatigue

- Headache

- Hypoglycemia

- Hyperglycemia

- Muscle pain

- Sore throat

- Sinusitis

- Upper respiratory infection

- Weight gain

Contraindications for thiazolidinediones (TZDs) are as follows:

- Allergy to thiazolidinediones (TZDs)

- Chronic kidney impairment

- Liver impairment
- Congestive heart failure
- Increased risk of pregnancy in premenopausal women; may cause ovulation to continue
- Pregnancy
- Breast feeding

The only special consideration noted for thiazolidinediones (TZDs) is that an individual's licensed HCP should be notified immediately if the following symptoms occur:

- Weight gain over five (5) pounds
- Sudden onset of edema (swelling)
- Shortness of breath

Refer to Table 22-4 for a list of selected thiazolidinediones (TZDs) by generic and brand names with dosage information.

Alpha Glucosidase Inhibitors

Alpha glucosidase inhibitors such as acarbose (Precose) are also used to treat Type 2 diabetes.

Adverse reactions:

- Abdominal cramping
- Diarrhea
- Gas
- Fever
- Hives
- Rash

The only special consideration for this medication is that acarbose (Precose) must be taken with the first bite of food at each meal.

Refer to Table 22-4 for dosage information on acarbose (Precose).

Meglitinides

Meglitinides stimulate the cells in the pancreas to make insulin. Nateglinide (Starlix) and repaglinide (Prandin) are meglitinides. Meglitinides may be used alone or with metformin (Glucophage).

Adverse reactions:

- Constipation
- Diarrhea
- Dyspepsia (upset stomach)
- Headache
- Hypoglycemia

- Joint pain

- Nausea

- Sinusitis

- Upper respiratory infection

- Vomiting

Contraindications for meglitinides are as follows:

- Diabetic coma

- Impaired liver function

- Pregnancy

- Breast feeding

The only special considerations for meglitinides is the following:

- Administer before meals to increase absorption of the medication.

Refer to Table 22-4 for a list of selected meglitinides by generic and brand names with dosage information.

Medications Used to Treat Hypoglycemia

An individual having symptoms of early hypoglycemia may be treated with a concentrated glucose food item such as a piece of hard candy, a sugar cube, or orange juice. The individual should then be fed a snack such as a turkey sandwich with a glass of skim milk. For acute, severe hypoglycemia, also known as insulin shock, medications may be administered. Refer to Table 22-3 for signs and symptoms of hypoglycemia. Medications for the treatment of severe hypoglycemia include the following:

- Diazoxide (Proglycem)

- Glucose (Glucose, Insta-Glucose)

Adverse reactions to diazoxide (Proglycem) include:

- Abdominal pain

- Allergic reaction to diazoxide (Proglycem)

- Anorexia

- Constipation

- Edema

- Nausea and vomiting

- Tachycardia

PITUITARY GLAND

Pituitary hormones are administered by licensed health care providers to determine diagnosis of adrenocortical insufficiency and for treatment.

THYROID
Thyroid Medications

Thyroid hormones are used for:

- Replacement therapy

- Treatment after the thyroid gland has been surgically removed or the gland has undergone radiological treatment to destroy its cells

Treatment needs to continue for the life of the individual. Lab work should be done periodically by the individual's licensed HCP to (1) make the needed adjustments in the individual's dose throughout the his lifetime and (2) monitor for toxic effects of the medication. Levothyroxine is a thyroid medication.

Adverse reactions of thyroid medication are usually due to an overdose resulting in toxicity. Signs and symptoms of toxicity are as follows:

- Arrhythmias

- Change in appetite, increase or decrease

- Diarrhea

- Fever

- Headache

- Heat intolerance

- Hypertension

- Insomnia

- Menstrual irregularities

- Nausea

- Nervousness

- Palpitations

- Sweating

- Tachycardia

- Weight loss

Contraindications for thyroid medications are as follows:

- Angina

- Hypertension

- MI

- Adrenal insufficiency

- Diabetes

- Individuals with normal thyroid function

- For weight reduction

- Use in elderly adults

Table 22-5 Thyroid and Antithyroid Medications by Generic and Brand Names with Dosage Information

GENERIC NAME	BRAND NAME	DOSAGE INFORMATION
Thyroid Medications		
levothyroxine	Synthroid, Levothroid, Levoxyl	Oral 25–200 mcg daily
thyroid	Armour Thyroid	Oral 60–180 mg daily
Antithyroid Medications		
methimazole	Tapazole	Oral tablets, 5–30 mg daily in divided doses
propylthiouracil	PTU	Oral tablets, 100–150 mg daily in divided doses
potassium iodide	Iostat, Thyro-Block	Oral tablets, 130 mg daily for treatment of radiation emergencies

Based on Woodrow, R. (2007). *Essentials of pharmacology for health occupations* (5th ed.), Table 23-2. Clifton Park, NY: Delmar, Cengage Learning.

Special considerations for thyroid medications include the following:

- Administer this medication at least thirty (30) minutes before breakfast. Do not skip doses.

- Do not change from one brand of medication to another or change from a brand-name medication to a generic name medication without first obtaining the individual's licensed HCP's approval.

- Do not administer thyroid hormones with OTC medications, herbal medications, and foods that contain iodine unless otherwise ordered by the licensed health care provider.

- Observe the individual closely. If nervousness, tremors, or irritability are observed, notify the individual's licensed health care provider.

Refer to Table 22-5 for a list of selected thyroid medications by generic and brand names with dosage information.

Antithyroid Medications

Antithyroid hormones are used for:

- Treatment of hyperthyroidism
- Preparation for removal of the thyroid
- Radioactive iodine therapy

Methimazole (Tapazole) and propylthiouracil (PTU) are antithyroid medications.

Adverse reactions:

- Blood dyscrasis
- Diarrhea
- Fever

- Headache
- Hives
- Itching
- Jaundice
- Loss of taste
- Muscle and joint pain
- Nausea
- Tingling in the extremities
- Vomiting

Contraindications for antithyroid medications are as follows:

- Pregnancy
- Breast feeding
- Liver diseases
- Prolonged therapy
- Individuals over forty (40) years of age

Special considerations for antithyroid medications include the following:

- Store the medication in a light-resistant container.
- Dilute (mix) the liquid iodine preparation with water or juice. Administer through a straw to decrease the unpleasant taste.
- Report signs of illness (fever, chills, sore throat, malaise, and so on) immediately to the individual's licensed HCP.
- Report any unusual reactions to the individual's licensed HCP.
- Do not administer with OTC medications, herbal medications, and foods that contain iodine unless otherwise ordered by the licensed health care provider.

Refer to Table 22-5 for a list of selected antithyroid medications by generic and brand names with dosage information.

SUMMARY

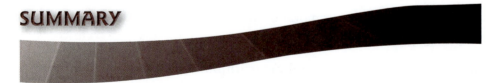

Endocrine system disorders may range from growth disorders to issues with unstable blood sugars, including diabetes mellitus. It is the UAP's responsibility to have a basic understanding of these illnesses and the medications used to treat them. This understanding will help the UAP give endocrine system medications safely and effectively.

WORKBOOK REVIEW

Go to the workbook and complete the exercises for Chapter 22.

REVIEW QUESTIONS

1. Adrenal corticosteroids:
   a. cure diseases caused by a deficiency (lack) of corticosteroids in the body
   b. must be administered along with other medications
   c. have no serious adverse reactions or side effects
   d. can safely be administered for prolonged periods of time
2. Hyperglycemia is a condition in which:
   a. there is too much sugar in the blood
   b. there is too little sugar in the blood
   c. the body is unable to use insulin
   d. the body produces normal amounts of insulin
3. Hypoglycemia is a condition in which:
   a. there is too much sugar in the blood
   b. there is too little sugar in the blood
   c. the body is unable to use insulin
   d. the body produces normal amounts of insulin
4. Diabetes mellitus is a condition in which:
   a. there is too much sugar in the blood
   b. there is too little sugar in the blood
   c. the body is unable to use insulin
   d. the body produces normal amounts of insulin
5. Insulin is used to treat:
   a. IDDM Type 1 diabetes
   b. hyperthyroidism
   c. NIDDM Type 2 diabetes
   d. hypoglycemia
6. Oral antidiabetic medications are used to treat:
   a. IDDM Type 1 diabetes
   b. hyperglycemia
   c. NIDDM Type 2 diabetes
   d. hypoglycemia

7. When giving oral antidiabetic medications, the UAP should remember the following points:
   a. blood sugar levels need to be monitored every other day
   b. these medications should be taken in the morning
   c. these medications should be taken between meals
   d. blood sugar levels need to be monitored weekly

8. Mild hypoglycemia may be treated with:
   a. candy, a sugar cube, or orange juice
   b. epinephrine
   c. oxygen
   d. insulin

9. Pituitary hormones:
   a. may be administered by UAPs with a written licensed HCP order
   b. are administered only by licensed health care providers
   c. are used to treat diabetes mellitus
   d. are used to treat thyroid disorders

10. When administering thyroid or antithyroid hormones, the UAP should:
    a. keep the medication with him at all times
    b. avoid OTC medications, herbal medications, and foods that contain iodine
    c. administer liquid preparations with a spoon at full strength
    d. administer the medication whenever he feels like it

Chapter 23
Medications for Treating Gastrointestinal Disorders

Learning Objectives

After reading this chapter and completing the review questions, you should be able to:

1. Spell and define terms.
2. Identify causes of gastrointestinal disorders.
3. Discuss the uses, adverse reactions, and special considerations for various gastrointestinal medications.

Key Terms

antiemetics

antiflatulents

emetics

emollients

erosive esophagitis

esophagitis

gastroesophageal reflux disease (GERD)

Helicobacter pylori

laxatives

peristalsis

pyrosis

rebound hyperacidity

ulcer

INTRODUCTION

There are many different types of gastrointestinal disorders. Gastrointestinal disorders range from indigestion and **pyrosis** (heartburn) to ulcers and **gastroesophageal reflux disease (GERD)**. As there are many types of disorders, there are also many types of gastrointestinal medications used to treat GI disorders.

Gastrointestinal medications discussed in this chapter fall into eight categories:

- Antacids
- Medications for the treatment of ulcers
- Medications for the treatment of inflammatory bowel disease
- Antidiarrhea medications

gastroesophageal reflux disease (GERD) A condition in which stomach acids travel back up into the esophagus causing inflammation and discomfort.

- Antiflatulents
- Laxatives
- Antiemetics
- Emetics

ANTACIDS

Antacids work by neutralizing hydrochloric acid in the stomach. Antacids are used to:

- Treat indigestion
- Treat heartburn
- Treat pain
- Promote healing of ulcers
- Manage esophageal reflux

Adverse reactions are varied based on the medication being given. However, frequent use may cause the following adverse reactions:

- Belching and flatus (with calcium carbonate- and sodium bicarbonate-based antacids)
- Constipation (with aluminum- or calcium carbonate-based antacids)
- Diarrhea (with magnesium-based antacids)
- Electrolyte imbalance
- Kidney complications
- Kidney stones
- Osteoporosis (with aluminum-based antacids)

Contraindications for antacids are as follows:

- Congestive heart failure
- Kidney disease
- History of kidney stones
- Cirrhosis of the liver
- Edema (swelling)
- Dehydration
- Electrolyte imbalance

Special considerations when using antacids include the following:

- Do not administer antacids within two (2) hours of administering other medications. Antacids interact and/or interfere with almost all other medications.
- Antacids should not be used for more than two (2) weeks. If ordered for an individual for a prolonged period of time, check with the

individual's licensed HCP to make sure the antacid should be administered for the extended length of time.

- Antacids are usually administered between meals and at bedtime.

- Tums and Rolaids can cause **rebound hyperacidity**, a reaction in which the body produces even more stomach acid.

- Notify the individual's licensed HCP if constipation or diarrhea develops when taking these medications.

- Give chewable tablets with eight (8) ounces of water. Remind the individual to chew the tablets thoroughly.

- Do not administer antacids to an individual who is taking any form of tetracycline. Notify the licensed health care provider if the individual has an order for both of these medications.

Table 23-1 gives a list of selected antacids by generic and brand names with dosage information.

Table 23-1 Antacids, Antiulcer Medications, Antidiarrhea Medications, and Antiflatulents by Generic and Brand Names with Dosage Information

GENERIC NAME	BRAND NAME	DOSAGE INFORMATION
Antacids		
aluminum	Amphojel	Suspension, 320 mg/5 ml
		Tablets, 300–600 mg
calcium carbonate	Tums	Tablets, 500–1,000 mg, also in liquid
aluminum-magnesium combinations	Riopan, Maalox, Gelusil, Mylanta	Suspension, tablets (with simethicone); dose varies with product
Medications for Ulcers and GERD		
H₂-Blockers		
cimetidine	Tagamet	200–300 mg every 6 hours oral
	Tagamet HB (OTC)	200 mg daily-twice a day oral (2 weeks maximum)
famotidine	Pepcid	20–40 mg oral tablets at bedtime
	Pepcid AC (OTC)	10 mg daily-twice a day (2 weeks maximum)
ranitidine	Zantac	150 mg tablets twice a day
	Zantac 75 (OTC)	75 mg daily to twice a day (2 weeks maximum)
Proton Pump Inhibitors		
esomeprazole	Nexium	20–40 mg daily sustained release capsules
lansoprazole	Prevacid	15–30 mg daily sustained release capsules
		SoluTab/suspension; 30 mg daily
omeprazole	Prilosec	20–40 mg every morning before meal, sustained release capsules
	Prilosec OTC	20 mg daily before meal sustained release tablet (2 weeks maximum)
pantoprazole	Protonix	20–40 mg daily sustained release tablet
rabeprazole	Aciphex	20 mg daily sustained release tablet

(continues)

Table 23-1 Antacids, Antiulcer Medications, Antidiarrhea Medications, and Antiflatulents by Generic and Brand Names with Dosage Information—*continued*

GENERIC NAME	BRAND NAME	DOSAGE INFORMATION
GI Protectants		
misoprostol	Cytotec	100–200 mcg three times a day with meals and at bedtime with food
sucralfate	Carafate	1 g 4 times a day (1 hour before meals and at bedtime), tablets, suspension
For Inflammatory Bowel Disease		
Salicylates		
mesalamine	Asacol	800 mg oral three times a day (up to 6 weeks), sustained release tablet
sulfasalazine	Rowasa	4 g rectally at bedtime (retain 8 hours; use 3–6 weeks), enema
	Azulfidine	500 mg tablet or enteric coated tablet
		500 mg–1 g four times a day
Antidiarrhea Medications		
diphenoxylate with atropine	Lomotil	Solution or tablets, 2.5–5 mg four times a day
kaolin and pectin	Kapectolin	Suspension, 15–30 ml after each Bowel Movement (max 120 ml/12 h)
loperamide	Imodium	Solution, tablet, capsule; 4 mg initially, 2 mg after each loose Bowel Movement (Prescription maximum 16 mg/day)
	Imodium A-D (OTC)	OTC maximum 8 mg/day × 2 days
Lactobacillus acidophilus	Lactinex, Bacid	2 capsules, 4 tablets, or 1 pkg granules three to four times a day
Antiflatulents		
simethicone	Mylicon	Suspension, tablets after meals and at bedtime
		160–500 mg daily in divided doses

Note: This is only a representative sample. Other products are available.

Based on Woodrow, R. (2007). *Essentials of pharmacology for health occupations* (5th ed.), Table 16-1. Clifton Park, NY: Delmar, Cengage Learning.

MEDICATIONS FOR TREATING ULCERS

An **ulcer** is a lesion caused by loss of tissue, usually combined with inflammation. In the GI tract, ulcers may affect the following areas:

- Esophagus
- Stomach
- Upper intestine

Causes of ulcers include the following:

- Excessive or strong acids
- Ingestion of medications
- A bacteria known as *Helicobacter pylori*

Medications used to treat ulcers include the following:

- Histamine H$_2$-blockers
- GI protectants
- Proton pump inhibitors
- Medications to treat *Helicobacter pylori* (*H. pylori*)

Histamine H$_2$-Blockers

Histamine H$_2$-blockers are used for short-term relief of the following disorders:

- Indigestion
- Heartburn
- Gastroesophageal reflux disease (GERD)
- Upper GI bleeding
- **Esophagitis**—inflammation of the lining of the esophagitis

Adverse reactions:

- Abdominal cramps
- Agitation
- Anxiety
- Confusion
- Constipation
- Depression
- Diarrhea
- Dizziness
- Drowsiness
- Erectile dysfunction—reversible with Tagamet
- Hallucinations
- Headache
- Insomnia
- Mental confusion, especially in elderly or fragile individuals (rarely occurs with Pepcid)
- Nausea
- Psychosis
- Rash
- Vomiting

Contraindications for histamine H$_2$-blockers are as follows:

- Allergy to histamine H$_2$-blockers
- Alcohol intolerance
- Impaired kidney function

- Liver disease

- Pregnancy

- Breast feeding

Special considerations for histamine H_2-blockers include the following:

- Administer medication with meals.

- Instruct individuals who are taking these medications to avoid caffeine, alcohol, strong spices, nicotine, black pepper, herbal medications, and OTC medications, especially if the herbal and OTC medications contain aspirin.

- Do not administer antacids to an individual who is taking any form of histamine H_2-blockers. Notify the individual's licensed HCP if she has an order for both of these medications.

Table 23-1 gives a list of selected histamine H_2-blockers by generic and brand names with dosage information.

GI Protectants

GI protectants protect the lining of the stomach. Sucralfate (Carafate) is used to treat an active ulcer. Sucralfate (Carafate) mixes with the acid in the stomach making a paste that sticks to the lining of the stomach protecting the ulcer. Misoprostol (Cytotec) (1) slows the release of stomach acid and (2) protects the lining of the stomach from the effect of certain medications.

Adverse reactions with sucralfate (Carafate) are rare but may include the following:

- Allergic reaction to sucralfate (Carafate)

- Constipation

- Itching

- Rash

There are no contraindications for sucralfate (Carafate).

The only special consideration for sucralfate (Carafate) is that the medication must be administered on an empty stomach.

Adverse reactions for misoprostol (Cytotec):

- Abdominal pain

- Constipation

- Diarrhea

- Dyspepsia (upset stomach)

- Flatulence (gas)

- Headache

- Incomplete miscarriage, with potential for dangerous uterine bleeding and maternal or fetal death

- Menstrual irregularities

- Nausea
- Vomiting

Contraindications for misoprostol (Cytotec) are as follows:

- Allergy to misoprostol (Cytotec)
- Women of childbearing age
- Pregnancy

Special considerations for misoprostol (Cytotec) are:

- Administer medication with food.
- When administering medication to a woman, administer the first dose of the medication on her second or third day of her normal menstrual cycle.
- Wait thirty (30) minutes after administering this medication to give an antacid.
- Avoid antacids that contain magnesium.

Table 23-1 gives a list of selected GI protectants by generic and brand names with dosage information.

Proton Pump Inhibitors

Proton pump inhibitors decreases secretion of gastric acid. Proton pump inhibitors are used for short-term relief of the following disorders:

- GERD
- Confirmed gastric and duodenal ulcer
- **Erosive esophagitis**
- Pyrosis (heartburn)

Adverse reactions:

- Abdominal pain
- Abnormal thinking
- Anxiety
- Asthma
- Constipation
- Cough
- Depression
- Diarrhea
- Dizziness
- GI hemorrhage
- Hair loss
- Headache
- Hives

erosive esophagitis
A condition in which stomach acids travel back up through the bottom of the esophagus causing irritation and tissue damage.

- Hyperglycemia (with Protonix)
- Hypertension
- Hypotension
- Itching
- Nausea
- Nosebleed
- Photosensitivity
- Rash
- Syncope
- Tinnitus
- Upper respiratory tract infection
- Vitamin B12 deficiency with long-term use, especially in elderly individuals
- Vomiting

Contraindications for proton pump inhibitors are as follows:

- Allergy to proton pump inhibitors
- Liver disease
- Pregnancy
- Breast feeding

Special considerations for proton pump inhibitors include the following:

- Administer medication thirty (30) to sixty (60) minutes before a meal, preferably in the morning.
- When administering Nexium, administer one (1) hour before or two (2) hours after a meal.
- Do not crush or cut capsules or tablets. Instruct the individual not to chew capsules or tablets. If the individual cannot swallow the medication whole, contact the individual's licensed HCP. A licensed HCP order may be obtained permitting the capsule to be opened and the medication sprinkled then mixed into one (1) tablespoon of cool applesauce. If the medication is administered in applesauce, the individual will need to drink a full glass of water immediately after eating the tablespoon of applesauce mixed with the medication.
- When administering orally disintegrating (melting) tablets, place tablet on the individual's tongue. Allow the tablet to disintegrate (melt) until the parts can be swallowed.
- When administering oral suspension, empty packet of medication into a glass with two (2) tablespoons of water. Mix well. Have the individual immediately drink all of the suspension.

- GI upset may be decreased by eating small frequent meals and drinking plenty of fluids.

Table 23-1 gives a list of selected proton pump inhibitors by generic and brand names with dosage information.

Medications to Treat *Helicobacter Pylori*

Helicobacter pylori is an infection in the lining of the stomach that is related to stomach and peptic ulcers as well as stomach cancer (Myers, 2006). *Helicobacter pylori* is also known as *H. pylori*. *H. pylori* is treated with a combination of three medications over a fourteen (14)-day period. The combination of medications includes antibiotics for treatment of the infection.

Medications are ordered in multipacks. Two such multipacks frequently ordered are as follows:

- Prevpac, which includes amoxicillin, clarithromycin (both antibiotics), and Prevacid
- Helidac pack, which includes tetracycline, metronidazole (an antibacterial and antiprotozoal), and bismuth salicylate

Both Prevacid and bismuth salicylate are antiulcer medications.

Adverse reactions, contraindications, and special considerations for the above antibiotics, antibacterial, and antiprotozoal may be found in Chapter 19.

MEDICATIONS FOR TREATMENT OF INFLAMMATORY BOWEL DISEASE

Inflammatory bowel disease is a chronic condition of the gastrointestinal tract. Two types of inflammatory bowel disease are (1) ulcerative colitis and (2) Crohn's disease. Ulcerative colitis involves inflammation of the inner lining of the colon and rectum. Crohn's disease may involve inflammation anywhere in the gastrointestinal tract from the mouth to the rectum. Signs and symptoms for both ulcerative colitis and Crohn's disease are as follows:

- Abdominal pain/cramping
- Diarrhea
- Fever
- Rectal bleeding
- Weight loss

The severity of an individual's symptoms depends upon the progression of her disease. The more severe her disease is, the more severe her symptoms will be (Asacol, 2009).

Salicylates are the medication of choice for treatment of inflammatory bowel disease. Most individuals do well on salicylates. Salicylates are safe for long-term use.

Adrenal corticosteroids may be used to treat an individual who is unable to take salicylates or for whom salicylates do not adequately control her symptoms. Refer to Chapter 22 for additional information on adrenal corticosteroids.

Adverse reactions for salicylates:

- Abdominal cramps/pain
- Anaphylaxis
- Anxiety
- Anorexia
- Depression
- Diarrhea
- Dizziness
- Drowsiness
- Dry mouth
- Fatigue
- Hallucinations
- Headache
- Hives
- Insomnia
- Itching
- Jaundice
- Nausea
- Orange-yellow urine with sulfasalazine (Azulfidine)
- Photosensitivity
- Seizures
- Stevens-Johnson syndrome
- Vertigo
- Vomiting
- Weakness

Contraindications to salicylates are as follows:

- Allergy to salicylates
- Allergy to sulfonomides
- Kidney impairment
- Liver impairment
- Urinary tract obstruction
- Intestinal obstruction
- Pregnancy
- Breast feeding

Special considerations for salicylates include the following:

- Administer after meals. Space doses evenly throughout the day.

- Administer with a full glass of water.

- Do not crush or cut extended-release tablets. Instruct the individual not to chew extended-release tablets.

- When administering mesalamine (Rowasa, Asacol) rectally, have the individual hold the suppository for one (2) to three (3) hours to obtain the best effect of the medication.

- Offer individual plenty of fluids.

- Do not administer OTC and herbal medications unless they are ordered by the individual's licensed HCP.

Table 23-1 gives a list of selected salicylates used to treat inflammatory bowel disease by generic and brand names with dosage information.

ANTIDIARRHEA MEDICATIONS

Diarrhea is frequent passing of loose, watery stools. Diarrhea is (1) a symptom of many different medical conditions and (2) often an adverse reaction to a medication. Regarding treatment, it is often more important to find the underlying cause of the diarrhea than to treat the symptom. However, when the cause is unknown, it is beneficial to treat the symptom to (1) prevent dehydration and electrolyte imbalance and (2) give the individual some relief (Myers, 2006).

Antidiarrhea medications decrease the number of loose, watery stools an individual is having. Antidiarrhea medications may work in several ways, including the following:

- Causing a drying effect by absorbing fluid and protecting the bowel

- Slowing **peristalsis** (the rhythmic, involuntary movement in the GI tract that moves food from the esophagus to the rectum)

- Reestablishing the normal flora in the intestines

Kaolin and Pectin

Kaolin and Pectin causes a drying effect by absorbing fluid and protecting the bowel.

Adverse reactions:

- Constipation

- Fecal impaction

The only contraindication for Kaolin and Pectin is bowel obstruction.

The only special consideration for Kaolin and Pectin is to administer the medication two (2) to three (3) hours before or after other oral medications.

Diphenoxylate with Atrophine (Lomotil) and Loperamide (Imodium)

Diphenoxylate with Atrophine (Lomotil) and Loperamide (Imodium) slow peristalsis.

Adverse reactions:

- Abdominal distention
- Blurred vision
- Confusion
- Constipation
- Dizziness
- Dry eyes
- Dry mouth
- Flushing
- Headache
- Insomnia
- Lethargy
- Nausea
- Nervousness
- Urinary retention
- Vomiting

Contraindications for Diphenoxylate with Atrophine (Lomotil) and Loperamide (Imodium) are as follows:

- Allergy to Diphenoxylate with Atrophine (Lomotil) and Loperamide (Imodium)
- Abdominal pain of unknown cause
- Diarrhea caused by infection or poisoning
- Obstructive jaundice
- Glaucoma
- Use of MAOIs
- Pregnancy
- Breast feeding
- Colitis related to broad-spectrum antibiotics
- Ulcerative colitis
- Cirrhosis
- Use with caution in elderly individuals

Special considerations for Diphenoxylate with Atrophine (Lomotil) and Loperamide (Imodium) include the following:

- Diphenoxylate with Atrophine (Lomotil) and Loperamide (Imodium) should be used on a short-term basis only.

- Do not exceed ordered doses.
- Offer an individual plenty of fluids.
- Do not confuse *lomotil* with *lamictal*.
- Administer with food if GI upset occurs.

Lactobacillus Acidophilus (Lactinex)

Lactobacillus acidophilus (Lactinex) is used to treat simple diarrhea caused by antibiotics, infection, irritable bowel, colostomy, and amebiasis. *Lactobacillus acidophilus* (Lactinex) reestablishes the normal flora in the bowel.

There are no adverse reactions for *Lactobacillus acidophilus* (Lactinex).

Contraindications for *Lactobacillus acidophilus* (Lactinex) are as follows:

- An individual with a high fever
- An individual with an allergy to milk products
- Long-term use
- Individuals with prosthetic heart valves or valvular disease—there is a risk of infection

The only special consideration for *Lactobacillus acidophilus* (Lactinex) is that the medication (capsules, tables, or granules) may be taken or mixed with food, including cereal, juice, or water.

Table 23-1 gives a list of selected antidiarrhea medications by generic and brand names with dosage information.

ANTIFLATULENTS

Antiflatulents break up gas bubbles in the GI tract. Antiflatulents are used to treat (1) the symptoms of gastric bloating and (2) pain from flatus after surgery.

There are no adverse reactions, contraindications, or special considerations with antiflatulents.

Table 23-1 gives additional information on antiflatulents, including generic and brand names with dosage information.

LAXATIVES

Laxatives are medications that aid the body in the elimination of waste. Laxatives are used (1) to treat constipation, (2) to prepare for diagnostic testing, and (3) to prepare for surgery. There are six categories of laxatives:

- Bulk-forming laxatives
- Stool softeners
- Emollients
- Saline laxatives
- Stimulant laxatives
- Osmotic laxatives

Bulk-Forming Laxatives

Bulk-forming laxatives are used to treat simple constipation. Bulk-forming laxatives are:

- The treatment of choice for elderly individuals
- The treatment of choice for laxative-dependent individuals
- Useful in treating individuals with diverticulosis
- Used in treating individuals with chronic, watery diarrhea

Contraindications for bulk-forming laxatives are as follows:

- Acute abdominal pain
- Appendicitis
- Dysphagia (difficulty swallowing)
- Esophageal obstruction
- Fecal impaction
- Intestinal obstruction
- Nausea
- Vomiting

Special considerations for bulk-forming laxatives include the following:

- Dissolve the medication in one full glass of water or juice. Administer immediately when dissolved. Follow with a second full glass of water or juice.

Table 23-2 gives a list of selected bulk-forming laxatives by generic and brand names with dosage information.

Table 23-2 Laxatives and Antiemetics by Generic and Brand Names with Dosage Information and Onset of Action

GENERIC NAME	BRAND NAME	DOSAGE INFORMATION	ONSET OF ACTION
Laxatives			
Bulk-forming (psyllium)	Metamucil, Konsyl-D, Fiberall, others	Powder, 1 teaspoon, dissolved in full glass of fluid one–three times a day	12–72 hrs
Stool softener (docusate)	Surfak, Dialose, Colace, others	Oral capsules, liquid 50–300 mg daily	12–72 hrs
Emollient			
mineral oil	Kondremul, Fleet	5–45 ml oral daily; 60–120 ml rectal daily	oral onset 6–8 hrs
Saline laxative			
magnesium hydroxide	Milk of Magnesia	Suspension, 15–60 ml daily	0.5–3 hrs
Stimulant laxatives			
cascara sagrada		5 ml single dose	0.25–8 hrs
senna	Senokot	8.6 mg tablet, 1–2 twice a day or 10–15 ml syrup twice a day	

Table 23-2 Laxatives and Antiemetics by Generic and Brand Names with Dosage Information and Onset of Action—continued

GENERIC NAME	BRAND NAME	DOSAGE INFORMATION	ONSET OF ACTION
bisacodyl	Dulcolax	5–15 mg tablets	
	Correctol	10 mg suppository	
Osmotic laxatives			
glycerin	Colace suppository	1–2 suppositories as needed	15–60 mins
	Enema	5–15 ml rectal as needed	
lactulose	Cephulac, Enulose	15–60 ml oral daily	24–48 hrs
polyethylene glycol	Miralax	17–34 g (1–2 capfuls) in 8 oz liquid daily	1–2 days
sorbitol	D-Glucitol	30–150 ml oral of 70% solution	
		120 ml rectal of 25%–30% solution	
Antiemetics			
dimenhydrinate	Dramamine	Oral, every 4–6 hrs as needed for motion sickness (max 400 mg PO)	
meclizine	Antivert	25–50 mg daily, one hour before motion (repeat every 2 hours as needed)	
		25–100 mg in divided doses/Meniere's Disease	
metoclopramide	Reglan	Oral, dose varies with condition	
prochlorperazine	Compazine	5–10 mg oral, four times a day; 25 mg suppository twice a day	
promethazine	Phenergan	Tablets, syrup, suppository 25 mg	
scopolamine	Transderm-Scop	0.5 mg patch every 72 hours for motion sickness	
trimethobenzamide	Tigan	Oral 300 mg, suppository 100–200 mg 3–4 times a day	
Antiemetics (Preoperative or with Chemotherapy)			
dolasetron	Anzemet	Administered IV by licensed HCP only	
ondansetron	Zofran	16 mg oral	

Note: This is only a representative sample. Others are available.

Based on Woodrow, R. (2007). *Essentials of pharmacology for health occupations* (5th ed.), Table 16-2. Clifton Park, NY: Delmar, Cengage Learning.

Stool Softeners

Stool softeners soften stools making passage of the stool easier.

Adverse reactions are uncommon with the exception of the following:

- Mild abdominal cramping
- Rash

Contraindications for stool softeners are as follows:

- Acute abdominal pain
- Prolonged use without medical supervision

Special considerations for stool softeners include the following:

- Notify the individual's licensed HCP immediately if the individual experiences diarrhea or abdominal pain.
- Offer the individual plenty of fluids.

Table 23-2 gives additional information on selected stool softeners, including generic and brand names and dosage information.

Emollients

Emollients lubricate the bowel helping with the passage of stool from the body. Mineral oil is an emollient. Mineral oil may be administered orally or rectally in the form of an enema.

Adverse reactions:

- Anal irritation due to leakage of oil from the rectum
- Malabsorption of vitamins A, D, E, and K with prolonged use

Contraindications for emollients are as follows:

- Bedridden, fragile, or elderly individuals
- Dysphagia (difficulty swallowing)
- Gastric retention
- Hiatal hernia
- Pregnancy
- Prolonged use
- Use along with stool softeners

The only special consideration for emollients is the avoidance of frequent or prolonged use.

Table 23-2 gives additional information on selected emollients, including generic and brand names and dosage information.

Saline Laxatives

Saline laxatives should be used only in single doses and infrequently with an order from the individual's licensed HCP. If an individual is experiencing more frequent episodes of constipation or chronic constipation, the individual's licensed HCP should be notified.

Adverse reactions:

- Cardiac complications
- Confusion
- Edema (swelling)
- Electrolyte imbalance
- Liver complications

- Renal (kidney) complications
- Sedation
- Weakness

Contraindications for saline laxatives are as follows:

- Long-term use
- Congestive heart failure
- Other cardiac disease
- Edema (swelling)
- Cirrhosis
- Kidney disorders
- Use of diuretics
- Acute abdominal pain
- Colostomy

The only special consideration for saline laxatives is the avoidance of frequent or prolonged use.

Table 23-2 gives additional information on selected saline laxatives, including generic and brand names and dosage information.

Stimulant Laxatives

Stimulant laxatives are used for the following:

- Before surgery
- Before diagnostic testing
- After diagnostic testing for such reasons as to remove barium from the bowel

Stimulant laxatives are habit forming and may result in laxative dependency. Therefore, these medications should not be used on a frequent or regular basis to relieve constipation. Stimulant laxatives are available in oral form, as suppositories, and as enemas.

Adverse reactions:

- Abdominal cramps/discomfort
- Discoloration of urine with senna and cascara
- Electrolyte imbalance with prolonged use
- Loss of normal bowel function with prolonged use
- Nausea (frequent)
- Rectal or colonic irritation with suppositories

Contraindications for stimulant laxatives are as follows:

- Acute abdominal pain or cramping
- Ulcerative colitis
- Pregnancy

- Breast feeding

- Long-term use

Special consideration for stimulant laxatives is the avoidance of frequent or prolonged use.

Table 23-2 gives additional information on selected stimulant laxatives, including generic and brand names and dosage information.

Osmotic Laxatives

Osmotic laxatives draw water from the surrounding tissue into the stool stimulating the body to pass the stool out of the body. Osmotic laxatives are administered orally or rectally by suppository or enema.

Adverse reactions:

- Abdominal cramps

- Abdominal distention

- Diarrhea

- Flatulence (gas)

- Hyperglycemia in diabetic individuals

- Rectal irritation

Contraindications for osmotic laxatives are as follows:

- Individuals on a low-galactose diet

- Pregnancy

- Breast feeding

- Use with caution in elderly individuals

Special considerations for osmotic laxatives include the following:

- Do not administer along with other laxatives.

- Dissolve the contents of single-use packet in four (4) ounces of water or juice.

- Dilute syrup with water or juice to mask the taste.

- Offer individuals plenty of fluids.

Table 23-2 gives additional information on selected stimulant laxatives including generic and brand names and dosage information.

ANTIEMETICS

Antiemetics are used to:

- Treat vertigo

- Treat motion sickness

- Prevent nausea and vomiting

- Stop vomiting

Meclizine (Antivert)

Meclizine (Antivert) is an antihistamine used as an antiemetic.
Adverse reactions:

- Anxiety, especially with elderly individuals
- Blurred vision
- Confusion, especially with elderly individuals
- Depression
- Drowsiness
- Dry mouth
- Extrapyramidal reactions—refer to Chapter 16 for additional information
- Restlessness, especially with elderly individuals
- Sedation
- Vertigo
- Weakness

Contraindications for meclizine (Antivert) are as follows:

- Allergy to meclizine (Antivert)
- Pregnancy
- Breast feeding
- Use with fragile or elderly individuals
- Glaucoma
- Prostate disorders
- Arrhythmias
- Hypertension
- Seizures
- COPD
- Asthma

Special considerations for meclizine (Antivert) include the following:

- Tablets may be chewed or swallowed whole.
- Dry mouth may be relieved with hard candy or frequent sips of fluid.

Metoclopramide (Reglan)

Metoclopramide (Reglan) is an antiemetic used in the prevention of nausea and vomiting in individuals undergoing chemotherapy.
Adverse reactions:

- Anxiety
- Constipation

- Depression—can be severe

- Diarrhea

- Drowsiness

- Extrapyramidal reactions—refer to Chapter 16 for additional information

- Fatigue

- Hypertension

- Hypotension

- Insomnia

- Nausea

- Restlessness

- Use with caution with elderly individuals—not for long-term use with these individuals

Contraindications for Metoclopramide (Reglan) are as follows:

- Allergy to Metoclopramide (Reglan)

- Parkinson's disease

- GI obstruction, perforation, or hemorrhage

- History of seizures

Special considerations for Metoclopramide (Reglan) include the following:

- Mix oral solution in water, juice, carbonated beverage, or semi-solid food (such as applesauce or pudding) just before administering medication.

- Administer medication thirty (30) minutes before meals.

- Report involuntary movements of the face, eyes, or limbs to the individual's licensed HCP.

Table 23-2 gives a list of antiemetics by generic and brand names with dosage information.

EMETICS

Emetics are medications used to induce vomiting in an individual who has taken an overdose of oral drugs or has ingested certain poisons. Emetics should *not* be used in the following circumstances:

- An individual who is in shock

- An individual who is semiconscious or unconscious

- An individual who has ingested a caustic substance such as lye or acid

A common OTC emetic is syrup of ipecac. Syrup of ipecac will usually cause vomiting within twenty (20) minutes. Syrup of ipecac may be given a second time if the individual has not vomited in that period of time. After the vomiting has stopped, activated charcoal can be given to absorb the remaining poison.

Note: **As with all medications, a licensed health care order is needed for the administration of the syrup ipecac.**

SUMMARY

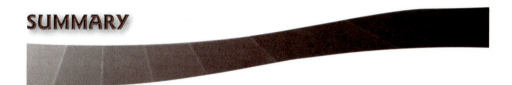

There are many disorders that can affect the GI system. Most or all of these disorders may cause significant discomfort in the body. GI disorders may also affect an individual's nutritional intake. This may cause additional health problems. It is the UAP's responsibility to have a basic understanding of these illnesses and the medications used to treat them. This understanding will help the UAP to give gastrointestinal medications safely and effectively.

WORKBOOK REVIEW

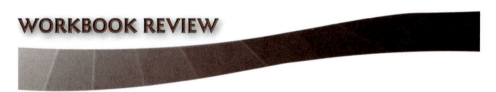

Go to the workbook and complete the exercises for Chapter 23.

REVIEW QUESTIONS

1. Pyrosis is:
   a. another name for heartburn
   b. another name for indigestion
   c. another name for dyspepsia
   d. a type of antacid
2. Antacids work to:
   a. cause indigestion
   b. neutralize stomach acids
   c. minimize abdominal cramps
   d. stop diarrhea
3. Administer antacids:
   a. before meals
   b. two hours from administering other medications
   c. with Tagamet
   d. with milk

4. An ulcer is:
   a. a condition seen primarily in middle-aged men
   b. caused by Tums or Rolaids
   c. a condition of irritation and tissue damage in the esophagus caused by stomach acid
   d. a lesion caused by loss of tissue, usually combined with inflammation

5. An individual who has an ulcer should:
   a. avoid caffeine and alcohol
   b. eliminate fruits and vegetables from her diet
   c. limit daily exercise
   d. monitor her blood pressure daily

6. Erosive esophagitis is:
   a. a condition seen primarily in middle-aged men
   b. caused by Tums or Rolaids
   c. a condition of irritation and tissue damage in the esophagus caused by stomach acid
   d. the same as rebound hyperacidity

7. Laxatives are used to:
   a. relieve constipation
   b. relieve symptoms of an ulcer
   c. relieve diarrhea
   d. prevent vomiting

8. One result of laxative abuse is:
   a. fecal impaction
   b. persistent diarrhea
   c. lack of response from the colon to the urge to have a bowel movement
   d. nausea and vomiting

9. Diarrhea is:
   a. the frequent passing of loose, watery stools
   b. easily controlled by decreasing the amount of liquids one drinks daily
   c. always caused by an infection
   d. more a nuisance than a serious concern

10. Emetics are:
    a. medications used to stop vomiting
    b. medications used to induce vomiting
    c. medications used to treat diarrhea
    d. medications used to treat ulcers

11. An individual's licensed HCP may order an emetic for an individual who:
    a. is in shock
    b. is semiconscious or unconscious
    c. has taken an overdose of oral drugs
    d. has ingested a caustic substance

Chapter 24
Medications for Treating Musculoskeletal Disorders

Learning Objectives

After reading this chapter and completing the review questions, you should be able to:

1. Spell and define terms.
2. Discuss the uses, adverse reactions, and special considerations for various medications used to treat musculoskeletal system disorders.

Key Terms

gout	muscle spasms	osteoporosis	spondylitis
inflammation	myasthenia gravis	peritonitis	

INTRODUCTION

The musculoskeletal system gives the body structure and the ability to move. Disorders of this system primarily include pain and inflammation of joints and muscles, along with disorders that impact movement. Medications that are used to treat these disorders fall into five categories:

- Skeletal muscle relaxants
- Muscle stimulants
- Anti-inflammatory medications
- Medications to treat gout
- Medications to treat osteoporosis

SKELETAL MUSCLE RELAXANTS

Skeletal muscle relaxants are used to treat:

- Pain

- Abnormal contractions of the muscles

- Impaired mobility

- **Muscle spasms** caused by:

  - Strains and sprains

  - Injury or trauma

  - Disease

Muscle relaxants may have:

- An indirect effect on the spinal cord and brain with no direct effect on the skeletal muscle

- A direct effect on skeletal muscles

The type of muscle relaxant ordered by the individual's licensed HCP will be determined by the type of disorder the individual has. For instance, diazepam (Valium), which has an effect on the brain and spinal cord, may be ordered to treat an acute musculoskeletal disorder that causes significant pain. Dantrolene (Dantrium), which directly affects skeletal muscle, may be ordered to manage muscle spasms from multiple sclerosis or cerebral palsy.

Adverse reactions:

- Allergic reaction to skeletal muscle relaxants

- Ataxia (Impaired coordination)

- Bed-wetting at night

- Blurred vision

- Confusion

- Constipation

- Diarrhea

- Dizziness

- Drowsiness

- Dry mouth

- Headache

- Hypotension

- Nausea

- Nervousness

- Respiratory depression

- Slurred speech

- Tremor

muscle spasms
Involuntary contractions of one or more muscles, usually accompanied by pain and limited movement.

- Urinary frequency

- Urinary retention

- Vomiting

- Weakness

Contraindications for muscle relaxants are as follows:

- Muscular dystrophy

- Myasthenia gravis

- Pregnancy

- Breast feeding

- History of drug abuse

- Impaired kidney function

- Liver disorders

- Blood dyscrasias

- COPD

- Use in elderly individuals

Special considerations for muscle relaxants include the following:

- These medications may be given with meals.

- Do not give OTC medications, including antihistamines, decongestants, and cough medicines, and herbal medications with these medications unless the OTCs and herbal medications are ordered by the individual's licensed HCP.

- Do not suddenly discontinue these medications. If the medications are quickly stopped by the individual's licensed HCP, contact his licensed HCP to clarify the order for discontinuation of the medication. An individual who suddenly stops taking this medication may experience headache, insomnia, nausea, spasticity, and/or tachycardia.

- Instruct the individual not to drive while taking these medications.

- Skeletal muscle relaxants are for short-term use only. Use these medications only for as long as needed. Prolonged use could lead to physical and/or psychological dependence and withdrawal symptoms.

Table 24-1 gives a list of selected skeletal muscle relaxants by generic and brand names with dosage information.

Neuromuscular Blocking Medications (NMBAs)

Neuromuscular blocking medications (NMBAs) are a type of skeletal muscle relaxants. Neuromuscular blocking medications (NMBAs) are used in an acute care setting during surgical, endoscopic, and orthopedic procedures. These medications are only administered by anesthesiologists and

Table 24-1 Skeletal Muscle Relaxants by Generic and Brand Names with Dosage Information

GENERIC NAME	BRAND NAME	DOSAGE INFORMATION	COMMENTS
carisoprodol	Soma	Oral 350 mg three–four times a day	Caution with asthma; watch for abuse potential
cyclobenzaprine	Flexeril	Oral 15–30 mg/day in divided doses	For acute painful musculoskeletal conditions
diazepam	Valium	Oral 2–10 mg three–four times a day	Abrupt withdrawal after prolonged use may cause seizures
methocarbamol	Robaxin	Oral 4–8 g daily in divided doses	For acute painful musculoskeletal conditions
dantrolene	Dantrium	Oral 25–100 mg two to four times a day	For multiple sclerosis and cerebral palsy, not for trauma or rheumatic disorders
baclofen	Lioresal	Oral 10–20 mg three to four times a day	May be of some value with spinal cord injury or spinal cord diseases
tizanidine	Zanaflex	Oral 2–8 mg one to three times a day in 6–8 hour intervals	For increased muscle tone associated with spasticity, for example, multiple sclerosis or spinal cord trauma

Note: Representative sample; other products are available.

Based on Woodrow, R. (2007). *Essentials of pharmacology for health occupations* (5th ed.), Table 21-1. Clifton Park, NY: Delmar, Cengage Learning.

other specially trained licensed health care providers who are skilled in intubation and CPR. Individuals may have serious reactions to neuro-muscular blocking medications (NMBAs) including allergic reactions, respiratory arrest, and cardiac arrest.

MUSCLE STIMULANTS

The muscle stimulant anticholinesterase (Prostigmin) is used to treat symptoms of myasthenia gravis. **Myasthenia gravis** is a progressive musculoskeletal disorder with symptoms of chronic fatigue and muscle weakness, especially in the face and throat. The onset is gradual with eventual extension to other muscles, including the respiratory system.

Adverse reactions:

- Abdominal cramping
- Anaphylaxis
- Asthenia (loss of strength)
- Bradycardia
- Bronchospasm
- Cardiac arrest
- Diarrhea

- Dizziness
- Drowsiness
- Dyspnea (shortness of breath)
- Flushing
- Headache
- Hives
- Hypotension
- Joint pain
- Loss of consciousness
- Muscle cramps and spasms
- Nausea
- Rash
- Respiratory depression or arrest
- Tachycardia
- Urinary frequency
- Vision changes
- Vomiting

Contraindications for anticholinesterase (Prostigmin) are as follows:

- Allergy to cholinergics and bromide
- GI obstruction
- Urinary obstruction
- **Peritonitis** (inflammation of the lining of the abdominal wall)

Special considerations for anticholinesterase (Prostigmin) include the following:

- Administer medication one (1) hour before or two (2) hours after meals.
- Instruct individual to avoid driving while taking this medication.

ANTI-INFLAMMATORY MEDICATIONS

Inflammation is a protective response of the body to irritation or injury. Inflammation may be acute or chronic. The symptoms of inflammation include:

- Redness
- Warmth
- Swelling
- Pain
- At times, limited mobility (Myers, 2006)

Anti-inflammatory medications help to relieve the symptoms of inflammation but do not treat its cause. Anti-inflammatory medications may be used in the treatment of the following disorders:

- Muscle strains and sprains
- Bursitis
- Gout
- Rheumatoid arthritis
- Osteoarthritis
- **Spondylitis** (inflammation of the vertebrae)
- Gout
- Dermatitis
- Colitis

Analgesics

Analgesics are used to treat many types of inflammation during its acute stage. Additional information on analgesics may be found in Chapter 17.

Corticosteroids

Corticosteroids are used to treat many types of inflammation during its acute stage. Because of the serious side effects of corticosteroids, these medications are used only for short-term treatment. Additional information on corticosteroids may be found in Chapter 22.

Nonsteroidal Anti-Inflammatory Medications (NSAIDs)

Nonsteroidal anti-inflammatory medications (NSAIDs) may be used to treat mild to moderate pain. The most common adverse reactions are:

- Allergic reaction to NSAIDs
- Blood dyscrasias
- Bronchospasm, especially with aspirin
- Constipation
- Diarrhea
- Dizziness
- Drowsiness
- Fatigue
- GERD
- GI bleeding, especially in fragile and elderly individuals who may suffer a "silent bleed" leading to a fatal GI event
- Headache
- Hearing loss

- Heartburn
- Light-headedness
- Liver toxicity
- Nausea
- Rash
- Tinnitus
- Ulcers in the GI tract
- Visual disturbances
- Vomiting

Contraindications for nonsteroidal anti-inflammatory medications (NSAIDs) are as follows:

- Allergy to aspirin
- Asthma
- Congestive heart failure
- Gastric ulcers
- Inflammatory bowel disease
- GI bleeding
- Hypertension
- Blood dyscrasias
- Thyroid disease
- GERD
- Kidney disease
- Liver impairment
- Pregnancy
- Breast feeding
- Use cautiously in fragile and elderly individuals

Special considerations for nonsteroidal anti-inflammatory medications (NSAIDs) include the following:

- Administer medication with food to decrease GI upset.
- Administration of NSAIDs should be stopped one (1) week before surgery. If medication has not been stopped, contact the individual's licensed HCP for orders.
- If the individual is taking both NSAIDs and aspirin or acetaminophen (Tylenol), notify the individual's licensed HCP. An individual should not be taking these medications at the same time unless specifically ordered by his licensed HCP.
- Do not crush or cut enteric-coated medications. Instruct the individual not to chew enteric-coated medications.

- Do not administer enteric coated medications with dairy products, such as milk or yogurt.

- Observe the individual for signs of bleeding, including the following:

  - Prolonged bleeding from cuts

  - Nosebleeds

  - Bleeding of gums after brushing the teeth

  - Increased menstrual bleeding

  - Unusual bruising

  - Red or dark brown urine

  - Red or tarry stools

If signs of bleeding occur, immediately notify the individual's licensed HCP.

Table 24-2 gives a list of selected NSAIDs by generic and brand names with dosage information.

Table 24-2 Nonsteroidal Anti-Inflammatory Medications and Cox-2 Inhibitors by Generic and Brand Names with Dosage Information

GENERIC NAME	BRAND NAME	DOSAGE INFORMATION
Nonsteroidal Anti-inflammatory Medications (NSAIDs)		
diclofenac	Voltaren	Oral 150–225 mg daily in divided doses
	Voltaren XR	Oral 100 mg one to two times a day
ibuprofen	Motrin, Advil (OTC)	Oral 200–800 mg four times a day
indomethacin	Indocin	Oral up to 200 mg daily in divided doses
	Indocin SR	Oral 75 mg one to two times a day
ketorolac	Toradol	Oral 20 mg once, then 10 mg every four to six hours for five days maximum
naproxen	Naprosyn, Anaprox, Aleve (OTC)	Oral 220–550 mg twice a day every 12 hours
oxaprozin	Daypro	Oral 600–1200 mg once daily
sulindac	Clinoril	Oral 150–200 mg twice a day
etodolac	Lodine	Oral 600–1200 mg daily in divided doses
	Lodine XL	Oral 400–1000 mg daily
meloxicam	Mobic	Oral 7.5–15 mg daily
nabumetone	Relafen	Oral 1,000–2,000 mg daily
COX-2 Inhibitor		
celecoxib	Celebrex	Oral 100–200 mg twice a day

Note: Other NSAIDs are available.

Based on Woodrow, R. (2007). *Essentials of pharmacology for health occupations* (5th ed.), Table 21-2. Clifton Park, NY: Delmar, Cengage Learning.

COX-2 Inhibitors

COX-2 inhibitors pose less risk for GI bleeding and cause fewer gastric problems, such as GI irritation and GI upset. However, over the past five (5) years or so, there has been concern over the safety of COX-2 inhibitors.

In 2004, rofecoxib (Vioxx) was voluntarily removed from the market. Individuals taking rofecoxib (Vioxx) had been shown to have twice the rate of myocardial infarction (MI) and stroke (CVA) compared to those taking a placebo. Later, Bextra was taken off the market because at times it caused severe skin reactions that proved fatal at times.

Celebrex currently has warnings for adverse cardiac effects similar to those for which Vioxx was removed from the market. Responsible licensed health care providers track information on these medications and others.

Adverse reactions:

- Abdominal pain
- Anaphylaxis
- Angina
- Constipation
- Diarrhea
- Dizziness
- Drowsiness
- Dry mouth
- Dyspepsia
- Fatigue
- Flatus
- GI bleeding
- Headache
- Insomnia
- Liver toxicity
- MI
- Nausea
- Nosebleed
- Rash
- Tachycardia
- Upper respiratory infection

Contraindications for Celebrex are as follows:

- Allergy to Celebrex, sulfonamides, and other NSAIDs
- Advanced kidney disease
- Severe liver impairment

- Allergy to aspirin

- Pregnancy

- Breast feeding

- Use with caution in elderly individuals

Special considerations for Celebrex include the following:

- Do not administer with an antacid. If there are orders for both medications, contact the individual's licensed HCP.

- Administer Celebrex with food or milk.

- Do not administer with other NSAIDs or aspirin. If the individual has orders for both medications, contact the individual's licensed HCP.

Table 24-2 gives additional information on Celebrex, including generic and brand name and dosage information.

Disease-Modifying Antirheumatic Medications (DMARDs)

Disease-modifying antirheumatic medications (DMARDs) are used to treat rheumatoid arthritis. Disease-modifying antirheumatic medications (DMARDs) may be able to slow the progression of the disease but do not cure the disease.

Adverse reactions:

- Allergic reaction to DMARDs

- Anemia

- Arrhythmias

- Deep-vein thrombosis

- Depression

- Diarrhea

- Diabetes mellitus

- Fatigue

- Gastric irritation

- Hair loss

- Headache

- Hives

- Hypertension

- Hypotension

- Injection site reaction

- Itching

- Kidney failure

- Liver toxicity

- Lymphoma

- Nausea
- Pneumonia
- Rash
- Seizures
- Serious infections
- Sinusitis
- Thrombophlebitis
- Upper respiratory tract infection
- Urinary tract infection
- Vomiting
- Weight gain

Contraindications for disease-modifying antirheumatic medications (DMARDs) are as follows:

- Allergy to DMARDs
- Pregnancy
- Breast feeding
- Heart failure
- Active infection, including chronic or localized infection
- Liver disease
- Latex allergy
- Use with caution in elderly individuals

Special considerations for disease-modifying antirheumatic medications (DMARDs) include the following:

- Administer Arava with or without food.
- Administer methotrexate orally one (1) hour before or two (2) hours after meals.
- For an individual on methotrexate, take the individual's temperature daily. Report fever to his licensed HCP.
- Refrigerate injectable medications and protect them from light.
- Monitor individual for signs and symptoms of infection (fever, productive cough, sore throat, burning on urination). If symptoms are noted, immediately notify the individual's licensed HCP.
- Offer the individual small, frequent servings of food and plenty of fluids to decrease GI upset.
- Arava and methotrexate may cause harm to a fetus. Instruct both male and female individuals to use contraception and to talk with the licensed HCP if pregnancy is suspected or planned.
- If the individual has an injection site reaction, apply cool compresses.

Table 24-3 Disease-Modifying Antirheumatic Medications (DMARDs) by Generic and Brand Names with Dosage Information

GENERIC NAME	BRAND NAME	DOSAGE INFORMATION
Adalimumab	Humira	Subcutaneous, 40 mg every 1–2 weeks
Etanercept	Enbrel	Subcutaneous, 25 mg twice a week
Infliximab	Remicade	Intravenously by licensed health care provider only
Leflunomide	Arava	Oral, 100 mg daily for three days, then 20 mg daily
Methotrexate	Rheumatrex	Oral, 7.5 mg weekly

Note: Representative sample only.

Source: Based on Broyles, Reiss, and Evans (2007), *Pharmacological aspects of nursing care* (7th ed.) table 12-2. Clifton Park, NY: Delmar, Cengage Learning.

- Instruct the individual to avoid crowds as well as individuals who are ill.

- Instruct the individual to avoid sun exposure, use sunscreen, and wear appropriate clothing when outdoors.

- Instruct the individual to avoid the use of alcohol.

Note: **Several of the disease-modifying antirheumatic medications (DMARDs), such as Enbrel, are given via subcutaneous injection. This method of medication administration is not taught in this manual. The UAP should only administer subcutaneous injections if this route of administration is permitted by his state regulations and workplace policies and after he has been given appropriate training in that technique.**

Table 24-3 gives a list of selected disease-modifying antirheumatic medications (DMARDs) by generic and brand names with dosage information.

MEDICATIONS USED TO TREAT GOUT

Gout is a metabolic disease that causes painful swelling of certain joints. The most common site is the great toe. Other joints that may be affected include the ankle, knee, and elbow. Treatment of acute symptoms usually includes medication, such as colchicine and indomethacin, and a diet low in purine-rich foods. Long-term treatment may include the medications probenecid (Benemid) and allopurinol (Zyloprim) (Myers, 2006).

Adverse reactions:

- Abdominal pain
- Blood disorders
- Diarrhea
- GI bleeding
- Hair loss

- Kidney impairment

- Nausea

- Neuropathy

- Rash

- Vitamin B12 malabsorption

- Vomiting

Contraindications for medications to treat gout are as follows:

- Allergy to gout medications

- Blood dyscrasias

- Serious GI disorders

- Serious cardiac disorders

- Serious kidney disorders

- Serious liver disorders

- Pregnancy

- Breast feeding

- Use with caution in fragile or elderly individuals

Special considerations for medications used for gout include the following:

- Offer individual one (1) to two (2) liters of fluid daily.

- Instruct individual to avoid alcohol, herbal teas, and caffeine.

- Assist individual in following diet low in purine-rich foods.

Table 24-4 gives a list of selected medications to treat gout by generic and brand names with dosage information.

Table 24-4 Medications to Treat Gout by Generic and Brand Names with Dosage Information

GENERIC NAME	BRAND NAME	DOSAGE INFORMATION
Allopurinol	Zyloprim	Oral, 200–800 mg/day
Colchicine		Oral, 0.6 mg
Probenicid	Benemid	Oral, 250 mg twice a day for one (1) week, then 500 mg twice a day, increasing dose, if needed to 2,000 mg a day in divided doses
Indomethacin	Indocin	50 mg up to four (4) times a day

Note: Representative sample only.

Source: Based on Broyles, Reiss, and Evans (2007), *Pharmacological aspects of nursing care* (7th ed.) table 13-1. Clifton Park, NY: Delmar, Cengage Learning.

MEDICATIONS TO TREAT OSTEOPOROSIS

Osteoporosis is a disease involving the loss of bone thickness and deterioration of bone tissue. The result is an increase in fractures, especially of the hip, spine, and wrist. Osteoporosis occurs most often in postmenopausal women, immobilized individuals, and individuals on long-term steroid treatment (Myers, 2006).

Medications used to prevent and treat osteoporosis include the following:

- Estrogens
- Selective estrogen-receptor modifiers (SERMs)
- Calcitonin-salmon
- Bisphosphonates

Estrogens

Postmenopausal osteoporosis prevention with estrogen, with or without progestin, helps to stop the loss of bone thickness and deterioration of bone tissue in postmenopausal women. To be effective, treatment must begin shortly after menopause. Because of the adverse effects of estrogen, estrogen should be used only when an individual is unable to take other medications for the treatment or prevention of osteoporosis. Refer to Chapter 27 for additional information on estrogen and progestin.

Selective Estrogen-Receptor Modifiers (SERMs)

Selective estrogen-receptor modifiers (SERMs) increase bone thickness and reduce fractures. In addition, selective estrogen-receptor modifiers (SERMs) do not have the risk that estrogen does for breast and endometrial cancers. Ralixifene (Evista) is a selective estrogen-receptor modifier (SERM).

Adverse reactions:

- Chest pain
- Deep-vein thrombosis
- Depression
- Diarrhea
- Dyspepsia
- Flatulence
- Hot flashes
- Infection
- Insomnia
- Joint pain
- Leg cramps
- Migraine

- Nausea
- Pneumonia
- Rash
- Sweating
- Thrombophlebitis
- Urinary tract infection
- Vaginal bleeding
- Vaginitis
- Vertigo
- Vomiting
- Weight gain

Contraindications for ralixifene (Evista) are as follows:

- Allergy to ralixifene (Evista)
- History of thromboembolic events
- Premenopausal women
- Pregnancy
- Breast feeding

Special considerations for ralixifene (Evista) include the following:

- Administer ralixifene (Evista) with or without food.
- Monitor individual for signs of deep-vein thrombosis and thrombophlebitis. If noted, immediately contact his licensed HCP.

Table 24-5 gives additional information on ralixifene (Evista), including generic and brand name and dosage information.

Calcitonin-Salmon (Miacalcin)

Calcitonin-salmon (Miacalcin) is a calcium-lowering hormone used to treat postmenopausal osteoporosis in women who are more than five (5) years past menopause. Calcitonin-salmon (Miacalcin) is a nasal spray.

Adverse reactions:

- Allergic reactions, including facial flushing, facial swelling, and anaphylaxis
- Altered taste
- Chest pain
- Diarrhea
- Dizziness
- Dyspnea (shortness of breath)
- Headache
- Nasal irritation

Table 24-5 Medications for Osteoporosis Prevention and Treatment by Generic and Brand Names with Dosage Information

GENERIC NAME	BRAND NAME	PREVENTION DOSE	TREATMENT DOSE	COMMENTS
Selective Estrogen-Receptor Modifiers				
raloxifene	Evista	Oral 60 mg daily	Oral 60 mg daily	Can be given without regard to meals
Calcitonin-Salmon				
calcitonin-salmon	Miacalcin	Not indicated	Intranasally 200 units daily	Alternate nostrils every day
Bisphosphonates				
alendronate	Fosamax	Oral 5 mg daily before meals	Oral 10 mg daily before meals	
		Oral 35 mg weekly before meals	Oral 70 mg weekly before meals	
ibandronate	Boniva		Oral 150 mg every month	
risedronate	Actonel	Oral 5 mg daily before meals	Oral 5 mg daily before meals	
		Oral 35 mg weekly before meals	Oral 35 mg weekly before meals	
			Oral 30 mg daily before meals for 2 months	

Based on Woodrow, R. (2007). *Essentials of pharmacology for health occupations* (5th ed.), Table 21-3. Clifton Park, NY: Delmar, Cengage Learning.

- Nausea

- Nosebleed

- Rash

- Urinary frequency

- Vomiting

- Weakness

Contraindications for calcitonin-salmon (Miacalcin) are as follows:

- Allergy to calcitonin-salmon (Miacalcin)

- Pregnancy

- Breast feeding

Special considerations for calcitonin-salmon (Miacalcin) include the following:

- When administering calcitonin-salmon (Miacalcin), bring nasal spray to room temperature.

- Administer calcitonin-salmon (Miacalcin) as one spray in one nostril daily. Alternate nostrils every day. Have individual blow nose before administering nasal spray.

- Administer at bedtime to decrease GI upset.
- Store unopened bottle of nasal spray in refrigerator. Once opened, store at room temperature in an upright position. Discard the unused portion of unrefrigerated bottle of nasal spray after thirty (30) days.

Table 24-5 gives additional information on calcitonin-salmon (Miacalcin), including generic and brand name and dosage information.

Bisphosphonates

Bisphosphonates directly act to (1) increase bone thickness at the hip and spine and (2) decrease first fractures and future fractures. Alendronate (Fosamax) and risedronate (Actonel) are bisphosphonates.

Adverse reactions:

- Abdominal pain
- Altered taste
- Anemia
- Chest pain
- Constipation
- Depression
- Diarrhea
- Dizziness
- Dry eyes
- Dyspepsia
- Esophagitis
- Flatulence
- Fluid overload
- Headache
- Hypertension
- Nausea
- Photosensitivity
- Rash
- Skin cancer
- Urinary tract infection
- Vomiting

Contraindications for bisphosphonates are as follows:

- Allergy to bisphosphonates
- Esophageal abnormalities
- Renal (kidney) insufficiency

- Low calcium
- Inability to sit upright for thirty (30) minutes after administration of the medication

Special considerations for bisphosphonates include the following:

- Administer medication first thing in the morning on an empty stomach with six (6) to eight (8) ounces of water, before first food, beverage, or medication of the day.
- Do not give food, other beverage, or oral medications for at least thirty (30) minutes after giving bisphosphonate.
- Keep individual upright for at least thirty (30) minutes after administering bisphosphonate.
- Do not administer with other NSAIDs or aspirin. If the individual has orders for both medications, contact the individual's licensed HCP.

Table 24-5 gives additional information on selected bisphosphonates including generic and brand name and dosage information.

SUMMARY

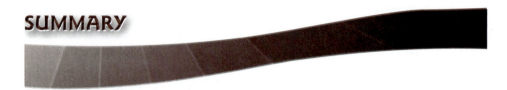

Musculoskeletal disorders can be debilitating and uncomfortable to the individual who experiences them. It is the UAP's responsibility to have a basic understanding of these illnesses and the medications used to treat them. This understanding will help the UAP to give musculoskeletal medications safely and effectively.

WORKBOOK REVIEW

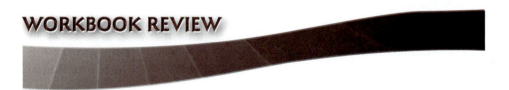

Go to the workbook and complete the exercises for Chapter 24.

REVIEW QUESTIONS

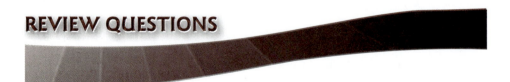

1. A muscle spasm is:
   a. an involuntary relaxation of a muscle
   b. an involuntary muscle contraction with pain and limitation of movement
   c. caused by inflammation
   d. not a common occurrence

2. An individual taking muscle relaxants:
   a. has to take them on an empty stomach
   b. can stop taking them suddenly without consequence
   c. should not take antihistamines, decongestants, or cough medicines unless they were ordered by the individual's licensed HCP
   d. all of the above

3. Myasthenia gravis is:
   a. a progressive musculoskeletal disorder with symptoms of chronic fatigue and muscle weakness
   b. another name for gout
   c. treated with neuromuscular blocking agents
   d. an adverse reaction to a muscle relaxant

4. Inflammation is:
   a. a burning sensation
   b. a protective response of the body to irritation or injury
   c. a symptom of an inability to move
   d. another name for a headache

5. Corticosteroids:
   a. may be used for long-term therapy
   b. are only used to treat rheumatic conditions and sprains
   c. are used for short-term therapy only
   d. are used to treat osteoporosis only

6. Use of NSAIDs may cause:
   a. back pain
   b. dizziness
   c. GI bleeding
   d. hoarseness

7. Celebrex:
   a. has only rare, mild side effects
   b. is safe to use for all individuals
   c. has a warning for adverse cardiac effects similar to those for which Vioxx was removed from the market
   d. can be safely administered with antacids, other NSAIDs, and aspirin

8. Gout causes inflammation primarily in the:
   a. joint of the big toe
   b. muscles of the back
   c. the shoulders
   d. all of the above

9. Examples of medications used to treat gout include:
   a. erythromycin
   b. Sudafed
   c. allopurinol
   d. Topamax

10. Osteoporosis:
    a. results in an increase in fractures, especially of the hip, spine, and wrist
    b. affects individuals of all ages
    c. affects men and women equally
    d. is easily cured

Chapter 25
Medications for Treating Respiratory Disorders

Learning Objectives

After reading this chapter and completing the review questions, you should be able to:

1. Spell and define terms.
2. Identify causes of respiratory disorders.
3. Discuss the uses, adverse reactions, and special considerations for various respiratory medications.

Key Terms

allergy

asthma

bronchitis

emphysema

epigastric
distress

rebound nasal
congestion

INTRODUCTION

Respiratory disorders may be caused by allergies, microorganisms such as bacteria or viruses, fungi, environmental factors, and/or heredity factors. Respiratory disorders include the following:

- Upper respiratory infections, including the common cold
- Pneumonia
- **Asthma**
- **Bronchitis**
- **Emphysema**

This chapter discusses various respiratory disorders and the medications used to treat them.

asthma
A chronic disorder of the bronchial airways that results in narrowed, inflamed, and sensitive bronchial tubes.

bronchitis
Chronic inflammation of the lining of the air passages in the lungs.

emphysema
A chronic respiratory disease with damage to the air sacs in the lungs, causing loss of elasticity and decrease in the exchange of oxygen and carbon dioxide.

rebound nasal congestion
A reaction to overuse of a nasal spray or decongestant in which the nose becomes more congested.

DECONGESTANTS

Decongestants shrink the swollen linings of the respiratory tract and open nasal passages. Decongestants are used to relieve symptoms of nasal congestion caused by:

- Upper respiratory tract infection such as the common cold
- Allergies
- Sinusitis

Adverse reactions:

- Anorexia
- Anxiety
- Arrhythmias
- Asthma
- Cerebral hemorrhage
- Dizziness
- Drowsiness
- Dry mouth
- Fear
- Hallucinations
- Headache
- Hypertension
- Insomnia
- Irritation of the lining of the nose
- Nervousness
- Palpitations
- **Rebound nasal congestion**
- Seizures
- Tremors

Contraindications for decongestants are as follows:

- Allergy to decongestants or other sympathomimetics
- Alcohol intolerance
- Hypertension
- Severe coronary artery disease (CAD)
- Use of MAOIs
- Hyperthyroidism
- Diabetes mellitus
- Glaucoma

- Ventricular tachycardia
- Pregnancy
- Breast feeding
- Use with caution in elderly individuals

Special considerations for using decongestants include the following:

- Administer at least two (2) hours before bedtime to decrease insomnia.
- Administer exactly as ordered. Do not exceed dosage. Decongestants are used as short-term treatment only because rebound congestion may occur within a few days.
- Do not crush or cut extended-release tablets or capsules. Instruct individual not to chew extended-release tablets or capsules.
- Notify the individual's licensed health care provider if she complains of dizziness, insomnia, irregular heartbeat, or tremors while taking the medication.
- Do not administer to an individual who is receiving MAOIs, antihypertensive medications, or tricyclic antidepressants without first contacting the individual's licensed health care provider.
- Do not give OTC medications or herbal medications unless the OTC and herbal medications are ordered by the individual's licensed HCP.
- Instruct the individual not to drive while taking these medications.

Table 25-1 gives a list of selected decongestants by generic and brand names with dosage information.

ANTIHISTAMINES

Antihistamines relieve **allergy** symptoms, including the following:

- Red and watery eyes
- Itching
- Hives
- Reactions to insect stings or plant poisons
- Contact dermatitis

Antihistamines are grouped into two categories:

- First generation, which have anticholinergic effects
- Second generation, which do not have anticholinergic effects compared to the first-generation antihistamines

Adverse reactions to first generation antihistamines:

- Anorexia
- Constipation
- Decreased coordination

allergy
An individual's hypersensitivity to a substance that causes a physical reaction.

Table 25-1 Antihistamines and Decongestants by Generic and Brand Names with Dosage Information

GENERIC NAME	BRAND NAME	DOSAGE INFORMATION
Antihistamines		
First Generation		
chlorpheniramine	Chlor-Trimeton, Aller-Chlor	Elixir 2 mg/5 ml every 4–6 hours
		Tablets 4 mg every 4–6 hours
		Extended release tablets 8–12 mg twice a day
clemastine	Tavist Allergy	Tablets 1.34–2.68 mg 2–3 times a day
diphenydramine	Diphenhist	Elixir 25–50 mg every 4–6 hours
	Benadryl Allergy	Tablets 25–50 mg every 4–6 hours
promethazine	Phenergan	Elixir 6.25–25 mg/5 ml every 4–6 hours
Second Generation		
cetirizine	Zyrtec	Tablets 5–10 mg/day, syrup 5 mg/5 ml
desloratadine	Clarinex	Syrup, tablets 5 mg daily
fexofenadine	Allegra	Tablets 30–60 mg twice a day, 180 mg/day
loratadine	Claritin, Alavert	Syrup, tabs 5 mg daily
Decongestants		
oxymetazoline	Afrin, Allerest	Solution 0.025%–0.05% 2–3 sprays, drops every 12 hours
phenylephrine	Neosynephrine, Nostril	Solution 0.125%–1% 1–3 drops/sprays every four hours
pseudoephedrine	Sudafed, Efidac	Solution or tabs 30–60 mg every 4–6 hours
		Tablets extended release 120 mg every 12 hours or 240 mg every 24 hours

Note: This is a representative list.

Based on Woodrow, R. (2007). *Essentials of pharmacology for health occupations* (5th ed.), Table 26-4. Clifton Park, NY: Delmar, Cengage Learning.

- Dizziness
- Drying of eyes, ears, nose, and throat
- Impaired coordination
- Insomnia
- **Epigastric distress** (heartburn)
- Hypotension, especially in elderly individuals
- Nausea
- Sedation
- Sleepiness
- Thickening of bronchial secretions (phlegm)
- Tremors
- Urinary retention
- Visual disorders

- Vomiting
- Weakness

Contraindications for first-generation antihistamines are as follows:

- Asthma
- COPD
- Cardiovascular disorders
- Benign prostatic hypertrophy
- Pregnancy
- Breast feeding
- Seizure disorders
- Use with elderly individuals

Special considerations when giving a first-generation antihistamine include the following:

- Instruct the individual to avoid the use of alcohol. Use of alcohol with antihistamines may cause significant drowsiness.
- Do not administer to an individual who is receiving MAOIs or anticoagulants without first checking with the individual's licensed health care provider.
- Offer individual plenty of fluids.
- Instruct the individual not to drive or use machinery while taking these medications.
- Prolonged use of antihistamines should be avoided. If the individual continues to have symptoms after two (2) weeks, contact the individual's licensed HCP.

Adverse reactions of second generation antihistamines are usually mild:

- Drowsiness
- Dyspepsia
- Fatigue
- Headache
- Nausea
- Upper respiratory tract infection
- Viral infection

Contraindications for second-generation antihistamines are as follows:

- Allergy to second-generation antihistamines or their components
- Kidney impairment
- Liver impairment

- Pregnancy
- Breast feeding
- Use with erythromycin
- Use cautiously in elderly individuals

Special considerations for second generation antihistamines include the following:

- Do not administer fexofenadine (Allegra) with apple juice, orange juice, or grapefruit juice.
- Do not administer antacids within two (2) hours of administering fexofenadine (Allegra).
- Administer loratadine (Claritin) once a day on an empty stomach. Administer rapidly disintegrating (melting) tablet on the tongue and allow to melt. May administer with or without water.
- Once opening foil pouch of loratadine (Claritin) disintegrating tablets, use within six (6) months or discard. Immediately discard individual blister packet after opening.
- If the individual will be undergoing diagnostic skin testing for allergies, obtain an order from her licensed HCP to stop medication four (4) days before testing.
- Offer the individual plenty of fluids.
- Instruct the individual not to drive or use machinery while taking these medications.

Table 25-1 gives a list of selected antihistamines by generic and brand names with dosage information.

ANTITUSSIVES

Antitussive medications prevent coughing in an individual who does not need to have a productive cough. Antitussive medications allow an individual to sleep better, decreasing fatigue. There are two categories of antitussive medications:

- Narcotic antitussives
- Nonnarcotic antitussives

Adverse reactions for narcotic antitussives:

- Constipation
- Dizziness
- Nausea
- Orthostatic hypotension
- Physical and/or psychological dependence with long-term use
- Respiratory depression

- Sedation

- Urinary retention

- Vomiting

Contraindications for narcotic antitussives are as follows:

- Allergy to narcotic antitussives or its components

- Liver disease

- Kidney disease

- Asthma

- COPD

- Hypothyroidism

- Pregnancy

- Breast feeding

- Alcoholism

- History of drug abuse

- Use in elderly individuals

Special considerations for narcotic antitussives include the following:

- *Warning:* Narcotic antitussives, which contain codeine, may cause physical and/or psychological dependence.

- When administering a solid antitussive medication in the form of lozenges, instruct the individual not to chew the medication. The medication must dissolve in her mouth so that the medication can numb the throat.

- Do not administer liquid antitussives with water. This could weaken their effect.

- Instruct the individual to avoid the use of alcohol while taking these medications.

- Instruct the individual to move slowly when sitting or standing to avoid dizziness from sudden change in blood pressure.

- Instruct the individual not to drive or use machinery while taking these medications.

Table 25-2 gives a list of selected narcotic antitussives by generic and brand names with dosage information.

Nonnarcotic antitussives have fewer adverse reactions compared to narcotic antitussives. Nonnarcotic antitussives (1) do not depress respirations and (2) do not cause physical and/or psychological dependence.

Adverse reactions for nonnarcotic antitussives:

- Dizziness

- Nausea

Table 25-2 Antitussives by Generic and Brand Names with Dosage Information

GENERIC NAME	BRAND NAME	DOSAGE INFORMATION	COMMENTS
Narcotic			
codeine	Tussi-Organidin NR Robitussin AC	Solutions or tablets 10–20 mg every 4–6 hours	Any cough medicine containing a controlled substance is not for extended use; can develop physical dependence and tolerance; watch for side effects
hydrocodone bitartrate	Hydromet Hycodan, Lorcet	Syrup or tablets 5–10 mg every 4–6 hours	
Nonnarcotic			
benzonatate	Tessalon	Capsules 100–200 mg three times a day	Swallow caps whole
dextromethorphan	Benylin, Robitussin DM	Solution 10–20 mg every 4 hours Solution 30 mg every 6–8 hours	
diphenhydramine	Benadryl	Capsules 25 mg every 4–6 hours	Anticholinergic effects, especially drying

Based on Woodrow, R. (2007). *Essentials of pharmacology for health occupations* (5th ed.), Table 26-3. Clifton Park, NY: Delmar, Cengage Learning.

- Sedation
- Vomiting

Contraindications for nonnarcotic antitussives are as follows:

- Allergy to nonnarcotic antitussives
- Chronic productive cough
- MAOI use
- Diabetes mellitus
- Pregnancy
- Breast feeding

Special considerations for nonnarcotic antitussives include the following:

- When administering a solid antitussive medication in the form of lozenges, instruct the individual not to chew the medication. The medication must dissolve in her mouth so that the medication can numb the throat.
- Do not administer liquid antitussives with water. This could weaken their effect.

Table 25-2 gives a list of selected nonnarcotic antitussives by generic and brand names with dosage information.

EXPECTORANTS

Expectorants are used to:

- Help loosen mucus
- Liquify bronchial secretions
- Remove phlegm (sputum)

Adverse reactions:

- Diarrhea
- Dizziness
- Drowsiness
- Headache
- Hives
- Nausea
- Rash
- Runny nose
- Vomiting

Contraindications for expectorants are as follows:

- Allergy to expectorants or its components
- Alcohol intolerance
- Diabetes mellitus
- Cough lasting more than one (1) week
- Cough with fever, rash, or headache
- Pregnancy

Special considerations when taking expectorants include the following:

- Administer with a full glass of water.
- Teach the individual how to cough up secretions:
  - Sit the individual in an upright position.
  - Put on gloves.
  - Instruct the individual to take several slow, deep breaths.
  - Instruct the individual to place a tissue over her mouth. If she is unable, hold a tissue over her mouth for her.
  - Instruct the individual to cough into the tissue.
- Note the color, amount, and character of the secretions. Document this information in the individual's progress note.
- Encourage fluid intake.

Table 25-3 gives a list of selected expectorants by generic and brand names with dosage information.

Table 25-3 Expectorants by Generic and Brand Names with Dosage Information

GENERIC NAME	BRAND NAME	DOSAGE INFORMATION
Expectorants		
guaifenesin	Mucinex	Extended release tablets 600–1200 mg, once to twice a day
	Robitussin	Solution 1–2 tsp every 3–4 hours

Note: This is only a representative sample.

Based on Woodrow, R. (2007). *Essentials of pharmacology for health occupations* (5th ed.), Table 26-2. Clifton Park, NY: Delmar, Cengage Learning.

BRONCHODILATORS

Bronchodilators relieve spasms in the air passages of the lungs and increase the aeration of the lungs. Bronchodilators may be used in the treatment of the following respiratory disorders:

- Asthma
- Bronchitis
- Emphysema
- COPD

Bronchodilators are available as inhalants or oral medications. Bronchodilators may be categorized as:

- Sympathomimetics
- Parasympatholytics
- Xanthine

Sympathomimetics (Adrenergics)

Sympathomimetics (adrenergics) are strong bronchodilators. Although effective at improving an individual's ability to breath, sympathomimetics have serious side effects. When administering these medications, an individual's licensed HCP orders need to be followed closely.

Adverse reactions:

- Anaphylaxis
- Angina
- Anorexia
- Arrhythmias
- Dizziness
- Dry mouth
- Flushing
- Headache
- Hives
- Hyperglycemia

- Hypertension
- Insomina
- Nausea
- Nervousness
- Palpitations
- Rash
- Sweating
- Tachycardia
- Tremors
- Vomiting

Contraindications for sympathomimetics are as follows:

- Allergy to sympathomimetics
- Cardiovascular disorders, including hypertension
- Kidney disorders
- Glaucoma
- Diabetes mellitus
- Seizure disorders
- Hyperthyroidism
- Pregnancy
- Breast feeding
- Use with caution in elderly individuals

Special considerations for sympathomimetics include the following:

- Administration of the first dose should be observed by a licensed health care provider.
- Do not crush or cut extended-release capsules or tablets. Instruct the individual not to chew extended-release capsules or tablets.
- Do not give with food.
- If evening dose of sympathomimetics is ordered, administer several hours before bedtime to decrease insomnia.
- Instruct the individual to limit intake of caffeine-containing foods and beverages.
- Do not administer OTC medications or herbal medications unless the OTC and herbal medications are ordered by the individual's licensed HCP.
- Do not change the brand of medication or change to a generic medication without first contacting the individual's licensed HCP.

- Offer the individual plenty of fluids.
- These medications may cause sudden bronchospasms. If this happens, hold the medication and immediately notify the individual's licensed health care provider.

Note: If the UAP is unable to reach the individual's licensed HCP, the UAP should send the individual to be evaluated at a medical care center or emergency center. UAPs should not hold a medication without a licensed health care provider's order to do so unless it is an urgent situation. Even then, the medication should be held no longer than for a brief period of time. The UAP needs to check her specific workplace policy and state regulations for guidelines to follow in such a situation.

Table 25-4 gives a list of selected sympathomimetics by generic and brand names with dosage information.

Parasympatholytics (Anticholinergics)

Parasympatholytics (anticholinergics) cause local bronchodilation. Ipratropium bromide (Atrovent) is used for long-term treatment of bronchial spasms and wheezing in individuals who have COPD, including chronic bronchitis and emphysema.

Table 25-4 Sympathomimetics by Generic and Brand Names with Dosage Information

GENERIC NAME	BRAND NAME	DOSAGE INFORMATION
Sympathomimetics		
albuterol sulfate	Proventil, Proventil HFA	MDI 1–2 puffs every 4–6 hours
		Inhalation solution 0.5 ml 0.5% sol/3 ml normal saline
		Tablets 2–4 mg every 6–8 hours
	Volmax	Extended release tablets 4–8 mg every 12 hours
epinephrine	Primatene, Adrenalin	MDI 1–2 puffs every 3–4 hours
isoproterenol	Isuprel	MDI 1–2 puffs every 4–6 hours
		Inhalation solution 0.5 ml 0.5% sol/3 ml normal saline three times a day
levalbuterol	Xopenex	Inhalation solution 0.63–1.25 mg every 6–8 hours
metaproterenol sulfate	Alupent	Tablets 10–20 mg 3–4 times a day
		Aerosol 0.3 ml 5% sol/3 ml normal saline 3–4 times a day
		MDI 2–3 puffs every 3–4 hours
salmeterol	Serevent Diskus	Powder for inhalation, 1 puff every 12 hours
terbutaline sulfate	Brethine	Tablets 2.5–5 mg every 6 hours while awake

Based on Woodrow, R. (2007). *Essentials of pharmacology for health occupations* (5th ed.), Table 26-1. Clifton Park, NY: Delmar, Cengage Learning.

Adverse reactions:

- Agitation
- Blurred vision
- Chest pain
- Confusion
- Dizziness
- Drowsiness
- Dry mouth
- Headache
- Hypotension
- Nasal dryness
- Nausea
- Nervousness
- Nosebleed
- Palpitations
- Rash
- Sore throat
- Thickened secretions and mucus plugging
- Vomiting

Contraindications for parasympatholytics are as follows:

- Allergy to parasympatholytics or its components
- Unstable cardiac status
- History of myocardial infarction (heart attack)
- Prostatic hypertrophy
- Glaucoma
- Urinary retention
- Pregnancy
- Breast feeding
- Use with caution in elderly individuals

Special considerations for parasympatholytics include the following:

- Administer by inhalation or intranasal as per licensed HCP order.
- When using a nasal pump, prime pump with seven pumps to initiate pump. Administer two pumps if pump has not been used for twenty-four (24) hours.
- When using aerosol inhaler, prime new inhaler with three (3) sprays. Also prime inhaler with three (3) sprays if inhaler has not been used for twenty-four (24) hours.

- Have individual rinse mouth after each dose to decrease throat irritation and dryness.

- Do not administer OTC medications or herbal medications unless the OTC and herbal medications are ordered by the individual's licensed HCP.

- Do not change the brand of medication or change to a generic medication without first contacting the individual's licensed HCP.

- Offer individual plenty of fluids.

Table 25-5 gives a list of selected parasympatholytics by generic and brand names with dosage information.

Table 25-5 Parasympatholytics, Xanthines, Corticosteroids, and Asthma Medications by Generic and Brand Names with Dosage Information

GENERIC NAME	BRAND NAME	DOSAGE INFORMATION
Parasympatholytics		
ipratropium bromide	Atrovent	MDI 1–2 puffs 4 times a day
		Aerosol 1 unit dose (500 mcg/2.5 ml normal saline 4 times a day)
		Nasal solution 0.03–0.06% each nostril 3–4 times a day
ipratropium/albuterol	Combivent	MDI 2 puffs 4 times a day
	DuoNeb	Nebulizer solution 1 vial (3 ml) 4 times a day
tiotropium	Spiriva	Powder for inhalation, 18 mcg daily
Xanthines		
aminophylline	Aminophylline	Administered by licensed HCP only
theophylline	Uniphyl	Oral extended release tablet 100–600 mg daily
	Theo-24	Oral extended release capsule 100–300 mg daily
Corticosteroids (inhaled and intranasal)		
beclomethasone	QVAR	MDI 1–2 puffs twice a day
	Beconase AQ	Spray 1–2 sprays each nostril once to twice a day
budesonide	Pulmicort Turbuhaler	Powder for inhalation, 1–2 puffs (200–400 mcg) twice a day
	Pulmicort Respules	Nebulizer suspension 0.25 mg once to twice a day
	Rhinocort Aqua	Aerosol 1–2 inhalations each nostril daily
fluticasone	Flovent	MDI 2–4 puffs twice a day
	Flonase	Spray 2 sprays each nostril daily
w/salmeterol	Advair Diskus	Powder for inhalation, 1 inhalation every 12 hours
flunisolide	Aerobid	MDI 2 puffs twice a day
	Nasalide, Nasarel	Spray 2 sprays each nostril 2–3 times a day
mometasone	Nasonex	Spray 2 sprays each nostril daily
triamcinolone	Azmacort	MDI 2 puffs 3–4 times a day
	Nasacort AQ	Inhaler, 2 puffs each nostril daily

(continues)

Table 25-5 Parasympatholytics, Xanthines, Corticosteroids, and Asthma Medications by Generic and Brand Names with Dosage Information—*continued*

GENERIC NAME	BRAND NAME	DOSAGE INFORMATION
Medications for Treatment of Asthma		
cromolyn sodium	Intal	Inhalant solution 20 mg per treatment
		MDI 2 puffs four times a day
	Nasalcrom	Inhaler, 1 spray each nostril 3–4 times a day
montelukast	Singulair	Oral tablets 5–10 mg daily
zafirlukast	Accolate	Oral tablets 10–20 mg twice a day

Note: This is a representative list. Other products are available.

Based on Woodrow, R. (2007). *Essentials of pharmacology for health occupations* (5th ed.), Table 26-1. Clifton Park, NY: Delmar, Cengage Learning.

Xanthines

Xanthines require frequent blood test to monitor therapeutic blood levels of the medications. In addition, Xanthines have significant adverse effects and interactions with other medications. For these reasons, Xanthines are no longer used as often as they once were.

Adverse reactions:

- Abdominal cramps
- Anorexia
- Arrhythmias
- Diarrhea
- Headache
- Hypergylcemia
- Insomnia
- Irritability
- Nausea
- Nervousness
- Palpitations
- Seizures that may be fatal
- Tachycardia
- Tremors
- Urinary frequency
- Vomiting

Contraindications for xanthines are as follows:

- Cardiovascular disorders, including hypertension
- Kidney disorders
- Liver disease

- COPD
- Liver impairment
- Diabetes mellitus
- Peptic ulcer
- Glaucoma
- Pregnancy
- Breast feeding
- Individuals receiving flu vaccine
- Individuals with flu
- Use with caution in elderly individuals

Special considerations for xanthines include the following:

- Administer oral forms of xanthines with a full glass of water on an empty stomach. If GI upset occurs, administer with meals.
- Do not administer OTC medications or herbal medications unless the OTC and herbal medications are ordered by the individual's licensed HCP.
- Offer the individual small, frequent meals and plenty of fluids.
- Do not change the brand of medication or change to a generic medication without first contacting the individual's licensed HCP.

Table 25-5 gives a list of selected xanthines by generic and brand names with dosage information.

CORTICOSTEROIDS

Corticosteroids are used to treat asthma and some forms of COPD. In an acute health care setting, licensed HCPs may administer corticosteroids intravenously. In other settings, corticosteroids are administered as inhalants by **metered dose inhaler (MDI)** or aerosol.

Adverse reactions:

- Asthma symptoms
- Bronchospasm
- Cough
- Diarrhea
- Dizziness
- Dry mouth
- Headache
- Hoarseness
- Nasal burning and irritation
- Nasal congestion
- Nausea
- Nosebleed

- Oral fungal infections
- Sore throat
- Vomiting

Contraindications for corticosteroids administered intranasal and by inhalation are as follows:

- Allergy to corticosteroids or milk proteins
- Bacterial infections
- Cirrhosis
- Congestive heart failure
- Diabetes mellitus
- Fungal infections
- Hypertension
- Hypothyroidism
- Kidney failure
- Primary treatment of acute episodes of asthma
- Pregnancy
- Breast feeding
- Viral infections
- Use with caution in elderly individuals

Special considerations for corticosteroids administered intranasal and by inhalation include the following:

- Instruct the individual to rinse her mouth with water after each administration of corticosteroids. Rinsing her mouth helps to prevent oral fungal infections.
- Instruct the individual to stay away from crowds as well as individuals who are ill.
- Instruct the individual not to smoke while taking corticosteroids.
- Monitor individual for signs and symptoms of infection (fever, cough, sore throat). If noted, immediately contact the individual's licensed HCP.

Table 25-5 gives a list of selected corticosteroids administered intranasal and by inhalation by generic and brand names with dosage information.

MEDICATIONS FOR THE TREATMENT OF ASTHMA
Antileukotrienes

Antileukotrienes help to control the inflammation associated with asthma. Antileukotrienes are used for the prevention, treatment, and management of asthma.

Adverse reactions:

- Abdominal pain
- Asthenia (loss of strength)
- Back pain
- Cough
- Diarrhea
- Dizziness
- Dyspepsia (upset stomach)
- Fatigue
- Fever
- Flu
- Headache
- Infection
- Joint pain
- Nasal congestion
- Nausea
- Rash
- Vomiting

Contraindications for antileukotrienes are as follows:

- Acute asthma attacks
- Allergy to antileukotrienes or their components
- Pregnancy
- Breast feeding
- Individuals older than 55 years
- Liver disease

Special considerations for antileukotrienes include the following:

- Administer zafirlukast (Accolate) one (1) hour before or two (2) hours after a meal.
- Admininster montelukast sodium (Singulair) with or without food. If ordered by the individual's licensed HCP, mix medication granules with applesauce or ice cream then administer.
- If montelukast sodium (Singulair) is ordered once daily, administer in the evening.
- Continue to administer medication exactly as prescribed even if the individual is symptom free.
- Offer the individual small, frequent meals and plenty of fluids to decrease GI upset if it occurs.

Table 25-5 gives a list of selected antileukotrienes by generic and brand names with dosage information.

Cromolyn Sodium

Cromolyn sodium is used for prevention of asthma attacks, including the prevention of bronchospasms brought on by exercise. Cromolyn sodium is administered by inhalation or intranasal.

Adverse reactions:

- Allergic reactions, including anaphylaxis
- Altered taste
- Bronchospasm
- Cough
- Diarrhea
- Difficult or painful urination
- Dizziness
- Drowsiness
- Headache
- Hives
- Muscle pain
- Nausea
- Nasal burning and irritation
- Nosebleed
- Rash
- Sneezing
- Sore throat
- Stinging of eyes
- Urinary frequency

Contraindications for cromolyn sodium are as follows:

- Allergy to cromolyn sodium
- Acute asthma attacks
- Kidney impairment
- Liver impairment
- Pregnancy
- Breast feeding

Special considerations for cromolyn sodium include the following:

- Administer oral form of cromolyn sodium thirty (30) minutes before meals and at bedtime.
- Before administering medication by inhalation, shake canister gently.

- Do not immerse canister of inhalant medication in water.

- Prepare nebulizer as trained. Have individual rinse her mouth after each administration of inhalant medication. Refer to Chapter 7 for additional information on use of nebulizer and IPPB machine.

Note: **If the UAP has never used a nebulizer or IPPB machine, she will need training on how to use them before giving the medication.**

- Before administering nasal spray, have the individual blow her nose. After each administration of intranasal medication, have the individual rinse her mouth and perform frequent mouth care.

- Do not expose inhalant or nasal medications to direct sunlight.

Table 25-5 gives additional information on cromolyn sodium by generic and brand name with dosage information.

SMOKING CESSATION

According to Medline Plus, smoking harms almost every organ in the body. Cigarette smoking accounts for over 30% of all cancer deaths, including 87% of lung cancer deaths. Cigarette smoking is also responsible lung disease, heart and blood vessel disease, stroke, and cataracts. Women who smoke have a greater chance of having problems during pregnancy and/or having a baby die from sudden infant death syndrome (SIDS) (Medline Plus, 2009b).

According to the American Cancer Society, smoking is the single most preventable cause of death in our society. Each year about 443,600 people in the United States die from illnesses related to tobacco use. Smoking cigarettes kills more Americans than alcohol, car accidents, suicide, AIDS, homicide, and illegal drugs combined (American Cancer Society, 2009b).

Smoking cessation may be aided by the use of gums, patches, inhalers, sprays, or prescription medications. Success in quitting is aided by an individual attending a support group and/or a behavior modification program.

Adverse reactions:

- Allergic reaction

- Altered taste

- Anxiety

- Cardiac irritability

- Chewing problems from chewing nicotine gum

- Depression

- Dizziness

- Drowsiness

- Headache

- Hyperglycemia

- Hypertension

- Hypotension
- Insomnia
- Light-headedness
- Mouth irritation
- Nausea
- Nervousness
- Palpitations
- Seizures
- Skin irritation from patches
- Tachycardia
- Throat irritation from gum
- Tremors
- Vomiting

Contraindications for smoking cessation products are as follows:

- Allergy to smoking cessation products or their components
- Individuals with dental problems, including gum disease
- History of drug abuse or overdependence on medications
- Kidney impairment
- Liver impairment
- Unstable cardiovascular status
- Pregnancy
- Breast feeding
- Seizure disorder for bupropion hydrocloride (Zyban, Wellbutrin)
- Anorexia
- MAOI use for bupropion hydrocloride (Zyban, Wellbutrin)
- Acute alcohol or sedative withdrawal for bupropion hydrocloride (Zyban, Wellbutrin)
- Use with caution in elderly individuals

Special considerations for smoking cessation products include the following:

- *Warn individual not to smoke while using these products.*
- Do not cut or crush extended-release tablet. Instruct the individual not to chew extended-release tablet.
- Administer bupropion hydrocloride (Zyban, Wellbutrin) several hours before bedtime to decrease insomnia.
- Do not abruptly stop bupropion hydrocloride (Zyban, Wellbutrin).
- Instruct the individual to avoid the use of alcohol.

Table 25-6 Smoking Cessation Products by Generic and Brand Names with Dosage Information

GENERIC NAME	BRAND NAME	DOSAGE INFORMATION
nicotine	Nicorette	1 piece of gum whenever urge to smoke
		Daily maximum of 2 mg pieces = 30
		Daily maximum of 4 mg pieces = 15
	Nicoderm CQ, Habitrol	1st dose 21 mg patch/day, for 4–8 wk
		2nd dose 14 mg patch/day, for 2–4 wk
		3rd dose 7 mg patch/day, for 2–4 wk
	Nicotrol inhaler	24–64 mg (6–12 cartridges) daily for up to 12 wk, then gradual reduction in dose for up to 12 wk
bupropion	Zyban	Sustained release tablets 150 mg daily for 3 days, then 150 mg twice a day for 7–12 wk
	Wellbutrin	
	Wellbutrin SR	
varenicline tartrate	Chantix	0.5 mg daily for days 1–3, 0.5 mg days 4–7, 1 mg days 8 through end of 12 week treatment regime

Based on Woodrow, R. (2007). *Essentials of pharmacology for health occupations* (5th ed.), Table 26-5. Clifton Park, NY: Delmar, Cengage Learning.

- Offer individual plenty of fluids.
- Encourage the individual to perform frequent mouth care.

Table 25-6 gives a list of selected smoking cessation products by generic and brand name with dosage information.

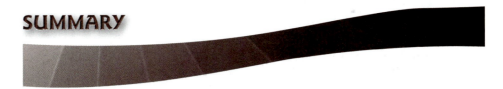

SUMMARY

Respiratory disorders can range from the common cold to allergies and asthma. It is the UAP's responsibility to have a basic understanding of these illnesses and the medications used to treat them. This understanding will help the UAP to give respiratory medications safely and effectively.

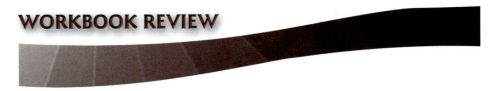

WORKBOOK REVIEW

Go to the workbook and complete the exercises for Chapter 25.

REVIEW QUESTIONS

1. Upper respiratory infections include:
   a. pneumonia
   b. the common cold
   c. emphysema
   d. COPD

2. Asthma is:
   a. another name for bronchitis
   b. a type of allergy
   c. a chronic disorder of the bronchial airways
   d. treated with antihistamines

3. An allergy is:
   a. a condition that only occurs in the spring
   b. the same as a cold
   c. an individual's hypersensitivity to a substance that causes a physical reaction
   d. caused by a virus or bacteria

4. Decongestants provide relief of:
   a. hives
   b. itching
   c. nasal congestion
   d. tuberculosis

5. Rebound nasal congestion is:
   a. a reaction to an overuse of a nasal spray or decongestant, which causes further congestion
   b. caused by being hit in the nose
   c. a result of seasonal allergies
   d. a symptom of a cold

6. Antitussives are used to treat symptoms of:
   a. a cold
   b. seasonal allergies
   c. rebound nasal congestion
   d. persistent cough

7. When using expectorants, an individual should cough up secretions when:
   a. lying down
   b. sitting upright
   c. standing up
   d. she gets out of the shower

8. If a bronchodilator causes a sudden bronchospasm in an individual, the UAP should:
   a. hold the medication and call the individual's licensed HCP
   b. offer a glass of water
   c. help the individual to stand up and walk around
   d. observe the individual for twenty-four (24) hours and keep giving the medication as ordered

9. When administering corticosteroids intranasal or by inhalation:
   a. continue to administer the medication until the medication is gone
   b. encourage the individual to remain active, including attending her work, day program, and/or other group social activities
   c. instruct the individual that she may continue to smoke while taking corticosteroids
   d. instruct the individual to rinse her mouth with water after each administration of corticosteroids

10. Antileukotrienes are:
   a. safe for individuals over 55 years of age
   b. safe to take when pregnant and when breast feeding
   c. to be continued exactly as prescribed even if the individual is symptom free
   d. used for long-term treatment of COPD

Chapter 26
Medications for Treating Urinary System Disorders

Learning Objectives

After reading this chapter and completing the review questions, you should be able to:

1. Spell and define terms.
2. Discuss the uses, adverse reactions, and special considerations for various urinary system medications.

Key Terms

ascites

benign prostatic
   hypertrophy (BPH)

cystitis

cystoscopy

diuresis

diuretics

Escherichia coli (E. coli)

hyperkalemia

hypochloremia

hypokalemia

nocturia

stomatitis

urinary tract infection
   (UTI)

INTRODUCTION

The urinary system is responsible for (1) removing liquid waste from the body, (2) managing blood chemistry, and (3) managing fluid balance. The urinary system is made up of the following:

- Kidneys
- Ureters
- Bladder
- Urethra

cystitis
Inflammation of the urinary bladder.

urinary tract infection (UTI)
An infection of one or more parts of the urinary system, most commonly caused by *Escherichia coli* (*E. coli*).

Common disorders of the urinary system include the following:

- **Cystitis**
- Kidney stones
- Nephritis
- Renal failure (kidney failure)
- Urinary incontinence
- **Urinary tract infection (UTI)**

Medications used to treat disorders of the urinary system include the following:

- Diuretics
- Urinary system antibacterials
- Urinary system antiseptics
- Antispasmodics
- Cholinergics
- Urinary analgesics
- Medications for the treatment of **benign prostatic hypertrophy (BPH)**

benign prostatic hypertrophy (BPH)
A noncancerous, noninflammatory enlargement of the prostate, most common in men over 50 years of age.

diuretics
Medications that increase urine output and relieve or prevent edema.

Refer to Chapter 12 for additional information on the urinary system.

DIURETICS

Diuretics increase urine output and relieve or prevent edema.

Five categories of diuretics will be discussed in this chapter. These are as follows:

- Thiazide diuretics
- Loop diuretics
- Potassium-sparing diuretics
- Osmotic diuretics
- Carbonic anhydrase diuretics

Thiazide Diuretics

Thiazide diuretics are used to treat the following disorders:

- Edema from many illnesses including congestive heart failure and cirrhosis
- Hypertension
- **Diuresis**
- Prevention of kidney stones
- Electrolyte imbalance

diuresis
An excessive production of urine in the body.

Adverse reactions:

- Anorexia
- Anaphylaxsis
- Confusion
- Dehydration
- Diarrhea
- Dizziness
- Drowsiness
- Fatigue
- Headache
- Electrolyte imbalance
- Hives
- Hypergylcemia
- **Hypochloremia** (a low level of chloride in the blood)
- **Hypokalemia** (a low level of potassium in the blood)
- Jaundice
- Kidney failure
- Insomnia
- Muscle cramps, spasm, or weakness
- Nausea
- **Nocturia** (a condition of more frequent urination, especially at night)
- Orthostatic hypotension
- Photosensitivity with fever
- Polyuria (frequent urination)
- Postural hypotension
- Rash
- Vertigo
- Vomiting
- Weakness

Contraindications for thiazide diuretics are as follows:

- Allergy to thiazide diuretics or sulfonamide
- Diabetes mellitus
- History of gout
- Kidney impairment
- Liver impairment
- Electrolyte imbalance

- Gout
- Systemic lupus erythematosus
- Bipolar disorder
- Prolonged use
- Pregnancy
- Breast feeding
- Use with elderly individuals

Special considerations when using thiazide diuretics include the following:

- Notify the individual's licensed health care provider if adverse reactions occur.
- Administer thiazide diuretics with food or milk to decrease GI upset.
- Administer thiazide diuretics in the morning so that medication does not disturb an individual's sleep.
- Offer the individual potassium-rich foods.
- Offer the individual plenty of fluids.
- Weigh the individual daily, on the same scale and wearing the same clothes. Report a sudden or significant weight gain or loss to the individual's licensed HCP.
- Remind the individual to move slowly during body position changes, such as sitting from lying down or standing from sitting.
- Instruct the individual to avoid the use of alcohol.
- Do not administer OTC medications or herbal medications unless the OTC and herbal medications are ordered by the individual's licensed HCP.

Table 26-1 gives a list of selected thiazide diuretics by generic and brand names with dosage information.

Loop Diuretics

Loop diuretics are used to treat the following disorders:

- Hypertension if thiazide diuretics are ineffective
- Edema due to kidney impairment or liver disease
- Congestive heart failure
- **Ascites** due to cancer or cirrhosis

ascites
An abnormal collection of fluid in the abdomen.

Adverse reactions to loop diuretics are similar to those for thiazide diuretics. In addition, loop diuretics may also cause:

- Allergic reactions to loop diuretics
- Blood dyscrasias with prolonged use

Table 26-1 Diuretics by Generic and Brand Names with Dosage Information

GENERIC NAME	BRAND NAME	DOSAGE INFORMATION
Thiazide and Related Diuretics		
indapamide	Lozol	2.5–5 mg daily oral
hydrochlorothiazide	Esidrix, HydroDIURIL	25–50 mg daily oral three times a day
metolazone	Zaroxolyn	5–20 mg daily oral
Loop Diuretics		
furosemide	Lasix	20–80 mg daily, oral
bumetanide	Bumex	0.5–2 mg daily, oral
torsemide	Demadex	5–20 mg daily, oral
		dosage not to exceed 200 mg/day
Potassium-Sparing Diuretics		
spironolactone	Aldactone	50–100 mg daily oral
triamterene	Dyrenium	100 mg oral twice a day after meals
Combination Potassium-Sparing and Thiazide Diuretics		
spironolactone and hydrochlorothiazide	Aldactazide	25–100 mg daily oral
triamterene and hydrochlorothiazide	Dyazide, Maxzide	1 capsule or tablet daily oral
Osmotic Agents		
mannitol	Osmitrol	IV Administered only by licensed HCP
urea	Ureaphil	IV Administered only by licensed HCP

Note: This is a representative list.

Based on Woodrow, R. (2007). *Essentials of pharmacology for health occupations* (5th ed.), Table 15-1. Clifton Park, NY: Delmar, Cengage Learning.

- Blurred vision
- Fever
- Fluid and electrolyte imbalance, including dehydration, chest pain, and circulatory collapse
- Hearing loss
- Itching
- Photosensitivity
- Purpura (small hemorrhages in the skin)
- Tinnitus

Contraindications for loop diuretics are as follows:

- Allergy to sulfonamides
- Cirrhosis and other liver diseases
- Kidney impairment

- Dehydration
- Electrolyte imbalance
- Individuals taking digitalis
- Diabetes mellitus
- History of gout
- Pregnancy
- Breast feeding
- Use with caution in elderly individuals

Special considerations for loop diuretics include the following:

- Notify the individual's licensed health care provider if adverse reactions occur.
- Administer loop diuretics with food to decrease GI upset.
- Administer loop diuretics in the morning so the medication does not disturb sleep. If a second dose is ordered, administer in the afternoon.
- Offer the individual potassium-rich foods.
- Offer the individual plenty of fluids.
- Weigh the individual daily, on the same scale and wearing the same clothes. Report a sudden or significant weight gain or weight loss to the individual's licensed HCP.
- Remind the individual to move slowly during body position changes, such as sitting from lying down or standing from sitting.
- Instruct the individual to avoid the use of alcohol.
- Do not administer OTC medications or herbal medications unless the OTC and herbal medications are ordered by the individual's licensed HCP.
- Instruct the individual to avoid exposure to sunlight, use sunscreen, and wear appropriate clothing when outdoors.
- Do not administer loop diuretics to an individual who is receiving lithium. Notify the individual's HCP that the individual has orders to receive both medications.

Table 26-1 gives a list of selected loop diuretics by generic and brand names with dosage information.

Potassium-Sparing Diuretics

Potassium-sparing diuretics are administered when potassium depletion poses a danger for an individual. Potassium-sparing diuretics in combination with thiazide diuretics are very effective in treating the following:

- Cirrhosis of the liver
- Severe heart failure

Adverse reactions:

- Anaphylaxis
- Dehydration
- Diarrhea
- Dry mouth
- Fatigue
- Headache
- Jaundice
- Kidney stones
- Hyperglycemia
- **Hyperkalemia** (a high level of potassium in the blood)
- Hypotension
- Nausea
- Photosensitivity
- Vomiting
- Weakness
- Weight loss (significant)

Contraindications for potassium-sparing diuretics are as follows:

- Allergy to potassium-sparing diuretics
- Hyperkalemia
- Severe liver disease
- Severe kidney impairment
- Use of other potassium-sparing diuretics
- Use of potassium supplements

Special considerations when taking potassium-sparing diuretics include the following:

- Administer triamterene (dyrenium) after meals.
- Administer spironolactone (Aldactone) with food.
- Administer last dose of the day in early evening to prevent disturbance of sleep.
- Instruct the individual to avoid potassium-rich foods, potassium supplements, alcohol, licorice, and salt substitutes.
- Offer the individual plenty of fluids.
- Weigh the individual daily, on the same scale and wearing the same clothes. Report a sudden or significant weight gain or weight loss to the individual's licensed HCP.
- Remind the individual to move slowly during body position changes, such as sitting from lying down or standing from sitting.

- Do not give OTC medications or herbal medications unless the OTC and herbal medications are ordered by the individual's licensed HCP.

- Instruct the individual to avoid exposure to sunlight, use sunscreen, and wear appropriate clothing when outdoors.

- Inform male individuals that medication may cause breast enlargement.

- Observe the individual for signs of hyperkalemia. Signs and symptoms of hyperkalemia include the following:

  - Cardiac arrest

  - Diarrhea

  - Muscle weakness

  - Nausea

  - Slow, irregular pulse

- If cardiac arrest occurs, immediately call 911 or the local emergency medical service number. If trained in CPR, begin CPR. Once the individual is at the medical care center or emergency room, notify the individual's licensed HCP.

- Notify the individual's HCP immediately if other adverse reactions occur.

Table 26-1 gives a list of selected potassium-sparing diuretics by generic and brand names with dosage information.

Osmotic Diuretics

Osmotic diuretics are used to treat acute renal failure, intracranial pressure, and intraocular pressure and to promote the removal of toxins from the body in the case of drug poisoning. Osmotic diuretics are administered in acute care settings only by licensed health care providers.

Table 26-1 gives a list of selected osmotic diuretics by generic and brand names.

Carbonic Anhydrase Inhibitor Diuretics

Carbonic anhydrase inhibitor diuretics are used in combination with other medications to treat glaucoma. Additional information on carbonic anhydrase inhibitors (CAIs) may be found in Chapter 15, including information on adverse effects, contraindications, and special considerations for administration.

URINARY ANTIBACTERIALS

Sulfonamides are a urinary antibacterial used to treat urinary tract infections.

Adverse reactions:

- Allergic reactions, including anaphylaxis that may be fatal

- Anorexia

- Anxiety
- Ataxia
- Blood dyscrasias
- Conjunctivitis (an inflammation of the mucous membrane that lines the eyelids and covers the eye)
- Depression
- Dermatitis
- Diarrhea
- Drowsiness
- Dry mouth
- Hallucinations
- Hair loss
- Headache
- High fever
- Hives
- Insomnia
- Itching
- Kidney damage and failure
- Jaundice
- Liver toxicity
- Nausea
- Rash
- Seizures
- **Stomatitis** (inflammation inside the mouth)
- Tinnitus
- Vertigo
- Vomiting

Contraindications for urinary antibacterials are as follows:

- Allergy to sulfonamides, trimethoprim, sulfonylureas, thiazide diuretics, or loop diuretics
- Kidney impairment
- Liver impairment
- Pregnancy
- Breast feeding
- Urinary obstruction
- Bronchial asthma
- Blood dyscrasias

- History of multiple allergies
- Use with caution in elderly individuals

Special considerations for urinary antibacterials include the following:

- Observe the individual for signs and symptoms of superinfection (high fever, sore throat, cough). If noted, immediately contact the individual's licensed HCP.
- Administer sulfonamides as ordered along with a full glass of water.
- Administer medication with food to decrease GI upset.
- Offer the individual plenty of fluids.
- Make sure the individual takes the entire prescription as ordered by the licensed health care provider in order to avoid reinfection.
- Observe and document the color and character of the individual's urine. *Note: Some sulfonamides may cause the urine to have an orange-yellow discoloration.*
- Instruct the individual to avoid direct sunlight, use sunscreen, and wear appropriate clothing when outdoors.
- Notify the individual's licensed HCP immediately if adverse reactions occur.
- Do not administer herbal medications or OTC medications containing aspirin and vitamin C without specific orders from the individual's licensed HCP. These should not be taken with sulfonamides.

Table 26-2 gives a list of selected urinary antibacterials by generic and brand names with dosage information.

URINARY ANTI-INFECTIVES

Urinary anti-infectives are used to treat acute and chronic upper and lower urinary tract infections.

Adverse reactions:

- Anaphylaxis
- Anemia
- Anorexia
- Asthma attacks
- Confusion
- Constipation
- Delirium
- Diarrhea
- Discolored urine (brown)

Table 26-2 Urinary Antibacterials and Urinary Anti-Infectives by Generic and Brand Names with Dosage Information

GENERIC NAME	BRAND NAME	DOSAGE INFORMATION
Urinary antibacterials		
Sulfisoxazole	Gantrisin	Oral, 2–4 mg initially, then 4–8 mg daily in 4–6 equally divided doses
Cotrimoxazole	Bactrim	Oral, tablet and suspension
	Septra	50–100 mg every 12 hours or 15–20 mg/kg/day in divided doses
Urinary anti-infectives		
Trimethoprim	Trimpex	Oral, tablet
	Proloprim	100 mg every 12–24 hours
	Primsol	
Nitrofurantoin	Furadantin	Oral, tablet, capsule, suspension
	Macrodantin	50–100 mg four times a day
Ciprofloxacin	Cipro	Oral, 250–500 mg every 12 hours
	Cipro XR	Oral, 500–1,000 mg daily
Norfloxacin	Noroxin	Oral, 400 mg every 12 hours for three days; may administer for up to 21 days for complicated UTIs

Based on Schull, P. D. (2007). *Premier 2008 edition nursing spectrum drug handbook.* USA: Nursing Spectrum.

- Dizziness
- Drowsiness
- Eyes: burning, stinging, irritation, itching, tearing, and redness
- Hair loss
- Headache
- Hepatitis
- Hives
- Hyperglycemia
- Itching
- Muscle weakness
- Nausea
- Numbness and weakness of lower extremities
- Orthostatic hypotension
- Photosensitivity
- Rash
- Respiratory distress with prolonged use
- Stevens-Johnson syndrome
- Superinfection

- Vertigo
- Vomiting

Contraindications for urinary anti-infectives are as follows:

- Allergy to urinary anti-infectives
- Liver impairment
- Kidney impairment
- Diabetes mellitus
- Anemia
- Electrolyte imbalance
- Asthma
- Pregnancy
- Breast feeding
- Use with caution in elderly individuals, individuals of color, and individuals of Mediterranean or Near Eastern descent

Special considerations for using urinary anti-infectives include the following:

- Administer nitrofurantoin (Macrodantin) at regular intervals around the clock with food or milk to decrease GI upset.
- Administer ciprofloxacin (Cipro, Cipro XR) two (2) hours after a meal. Do not administer with dairy products or caffeinated beverages. Instruct individual not to chew medications, including extended-release and microcapsules in suspension.
- Administer norfloxacin (Noroxin) on an empty stomach with a full glass of water one (1) hour before or two (2) hours after a meal.
- Avoid the use of antacids.
- Instruct the individual to avoid the use of alcohol.
- Offer plenty of fluids.
- Make sure the individual takes the entire prescription as ordered by the licensed health care provider in order to avoid reinfection.
- Observe and document the color and character of the individual's urine. *Note: Some sulfonamides may cause the urine to have a brown discoloration.*
- Instruct the individual to avoid direct sunlight, use sunscreen, and wear appropriate clothing when outdoors.
- Notify the individual's licensed HCP immediately if adverse reactions occur.
- Administer the medications as ordered to maintain the proper amount of medication in the bloodstream.

Table 26-2 gives a list of selected urinary anti-infectives by generic and brand names with dosage information.

ANTISPASMODICS

Antispasmodics prevent spasms of the urinary bladder. By doing so, antispasmodics relieve urinary urgency, nocturia, and urinary incontinence.

Adverse reactions:

- Allergic reactions
- Blurred vision
- Chest pain
- Confusion
- Constipation
- Diarrhea
- Dizziness
- Dry mouth
- Drowsiness
- Dry skin
- Headache
- Hives
- Hot flashes
- Hypotension
- Infection
- Nausea
- Palpitations
- Rash
- Tachycardia
- Urinary retention
- Urinary tract infection
- Vertigo
- Vomiting
- Weight gain

Contraindications for antispasmodics are as follows:

- Allergy to antispasmodics
- Liver disease
- Kidney disease
- Urinary or gastric retention
- Glaucoma
- Urinary obstruction
- Intestinal obstruction

- Myasthenia gravis
- Acute hemorrhage with shock
- Hyperthyroidism
- Ulcerative colitis
- Cardiovascular disease
- Prostatic hypertrophy
- Pregnancy
- Breast feeding
- Use with elderly individuals

Special considerations for antispasmodics include the following:

- Administer antispasmodics with food.
- Do not crush or break tablets. Instruct the individual not to chew tablets.
- Apply transdermal patch to dry, intact skin on abdomen, hip, or buttock. Change area of application with each medication administration. Do not cut or puncture transdermal patch.
- Instruct the individual to avoid the use of alcohol.
- Instruct the individual not to drive or use machinery while taking these medications.
- Offer the individual plenty of fluids.

Table 26-3 gives a list of selected antispasmodics by generic and brand names with dosage information.

CHOLINERGICS

Bethanechol (Urecholine) is used to treat nonobstructive urinary retention. Bethanechol (Urecholine) causes the bladder to contract, forcing the bladder to pass urine.

Adverse reactions:

- Abdominal cramping
- Bradycardia
- Constriction of airway passages
- Diarrhea
- Flushing
- Headache
- Hypothermia
- Nausea
- Orthostatic hypotension
- Salivation

Table 26-3 Antispasmodics and Other Urinary System Medications by Generic and Brand Names with Dosage Information

GENERIC NAME	BRAND NAME	DOSAGE INFORMATION
Antispasmodic		
propantheline	Pro-Banthine	Oral 7.5–30 mg three times a day on empty stomach
tolterodine	Detrol	Oral 1–2 mg twice a day
	Detrol LA	Oral 2–4 mg daily
oxybutynin	Ditropan	Oral 5 mg 2–3 times a day
	Ditropan XL	Oral 5–30 mg daily
	Oxytrol patch	3.9 mg, change every 2–3 days
hyoscyamine	Cystospaz, Levsin	0.125–0.25 mg oral, sublingual 3–4 times a day
flavoxate	Urispas	Oral 100–200 mg 3–4 times a day
Cholinergic		
bethanechol	Urecholine	Oral
		Dose according to condition
		Administer on empty stomach
Urinary Analgesic		
phenazopyridine	Pyridium, Azo Standard	Oral 200 mg three times a day after meals
Medications for BPH		
Antiandrogen		
finasteride	Proscar	Oral 5 mg daily
dutasteride	Avodart	Oral 0.5 mg daily
Alpha-Blockers		
doxazosin	Cardura	Oral 1–8 mg at bedtime
tamsulosin	Flomax	Oral 0.4–0.8 mg daily after meals
terazosin	Hytrin	Oral 5–10 mg at bedtime

Note: This is a sample list of available medications.

Based on Woodrow, R. (2007). *Essentials of pharmacology for health occupations* (5th ed.), Table 15-2. Clifton Park, NY: Delmar, Cengage Learning.

- Sweating
- Tachycardia
- Urinary urgency
- Vomiting

Contraindications for Bethanechol (Urecholine) are as follows:

- Sensitivity to cholinergics
- Hyperthyroidism
- Obstruction of GI tract
- Obstruction of urinary tract
- Peptic ulcer disease

- Irritable bowel syndrome

- Asthma

- Cardiovascular disease

- Bradycardia

- Hypotension

- Hypertension

- Parkinson's disease

- Seizure disorder

- Pregnancy

- Breast feeding

Special considerations for bethanechol (Urecholine) include the following:

- Administer bethanechol (Urecholine) on an empty stomach one (1) hour before or two (2) hours after a meal.

- Remind the individual to move slowly during body position changes, such as sitting from lying down or standing from sitting.

Additional information on bethanechol (Urecholine) may be found in Table 26-3.

URINARY ANALGESICS

Phenazopyridine (Pyridium) is used to treat the burning, pain, discomfort, and urinary urgency related to the following:

- Cystitis

- Injury or trauma

- Irritation from procedures such as **cystoscopy**

- Surgery

Phenazopyridine (Pyridium) does not cure the cause of the discomfort. Phenazopyridine (Pyridium) is used for relief of symptoms only. An antibacterial medication is usually ordered along with Phenazopyridine (Pyridium).

Adverse reactions:

- Allergic reaction

- Contact lens staining

- Discolored tears and urine, bright orange

- Headache

- GI disturbances

- Itching

- Kidney damage

- Liver impairment

cystoscopy
The direct visualization of the urinary tract and bladder with use of a scope inserted into the urethra.

- Rash
- Vertigo

Contraindications for phenazopyridine (Pyridium) are as follows:

- Allergy to phenazopyridine (Pyridium)
- Renal (kidney) insufficiency
- Hepatitis
- Pregnancy
- Breast feeding

Special considerations for phenazopyridine (Pyridium) include the following:

- Administer phenazopyridine (Pyridium) with or after meals.
- Instruct the individual that phenazopyridine (Pyridium) may stain his contact lenses.
- Offer the individual plenty of fluids.

Additional information on phenazopyridine (Pyridium) may be found in Table 26-3.

MEDICATION FOR THE TREATMENT OF BENIGN PROSTATIC HYPERTROPHY (BPH)

Benign prostatic hypertrophy (BPH) is the noncancerous, noninflammatory enlargement of the prostate. The condition is most common in men over 50 years of age. Signs and symptoms of benign prostatic hypertrophy include the following:

- Urinary urgency
- Urinary frequency
- Urinary hesitancy
- Painful urination
- Nocturia

Two classes of medications used to treat benign prostatic hypertrophy (BPH) are (1) antiandrogens and (2) alpha blockers.

Antiandrogens

Antiandrogens decrease the size of the prostate, thereby decreasing the symptoms of BPH and the urinary obstruction caused by enlargement of the prostate. Antiandrogens are not curative. These medications only offer relief of symptoms from the disorder.

Adverse reactions:

- Breast tenderness and enlargement
- Decreased semen
- Decreased sex drive

- Dizziness
- Dyspepsia (upset stomach)
- Headache
- Impotence
- Lip swelling
- Rash

Contraindications for antiandrogens are as follows:

- Allergy to antiandrogens
- Use with women
- Liver impairment
- Use with elderly individuals

Special indications for antiandrogens include the following:

- Wear gloves when handling and administering antiandrogens. Medication may be absorbed through the UAP's skin.
- Do not handle antiandrogens if you are pregnant or may become pregnant.
- Do not open or crush capsule.
- Administer with a full glass of water.
- May administer with or without food.
- Do not administer medication if the capsule is cracked or leaking.
- Explain to the individual that sexual effects will eventually subside.

Table 26-3 gives a list of selected antiandrogens by generic and brand names with dosage information.

Alpha Blockers

Alpha blockers relax the muscles in the neck of the bladder, thereby decreasing the symptoms of BPH and increasing the passing of urine. Alpha blockers are not curative. These medications only offer relief of symptoms from the disorder.

Adverse reactions:

- Arrhythmias
- Blurred vision
- Chest pain
- Decreased semen
- Decreased sex drive
- Diarrhea
- Dizziness

- Drowsiness
- Dry mouth
- Fatigue
- Fever
- Headache
- Impotence
- Itching
- Nasal congestion
- Nausea
- Orthostatic hypotension
- Palpitations
- Rebound hypertension
- Shortness of breath
- Syncope
- Vomiting
- Weakness
- Weight gain

Contraindications for alpha blockers are as follows:

- Allergy to alpha blockers
- Prostate cancer
- Liver disease
- Dehydration
- Pregnancy
- Breast feeding

Special considerations for alpha blockers include the following:

- Do not suddenly stop terazosin hydrochloride (Hytrin). Terazosin hydrochloride (Hytrin) must be gradually decreased by the individual's licensed HCP.
- Administer terazosin hydrochloride (Hytrin) at the same time every day with or without food.
- Administer tamsulosin hydrochloride (Flomax) thirty (30) minutes after the same meal every day.
- Do not break or crush capsule. Instruct the individual not to chew the capsule.
- Do not administer herbal medications or OTC medications, especially NSAIDs and aspirin, without first contacting the individual's licensed HCP.

- Remind the individual to move slowly during body position changes, such as sitting from lying down or standing from sitting.
- Instruct the individual to avoid alcohol.

Table 26-3 gives a list of selected alpha blockers by generic and brand names with dosage information.

SUMMARY

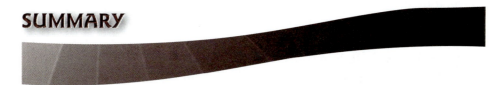

Urinary system disorders can be debilitating and uncomfortable to the individual who experiences them. It is the UAP's responsibility to have a basic understanding of these illnesses and the medications used to treat them. This understanding will help the UAP give urinary system medications safely and effectively.

WORKBOOK REVIEW

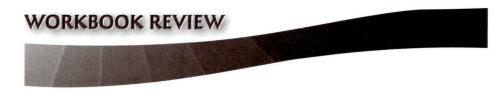

Go to the workbook and complete the exercises for Chapter 26.

REVIEW QUESTIONS

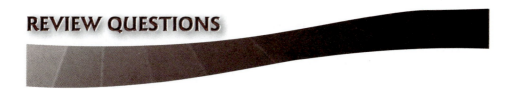

1. The urinary system is responsible for:
   a. removing carbon dioxide from the body
   b. carrying nutrients to the body's organs
   c. removing liquid waste from the body
   d. carrying nerve impulses to and from the brain
2. Disorders of the urinary system include:
   a. hepatitis
   b. diabetes
   c. HIV/AIDS
   d. urinary incontinence

3. Cystitis is:
   a. inflammation of the bladder
   b. another name for diuresis
   c. a lack of urine production
   d. a growth of cysts in the bladder

4. Diuresis is:
   a. lack of urine production
   b. excessive urine production
   c. another name for edema
   d. a medication used to reduce fluid volume in the body

5. Thiazide diuretics and loop diuretics are used to treat:
   a. seizure disorders
   b. Parkinson's disease
   c. breast cancer
   d. congestive heart failure

6. Urinary antibacterials and urinary anti-infectives are used to treat:
   a. urinary tract infections
   b. seizure disorders
   c. multiple sclerosis
   d. myasthenia gravis

7. Urinary analgesics treat pain, discomfort, and burning from:
   a. MRI
   b. mammograms
   c. cystitis and urinary surgery
   d. lab tests such as urine culture

8. Benign prostatic hypertrophy:
   a. affects men of all ages
   b. is a malignant (cancerous) growth of the Cowper's gland
   c. causes severe pain and the passing of large amounts of urine
   d. is a noncancerous, noninflammatory enlargement of the prostate

9. Medications used to treat benign prostatic hypertrophy (BPH) include:
   a. osmotic diuretics and loop diuretics
   b. carbonic anhydrase inhibitor diuretics
   c. antiandrogens and alpha blockers
   d. nitrate preparations

10. Medications that may discolor urine include:
   a. anti-infectives and pyridium
   b. Dilantin and Elavil
   c. aspirin and Cipro
   d. loop diuretics

Chapter 27
Medications Treating Reproductive System Disorders

Learning Objectives

After reading this chapter and completing the review questions, you should be able to:

1. Spell and define terms.
2. Discuss the uses, adverse reactions, and special considerations for various medications used to treat reproductive system disorders.
3. State four possible causes of erectile dysfunction.
4. State the risks and benefits of hormone replacement therapy.

Key Terms

amenorrhea

erectile dysfunction

hirsutism

hormone replacement therapy (HRT)

hypercalcemia

menopause

INTRODUCTION

The reproductive system is responsible for the production of (1) reproductive cells (sperm in males and the ovum in females) and (2) hormones that are responsible for sex characteristics (testosterone in males and estrogen and progesterone in females). The reproductive system is made up of the following organs:

MALE REPRODUCTIVE ORGANS	FEMALE REPRODUCTIVE ORGANS
Testes	Vulva
Epididymis	Clitoris
Vas deferens	Ovaries
Seminal vesicles	Fallopian tubes
Ejaculatory duct	Uterus
Prostate gland	Vagina
Cowper's gland	
Penis	

Common conditions of the reproductive system include the following:

- Cancers: prostate, testes, breast, uterus, ovary
- Erectile dysfunction (impotence)
- Hormone replacement
- Abnormal uterine bleeding
- Infertility
- Threatened or habitual miscarriage
- Menopause
- Prevention of pregnancy

Medications used to treat conditions of the reproductive system include the following:

- Estrogens
- Progestins
- Oral contraceptives
- Androgens
- Medications for treating impotence

Refer to Chapter 12 for additional information on the reproductive system.

MALE HORMONES
Androgens

Androgens are released mainly from the testes. Testosterone is an androgen.

Uses of testosterone include the following:

- In males:
  - Impotence
  - Low sperm production

- "Male" menopause
- Congenital disorders such as delayed puberty in males
- Injury or trauma
- Tumor
- Radiation therapy
- Surgery of the testicles
- In females:
  - Palliative treatment of advanced, metastatic breast cancer
  - Endometriosis
  - Fibrocystic breast disease

Adverse reactions:

- Acne
- Allergic reaction
- Anxiety
- Bleeding
- Changes in sex drive
- Decreased HDL cholesterol
- Depression
- Dizziness
- Edema
- Hair loss
- Headache
- Heart failure
- Hepatitis
- **Hirsutism** (increased growth of facial and body hair)
- Hyperkalemia
- Hypoglycemia
- Increased LDL cholesterol
- Increased oiliness of skin and hair
- Insulin resistance
- Jaundice
- Male-pattern baldness
- Memory loss
- Nausea
- Sleep apnea
- Stroke (CVA)
- Urinary tract infection

- Vertigo
- Vomiting

Additional adverse reactions in males:

- Benign prostatic hypertrophy (BPH)
- Breast enlargement and tenderness
- Frequent or persistent erections
- Low sperm production
- Sterility

Additional adverse reactions in females:

- **Amenorrhea** (without a menstrual cycle)
- Clitoral enlargement
- Deepening of the voice
- Hirsutism (increased growth of facial and body hair)
- Male-pattern baldness
- Menstrual irregularities

Contraindications for testosterone are as follows:

- Allergy to testosterone or its components
- Cardiac disease
- Kidney disease
- Liver disease
- Males with breast cancer
- Males with suspected prostate cancer
- Diabetes mellitus
- Sleep apnea
- **Hypercalcemia** (high level of calcium in the blood)
- Pregnancy
- Breast feeding

Special considerations for testosterone include the following:

- Administer gel as ordered to clean, dry, intact skin on shoulder, upper arm, or abdomen.
- Administer buccal medication above upper incisor tooth. Have individual hold medication in place for thirty (30) seconds to ensure medication stays in place. Rotate sides of mouth with each administration of buccal medication.
- Instruct individual to be careful not to dislodge (displace) buccal medication, especially when eating, brushing teeth, or rinsing mouth with mouthwash. If buccal medication falls off, discard the medication. Apply a new dose of the buccal medication. Keep the new application of buccal medication in place until the next dose

is due to be administered. If the buccal medication continues to fall off, notify the individual's licensed HCP.

- Transdermal patch may be applied directly to the scrotum in a male. Apply daily to clean, dry skin. To prevent irritation to the skin of the scrotum, apply transdermal patch to a different area each time patch is applied, waiting at least one (1) week before reusing the same site.

- Notify the individual's licensed HCP if the individual has gained five (5) or more pounds in one (1) week.

- Report adverse reactions to the individual's licensed HCP.

Note: Caution the individual against using testosterone and other androgens to build muscle strength or to improve the physical appearance of their body. Abuse and illegal use of androgens may lead to serious side effects, including sterility and psychosis with delusions, paranoia, depression, mania, and aggression with violence.

Table 27-1 gives a list of androgens by generic and brand names along with dosage information and uses.

ERECTILE DYSFUNCTION (ED)

erectile dysfunction
The inability for a male to achieve or maintain an erection; also called impotence.

Erectile dysfunction (ED) occurs when a man has trouble getting or keeping an erection. Erectile dysfunction (ED) becomes more common as an individual gets older. However, erectile dysfunction (ED) is not a natural part of aging (Medline Plus, 2009a).

Table 27-1 Androgens and Phosphodiesterase (PDE) Inhibitors by Generic and Brand Names with Dosage Information and Uses

GENERIC NAME	BRAND NAME	DOSAGE INFORMATION	USES
Androgens			
danazol	Danocrine	Oral 100–400 mg twice a day	Endometriosis, fibrocystic breast disease
methyltestosterone	Android, Testred	Oral 10–50 mg/day Buccal 25–100 mg/day	Advanced breast cancer
nandrolone	Deca-Durabolin	50–200 mg every 1–4 weeks	Anemia from renal disease
oxandrolone	Oxandrin	Oral 2.5–20 mg/day in divided doses	Treatment of advanced breast cancer
testosterone	Depo-Testosterone	Pellet implant, buccal; dose varies	
	Testoderm, Androderm, AndroGel	Patch, Transdermal gel	
testosterone in combination with estrogen	Estratest	Oral dose varies	Menopausal symptoms if estrogen alone is insufficient

(continues)

Table 27-1 Androgens and Phosphodiesterase (PDE) Inhibitors by Generic and Brand Names with Dosage Information and Uses—*continued*

GENERIC NAME	BRAND NAME	DOSAGE INFORMATION	USES
Phosphodiesterase (PDE) Inhibitors			
sildenafil	Viagra	Oral 50 mg 1 hour before sexual activity (maximum frequency once daily)	Treatment of erectile dysfunction (has no effect in the absence of sexual stimulation)
tadalafil	Cialis	Oral 10 mg before sexual activity (maximum frequency every 48 hours)	Onset of action is 30–45 minutes; duration is up to 36 hours
vardenafil	Levitra	Oral 10 mg 1 hour before sexual activity (maximum frequency once daily)	

Based on Woodrow, R. (2007). *Essentials of pharmacology for health occupations* (5th ed.), Table 24-1. Clifton Park, NY: Delmar, Cengage Learning.

According to the National Kidney and Urological Disease Information Clearinghouse (NKUDIC), possible causes of erectile dysfunction (ED) are as follows:

- The most common cause of erectile dysfunction (ED) is damage to nerves, arteries, smooth muscles, and fibrous tissues, usually as a result of disease. Diseases include the following:
  - Diabetes mellitus
  - Kidney disease
  - Chronic alcoholism
  - Multiple sclerosis
  - Atherosclerosis
  - Vascular disease
  - Neurologic disease
- Lifestyle choices that contribute to heart disease and vascular problems, such as the following:
  - Smoking
  - Being overweight
  - Being physically unfit due to lack of exercise
- Surgery, especially radical prostate and bladder surgery for cancer
- Injury to the penis, spinal cord, prostate, bladder, and pelvis

- Medicines for high blood pressure, antihistamines, antidepressants, tranquilizers, appetite suppressants, and cimetidine (Tagamet), an ulcer drug.

- Psychological factors such as stress, anxiety, guilt, depression, low self-esteem, and fear of sexual failure

- Smoking

- Hormonal abnormalities, such as not enough testosterone (National Kidney and Urological Disease Information Clearinghouse, 2009)

Medications used to treat erectile dysfunction (ED) are called phosphodiesterase (PDE) inhibitors. Phosphodiesterase (PDE) inhibitors include the following medications:

- Sildenafil citrate (Viagra)

- Vardenafil (Levitra)

- Tadalafil (Cialis)

Adverse reactions:

- Angina

- Diarrhea

- Dizziness

- Dyspepsia

- Flushing

- Headache

- Hypotension

- Insomnia

- Itching

- Nasal congestion

- Nausea

- Orthostatic hypotension

- Palpitations

- Prolonged or persistent erections

- Rash

- Rhinitis

- Shortness of breath

- Sweating

- Syncope

- Tachycardia

- Urinary tract infection

- Vision changes
- Vomiting

Contraindications for phosphodiesterase (PDE) inhibitors are as follows:

- Allergy to phosphodiesterase (PDE) inhibitors
- Use of nitrates, antihypertensives, erythromycin, ketoconazole, itraconazole, saquinavir, or alpha-adrenergic agonists
- Serious cardiovascular disease
- Hypotension or hypertension, uncontrolled
- Heart failure
- Kidney impairment
- Liver impairment
- Bleeding disorder
- Active peptic ulcer disease
- Penile deformity
- Sickle cell anemia
- Multiple myeloma
- Leukemia
- Individuals older than 65 years of age

Special considerations for phosphodiesterase (PDE) inhibitors include the following:

- *Warning:* Individuals who are already at risk of cardiac disorders may experience a heart attack (MI), sudden cardiac death, arrhythmia, cerebrovascular hemorrhage, TIA, and/or hypertension when taking phosphodiesterase (PDE) inhibitors.
- Administer thirty (30) minutes to four (4) hours before sexual activity with or without food.
- Do not exceed prescribed dose.
- Do not administer more than one dose daily.
- *Never* administer phosphodiesterase (PDE) inhibitors with nitrates. May cause fatal hypotension.
- Instruct the individual to report a painful erection or an erection lasting more than four (4) hours to his licensed HCP.
- Instruct individual to avoid a high-fat diet. A high-fat diet may interfere with the effectiveness of phosphodiesterase (PDE) inhibitors.
- Instruct individual to change positions slowly.

Table 27-1 gives a list of phosphodiesterase (PDE) inhibitors by generic and brand names along with dosage information and uses.

FEMALE HORMONES
Estrogen

Estrogens are released mainly from the ovaries. Uses of estrogens include the following:

menopause
The time when a woman's ovaries stop working and menstruation stops.

- Relief of symptoms of **menopause**
- Contraceptives, including for menstrual irregularities and pain during menstruation
- Surgical removal of the ovaries
- Osteoporosis
- After rape or incest to prevent pregnancy
- Palliative treatment of advanced breast cancer in males

For additional use of estrogen and hormone replacement therapy, see the section "Hormone Replacement Therapy (HRT)."

Adverse reactions:

- Anorexia
- Acne (may improve or worsen)
- Constipation
- Depression
- Diarrhea
- Dizziness
- Edema
- Fluid retention
- Gallbladder disease
- Headache, especially migraine
- Hives
- Hypercalcemia
- Hyperglycemia
- Hypertension
- Increased appetite
- Increased risk for blood clotting disorders
- Increased triglycerides
- Iron deficiency
- Itching
- Jaundice
- Myocardial infarction (MI, heart attack)
- Nausea

- Skin discolorations
- Stroke (CVA)
- Visual changes
- Vomiting
- Weight gain

Additional adverse reactions in males:

- Breast tenderness and enlargement
- Decreased sex drive
- Erectile dysfunction
- Shrinkage of the testicles

Additional adverse reactions in females:

- Abdominal cramps
- Amenorrhea (without a menstrual cycle)
- Breakthrough or irregular bleeding
- Breast tenderness and enlargement
- Bloating
- Decreased sex drive
- Fungal vaginal infections
- Uterine cancer
- Undiagnosed vaginal bleeding

Contraindications for estrogens are as follows:

- Allergy to estrogens or its components
- Blood clotting disorders
- Cardiovascular disease, including hypertension, stroke (CVA) and myocardial infarction (MI, heart attack)
- Liver disease
- Gallbladder disease
- Breast cancer, except for palliative treatment
- Visual changes, including worsening of nearsightedness and astigmatism
- Severe headache, including migraines
- Shortness of breath
- Chest or calf pain
- Seizure disorder
- Asthma
- Kidney disease

- Surgery—estrogens should be stopped four (4) weeks before surgery if possible
- Pregnancy
- Breast feeding
- Diabetes mellitus
- Prolonged, continued use in high-doses
- Heavy smokers

Special considerations for estrogen include the following:

- Administer esterified estrogens (Estratab, Ogen) with food or fluids.
- Place transdermal patch on clean, dry, intact skin.
- Notify the individual's licensed HCP if there is a weight gain of five (5) pounds or more in one (1) week.
- Report the adverse reactions to the individual's licensed HCP.
- Advise the individual that estrogens may cause contact lens intolerance.

Table 27-2 gives a list of selected estrogens by generic and brand names along with dosage information and uses.

Table 27-2 Estrogens, Progestins, and Contraceptives by Generic and Brand Names with Dosage Information and Uses

GENERIC NAME	BRAND NAME	DOSAGE INFORMATION	USES
Estrogens			
estradiol	Estrace	Oral, intravaginal	Menopause, prostate cancer, breast cancer, uterine bleeding
	Estrasorb, EstroGel	Topical, emulsion, gel	Only for menopausal symptoms
	Estraderm, Vivelle, Depo-Estradiol	Transdermal, dose varies	
conjugated estrogens	Premarin	Oral, vaginal cream; dose varies with condition and symptoms	Breast engorgement, prostate cancer, menopausal symptoms
esterified estrogens	Estratab, Ogen	Oral, vaginal cream; dose varies with condition	Prostate cancer, menopausal symptoms; uterine bleeding
Progestins			
medroxyprogesterone	Provera Depo-Provera	Oral tablets administered by licensed HCPs only	Abnormal uterine bleeding, menopausal symptoms, contraception
megestrol acetate	Megace	Oral 160–800 mg daily in divided doses	Endometrial and breast cancer, anorexia, and cachexia of AIDS

(continues)

Table 27-2 Estrogens, Progestins, and Contraceptives by Generic and Brand Names with Dosage Information and Uses—*continued*

GENERIC NAME	BRAND NAME	DOSAGE INFORMATION	USES
Estrogen-Progestin Combinations			
conjugated estrogens/ medroxyprogesterone	Premphase, Prempro	Oral, dose varies	For menopausal symptoms
estradiol/norethindrone	CombiPatch	Transdermal, 1 patch every 3–4 days	For menopausal symptoms
Contraceptive Agents			
Monophasic Preparations			
50 mcg estrogen	Ovral	Oral	Contain the same proportion of estrogen and progesterone in each tablet
	Ovcon-50		
35 mcg estrogen	Norinyl 1/50	Oral	
	Norinyl 1/35		
	Brevicon		
	Ortho-Cyclen		
30 mcg estrogen	Lo-Ovral	Oral	
	Loestrin		
	Yasmin		
20 mcg estrogen	Loestrin	Oral	
	Ortho Evra	Transdermal	1 patch every 7 days for 3 week cycle
Biphasic Preparation			
35 mcg estrogen	Ortho-Novum 10/11	Oral	
	Neocon 10/11		
Triphasic Preparations			
	Seasonale/Triphasil	Oral, dose varies	
	Ortho-Novum 7/7/7		
	Tri-Cyclen		
Progestin-Only Preparations			
	Micronor/Ovrette	Oral	
	Depo-Provera	150 mg every 3 months, administered only by a licensed HCP	

Note: List of brand names is a sample only of available contraceptives. There are too many contraceptives available to list.

Based on Woodrow, R. (2007). *Essentials of pharmacology for health occupations* (5th ed.), Table 24-2. Clifton Park, NY: Delmar, Cengage Learning.

Progestins

Progestins are synthetic medications that act like the female hormone progesterone. Uses of progestins include the following:

- Amenorrhea
- Abnormal uterine bleeding
- Contraception
- Relief of symptoms of menopause, in combination with estrogens
- Treatment for advanced and metastatic breast cancer and uterine cancer
- Management of sexual deviancy in males, especially pedophilia and sexual sadism

Adverse reactions:

- Abdominal pain
- Acne
- Allergic reaction, including anaphylaxis
- Appetite changes
- Amenorrhea
- Bloating
- Blood clotting disorders
- Breakthrough bleeding and spotting
- Breast secretions
- Breast tenderness and enlargement
- Decrease in bone thickness possible with prolonged use
- Depression
- Drowsiness
- Fatigue
- Fluid retention
- Headache including migraine
- Hives
- Hyperglycemia
- Itching
- Insomnia
- Jaundice
- Leg cramps
- Menstrual irregularities

- Migraine headache

- Moodiness

- Nausea

- Rash

- Vision changes, including double vision

- Weight gain

Contraindications for progestins are as follows:

- Allergy to progestins or their components

- History of depression

- History of blood clotting disorder, especially with smoking

- History of stroke (CVA)

- Liver disease or impairment

- Undiagnosed vaginal bleeding

- Pregnancy

- Breast feeding

- Cancers of the breast, cervix, uterus, and vagina

- Asthma

- Seizure disorders

- Migraine headaches

- Diabetes mellitus

- Cardiac disease

- Kidney disease or impairment

Special considerations for progestins include the following:

- Notify the individual's licensed HCP if there is a weight gain of five (5) or more pounds in one (1) week.

- If the individual complains of adverse reactions, contact the individual's licensed HCP.

Table 27-2 gives a list of selected progestins by generic and brand names along with dosage information and uses.

HORMONE REPLACEMENT THERAPY (HRT)

Because of menopause, surgery, or disease, a woman's body stops producing estrogen and progesterone. Medications for **hormone replacement therapy (HRT)** are used to replace or maintain a level of estrogen and/ or progesterone. According to the National Institutes of Health, the benefits and risks of HRT are as follows:

- Benefits:

  - Relief of menopausal symptoms

  - Prevention of bone loss and osteoporosis

- Risks:
  - Increased risk of endometrial cancer
  - Increased risk of breast cancer
  - Increased risk of heart attack, stroke, and blood clots
  - Increased risk of Alzheimer's disease
  - Increase of urinary incontinency (National Institutes of Health, 2009)

The U.S. Food and Drug Administration (FDA) has approved HRT treatment for (1) moderate to severe hot flashes and night sweats and (2) moderate to severe vaginal dryness and osteoporosis related to menopause. Because HRT has risks for serious side effects, women and their licensed HCPs need to weigh the benefits and risks of HRT before starting treatment and frequently during treatment.

In addition, the FDA has made the following recommendations:

- If HRT is prescribed only for vaginal symptoms, the FDA recommends that licensed HCPs consider the use of topical vaginal products for symptom relief.

- If used for the treatment of osteoporosis, the FDA recommends that licensed HCPs weigh the benefits and risks and, if possible, choose an alternative treatment to HRT.

- HRT is not approved for the treatment of Alzheimer's disease. In fact, it has been shown to increase the risk for dementia.

- HRT treatment should be used at the lowest doses for the shortest period of time (National Health and Blood Institute, 2009).

CONTRACEPTIVES

Contraceptives are available as a (1) combination product of estrogen and progesterone or (2) progestin-only product. Contraceptives may be administered orally or by transderm patch.

Contraceptives have numerous uses including the following:

- Prevention of pregnancy
- Treatment of other medical conditions including the following:
  - Acne
  - Painful menstrual cycles
  - Heavy bleeding during menstrual cycles
  - Irregular menstrual cycles
  - Endometriosis
- Protective effect against pelvic inflammatory disease
- Positive effects against other diseases and disorders

Adverse reactions:

- Breast tenderness and enlargement
- Breakthrough bleeding (spotting)

- Changes in sex drive
- Depression (may be severe)
- Facial discoloration
- Fluid retention
- Migraine headaches
- Mood changes
- Nausea
- Light menstrual flow
- Vision changes, including loss of vision
- Weight gain or loss

Contraindications for the use of contraceptives are as follows:

- Blood clotting disorder
- Breast cancer
- Estrogen-sensitive cancer
- Cervical cancer
- Migraine headaches
- Sickle cell anemia
- Undiagnosed vaginal bleeding
- Cardiovascular disease, including hypertension, stroke (CVA), angina, and heart attack
- Diabetes mellitus
- Liver disease or impairment
- Pregnancy
- Breast feeding
- Use with caution in women over 35 years of age who smoke

Special considerations with the use of contraceptives include the following:

- Administer oral contraceptives at the same time every day.
- Instruct the individual to use backup contraception (birth control) when taking other medications, such as antibiotics, that may decrease the effectiveness of her oral contraceptive (birth control pill).
- Notify the individual's licensed HCP if there is a weight gain of five (5) or more pounds in one (1) week.
- If the individual complains of adverse reactions, contact the individual's licensed HCP.

Table 27-2 gives a list of selected oral contraceptives by generic and brand names with dosage information and uses.

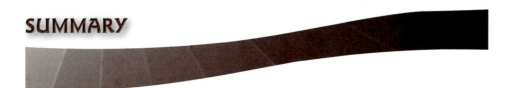

SUMMARY

Reproductive system conditions can range from structural disorders to sexual disorders. It is the UAP's responsibility to have a basic understanding of these illnesses and the medications used to treat them. This understanding will help the UAP to give reproductive system medications safely and effectively.

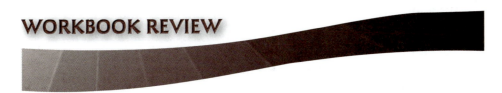

WORKBOOK REVIEW

Go to the workbook and complete the exercises for Chapter 27.

REVIEW QUESTIONS

1. The reproductive system is responsible for:
   a. the production of reproductive cells and hormones that are responsible for sex characteristics
   b. removing wastes from the body
   c. removing carbon dioxide from the body
   d. carrying nutrients to the body's organs
2. Testosterone is a male hormone used to:
   a. treat male-pattern baldness
   b. treat depression
   c. reduce the severity of symptoms in some women with metastatic breast cancers
   d. decrease blood cholesterol levels
3. Erectile dysfunction may be caused by:
   a. too much exercise
   b. high sugary foods
   c. lack of sleep
   d. vascular diseases and diabetes
4. Estrogen hormones are used to treat:
   a. symptoms of menopause and premature menopause
   b. impotence
   c. ovarian cancer
   d. a diabetes

5. For a woman taking estrogen or progesterone, her licensed health care provider should be notified *immediately* if she has:
   a. a sudden shortness of breath and severe headache
   b. aching feet
   c. a weekly weight gain of two (2) pounds
   d. backache

6. Progestins are used to treat:
   a. asthma
   b. abnormal uterine bleeding
   c. vaginal candidiasis
   d. infertility

7. When an individual is taking progesterone and complains of difficulty breathing and blurred vision, the UAP should:
   a. tell the individual to take deep breaths
   b. call the individual's licensed HCP immediately
   c. observe the individual for twenty-four (24) hours
   d. all of the above

8. Hormone replacement therapy (HRT) is used to:
   a. increase female hormone levels
   b. decrease female hormone levels
   c. suppress female hormone levels
   d. help the body produce female hormones

9. A *benefit* of HRT is:
   a. the relief of menopausal symptoms
   b. the ability to maintain an erection
   c. a decrease in the risk of heart and vascular diseases
   d. an increase in the risk of developing Alzheimer's disease

10. A contraindication for the use of contraceptives is:
   a. dermatitis
   b. heart attack or stroke
   c. asthma
   d. depression

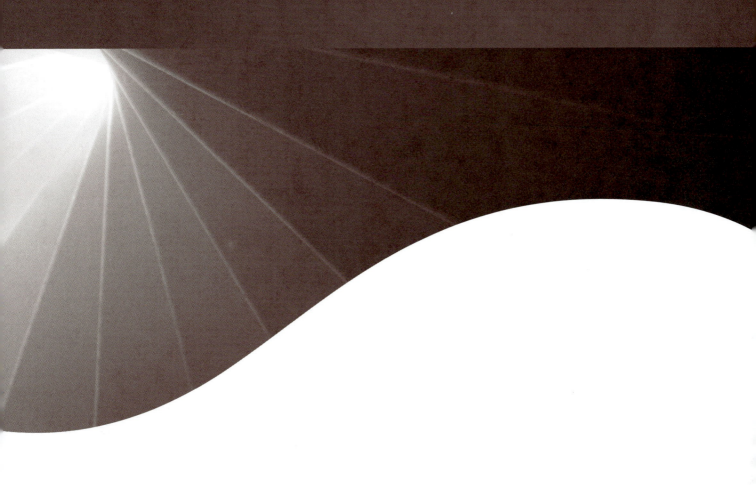

MODULE V
Communication
and
Documentation

Chapter 28
Role of the Unlicensed Assistive Personnel (UAP) in Medication Administration

Learning Objectives

After reading this chapter and completing the review questions, you should be able to:

1. Spell and define terms.
2. Explain the role of the UAP in medication administration.
3. List the key ingredients to a good relationship.
4. Briefly describe the communication process.
5. List five possible barriers to effective listening and communication.
6. List the four senses used in medication administration.
7. Describe the difference between subjective observation and objective observation.
8. Briefly describe three possible objective observations for each of the body's systems.
9. List the four questions that must be answered in order to report effectively.
10. Provide three examples of an emergency situation.
11. Provide three examples of a nonemergency situation.
12. Describe two situations when verbal reports are used to communicate with others.
13. State two pieces of information that should be included in a written report.
14. List ten guidelines for charting.

Key Terms

aphasia	communication book	objective observation	stethoscope
assessment	function	observation	subjective observation
body language	mute	senses	wheezing
communication			

INTRODUCTION

Medication administration by UAPs is a basic task. The UAP follows the directions and instructions of licensed health care providers. Based upon the directions provided he gives (administers) the medication as ordered. At no time does he make an **assessment** of the individual's condition. If there is a change in the individual's condition, the change is immediately reported to the individual's licensed health care provider (HCP) and/or the UAP's supervisor per state regulation and/or workplace policy. Evaluations or outcomes of the effects of a medication on the individual are also not made by a UAP. Changes in a medication order are made only by licensed health care providers.

assessment
An evaluation.

The assessments and evaluations made for medication administration are made by the individual's licensed health care provider. Such a provider may be an LPN, an RN, a nurse practitioner, a nurse midwife, a pharmacist, a physician assistant, a dentist, a podiatrist, a physician, a doctor, or other licensed health care providers. Each state's regulations will determine the types of licensed health care providers who will be involved in the day-to-day practice of medication administration. Again, it is the UAP's responsibility to know his state regulations and their effect on his scope of function.

Because the UAP has a close day-to-day relationship with the individual for whom he is caring, the UAP is an important individual. Unlike the licensed health care provider, the UAP is able to observe the individual up close in all activities. The UAP comes to know the individual very well and is able to tell if there is even a small change. No one else is able to observe and report on this individual the way the UAP can. The quality of care that this individual will receive will only be as good as the information that the UAP and/or his supervisor will provide to the licensed health care providers.

BUILDING RELATIONSHIPS

Good relationships with the individual for whom one is caring, with his family and friends, with the individual's licensed HCPs, and with one's peers and supervisor play an important role in the quality of care an individual receives. Good relationships lay the fertile ground for the development of trust among all individuals involved in the caregiving process.

Trust is the foundation upon which the UAP will rely upon from day to day. Trust opens the door for effective communication. Without trust, the UAP is unable to share the information he gathers from and about an individual with the individual's licensed HCP, with other staff, and with supervisors.

Good relationships include trust, teamwork, appreciation for others, a willingness to help each other when needed, initiative, and effective communication.

Communication

Communication is a two-way process in which individuals share information. Communication occurs in three main ways:

- Oral
- Written
- Nonverbal through **body language** (using one's body to communicate a message)

To communicate effectively:

- One individual needs to send a message
- A second individual needs to:
  - Listen to the message
  - Receive the message
  - Respond to the message
  - Acknowledge that he understands the message

The UAP may experience difficulty at times when attempting to communicate with others. This may be due to one or more of the following barriers:

- A language barrier, each individual may speak a different language (an interpreter may be needed)
- Cultural differences
- Hearing impairment or loss
- Visual impairment or blindness
- **Aphasia** (difficulty expressing oneself or understanding communication or language)
- **Mute** (inability to speak because of a physical defect or emotional problem)
- Disorientation or confusion
- Use of medical words or jargon (licensed HCPs have a "medical language" that may be confusing or intimidating to the UAP)

Whether the UAP is communicating with an individual, the individual's licensed HCP, or a fellow staff person, it is the UAP's responsibility to communicate effectively. If the UAP is having difficulty, then it is the UAP's responsibility to contact his supervisor to ask for assistance. If available, the UAP may wish to attend in-services and other training on effective communication skills, communication with individuals with special needs, or other such topics.

Being able to communicate effectively allows the UAP to fulfill his duty to observe, report, and record any changes noted in the individuals he is caring for.

OBSERVATION

An individual has five **senses**: seeing, hearing, smell, taste, and feeling. An **observation** is made using four of these senses—seeing, hearing, smelling, and feeling. Observing and reporting physical, emotional, and behavioral changes are important in understanding an individual's health condition.

There are two types of observations: objective and subjective. An **objective observation** is one that is factual or measurable in some way. For example, blood pressure, temperature, and blood in the urine are measurable. A **subjective observation** is a statement or complaint by an individual, such as "I have pain in my shoulder" or "I feel sick to my stomach."

An individual uses his senses to make observations:

- He uses his *eyes* to *see*:

  - An individual vomiting

  - Blood in an individual's urine

  - Bruises or breaks in an individual's skin

  - An individual crying

  - A change in the way an individual walks

- He uses his *ears* to *hear*:

  - **Wheezing** when the individual breathes

  - A pulse or blood pressure with a **stethoscope**

  - An individual saying, "I am very tired today"

- He uses his *nose* to *smell*:

  - Body odor

  - Stool or urine when an individual is incontinent

- He uses his *hands and fingers* to *feel*:

  - A lump in an individual's breast

  - An individual's pulse

  - The warmth or coolness of an individual's skin

Remember that observations must be:

- Accurate and timely

- Reported to the licensed health care provider and/or the UAP's supervisor when noticed

- Documented in the individual's record by the UAP

observation
A fact that becomes known to an individual either through the use of his senses or by the reporting of the individual experiencing the problem.

objective observation
An observation made through the use of one's senses.

subjective observation
An observation made through information reported by the individual experiencing the problem.

wheezing
Difficulty breathing, specifically a whistling noise made when breathing.

stethoscope
An instrument used to hear sounds in the body, for example, heart and lung sounds.

Initial Observations

To make accurate observations, the UAP must first know what is expected or normal for the individual for whom he is caring. For this reason, it is important for the UAP to receive a report from the staff going off duty. If he has never cared for the individual before, the UAP should also read the individual's record or the **communication book** to know the individual's background.

Try to set up a routine way of making observations. Always keep in mind the age of the individual and the illnesses or problems the individual may have. It might be helpful to think of the body as a set of systems. Go through each system in a logical manner:

- Skin and nails (integumentary system):
  - Change in color: flushed, pale, yellow skin (jaundiced), bluish (cyanotic), pink
  - Change in temperatures: warm, cool, hot
  - Changes in moisture: dry, moist, sweating (perspiring)
  - Changes in appearances: rashes, bruises, scars, pressure ulcers or sores, redness, swelling (edema), cuts, bleeding, shiny, oily, calloused, wrinkled, itchy

Note: **When checking the skin, be sure to check in skin folds and under breasts.**

- Muscles, bones, and joints (musculoskeletal system):
  - Posture: stooped or bent over
  - Body alignment: curled up in bed, lying straight
  - Mobility: ability to move in bed, to get out of bed, to stand, to walk, change in walking pattern, limping, refusal to walk, ability to maintain balance
  - Range of motion: ability to move all joints
- Heart, blood vessels, and blood (cardiovascular system):
  - Blood pressure
  - Pulse: strength, regularity, rate
  - Skin: see "Skin and Nails"
  - Nails: see "Skin and Nails"
- Nose, throat, windpipe (trachea), bronchi, and lungs (respiratory system):
  - Respirations (breathing): rate, regularity, depth, difficulty in breathing, shortness of breath when active or while still, wheezing, gasping, snoring, or other noise
  - Cough: how often, loose, productive, color and consistency of phlegm (sputum)
  - Nose: red, swollen, running, bleeding, rubbing

communication book
A written form of communication used by staff to report on the condition of the individuals for whom they are caring.

- Brain, spinal cord, and nerves (nervous system):
  - Mental status: knows time, place, and individual(s)
  - Has the ability to talk and make gestures
  - Headaches
  - Convulsions (seizures)
- Eyes, ears, nose, and sense of touch (senses):
  - Eyes: reddened, dull, cloudy, bloodshot, yellow, dry, watery, drainage, crusty, puffy, bruised, burning, blurring, double vision, spots
  - Ears: drainage, painful, swollen, rubbing, hitting, ringing, buzzing, itching
  - Nose: drainage, bleeding
  - Sense of touch: ability to feel pressure and pain
- Kidneys, ureters, bladder, and urethra (urinary system):
  - Urination: frequency, ability to hold urine, urinary incontinence, complaints of burning or pain, leaking of urine
  - Urine: color, clarity, odor, presence of blood or mucus, change in color (dark or light), small amount
- Mouth, teeth, throat, food pipe (esophagus), stomach, large and small intestines, gallbladder, liver, and pancreas (gastrointestinal system):
  - Full or partial dentures
  - Dental cavities (caries)
  - Gums: swollen, bleeding, blistered, sores
  - Lips: pale, blue (cyanotic), dry, cracked, swollen, bleeding, blisters
  - Tongue: dry, cracked, coated (white), raw, swollen, painful
  - Appetite: amount of fluids and food eaten, tolerance to food, burping or belching
  - Eating: difficulty chewing or swallowing
  - Stomach: nausea and/or vomiting, gas, increased size of stomach (bloating), pain, cramps
  - Bowel elimination: frequency, amount, consistency, color of stools (light, green, dark red, black), diarrhea, constipation, incontinence, gas, difficulty in passing stool, no bowel movement for three (3) days
- Glands (endocrine system):
  - Signs and symptoms of diabetes
  - Low blood sugar (hypoglycemia)
  - High blood sugar (hyperglycemia)

Note: For signs and symptoms for hypoglycemia and hyperglycemia, refer to Table 22-3 in Chapter 22.

- Breast, vagina, ovaries, testes, penis (reproductive system):
  - Female:
    - Breasts: lumps, drainage from the nipples, rash, redness, pain
    - Menstrual periods: frequency, amount, odor, type of bleeding, clots, cramping
    - Vaginal discharge: type, odor, color
  - Male:
    - Testes: lumps, feeling of heaviness, pain
    - Penis: drainage, including type and color

function
One's ability to do his daily tasks such as eating, dressing, bathing, and toileting.

Besides watching for how the body is working, the UAP will also have to observe for pain, behavior, and an individual's ability to **function**:

- Pain: type of pain (sharp, dull, aching), location of the pain, related to specific activities, constant or comes and goes (intermittent), time pain started

- Behavior: more active, less active, abusive to self or others, crying, drowsy, sleepy, shouting/yelling, unusually angry or quiet, unable to concentrate, restless, pacing, sleeping too much

- Function: ability to complete daily tasks like bathing or dressing himself, ability to move around

Observations must be reported in a factual way. The UAP must tell what he sees, hears, smells, or feels. His opinion or what he thinks should never be part of what he reports. Remember to tell just the facts.

REPORTING

Because the UAP cares for individuals daily, his careful observations and reporting of those observations will determine the quality of care the individual receives.

To report effectively, the UAP needs to know four things:

1. What to report

2. Whom to report to

3. When to report

4. How to report

What to Report and Whom to Report To

Any change in an individual's physical, emotional, or behavioral condition needs to be reported to the individual's licensed health care provider and/or the UAP's supervisor per state regulation and/or workplace policy. It is not the UAP's decision what to report or what not to report.

The responsibility of the UAP is to observe, record his observations, and report. It is not his responsibility to interpret or explain the changes that he observes. Remember, *all* changes must be reported to the appropriate individual. Observation and reporting guidelines are provided in Table 28-1.

Table 28-1 Observation and Reporting Guidelines

GENERAL SIGNS AND SYMPTOMS OF ILLNESS THAT SHOULD BE REPORTED TO THE INDIVIDUAL'S LICENSED HEALTH CARE PROVIDER AND/OR THE UAP'S SUPERVISOR		
Chest pain	Nausea or vomiting	Lethargy
Shortness or breath	Diarrhea	Unusual drainage
Difficulty breathing	Cyanosis or change in color	Changes in vital signs
Weakness or dizziness	Change in mental status	Increased sweating
Headache	Increased thirst	Bleeding
Pain		

SYSTEM OR PROBLEM	OBSERVATION TO REPORT	SYSTEM OR PROBLEM	OBSERVATION TO REPORT
Signs/ Symptoms or Infection	Elevated temperature Sweating Chills Skin is hot or cold to the touch Skin is flushed, red, gray, or blue Inflammation of the skin (redness, edema, warmth, or pain) Drainage from sores or body cavities Any unusual body discharge like mucus or pus	Respiratory System	Respiratory rate is below 12 or above 24 Irregular respirations Noisy respirations Difficulty breathing Shortness of breath Gasping for breath Wheezing Coughing Blue color of lips, nail beds or mucous membranes
Pain	Chest pain Pain that spreads Pain with movement Pain during urination Pain when having a bowel movement (Remember that pain is *not* normal. All complaints of pain need to be reported.)	Integumentary System	Rash Redness in the skin that does not go away within 30 minutes after pressure is relieved New, abnormally dark areas in an individual with dark skin Pressure sores, blisters Skin Irritation Bruises Skin discoloration Swelling Lumps Abnormal sweating Skin is hot or very cool to the touch Open areas or skin breakdown

Table 28-1 Observation and Reporting Guidelines—*continued*

SYSTEM OR PROBLEM	OBSERVATION TO REPORT	SYSTEM OR PROBLEM	OBSERVATION TO REPORT
Circulatory System	Pulse is below 60 or above 100	Integumentary System *(continued)*	Drainage
	Blood pressure is below 100/60 or above 140/90		Foul odor
	Unable to feel a pulse or hear a blood pressure		Complaints of numbness, burning, tingling, itching
	Chest pain that spreads to the neck, jaw, or arm		Signs of Infection
			Unusual color (blue or gray) of the skin, lips, nail beds, roof of the mouth
	Shortness of breath		
	Headache, dizziness, weakness, or vomiting		Scrapes, skin tears, cuts, skin growths
	Cold, blue, or gray appearance		Dry skin
	Cold, blue painful feet or hands		Sunken, dark appearance around the eyes
	Difficulty breathing or abnormal breathing		
	Feeling faint or lightheaded		
Gastrointestinal System	Sores or ulcers inside the mouth	Nervous System	Becomes confused, less alert
	Difficulty chewing or swallowing food		Feeling faint or lightheaded
	Unusual bowel movements		Becomes more and more lethargic
	Blood, mucus, or other unusual materials in the stool		Loss of feeling
			Numbness, tingling
	Unusual color of the stool		Change in size of pupil, pupils are unequal
	Hard stool, difficulty having a bowel movement		
	Complaints of pain during a bowel movement		Involuntary body movement
			Loss of ability to move one's body
	Constipation		Loss or lack of coordination
	Diarrhea		
	Rectal bleeding	Musculoskeletal System	Pain
	Frequent belching (burping)		Deformity
	Changes in appetite		Swelling
	Excessive thirst		Unable to walk
	Complaints of indigestion or gas		Unable to move arms or legs
	Nausea or vomiting		Unable to move one or more joints
	Choking		Limited or abnormal range of motion
	Stomach pain		Jerky or shaky movements
	Stomach distention (bloating)		Weakness
	Vomitus or stool looks black, coffee-ground in appearance		Changes in the sense of feeling
			Changes in the ability to sit, stand, move, or walk
			Pain on movement

(continues)

Table 28-1 Observation and Reporting Guidelines—*continued*

SYSTEM OR PROBLEM	OBSERVATION TO REPORT	SYSTEM OR PROBLEM	OBSERVATION TO REPORT
Urinary System	Urinary output is low	Mental Status	Change in level of consciousness, awareness, alertness
	Fluid intake is low		Change in mood or behavior
	Fluid intake and urine output do not balance		Change in the ability to express oneself or to communicate
	Abnormal appearance of urine: dark, concentrated, red, cloudy		Increased drowsiness
	Unusual material floating in the urine: blood, pus, foreign matter, mucus		Sleepiness for no reason
	Complaints of difficulty urinating		Sudden confusion
	Complaints of pain, burning, frequency, urgency, pain in the lower back		Threats of harm to others or self
	Frequent urination in small amounts		
	Sudden incontinence		
	Swelling, signs of holding fluid		
	Sudden weight loss or weight gain		
	Breathing problems		
	Confusion		

Based on Hegner, B.R., Acello, B., and Caldwell, E. (2008). *Nursing assistant: a nursing process approach* (10th ed.), Table 8-2. Clifton Park, NY: Delmar, Cengage Learning.

When administering medications, UAPs do not make clinical assessments, medical decisions, or judgments based upon their observations. These assessments, decisions, and judgments require additional knowledge, critical thinking skills, and the experience of licensed health care providers.

When to Report

There are two basic types of situations to think about when reporting: emergency situations and nonemergency situations.

An emergency situation is any situation where an individual's life may be in danger. There may be a threat of serious or lasting injury. The situation is considered life threatening. These are some examples of emergency situations:

- An individual has chest pain that lasts more than two (2) minutes.

- An individual has a seizure (convulsion) that lasts more than two (2) minutes.

- An individual has an injury that will not stop bleeding.

- An individual has no pulse and/or no blood pressure.

- An individual cannot breathe or is having great difficulty breathing.
- An individual gets burned.
- An individual is choking.

In an emergency situation, the UAP needs to get help right away. If he is working in a setting with nurses or other licensed health care providers, he should stay with the individual. The UAP should call for help or send an individual to get help. If the UAP is trained in first aid, he should provide first aid treatment while he waits for help to arrive.

If the UAP is working in a community setting or in a setting where he is all alone, he should call 911 immediately or the emergency telephone number for his city or town. If he is trained in first aid, the UAP should provide first aid treatment while he waits for help to arrive.

After the individual is out of immediate danger and care is provided, the UAP would notify his supervisor and the individual's licensed health care provider of the situation. At this time, he would also complete any written documentation that is required by his state and employer.

A nonemergency situation is one where the health and safety of the individual may be of concern, but there is no threat of serious or lasting injury. These are some examples of nonemergency situations:

- An individual complains of indigestion or gas.
- An individual has mild diarrhea (two or more loose stools).
- An individual has difficulty sleeping.
- An individual has an upset stomach (nausea).
- An individual becomes sad, moody, or irritable.
- An individual has an earache.
- An individual has a sore throat and fever.

Nonemergency situations need to be reported when they occur or are observed; however, exactly when they are reported will depend on the individual's condition. For instance, if the problem should occur during the night, it may be reasonable to report it first thing the next morning. For example, if the individual awakens during the night with an earache, the UAP may report it first thing the next morning. If a problem requires the individual to be observed for a period of time, such as for a change in appetite or behavior, then the UAP may have to wait several days and report after he has collected the needed information. The UAP will need to refer to his state regulations and/ or workplace policy for the specific time period within which he is required to report.

How to Report

Reporting may be done in several ways:

- Verbally: in person or by telephone

- In writing: charting or documenting

A verbal (oral) report is one method used to pass information from one staff person to another. Through the use of verbal reports, staff are kept up to date on an individual's status and any changes in that individual's medications and/or other treatments. Verbal reports, therefore, are given often during a shift. Times when the UAP may use a verbal report to communicate with others are as follows:

- At the beginning and end of the shift

- When leaving the work area for breaks (such as lunch or coffee break) or for any other reason

- To report any unusual or new observation(s); this may be done in person or by telephone

The UAP should be specific when reporting his observations. If he is reporting a subjective observation (something an individual has told him), the UAP should repeat it exactly the way that individual told it to him. Here are some examples:

- Mr. Jones in Room 249 says it hurts every time he urinates.

- Mrs. Goldberg was wandering the hall and said she did not know where she was.

If he is reporting objective observations, the UAP should state exactly what he observed accurately and factually. Remember, he does not state his opinion. Here are some examples:

- Mrs. Smith's blood pressure is 142/86.

- Mr. Hernandez ate 50% of his lunch.

At the end of his shift, the UAP should report the following information:

- The condition of each individual he has cared for

- The care he gave to each individual

- Observations he made while caring for each individual

Whom the UAP reports to at the end of his shift will depend on the setting in which he works. If he is working in a long-term care facility, he will most likely report off to a nurse. If he is working in a community setting, he may be reporting off to another UAP.

CHARTING/DOCUMENTATION

Some work settings will require the UAP to record his observations in an individual's record and/or in a communication book. The individual's record is also called a medical record, document, or chart.

The process of writing in the individual's record is called charting or documenting.

A communication book or logbook is a written report that is completed by each shift on all individuals living in the setting where the UAP works. If his work setting uses a communication book, one of his responsibilities may be writing a report at the end of his shift on the individuals for whom he cared.

The information that is written in an individual's record and in a communication book includes the following:

- The care given to the individual(s) by the UAP
- Medications and treatments given to the individual(s) by the UAP
- The UAP's observations
- Any unusual circumstances that might have occurred
- Date and time of the entry
- Signature of the staff person making the entry

Medication administration will require the UAP to complete additional documentation. Some of the forms the UAP will learn to complete include:

- Medication administration records (Figures 28-1 and 28-2)
- Medication error reports
- Disposal forms
- Controlled substance count pages (Figure 28-3)
- Progress reports (Table 28-2)
- Other forms of documentation

Charting Guidelines

All of these forms and records are legal documents and may be used in court as evidence. It is therefore important that they be correct and legible. All charting, records, and forms must be in clear, simple, and accurate language. Entries must be printed or written carefully. There can be no misunderstanding of the meaning of each entry. The guidelines for charting are listed in Table 28-3. If the UAP follows these guidelines, he should have no problems. Also included in this chapter are guidelines for computerized charting (Table 28-4). Computerized charting is beginning to make its way into some work settings.

To simplify time entry, many work settings use international time to tell the difference between a.m. and p.m. (Table 28-5). With international time, the twenty-four (24) hours of each day are identified by the numbers 0100 (1:00 a.m.) through 2400 (12:00 a.m., midnight). The last two digits indicate the number of minutes of each hour (from 01 to 59). Thus, 0101 would be one (1) minute after 1:00 a.m., 1210 would be ten (10) minutes after 12 p.m. (noon), 1658 would be 4:58 p.m., and so on.

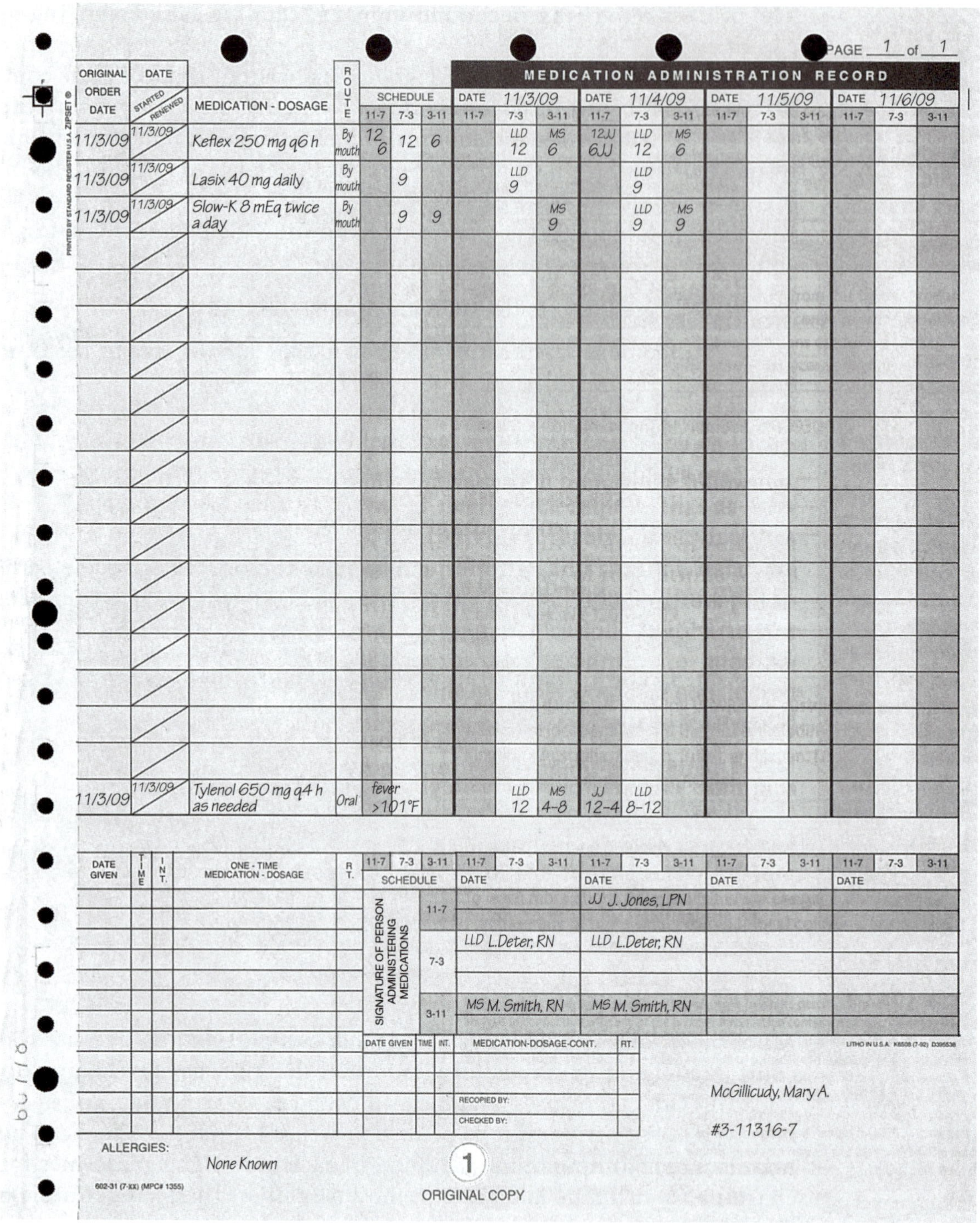

PAGE 1 of 1

MEDICATION ADMINISTRATION RECORD

ORIGINAL ORDER DATE	DATE STARTED / RENEWED	MEDICATION - DOSAGE	ROUTE	SCHEDULE 11-7	7-3	3-11	DATE 11/3/09 11-7	7-3	3-11	DATE 11/4/09 11-7	7-3	3-11	DATE 11/5/09 11-7	7-3	3-11	DATE 11/6/09 11-7	7-3	3-11
11/3/09	11/3/09	Keflex 250 mg q6 h	By mouth	12 6	12	6		LLD 12	MS 6	12JJ 6JJ	LLD 12	MS 6						
11/3/09	11/3/09	Lasix 40 mg daily	By mouth		9			LLD 9			LLD 9							
11/3/09	11/3/09	Slow-K 8 mEq twice a day	By mouth		9	9			MS 9		LLD 9	MS 9						
11/3/09	11/3/09	Tylenol 650 mg q4 h as needed	Oral	fever >101°F				LLD 12	MS 4-8	JJ 12-4	LLD 8-12							

DATE GIVEN	TIME	INT.	ONE - TIME MEDICATION - DOSAGE	RT.	SCHEDULE 11-7	7-3	3-11	DATE 11-7	7-3	3-11	DATE 11-7	7-3	3-11	DATE 11-7	7-3	3-11	DATE 11-7	7-3	3-11
					SIGNATURE OF PERSON ADMINISTERING MEDICATIONS		11-7		JJ J. Jones, LPN										
							7-3	LLD L.Deter, RN	LLD L.Deter, RN										
							3-11	MS M. Smith, RN	MS M. Smith, RN										

DATE GIVEN	TIME	INT.	MEDICATION-DOSAGE-CONT.	RT.

RECOPIED BY:

CHECKED BY:

McGillicudy, Mary A.

#3-11316-7

ALLERGIES: None Known

(1)

ORIGINAL COPY

602-31 (7-XX) (MPC# 1355)

LITHO IN U.S.A. K8508 (7-92) D395538

Figure 28-1 Medication Administration Record *(Delmar/Cengage Learning)*

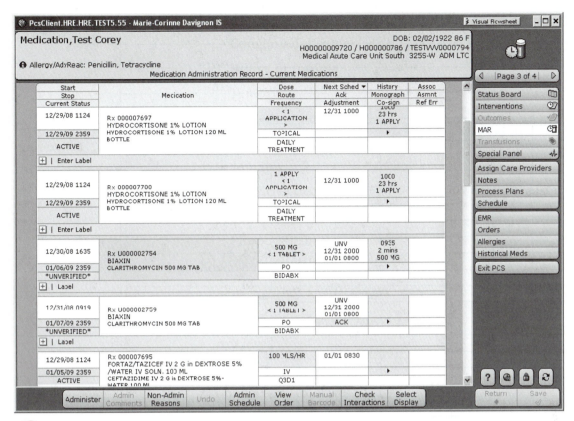

Figure 28-2 An electronic Medication Administration Record (eMAR) with the next scheduled date and time of Biaxin *(Copyright Hebrew Senior Life 2008)*

Table 28-2 Sample Progress Note

5/15/09 7 a.m.   C/O upset stomach. Did not eat breakfast. Temperature 98.8 orally. Color pale. Skin cool to touch. Does not want to get dressed. Reported to supervisor. P Smith, CNA

5/15/09 10 a.m.   Vomited small amount of yellow-green liquid. Temperature 99.0. Color flushed. Skin slightly warm to touch. Resting in bed. P Smith, CNA

5/15/09 12 p.m.   States he "feels better." Temperature 98.6. Color pink. Skin cool to touch. Taking small amounts of ice chips. No further vomiting. Continues to rest quietly in bed. P Smith, CNA

Based on Hegner, B.R., Acello, B., and Caldwell, E. (2008). *Nursing assistant: a nursing process approach* (10th ed), Figure 8-16. Clifton Park, NY: Delmar, Cengage Learning.

In addition to charting accurately and legibly, it is also very important that the UAP charts only that which he himself has done. The UAP must make sure that he never charts his work before completing it. He must also never chart work completed by another individual. Doing so would be considered fraudulent and is illegal.

Name:				( ) Original Entry or ( ) Transferred from Page No.			

Licensed Health Care Provider:	Pharmacy:	Rx No.	Rx Date:

Medication & Strength:	Rx No.	Rx Date:

Directions for use:	Rx No.	Rx Date:

Date	Time	Amount on Hand	Amount Used	Route	Amount Left	Staff Signature

MEDICATION DISCONTINUED/DISPOSED	MEDICATION TRANSFERRED
Discontinue Date: _____	New Page # _____
Removal Date: _____	
Signature Staff Removing: _____	Amount Transferred: _____
Signatures of Staff Destroying Medication: (2 signatures required) _____ _____	Signatures of Staff Verification: (2 signatures required) _____ _____

Figure 28-3 Controlled Substance Count Page *(Delmar/Cengage Learning)*

Table 28-3 Guidelines for Charting

1. Check for the right individual, right chart, right form, and right room before you start to record.

2. Fill out new headings on the forms completely.

3. Use the correct color of ink.

4. Never use pencil!

5. Date and time each entry when you record the entry.

6. Chart entries in the correct sequence.

7. Write entries in a brief, objective, and accurate format.

8. Use phrases instead of full sentences.

9. Print or write clearly.

10. Spell each word correctly.

11. Use only those abbreviations that are on your facility's approved list.

12. Leave no blank spaces.

13. Do not use the term *patient*, *resident*, or the individual's name.

14. Do not use ditto (") marks. Write out all words.

15. Sign each entry with your first initial, last name, and job title.

16. Never erase!

17. Never use erasable ink, correction tape, or correction fluid (Wite-Out®).

18. Make corrections by drawing one line through the mistake, then write your initials above or next to the error.

19. Chart only for yourself.

20. Chart only *after* you have completed the task.

21. Never sign for any procedure or observation that you did not do!

Source: Based on Hegner, Acello, and Caldwell (2008), *Nursing assistant: a nursing process approach* (10th ed), Figure 8-19. Clifton Park, NY: Delmar, Cengage Learning.

Table 28-4 Guidelines for Documentation on Computerized Medical Records

1. Do not be afraid of computerized charting.

2. When documenting on a specific individual, be sure you have entered the correct identification code.

3. Do not give your identification code or password to others.

4. Access only the information you are permitted to obtain.

5. Document only in the areas you are permitted to use.

6. Many computers have expert reminders or error codes on the screen. Read and follow the directions.

7. The procedure for late entry and addendum documentation will be different from a written system. Know and follow your facility policies for this type of charting.

8. Stay current. Attend in-service education programs to learn to use computerized charting and information systems.

Source: Based on Hegner, Acello, and Caldwell (2008), *Nursing assistant: a nursing process approach* (10th ed), Figure 8-19. Clifton Park, NY: Delmar, Cengage Learning.

Table 28-5 International Time

STANDARD CLOCK	INTERNATIONAL TIME	STANDARD CLOCK	INTERNATIONAL TIME
AM 12 midnight	2400	PM 12 noon	1200
1	0100	1	1300
2	0200	2	1400
3	0300	3	1500
4	0400	4	1600
5	0500	5	1700
6	0600	6	1800
7	0700	7	1900
8	0800	8	2000
9	0900	9	2100
10	1000	10	2200
11	1100	11	2300

Source: Based on Hegner, Acello, and Caldwell (2008), *Nursing assistant: a nursing process approach* (10th ed), Table 8-3. Clifton Park, NY: Delmar, Cengage Learning.

SUMMARY

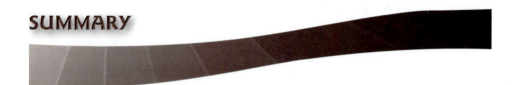

Careful observation takes practice. Changes in an individual's condition may be sudden and severe, such as a sudden collapse. Changes may be minor and more difficult to see, such as a disinterest in daily activities. Whatever those changes may be, one's role as a UAP is to observe, report, and record. The UAP is *not* responsible for interpreting or explaining changes in an individual's condition. He is responsible for reporting the changes to the individual's licensed health care provider and/or his supervisor.

Careful observation and clear reporting are the key to safe and effective care. Licensed health care providers depend on the UAP and the information he brings to them to provide quality care.

WORKBOOK REVIEW

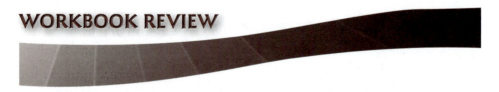

Go to the workbook and complete the exercises for Chapter 28.

REVIEW QUESTIONS

1. It is the UAP's job to:
   a. follow the directions and instructions of licensed health care providers
   b. make assessments of the individual's condition
   c. evaluate the effects of a medication
   d. change a medication order

2. The assessments and evaluations made for medication administration are made by the:
   a. family members
   b. UAP
   c. other individuals
   d. licensed health care providers

3. In working day to day with an individual, the UAP may:
   a. determine the causes for the changes in the individual's condition
   b. decide when a change in medication is necessary
   c. decide when an individual needs to be hospitalized
   d. observe and report changes in the individual's condition

4. An objective observation is:
   a. made using objects
   b. factual or measurable in some way
   c. an individual's statement or complaint
   d. one that can be made only by a licensed health care provider

5. A subjective observation is:
   a. an individual's statement or complaint
   b. made about the subject of a story or conversation
   c. factual or measurable in some way
   d. made by the individual's family members

6. In order to provide the best care possible to an individual:
   a. observations must be accurate, timely, and factual
   b. assumptions should be made from one's observations
   c. documentation should be completed in the individual's record by the UAP as soon as the UAP finds the time to complete it
   d. all of the above

7. If a UAP notices any change in an individual's physical, emotional, or behavioral condition, he should:
   a. call the individual's family
   b. change the individual's medication dosage
   c. report those changes to the individual's licensed health care provider and/or to the UAP's supervisor
   d. put the individual to bed

8. An example of an emergency situation is:
   a. an individual has no pulse and blood pressure
   b. an individual has difficulty sleeping
   c. an individual has an earache
   d. an individual becomes sad or moody

9. An example of a nonemergency situation is:
   a. an individual cannot breathe
   b. an individual gets burned
   c. an individual complains of indigestion or gas
   d. an individual has an injury that will not stop bleeding

10. In an emergency situation, the UAP should:
   a. send an individual to get help or call 911 or the emergency number for the town
   b. provide first aid treatment, even if he is not trained in it, while he is waiting for help
   c. immediately notify his supervisor and the individual's licensed health care provider
   d. complete any written documentation required while waiting for the ambulance to arrive

11. If a nonemergency situation should occur during the night, the UAP may:
   a. forget about reporting it
   b. report the situation the next morning unless the situation needs immediate attention
   c. tell another staff member about it
   d. call the individual's family

12. Verbal reports are given to other staff members:
   a. only at the end of one's shift
   b. when passing each other throughout the day
   c. to report the routine activities of the day
   d. to report any unusual or new observations

13. Written information in an individual's record or a communication book includes:
   a. the title of the books the individual read during the day
   b. the clothing the individual chose to wear
   c. any routine activities the individual completed, such as watching TV and performing his activities of daily living
   d. the care given by the UAP, including any medications and treatments that were given

14. When charting or writing information in an individual's record, it is important to:
   a. chart at the beginning of one's shift, before doing one's work
   b. chart what other staff members have done
   c. chart accurately and legibly
   d. print in large block letters

CLINICAL SCENARIOS

1. You are working in a group home on the 3 to 11 p.m. shift. Mary comes home from her day program at 4:00 p.m. and is unusually quiet. When you ask how she is, she yells, "Shut up!" and goes to her room. Usually Mary is very sociable and likes to tell you about her day. At dinner you notice that she has eaten less than half of her meal. When you're giving Mary her evening meds at 9:00 p.m., you notice her face is flushed. You take her temperature and see that it is 100.3°F.

   a. When do you report this, and to whom?

   b. Write a note for her medical record, describing this incident. Use today's date.

2. You are working the 7 a.m. to 3 p.m. shift in an assisted living facility. You notice at 7:30 a.m. that Fred hasn't come out for breakfast yet. When you enter his room to check on him, you smell a foul odor. As you approach his bed, you see that Fred has vomited on the floor. He is pale and sweating. When you call his name, he looks up at you. He tells you that his stomach and head hurt. What do you do now?

3. You are working with an individual in the kitchen at a day program. Suddenly you hear another individual yelling in pain. When you look to see what has happened, you see that Jack has burned his hand on a stove burner. Describe what you would do to deal with Jack's situation. Assume that you are trained in first aid.

4. While you are working the overnight shift, Sarah wakes up around 2:30 a.m. She tells you that she has an ache in her left ear. You check her record and see that she can have Tylenol, as needed, for earache. When you offer it to her, she takes it. She returns to bed around 2:45 a.m. and falls back to sleep. At around 5 a.m. she reawakens, still complaining of an earache. You don't observe any other signs of illness. She doesn't have a fever when you take her temperature.

   a. When do you report this, and to whom?

   b. Write a note for her medical record, describing this incident. Use today's date.

Chapter 29
Transcription of Health Care Provider Orders

Learning Objectives

After reading this chapter and completing the review questions, you should be able to:

1. Spell and define terms.
2. Explain the importance of accurate and complete documentation and transcription.
3. List the seven general principles of documentation and transcription.
4. Transcribe licensed health care provider's orders onto a medication sheet for a liquid form of medication and a solid form of medication.
5. Document medication administration onto an individual's medication sheet.
6. Write a progress note.
7. Discontinue a medication on a medication sheet.
8. Post and verify a transcribed order.
9. Complete a monthly quality review.

Key Terms

discontinuing

medication progress
   note

medication sheet

monthly quality
   review

oral suspension

posting

transcribe

verifying

INTRODUCTION

The different types of medication orders the UAP uses in administering medication are discussed in Chapter 5. This chapter discusses how the UAP writes the medication orders onto the medication sheets. The chapter uses sample forms to show how to transcribe, document, and write progress notes. Keep in mind that the forms used for these purposes are different from one work setting to another.

TRANSCRIPTION AND DOCUMENTATION

transcribe
To write down or to copy.

medication sheet
A form used to document medication administration.

The word **transcribe** means to write down or to copy. When used in the administration of medication, "transcription" means writing or copying information from a licensed health care provider's order form onto a **medication sheet**, record-keeping forms or charts, and staff communication books. It is essential that the information be transcribed accurately:

- To safeguard the health and safety of the individual receiving the medication

- To protect the UAP as caregiver

- Because it is the law—medical documentation sheets are legal documents

General principles of documentation and transcription include the following:

1. Each document must be legible (readable) so that others can read it.

2. Each document must be accurate when identifying *who*, *what*, *where*, and *when*.

3. Each document should contain only information that is important to the individual's medical needs and daily care.

4. Each document must be complete, without blank areas left to be filled in later.

5. Each document is written in ink. Pencil is *never* to be used.

6. The UAP should not use Wite Out®, correction tape, or correction fluid or write over mistakes. If the UAP makes an error, the UAP should draw a single line through the error in ink, then write her initials beside the error. The UAP then continues writing her documentation. Here is an example:

   ". . . was very ~~slippy~~ OBL sleepy after breakfast."

7. Each document describes objective observations, not subjective interpretations, of what has been observed. For example, write "Did not eat breakfast" rather than "Mary is acting funny this morning."

THE BASICS OF TRANSCRIPTION

Different workplaces have different documents for keeping records. However, no matter how different they are, each document must contain the following information:

- The individual's name

- Any allergies the individual may have—if she has none, write *NKA* (no known allergies)

- The date of the documentation

- Medications the individual is taking

- Space for indicating who gave the medications and when they were given, along with a space for documenting any unusual occurrences, such as refusal of medications or withholding medications for any reason

- Specific instructions or precautions about the medications

A section of a typical medication sheet used for documentation of daily medication administration may look like this:

MEDICATION OR TREATMENT		HOUR	1 (DATE)	2 (DATE)	3 (DATE)
Start date	Generic:				
	Brand:				
	Strength:				
	Amount:				
Stop date	Frequency:				
	Route:				
Special instructions/precautions:					

Each medication listed on an individual's medication record document should have listed:

- The brand and generic names of the medication

- Strength of the medication

- Dose and amount of the medication to be given

- Frequency and specific times for giving the medication

- The route by which the medication is given

- The *start date*—the date when the medication was or is to be first given

- The *stop date*—the date when the medication is to be stopped or discontinued, if this date is given

- Special instructions/precautions

Note: Not all states and/or workplace settings may require both the generic name and the brand name of a medication on the medication sheet.

Orders are only written by a licensed health care provider who is registered to prescribe medications with the state in which she works. Licensed health care providers may include physicians, physician's assistants, nurse practitioners, nurse-midwives, dentists, osteopaths, podiatrists, optometrists, and clinical nurse specialists in psychiatric/mental health nursing. Only such individuals with the proper credentials to do so may order medications.

BASIC TRANSCRIPTION
Medication Sheet

Below is a step-by-step description of how a licensed health care provider's order for medication is transcribed onto a medication sheet similar to the one seen earlier. Here is an order for Tylenol:

> Acetaminophen 325 mg 2 tabs by mouth q4h WA for right shoulder discomfort. Follow up with the licensed HCP in one week.

First, the UAP needs to interpret this order:

- *Acetaminophen* is the generic name of the medication Tylenol.

- *325 mg* is the strength of medication in each tablet.

- *2 tabs* is the amount of medication to give each time it is administered.

- *by mouth* is the route.

- *q4h WA* is the frequency, the abbreviation for "every four hours while awake."

- *Follow up with the licensed HCP in one one week* is a specific instruction.

Now the UAP enters this information onto the medication sheet that follows:

First, enter the *generic and brand names* of the medication. If the UAP is not sure of the generic or brand name of a medication, she should check the pharmacy label—it should have both names listed.

MEDICATION OR TREATMENT		HOUR	1	2	3
Start date	Generic: *acetaminophen* Brand: *Tylenol*				
	Strength:				
	Amount:				
Stop date	Frequency:				
	Route:				

Special instructions/precautions:

Now enter the *strength* of the medication—the medication available in each tablet.

MEDICATION OR TREATMENT		HOUR	1	2	3
Start date	Generic: acetaminophen				
	Brand: Tylenol				
	Strength: *325 mg*				
	Amount:				
Stop date	Frequency:				
	Route:				
Special instructions/precautions:					

Next, enter the *amount* of medication the individual is to take each time it is administered and the *frequency* of administration, or how many times a day it is to be given.

MEDICATION OR TREATMENT		HOUR	1	2	3
Start date	Generic: acetaminophen				
	Brand: Tylenol				
	Strength: 325 mg				
	Amount: *2 tablets*				
Stop date	Frequency: *q4h WA*				
	Route:				
Special instructions/precautions:					

Then enter the *route* by which the medication is to be given.

MEDICATION OR TREATMENT		HOUR	1	2	3
Start date	Generic: acetaminophen				
	Brand: Tylenol				
	Strength: 325 mg				
	Amount: 2 tabs				
Stop date	Frequency: q4h WA				
	Route: *by mouth*				
Special instructions/precautions:					

Finally, include any *special instructions or precautions* from the medication order.

MEDICATION OR TREATMENT		HOUR	1	2	3
Start date	Generic: acetaminophen				
	Brand: Tylenol				
	Strength: 325 mg				
	Amount: 2 tabs				
Stop date	Frequency: q4h WA				
	Route: by mouth				

Special instructions/precautions: Give only for right shoulder discomfort. Follow up with licensed HCP in one week.

Notice that this medication is to be given only for right shoulder discomfort. If the individual complains of pain elsewhere, such as in the back or leg, or if the individual should have a fever, the UAP could not give this medication. The licensed health care provider would have to give a new order for a medication to treat fever or to treat the complaints of back or leg pain.

Now that the order has been transcribed, it is important to set up a schedule for giving this medication. The column labeled "hour" is where this information is written. When deciding the specific times for giving medication, consider the following:

- The type of medication to be given
- The individual's daily schedule
- The schedule of the setting in which the UAP works

The medication must be given as ordered, which may not match the schedule of the UAP's workplace. For example, the UAP's workplace may routinely give medication every four (4) hours, and the licensed health care provider may write an order to give medication every six (6) hours or every two (2) hours. If there is a problem with the times medication is to be given, the UAP must check with her supervisor and the licensed health care provider to make sure that the medication schedule meets the medical needs of the individual getting the medication. Also, the UAP needs to make sure that the medication schedule that is set does not interfere with the individual's daily schedule, that is, work, recreation programs, regular outings or visits, and so on. Remember that medications given at times other than the workplace's regular schedule are more likely to be missed by relief and regular staff.

Look again at this order for Tylenol. Since the order indicates every four (4) hours while awake (q4h WA), it is fairly easy to set up a schedule starting with 8 a.m., and counting every four (4) hours until 8 p.m. The individual would receive Tylenol as ordered at 8 a.m., 12 p.m. (noon), 4 p.m., and 8 p.m. The medication sheet would look like this:

MEDICATION OR TREATMENT		HOUR	I	2	3
Start date	Generic: acetaminophen	8 AM			
	Brand: Tylenol				
	Strength: 325 mg	12 PM			
	Amount: 2 tabs	4 PM			
Stop date	Frequency: q4h WA	8 PM			
	Route: by mouth				

Special instructions/precautions: Give only for right shoulder discomfort. Follow up with the licensed HCP in one week.

The UAP may also see an order for a medication being given three times a day or given prn (as needed). In those cases, the UAP would enter the times as shown next. For an order written as follows:

> Acetaminophen 325 mg 2 tabs by mouth tid for left knee pain. Follow up with licensed HCP in 3 days.

MEDICATION OR TREATMENT		HOUR	I	2	3
Start date	Generic: acetaminophen	8 AM			
	Brand: Tylenol				
	Strength: 325 mg				
	Amount: 2 tabs	2 PM			
Stop date	Frequency: tid	8 PM			
	Route: by mouth				

Special instructions/precautions: Give only for left knee pain. Follow up with licensed HCP in 3 days.

For an order written as follows:

> Acetaminophen 325 mg 2 tabs by mouth q4h prn for temp greater than 101°F or headache. Notify the licensed HCP if temp lasts for more than 24 hr.

MEDICATION OR TREATMENT		HOUR	I	2	3
Start date	Generic: acetaminophen	P			
	Brand: Tylenol				
	Strength: 325 mg	R			
	Amount: 2 tabs	N			
Stop date	Frequency: q4h prn				
	Route: by mouth				

Special instructions/precautions: Give only if Temp > 101°F or for headache. Notify the licensed HCP if temp lasts more than 24 hours.

The next step in transcribing a medication order is to identify dates. In many work settings the *start date* is the date the medication was ordered by the licensed health care provider. The *stop date* is the day on which the UAP stops giving the medication. The stop date is not always specified in the order. A stop date is most likely given if the medication is for a specific issue, such as a ten(10)-day course of antibiotics for an infection. If no stop date is given, the UAP would write "cont." in that space, which is an abbreviation for "continuing." Workplace policies and state regulations for start and stop dates differ from one setting to another and one state to another. The UAP once again needs to know and follow the policies and regulations that apply to the setting in which she works.

If the licensed HCP writes an original order for Tylenol that was received on March 1 with no stop date, the order would read:

> Acetaminophen 325 mg 2 tabs by mouth q4h WA for right shoulder discomfort. Follow up with the licensed HCP in one week.

The sheet might look like this:

MEDICATION OR TREATMENT		HOUR	1	2	3
Start date 3/1/11	Generic: acetaminophen Brand: Tylenol	8 AM			
	Strength: 325 mg Amount: 2 tabs	12 PM			
Stop date	Frequency: q4h WA	4 PM			
Cont.	Route: by mouth	8 PM			

Special instructions/precautions: Give only for right shoulder discomfort. Follow up with licensed HCP in one week.

If the order contained a specific stop date of March 31, the order would read:

> Acetaminophen (Tylenol) 325 mg 2 tabs by mouth q4h WA for right shoulder discomfort for one month. Follow up with licensed HCP in one week.

The sheet might look like this:

MEDICATION OR TREATMENT		HOUR	1	2	3
Start date 3/1/11	Generic: acetaminophen Brand: Tylenol	8 AM			
	Strength: 325 mg Amount: 2 tabs	12 PM			
Stop date	Frequency: q4h WA	4 PM			
3/31/11	Route: by mouth	8 PM			

Special instructions/precautions: Give only for right shoulder discomfort. Follow up with licensed HCP in one week.

Not every start date is going to fall on the first of the month, however. A start date may occur on any day of the month. Indicating that on the medication sheet is a simple process. Simply block out the days before the start date on the medication sheet for that month.

Again using the order for Tylenol, the UAP may get a licensed health care provider's order to begin giving it on March 5 at 11 a.m. By the time the UAP returns to her facility, the first dose will be given at 12 p.m. Here is what the medication sheet would look like:

MEDICATION OR TREATMENT		HOUR	1	2	3	4	5	6	7
Start date 3/5/11	Generic: acetaminophen	8 AM	X	X	X	X	X		
	Brand: Tylenol	12 PM	X	X	X	X			
	Strength: 325 mg	4 PM	X	X	X	X			
Stop date Cont.	Amount: 2 tabs	8 PM	X	X	X	X			
	Frequency: q4h WA								
	Route: by mouth								

Special instructions/precautions: Give only for right shoulder discomfort. Follow up with licensed HCP in one week.

As with start dates, stop dates do not always occur at the end of the month. When there is a specific stop date, the documentation must show that the medication has been discontinued after the specific stop date. To do so, draw a diagonal line across the rest of the dates for that month and write "discontinued" and the date of the discontinuance. For an order that requires a medication to be discontinued on March 4, 2011, the medication sheet would look like this:

MEDICATION OR TREATMENT		HOUR	1	2	3	4	5	6	7
Start date 3/1/11	Generic: acetaminophen	8 AM					*discontinued 3/4/11*		
	Brand: Tylenol	12 PM							
	Strength: 325 mg	4 PM							
Stop date 3/4/11	Amount: 2 tabs	8 PM							
	Frequency: q4h WA								
	Route: by mouth								

Special instructions/precautions: Give only for right shoulder discomfort. Follow up with licensed HCP in one week.

The diagonal line would begin on the stop date, March 4, 2011, and run through the last date of the month, March 31, 2011, on the medication sheet. Some work settings will use arrows or draw a line using a yellow highlighter to indicate discontinuation of a medication. See the second sample:

MEDICATION OR TREATMENT		HOUR	1	2	3	4	5	6	7
Start date 3/1/11	Generic: acetaminophen	8 AM				—	—	—	—
	Brand: Tylenol	12 PM				—	—	—	—
	Strength: 325 mg	4 PM			*discontinued 3/4/11*				
	Amount: 2 tabs	8 PM				—	—	—	—
Stop date 3/4/11	Frequency: q4h WA								
	Route: by mouth								

Special instructions/precautions: Give only for right shoulder discomfort. Follow up with licensed HCP in one week.

Documenting on the Medication Sheet

Chapter 28 discusses the 10 guidelines for documentation. The guidelines stress the importance of accurate and factual documentation. Remember that all of the medical records the UAP uses in medication administration are legal documents. They may be used in a court of law at any time. The rule of thumb in health care is: "If the task is not documented, then the task has not been done."

The UAP will provide her signature and initials on the medication forms used in medication administration. Other staff members who administer medication will do so as well. It is, therefore, important that each staff person administering medication identify herself. Each time a UAP gives medication, she will write her initials on the medication sheet in the block next to the time that corresponds with the time and date that the medication is given. Here is an example:

MEDICATION OR TREATMENT		HOUR	1	2	3
Start date 3/1/11	Generic: acetaminophen	8 AM	PS	SR	
	Brand: Tylenol				
	Strength: 325 mg	12 PM	PS	SR	
	Amount: 2 tabs	4 PM	RM	RM	
Stop date Cont.	Frequency: q4h WA				
	Route: by mouth	8 PM	RM		

Special instructions/precautions: Give only for right shoulder discomfort. Follow up with the licensed HCP in one week.

SIGNATURE	INITIALS	SIGNATURE	INITIALS	SIGNATURE	INITIALS
Patricia Smith	PS				
Roberta Meyers	RM				
Samuel Roper	SR				

If the UAP were administering a medication with an order for "prn" medication, her entry would look a bit different. With a prn order, in addition to the UAP writing her initials, she must also include the time the medication was given. It would look something like this:

MEDICATION OR TREATMENT		HOUR	1	2	3
Start date 3/1/11	Generic: acetaminophen Brand: Tylenol	P	9 AM PS		
	Strength: 325 mg Amount: 2 tabs	R	1 PM PS		
Stop date Cont.	Frequency: q4h prn Route: by mouth	N	5 PM RM		

Special instructions/precautions: Give only if Temp > 101°F or for headache. Notify the licensed HCP if temp lasts more than 24 hours.

SIGNATURE	INITIALS	SIGNATURE	INITIALS	SIGNATURE	INITIALS
Patricia Smith	PS				
Roberta Meyers	RM				

The UAP may also have to indicate that a medication was not given for a variety of reasons. Here is an example of how to document a withheld medication on the medication sheet. In this example, the UAP still writes her initials in the box on the medication sheet. After entering them in the correct box, however, the UAP then circles them. The medication sheet would look like this:

MEDICATION OR TREATMENT		HOUR	1	2	3
Start date 3/1/11	Generic: acetaminophen Brand: Tylenol	8 AM	PS	(SR)	
	Strength: 325 mg Amount: 2 tabs	12 PM	PS	SR	
Stop date Cont.	Frequency: q4h WA	4 PM	RM	RM	
	Route: by mouth	8 PM	RM		

Special instructions/precautions: Give only for right shoulder discomfort. Follow up with licensed HCP in one week.

SIGNATURE	INITIALS	SIGNATURE	INITIALS	SIGNATURE	INITIALS
Patricia Smith	PS				
Roberta Meyers	RM				
Samuel Roper	SR				

In this example, staff person Samuel Roper withheld the 8 a.m. dose of medication. Additional documentation is needed when medication is withheld or has not been given as ordered for other reasons. See the next section, "Medication Progress Note."

Note: Different workplaces have different policies regarding documentation and may not use this method to indicate that a medication was withheld. This is just one example of how that may be documented.

Medication Progress Note

There will be times when the UAP attempts to give an individual medication, and for one reason or another the individual will not or cannot take it. For instance, this may be due to the individual's refusal to take the medication, a medication being held for special circumstances such as fasting for lab work, or the medication being unavailable. In such instances, the UAP will need to write a short note about the reason the medication was not taken by the individual. The UAP may also be asked to write notes about changes in symptoms or behaviors as observed over time. Usually there is a space on the back of the medication sheet for the UAP to write these notes. As with other documents, each work setting may have its own way to document this information, but all the notes contain similar information. The progress note may look like this:

DATE	TIME	MEDICATION AND DOSAGE	HELD	REFUSED	GIVEN	REASON	RESULT OR RESPONSE	SIGNATURE

Using the prn order for Tylenol, here is an example of how this form would be completed:

DATE	TIME	MEDICATION AND DOSAGE	HELD	REFUSED	GIVEN	REASON	RESULT OR RESPONSE	SIGNATURE
3/5/11	8 AM	Tylenol, 325 mg			X		Fever Still 103°F	P. Smith
3/5/11	12 PM	Tylenol, 325 mg			X		Fever 101.5°F	P. Smith
3/5/11	4 PM	Tylenol, 325 mg	X			c/o nausea	Fever 102.5°F Called Dr. Proctor's office and left message.	P. Smith

The UAP uses the **medication progress note** to document anything that needs to be tracked or monitored, such as responses to a medication, or to report anything unusual, such as refusal of medication.

Discontinuing a Medication

Discontinuing a medication was mentioned briefly earlier when talking about the stop date for a medication. Discontinuation of a medication is *only* decided by the individual's licensed health care provider(s). The UAP may not make that decision. Medication may be discontinued for a variety of reasons. Several of these reasons are:

- The individual may be taking an antibiotic for a specified period of time.

- The individual may have an adverse reaction to a newly prescribed medication.

- The licensed health care provider may feel that another medication would be better for the individual.

Sometimes the medication itself is not changed, but the dose, frequency, or route is changed. When this happens, this is also considered a new order. The old order must be discontinued. A new order must be transcribed. In the case of a prn medication, it is considered a new order if a new prn order is prescribed for new or different symptoms.

Whenever a medication is discontinued, it must be indicated on the medication sheet. The UAP must draw a single line diagonally through both the information box and the date columns and write "discontinued" and the date along the lines. It would look like this:

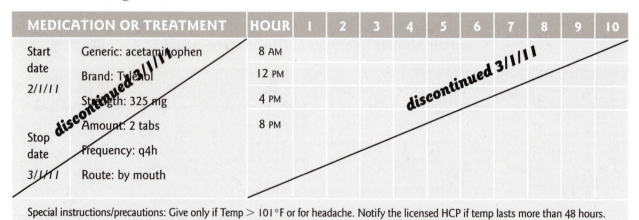

MEDICATION OR TREATMENT		HOUR	1	2	3	4	5	6	7	8	9	10
Start date 2/1/11	Generic: acetaminophen	8 AM										
	Brand: Tylenol	12 PM										
	Strength: 325 mg	4 PM										
	Amount: 2 tabs	8 PM										
Stop date 3/1/11	Frequency: q4h											
	Route: by mouth											

discontinued 3/1/11

Special instructions/precautions: Give only if Temp > 101°F or for headache. Notify the licensed HCP if temp lasts more than 48 hours.

In addition to completing the medication sheet in this manner, any change in an order should be verbally communicated to other staff, and a progress note should be written. The progress note would look like this:

DATE	TIME	MEDICATION AND DOSAGE	HELD	REFUSED	GIVEN	REASON	RESULT OR RESPONSE	SIGNATURE
3/1/11	8 AM	Tylenol 325 mg	X			Discontinued per licensed HCP order. Notified staff and documented on medication sheet.		*P. Smith*

medication progress note
A written note used to document events occurring during medication administration.

discontinuing
To stop a medication, done only with a licensed health care provider's order.

In some workplaces, a note is also written in the staff's communication book.

ADVANCED TRANSCRIPTION
Special Situations

Some medications are ordered to be given in unusual ways. For example, digoxin is prescribed at 0.25 mg for one (1) day, then 0.125 mg for the second day, 0.25 mg for the third day, 0.125 mg for the fourth day, and so on. This is because a dosage of 0.25 mg daily would quickly make the individual toxic, requiring medical intervention. The UAP may find similar situations with medications such as Tegretol, in which an order is received for one dose at one or more times of the day combined with a different dose at a different time during the day. Using this order for Tegretol as an example, the licensed health care provider's order reads:

Tegretol 200 mg by mouth bid and 100 mg by mouth daily at 4 p.m.

The UAP would need to use two separate sections of the medication sheet in order to transcribe this order correctly. Use one section for the 200 mg bid and the other for the 100 mg daily at 4 p.m.

MEDICATION OR TREATMENT		HOUR	1	2	3	4	5	6	7
Start date 3/1/11	Generic: *carbamazepine*	8 AM							
	Brand: *Tegretol*								
	Strength: *200 mg tablets*								
	Amount: *1 tablet*	8 PM							
Stop date	Frequency: *bid*								
Cont.	Route: *by mouth*								

Special instructions/precautions:

MEDICATION OR TREATMENT		HOUR	1	2	3	4	5	6	7
Start date 3/1/11	Generic: *carbamazepine*								
	Brand: *Tegretol*								
	Strength: *100 mg tablets*	4 PM							
	Amount: *1 tablet*								
Stop date	Frequency: *daily*								
Cont.	Route: *by mouth*								

Special instructions/precautions:

Note that two different strengths were used in these transcriptions; if the strength was ordered and transcribed as "200 mg tablets" for both, then the amount in the second transcription would be "1/2 tab," and the pharmacy would be expected to provide split tablets.

Transcribing Liquid Medication Orders

Transcribing an order for a liquid medication is very similar to transcribing an order for a solid, or pill form, medication. The difference lies in how the UAP transcribes the amount of the liquid ordered. The transcription is based on liquid measurements. Liquid measurements are discussed in detail in *Medication Administration: Math Module*. Here is a quick review, however, of how to measure liquids.

There are two basic systems for measuring liquids; one is in teaspoons (abbreviated as t) or tablespoons (abbreviated as T). These are often referred to as household measures. The other is in milliliters (mL) from the metric system. Here are some equivalents for the UAP to remember:

3 t = 1 T (3 teaspoons equals 1 tablespoon)

1 t = 5 mL (1 teaspoon equals 5 mL)

1 T = 15 mL (1 tablespoon equals 15 mL)

Remember that when measuring liquids, a medicine cup gives a much more accurate measurement than a standard household teaspoon or tablespoon. It is strongly advised that the UAP use a medicine cup whenever she is administering liquid medication.

When the UAP receives a licensed health care provider's order for a liquid medication, it will be given in milligrams, or mg, just like a pill form (this is the dose). However, there will be some changes in the wording. Liquid medications may be ordered as an **oral suspension**, which is a thick liquid that has to be shaken well before it is poured. The order may be written like this:

Penicillin VK by mouth suspension 250 mg by mouth tid × 10 days

The pharmacy label will have the strength written on it, just as for a pill. However, the strength will be written in a ratio of mg/mL: "Penicillin VK by mouth suspension 125 mg/5 mL." This means that there are 125 mg of medicine in 5 mL of liquid poured.

The pharmacy label will also have the amount written in the directions. However, instead of telling how many pills to give, the directions for a liquid medication will tell how many teaspoons, tablespoons, or mL to give. The directions would be written like this:

Take 2 teaspoons (10 mL) by mouth 3 times a day for 10 days.

oral suspension
A thick liquid medication that has to be shaken well before it is poured and administered.

The UAP would transcribe it on the medication sheet like this:

MEDICATION OR TREATMENT		HOUR	1	2	3
Start date 3/1/11	Generic: penicillin	8 AM			
	Brand: penicillin VK				
	Strength: 125 mg/5 cc	2 PM			
	Amount: 2 teaspoons/10 cc				
Stop date 3/11/11	Frequency: tid	8 PM			
	Route: by mouth				
Special instructions/precautions: Give only for 10 days.					

POSTING AND VERIFICATION OF ORDERS

All transcriptions of licensed health care provider's orders should be posted and verified by assigned staff (Figure 29-1). Each work setting, based upon its state regulations and policy, will determine if this procedure will be done and by whom. The steps for doing this procedure are as follows:

posting
The first step in a two-step process in transcribing medication orders onto a medication sheet.

verifying
The second step in a two-step process in transcribing medication orders onto a medication sheet.

1. The assigned staff member who transcribes the order places a check mark next to each medication order on the original licensed health care provider order form. This check mark should be easily distinguished from regular documentation. A check mark should be made next to each order transcribed.

2. When all orders have been transcribed from the licensed health care provider order form to the medication sheet, the staff member writes "Posted" along with the date, time, and her name at either the side or the bottom of the order form. This indicates that each order with a check mark next to it has been transcribed.

3. A second assigned staff member then reviews the transcribed orders. This staff member compares each order on the licensed health care provider order form to that on the medication sheet. When the review is completed, the staff member writes "Verified" along with the date, time, and her name next to the transcriber's name on the licensed health care provider order form. This indicates that all of the transcribed orders have been double-checked for accuracy and completeness.

4. Should the staff member administering the medication have any doubts about a medication order, she needs to check for the accuracy and completeness of the medication order before giving the medication to the individual. Remember that the staff member administering the medication is ultimately responsible for making sure the medication was transcribed correctly.

		ENTERED	FILLED	CHECKED	VERIFIED

NOTE: A NON-PROPRIETARY DRUG OF EQUAL QUALITY MAY BE DISPENSED - IF THIS COLUMN IS NOT CHECKED!

DATE	TIME WRITTEN	PLEASE USE BALL POINT - PRESS FIRMLY	✔	TIME NOTED	NURSES SIGNATURE
11/3/10	0815	Keflex 250 mg by mouth q6h ✔	✔	posted 11/3/10
			✔	at 8:30am
			✔	V. TENNY, R.N.
			✔	
		Codeine 30 mg by mouth q4h prn leg pain ✔	✔	
		Tylenol 650 mg by mouth q4h prn, temp 101°F ✔	✔	verified 11/3/10
		Lasix 40 mg by mouth daily ✔	✔	at 9:00am
		Slow-K 8 mEq by mouth bid ✔	✔	L. Deter, R.N.
		Digoxin 0.25 mg by mouth daily ✔	✔	
		J. Botte, M.D.		

AUTO STOP ORDERS: UNLESS REORDERED, FOLLOWING WILL BE D/C'D AT 0800 ON:

DATE	ORDER		
		☐ CONT	PHYSICIAN SIGNATURE
		☐ D/C ☐ CONT	PHYSICIAN SIGNATURE
		☐ D/C ☐ CONT	PHYSICIAN SIGNATURE
		☐ D/C	

CHECK WHEN ANTIBIOTICS ORDERED ☐ Prophylactic ☐ Empiric ☐ Therapeutic

Allergies:
None Known

PATIENT DIAGNOSIS
Diabetes, CAD

HEIGHT 5'5" WEIGHT 160lb

FORM 959-706 (9-XX) **PHYSICIANS ORDER** Reynolds + Reynolds LITHO IN U.S.A. K41814 (7-XX) D339380

McGillicudy, Mary A.
#3-11316-7

①

Figure 29-1 Verification and posting of licensed health care provider's orders. *(Delmar/Cengage Learning)*

MONTHLY QUALITY REVIEW OF ORDERS

Because transcription is done by human beings, there is always room for human error. In other words, there is always a chance that an error has been made in copying the licensed health care provider's order onto the medication sheet or in copying from one medication sheet to the next. This is true even if the medication orders are provided on a computerized sheet from a pharmacy or if the medication orders are transcribed by nursing.

To catch these errors before the wrong medication or dose is given to an individual, it is important that a **monthly quality review** be done of all medication sheets. During the monthly review, the orders on the medication sheets are compared with the orders on the licensed health care provider order form.

For example, consider an individual who is to take Synthroid daily for hypothyroidism. The medication does not get written on the medication sheet. The individual does not receive the medication for several months or more. Over time the UAP notices changes, including weight gain, excessive fatigue, slow thought process, muscle weakness, a hoarse or scratchy voice, and drying or loss of hair, in the individual. Although it is true that all of these symptoms may be the result of other causes, a review of the original licensed health care provider's order would show that the medication, Synthroid, was missing from the medication sheet.

To complete a monthly review of the licensed health care provider's orders, the UAP needs the original orders, completed medication sheets, and a checklist on which the UAP can compare and verify the accuracy of the transcriptions. Each facility will have its own method of completing a monthly review, but a checklist may look like this:

monthly quality review A monthly review of all medication orders.

Monthly Review of Orders for _____ (month and year)

Individual/Resident/Client: _____ (Individual's name)

Medication or Treatment	Date Ordered	Licensed Health Care Provider Ordering	Date Transcribed	Staff Member Transcribed	Accurate? Yes/No	Staff Member Reviewing

First, fill in the blanks at the top to indicate the month, year, and the name of the individual whose record is being reviewed.

Monthly Review of Orders for _____ June 2010 _____

Individual/Resident/Client: _____ Ruth Perkins _____

Medication or Treatment	Date Ordered	Licensed Health Care Provider Ordering	Date Transcribed	Staff Member Transcribed	Accurate? Yes/No	Staff Member Reviewing

Next, check the original licensed health care provider's orders and list each one in order in the left-hand column, along with the date it was ordered and the name of the physician who ordered it.

Monthly Review of Orders for ___June 2010___

Individual/Resident/Client: ___Ruth Perkins___

Medication or Treatment	Date Ordered	Licensed Health Care Provider Ordering	Date Transcribed	Staff Member Transcribed	Accurate? Yes/No	Staff Member Reviewing
Tylenol 325 mg by mouth prn	6/15/10	Dr. Proctor				
Ativan 1 mg bid by mouth	6/7/10	Dr. Proctor				

Now check the date of the transcription and the name of the staff member who did it by looking for the word "posted" along with the date and name of the staff member. Enter the dates and names in the appropriate columns.

Monthly Review of Orders for ___June 2010___

Individual/Resident/Client: ___Ruth Perkins___

Medication or Treatment	Date Ordered	Licensed Health Care Provider Ordering	Date Transcribed	Staff Member Transcribed	Accurate? Yes/No	Staff Member Reviewing
Tylenol 325 mg by mouth prn	6/15/10	Dr. Proctor	6/15/10	P. Smith		
Ativan 1 mg bid by mouth	6/7/10	Dr. Proctor	6/7/10	R. Miller		

Next, compare the order to the transcription for accuracy and indicate that in the appropriate column.

Monthly Review of Orders for ___June 2010___

Individual/Resident/Client: ___Ruth Perkins___

Medication or Treatment	Date Ordered	Licensed Health Care Provider Ordering	Date Transcribed	Staff Member Transcribed	Accurate? Yes/No	Staff Member Reviewing
Tylenol 325 mg by mouth prn	6/15/10	Dr. Proctor	6/15/10	P. Smith	Yes	
Ativan 1 mg bid by mouth	6/7/10	Dr. Proctor	6/7/10	R. Miller	Yes	

Finally, the UAP enters her name as the staff member doing the review.

Monthly Review of Orders for		June 2010				
Patient/Resident/Client:		Ruth Perkins				
Medication or Treatment	Date Ordered	Licensed Health Care Provider Ordering	Date Transcribed	Staff Member Transcribed	Accurate? Yes/No	Staff Member Reviewing
Tylenol 325 mg by mouth prn	6/15/10	Dr. Proctor	6/15/10	P. Smith	Yes	S. Roper
Ativan 1 mg bid by mouth	6/7/10	Dr. Proctor	6/7/10	R. Miller	Yes	S. Roper

Monthly quality reviews can be completed by any staff member familiar with the process of administering and documenting medications. The review can be done at any time of the day or night. Once the reviews are completed, they should also be reviewed by an appropriate manager or supervisor. This individual can then follow up as needed with staff members or licensed health care providers. This type of peer review is a good way of minimizing errors and guaranteeing the highest level of care for the individuals the UAP works with every day.

SUMMARY

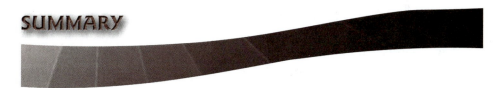

Transcribing and documenting are two of the basic skills required for medication administration. Not only do these skills provide accurate information to all staff members, but they are also a clear and concise way to communicate with staff members and licensed health care providers. Understanding how and when to use these tools provides a good basis for safe and effective administration of medication.

WORKBOOK REVIEW

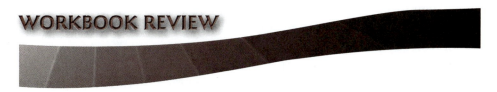

Go to the workbook and complete the exercises for Chapter 29.

REVIEW QUESTIONS

1. Accurate documentation and transcription:
   a. is done mainly for billing purposes
   b. serves the purpose of research
   c. eliminates the need for verbal communication between staff
   d. safeguards the health and safety of the individual receiving medication

2. Documentation and transcription principles include all of the following except:
   a. the document must be legible so that other people can read it
   b. the document should include only information related to the individual's medical needs and daily care
   c. it is okay to use Wite Out® and to document in pencil
   d. the document must include objective observations, not subjective statements

3. The start date on a medication order is:
   a. the date of the licensed HCP's visit
   b. the date when the medication was or is to be first given
   c. the date the order is written
   d. the first day of the month

4. The stop date on a medication order is:
   a. the last day of the month
   b. the date of the licensed HCP's visit
   c. the date of the transcription
   d. the date when the medication is to be stopped or discontinued

5. If an individual has an order for Tylenol to be given for fever and she asks for Tylenol because of knee pain:
   a. it is okay to give it to her
   b. you must get a new order from the licensed health care provider with specific instructions to give Tylenol for knee pain
   c. you can give it as long as you document why you did so
   d. you can give her another individual's pain medication

6. If medication is ordered to be given three times a day:
   a. you can give it whenever you have time
   b. you must give it at 8 a.m., 12 p.m., and 4 p.m.
   c. you must give it as ordered and documented on the medication sheet
   d. you can leave it up to the licensed health care provider to set the times

7. To document the discontinuation of a medication on a medication sheet, you:
   a. make a diagonal line across the dates after the stop date and write "discontinued" with the date along the diagonal line
   b. scratch out the rest of the dates with a black marker
   c. leave the dates blank after the stop date
   d. sign your name in all the boxes after the stop date
8. A medication progress note is written to:
   a. document changes in an individual's environment
   b. document subjective observations in response to medication
   c. all of these
   d. document a medication refusal
9. The process of transcribing and double-checking medication orders is called:
   a. documentation
   b. written orders
   c. posting and verifying
   d. all of the above
10. A monthly quality review:
   a. can be done by any staff member who knows how to administer and document medication
   b. must be done during the day
   c. does not minimize errors
   d. must be done by the licensed health care provider

CLINICAL SCENARIOS

1. When you are initially transcribing an order onto a medication sheet, what information must be included?
2. How do you document the administration of a prn medication on a medication sheet? Does this information need to be documented elsewhere? If so, where?
3. You try to give Mrs. Taylor her 4 p.m. medication, but she holds her mouth shut and will not take it. How do you document this on the medication sheet and in the medication progress note?

MODULE VI
Safety

Chapter 30
Additional Considerations

Learning Objectives

After reading this chapter and completing the review questions, you should be able to:

1. Spell and define terms.

2. List the four guidelines for the administration of an over-the-counter medication.

3. Demonstrate the administration of an over-the-counter medication.

4. Name three types of medication interactions.

5. List five types of adverse medication effects.

6. Explain two ways to prevent adverse medication interactions.

7. Explain the difference between psychological dependence and physical dependence.

8. Explain the difference between hypersensitivity and anaphylactic reaction.

9. Describe the four processes that undergo change as an individual ages.

10. List the Six Wrongs of medication administration and give an example of each.

11. Explain the four guidelines to prevent misinterpretation of a licensed health care provider's order.

12. Describe the four steps to follow should a medication error occur.

13. Complete a medication occurrence form.

14. Complete a drug incident report.

15. List four reasons a medication refusal may occur.

16. Explain the difference between an active medication refusal and a passive medication refusal.

17. List four ways to deal with a medication refusal.

Key Terms

absorption	excretion	medication refusals	psychological dependence
active refusal	hypersensitivity	metabolism	Six Wrongs
antagonism	idiosyncrasy	passive refusal	synergism
cumulative effect	medication error	physical dependence	teratogenic effect
dependence	medication loss	potentiation	
distribution	medication reconciliation		

INTRODUCTION

Over-the-counter (OTC) medications, use of nonmedical substances, medication interactions, use of medications in the elderly, adverse medication events, medication errors, medication losses, and **medication refusals** are all discussed in this chapter. Each of these topics could serve as a chapter in and of itself. This chapter merely presents a brief introduction to each topic.

USE OF OVER-THE-COUNTER MEDICATIONS

A general description of over-the-counter (OTC) medications and the labeling is discussed in Chapter 5. Even though these medications are easily purchased by individuals in drugstores, grocery stores, discount department stores, and pharmacies; on the Internet; and at other general locations, the UAP needs to remember that these medications are as powerful as prescription medications and therefore are not always safe. For that reason, it is important to tell the individual's licensed health care provider about the OTC medications that an individual is taking. In addition, it is important to observe an individual for interactions and/or side effects from OTC medications.

When administering OTC medications, the UAP will follow the same principles of medication administration as for prescription medications. These are:

- The Six Rights
- The Three Checks
- The basic guidelines for medication administration
- The four-step procedure for medication administration
- Handwashing
- Use of gloves

In addition, the guidelines below are to be followed:

- Obtain a written licensed health care provider's order for each OTC medication to be administered.
- Document OTC medications in the same manner as prescription medications.

- Store and lock OTC medications per state regulations and workplace policies.

- Report OTC medication errors just as prescription medication errors would be reported.

- Follow state regulations and workplace reporting policies.

USE OF NONMEDICAL SUBSTANCES

Nonmedical substances, such as alcohol, nicotine, and caffeine, affect the way the body works. The use of these legal drugs and any illegal drugs, such as marijuana, should be reported to the licensed health care provider. These drugs may interact with OTC, herbal, and prescription medications and may cause side effects, allergic reactions, and other problems.

MEDICATION INTERACTIONS

Whenever more than one medication is taken by an individual, it is possible that the combination of those medications will change the effect of each of the individual medications. One medication may increase, decrease, or cancel out the effects of the other. The following terms are used to describe medication interactions:

- **Synergism**: The action of two medications working together in which one medication helps the other for an effect that neither one could produce alone.

- **Potentiation**: The action of two medications in which one medication prolongs or multiplies the effect of the other medication.

- **Antagonism**: The opposing action of two medications in which one medication decreases or cancels out the effect of the other medication.

It is very important that the licensed health care provider knows *all* of the medications that an individual is taking, including OTC and herbal medications, in order to prevent unwanted medication interactions. On the other hand, the licensed health care provider may intentionally order two medications together because some medication interactions are wanted and beneficial.

ADVERSE EVENTS

Reactions to medications may be wanted or unwanted. Usually a medication has the expected effect. However, unexpected responses known as adverse effects can and do occur. These adverse effects may be dangerous and even life threatening at times.

Several of these effects are:

- **Teratogenic effect**: Administration of certain medications to pregnant women causes birth defects in newborns.

- **Idiosyncrasy**: A unique, unusual response to medication; for example, an individual takes a sleeping pill to help him sleep but instead gets overly excited and is awake all night.

- Tolerance: A decreased response to a medication that develops over time after repeated doses are given; to get the wanted effect, the dose of the medication has to be continually increased or the medication changed to a different medication.

- **Dependence**: An acquired need for a medication that may produce psychological and/or physical symptoms of withdrawal when the medication is discontinued.

- **Psychological dependence**: An acquired psychological need for a medication; no physical withdrawal other than anxiety occurs when the medication is discontinued.

- **Physical dependence**: The body's cells actually have a need for the medication; symptoms of physical withdrawal include retching, nausea, pain, tremors, and sweating when the medication is discontinued.

- **Hypersensitivity**: An allergic response to a medication; may be of varying severity.

Hypersensitivity may be mild with no immediate effects. A rash may appear after three (3) or four (4) days of taking a medication or may appear after taking a medication several times. Hypersensitivity is more likely to happen in individuals who are known to have other allergies.

Signs of hypersensitivity are:

- Flushing of skin

- Hives

- Itching

- Wheezing

Anaphylactic reaction is a sudden, severe, possibly fatal, allergic (hypersensitivity) reaction. Anaphylaxis occurs most commonly with antibiotics, X-ray dyes containing iodide, and certain foods. Signs of an anaphylactic reaction are:

- Swelling of eyes, lips, tongue, mouth

- Cyanosis (bluish skin)

- Laryngeal edema

- Shortness of breath

- Vascular collapse

- Shock

- Seizures

Treatment includes CPR, if needed, and medications such as epinephrine if ordered by the licensed health care provider. For the UAP working in a community health care setting, an emergency telephone call to the police and/or ambulance must be made immediately. Refer to Chapter 11 for additional information on anaphylaxis and for use of an Epipen.

Any knowledge of adverse reactions to medications must be included in the individual's medical history and medical record. This information may be helpful in preventing repeat episodes.

Individuals who have had an anaphylactic reaction to a substance should always wear a Medic-Alert tag or bracelet to identify the substance to which they are allergic. Individuals who have had a hypersensitivity reaction to a substance are at a higher risk for reactions to other substances and require close observation. Allergies should be listed on a card and carried in the individual's wallet.

Special considerations include:

- Take extreme caution when giving medication to an individual for the first time, especially if that individual has a history of other allergies.

- Never leave an individual who is experiencing an adverse reaction alone—not even for a moment! Call for help. Stay with the individual.

- If the reaction seems to be serious, call 911 or the emergency medical system (EMS) to get help.

- Once the individual is stable, the UAP must call the individual's licensed health care provider and his supervisor.

- Once the individual is cared for, the UAP needs to complete the required documentation.

USE OF MEDICATIONS IN THE ELDERLY

Today, individuals are living longer and taking more medications. The more medications an individual takes at one time, the greater the chance for adverse reactions. It is estimated that more than 200,000 adults over the age of 60 are hospitalized each year as a result of adverse reactions. Medication-related problems have been estimated to have caused as many as 106,000 deaths in 2000 (Woodrow, 2007). Since each individual ages differently, each individual will react differently to medications, including sensitivity to medications.

This makes medication administration among the elderly especially challenging. UAPs, therefore, need to be acutely aware of the medications that they are administering to the individuals for whom they are caring. UAPs need to make an extra effort to communicate well with licensed health care providers, pharmacists, coworkers, and other clinicians.

AGING

Aging is not a disease. Aging is a normal, gradual process that occurs in all individuals. Aging is cumulative. In other words, it begins when we are young and builds upon itself as we slowly age. Our actions and habits affect our health as we become older. What we eat and drink, whether we are active or inactive, whether we smoke or drink, and so on are all factors in determining how we age. By the age of 40 to 50 years, our lifestyles have begun to have a significant impact on our bodies and thus our health (Smith & Gove, 2005).

Each of us ages at our own pace. Each of our body systems also ages at its own rate. Most of the changes that an individual faces as he ages will not pose a problem for him. The changes will require him only to adapt. The older individual needs to get an adequate amount of sleep, have good nutrition with adequate fluids, remain mobile and active, and maintain a healthy weight. All individuals will need to receive preventive medical care. In addition, if the individual has a medical problem, such as hypertension or diabetes, the individual will need to see his licensed HCP on a regular basis and take his medication and treatments as ordered (Smith & Gove, 2005).

The UAP has the responsibility of understanding the aging process. The UAP should assist the individual in his care to:

- Adapt to his environment
- Remain safe
- Receive good nutrition with adequate fluids
- Remain mobile and active
- Maintain a healthy weight
- Obtain an adequate amount of sleep
- Obtain preventive medical care
- Receive medications and treatments as ordered (Smith & Gove, 2005)

Cumulative Effects of Medications

There are four processes in the body that undergo change as an individual ages. These are:

- Absorption
- Distribution
- Metabolism
- Excretion

Because of the changes that occur in these processes, medications build up in the systems of the elderly. This buildup leads to dangerous, or toxic, levels. This is known as a **cumulative effect** of medications. Cumulative effects of medications in the elderly are due to:

1. Inadequate **absorption**: The gastrointestinal tract is slowed, or the amount of fluids taken in by the individual is reduced.

2. Impaired **distribution**: The cardiovascular system works poorly; therefore, transportation of the medication throughout the body is inadequate.

3. Slower **metabolism**: The liver is unable to filter the medications as effectively as it once did.

4. Impaired **excretion**: The kidneys, the lungs, and/or the bowels are unable to remove wastes from the body as effectively as they once were able to.

cumulative effect
Increasing in effect.

absorption
The passage of substances across and into tissues.

distribution
The location of medications in various organs and tissues after administration.

metabolism
The chemical and physical changes continuously occurring in the body.

excretion
The process of removing substances from the body.

Because the buildup in the amount of a medication circulating in the body is often gradual, the side effects from the medication may not be easily recognized. Family, friends, individuals themselves, and even staff may think that the symptoms are due to "old age" or an illness. The best advice when starting a new medication in an older individual is, when possible, to start with the lowest effective dose and increase the dose slowly until the desired dose is reached.

Inappropriate Medication Use in the Elderly

In 1997, a group of physicians conducted a national survey of geriatric experts to determine the medications that were inappropriate for nursing home residents and adults 65 years of age and older. The results of this survey have come to be called *The Gray List.* In 2003 an updated and revised list was published called *Updating the Beers Criteria for Potentially Inappropriate Medications Use in Older Adults.* Table 30-1 provides a summary of both of these lists.

Table 30-1 Potentially Inappropriate Medications for Adults Sixty-Five (65) Years and Older

Adults over 65 should avoid these drugs completely unless noted otherwise.

GENERIC NAME	BRAND NAME	COMMENTS
Sedative-Hypnotics		
long-acting benzodiazepines—Prolonged daytime effects: sedation, dizziness, ataxia		
chlordiazepoxide	Librium, Limbitrol, Librax	
diazepam	Valium	
flurazepam	Dalmane	
meprobamate	Miltown	
short-acting benzodiazepines—Avoid long-term use; can be habit forming		
alprazolam	Xanax	No dose greater than 2 mg; do not exceed daily maximum
lorazepam	Ativan	No dose greater than 3 mg; do not exceed daily maximum
oxepam	Serax	No dose greater than 60 mg; do not exceed daily maximum
temazepam	Restoril	No dose greater than 15 mg; do not exceed daily maximum
triazolam	Halcion	No dose greater than 0.25 mg; do not exceed daily maximum
Antidepressants		
amitriptyline	Elavil	Anticholinergic effects
doxepin	Sinequan	Anticholinergic effects
fluoxetine	Prozac	Long half-life; potential for agitation
		Safer alternatives
Antipsychotics		
haloperidol	Haldol	Doses greater than 3 mg/day should be avoided (individuals with known psychotic disorders may receive higher doses)
thioridazine	Mellaril	Avoid doses greater than 30 mg/day (unless known psychotic disorder)

(continues)

Table 30-1 Potentially Inappropriate Medications for Adults Sixty-Five (65) Years and Older—*continued*
Adults over 65 should avoid these drugs completely unless noted otherwise.

GENERIC NAME	BRAND NAME	COMMENTS
Antihypertensives		
hydrochlorothiazide	Esidrix	Avoid greater than 50 mg doses
	HydroDIURIL	
methyldopa	Aldomet	
propranolol	Inderal	Other beta-blockers offer less Central Nervous System penetration
reserpine	Serpasil	
clonidine	Catapress	Potential for Central Nervous System adverse effects and orthostatic hypotension
Antiarrhythmic		
disopyramide	Norpace	May induce heart failure in older adults
		Anticholinergic; better alternatives
NSAIDs		
indomethacin	Indocin	Other NSAIDs cause less Central Nervous System and GI toxic reactions than these drugs
ketorolac	Toradol	
phenylbutazone	Butazolidin	
Oral Hypoglycemics		
chlorpropamide	Diabinese	Causes SIADH*
Analgesics		
meperidine	Demerol	May cause confusion
		Morphine is the better alternative to Demerol
propoxyphene	Darvon	Adverse Central Nervous System effects potentiated in older adults
	Darvocet N	
pentazocine	Talwin	
Platelet Inhibitors		
dipyridamole	Persantine	Only avoid short-acting; Extended Release acceptable
Histamine-2 Blockers		
cimetidine	Tagamet	Avoid doses greater than 900 mg/day
		Central Nervous System effects
Anti-infective		
nitrofurantoin	Macrodantin	Potential for kidney impairment
		Safer alternatives available
Antihistamines—*Nonanticholinergic* antihistamines are preferred for older adults		
chlorpheniramine	Chlor-Trimeton	All of these drugs have anticholinergic effects; use short-term only for conditions other than allergies
diphenhydramine	Benadryl, Tylenol PM	
hydroxyzine	Vistaril, Atarax	
promethazine	Phenergan	

Table 30-1 Potentially Inappropriate Medications for Adults Sixty-Five (65) Years and Older—*continued*

Adults over 65 should avoid these drugs completely unless noted otherwise.

GENERIC NAME	BRAND NAME	COMMENTS
Decongestants		
oxymetazoline	Afrin, Dristan, others	Avoid daily use greater than 2 weeks
phenylephrine	Neo-Synephrine	Avoid daily use greater than 2 weeks
pseudoephedrine	Sudafed	Avoid daily use greater than 2 weeks
Iron	Ferrous sulfate	Avoid doses greater than 325 mg/day
Antispasmodics—Avoid long-term use; risk for toxicity greater than potential benefit		
hyoscyamine	Cytospaz, Levsin, Levsinex	All of these have anticholinergic effects
belladonna alkaloids	Donnatal and others	
dicyclomine	Bentyl	
oxybutynin	Ditropan	Does not apply to Ditropan XL
tolterodine	Detrol	Does not apply to Detrol LA
Muscle Relaxants—All cause anticholinergic adverse side effects		
cyclobenzaprine	Flexeril	
orphenadrine	Norflex	
methocarbamol	Robaxin	
carisoprodol	Soma	
Antiemetics		
trimethobenzamide	Tigan	Can cause extrapyramidal effects

*SIADH, syndrome of inappropriate antidiuretic hormone secretion.

CNS effects include: anxiety, depression, confusion, disorientation, forgetfulness, hallucinations, nightmares.

Anticholinergic effects include: blurred vision, confusion, disorientation, dry mouth, dry eyes, constipation, palpitations, worsening of glaucoma, urinary retention.

Based on Woodrow, R. (2007). *Essentials of pharmacology for health occupations* (5th ed.), Table 27-1. Clifton Park, NY: Delmar, Cengage Learning.

In addition, in 1997, an article appeared in *Archives of Internal Medicine* titled "Explicit Criteria for Determining Potentially Inappropriate Use by the Elderly." The article added medications to *The Gray List*, including: digoxin (Lanoxin) if the dose is greater than 0.125 mg per day for an extended period of time, unless a heart irregularity is being treated.

A list of medications that may cause mental impairment in elderly individuals, including confusion, disorientation, hallucinations, and nightmares, follows:

Aldomet	Compazine
Artane	Corgard
Benadryl	Dalmane
Bentyl	Desyrel
Cogentin	Dilantin

(continues)

Ditropan	Quinidine
Donnatal	Reglan
Elavil	Sinemet
Halcion	Sinequan
Haldol	Tagamet
Inderal	Tegretol
Lopressor	Tenormin
Mellaril	Thorazine
Pamelor	Timoptic
Phenergan	Tofranil
Prednisone	Xanax
Pro-Banthine	

When administering medications, UAPs must be aware of their responsibility to prevent adverse reactions. This is even more so when administering medications to individuals who are residents in nursing homes and who are 65 years of age and older.

Special considerations for administering medications to these individuals are as follows:

- With each licensed HCP order for a new medication, the UAP should note (1) the diagnosis the medication will treat, (2) the individual's allergies, and (3) if there are any special instructions for administration of the new medication.

- The UAP needs to know the adverse effects, cumulative effects, and medication interactions of all of the medications he is administering.

- The UAP needs to question an unusual dose or change in an individual's medication. For example, an individual's medication has always been a white-colored tablet. The UAP refills the prescription. The container of medication delivered by the pharmacy now has red tablets in it. The UAP needs to call the pharmacy to determine if this is the correct medication. If the licensed health care provider has changed the dose of the medication, the UAP needs to call the licensed health care provider to get an explanation for the change in the dose of the medication. The UAP *never* administers a medication without having basic knowledge and understanding.

- The UAP should document (1) all adverse reactions noted, (2) his call(s) to the individual's licensed HCP reporting the reactions, and (3) the actions taken as follow-up to the call.

- The UAP should report an individual's adverse reactions to the supervisor on duty per workplace policy.

MEDICATION ERRORS

medication error
A medication is not given as prescribed by the licensed health care provider.

A **medication error** is when a medication is *not* given as prescribed by the licensed health care provider. A medication error has occurred when one of the Six Rights of medication administration has been violated. When this occurs, the Six Rights become the **Six Wrongs**:

- The *Wrong Individual* was given medication. An individual was given another individual's medication.

- The *Wrong Medication* was given to an individual. An individual may be given a medication that was never prescribed for him.

- The *Wrong Dose* of medication was given to the individual. The individual was prescribed to receive 250 mg of a medication and instead received 500 mg of that medication.

- A medication was given at the *Wrong Time* or not given at all. This includes a forgotten or missed medication. The time a medication is to be given is based on the licensed health care provider's order. As stated in Chapter 6, once a medication is transcribed and a time is assigned for administration, there is a one (1)-hour window for administration. The UAP has from half an hour before until half an hour after the assigned time to administer the medication. Any time outside this time frame is considered a medication error—*wrong time.*

Note: In some work settings, UAPs have from one (1) hour before until one (1) hour after the assigned time to administer medication.

- A medication was given by the *Wrong Route.* For example, drops were placed in the ear rather than in the nose.

- *Wrong Documentation:* Documentation was completed incorrectly. For instance, the UAP documents at 12:00 p.m. (1200) that an individual has received his medication. The individual, however, is not due to receive his medication until 4:00 p.m. (1600). The UAP forgets to administer the individual's medication and goes off duty at 10:00 p.m. (2200). The staff coming on duty believes the individual has received his medication. The individual never receives his medication.

Special circumstances surrounding medication errors include:

- Medication found on the floor does not necessarily indicate that a medication error has occurred. Follow the policies of the work setting and state regulations regarding the reporting of such an occurrence.

- It is important that individuals do not miss medication doses. Therefore, do not skip a dose without first consulting the licensed health care provider, one's supervisor, and/or the pharmacist. Under certain circumstances, missed medications may still be administered.

- If the UAP notices missing prescription medication, he must notify his supervisor immediately and report the missing medication to his state agency per state regulation. Missing OTC medication must be reported to his supervisor immediately and may require internal investigation.

- Events that are not within the UAP's control, such as an individual's refusal to take a medication, are not medication errors. However, these events should immediately be reported to the UAP's supervisor.

Prevention of Medication Errors

The main way to prevent medication errors is to follow the principles of medication administration, as taught in Chapters 6 and 7. However, medication errors may also occur when a medication order is misinterpreted. Below are guidelines to help prevent the misinterpretation of an order:

- Never leave the decimal point naked. In other words, write 0.2 mg instead of writing .2 mg. Not doing so may mean that the staff person administering a medication may accidentally overlook the decimal point and administer 2 mg of a medication rather than 0.2 mg of a medication. This may result in an overdose. *Remember, always place a zero before a decimal point.*

- Never place a decimal point and a zero after a whole number. The decimal point may be missed and the zero misinterpreted. For example, 5.0 mg may be read to mean 50 mg. The correct way is to write 5 mg. *Remember, always leave a whole number standing alone. Do not use a decimal point with the whole number.*

- Avoid using decimals whenever whole numbers can be used as alternatives. For example, 0.5 g can be expressed as 500 mg. *Remember, use whole numbers whenever possible. Avoid using decimals.*

- *If the UAP has difficulty interpreting the spelling of a medication name or the number for the dose in an order or if the dose seems inappropriate, he should always question the order.* This is not only his duty as a UAP but also his ethical and legal responsibility to be sure that the medications administered are safe. If a medication error results in legal action, the UAP could be held accountable even though the licensed health care provider's order was written incorrectly. Questioning the order will protect the UAP.

Note: Remember, it is the responsibility of the UAP to have basic knowledge and understanding of the medications he is administering. The UAP may use reference books and materials to look up information. He may ask the licensed health care provider and/or pharmacist questions about the medications.

Reporting of Medication Errors

Although medication errors should not happen, honest mistakes do occur. When a medication error does happen, follow the steps below:

- First, take care of the individual. Make sure that he is safe. If need be, call for help. Get emergency care if needed.

- Once the individual is stable, notify the supervisor. Call the individual's licensed health care provider.

- Stay with the individual. Follow the licensed health care provider's orders. Observe the individual for signs of difficulty or adverse reactions to the medication that was administered.

- Complete a written report. Each state and work setting will have an established protocol for reporting errors.

Figure 30-1 is a copy of a medication error reporting form from the Massachusetts Department of Public Health. The form, titled "Medication Occurrence Report," is used in the Massachusetts Medication Administration Program. This is a program in which UAPs, once trained and certified, administer medications to adults living and working in community residential, day, and work programs that are licensed by the Massachusetts Departments of Mental Health or Developmental Services. The form is used to track medication errors in these settings.

MEDICATION RECONCILIATION

medication reconciliation
A method used to compare the medications an individual is taking to the medications ordered by the individual's licensed HCP.

Medication reconciliation is a method used to compare the medications an individual is taking to the medications ordered by the individual's licensed HCP. This comparison is done every time there is a change in the individual's care. For instance, medication reconciliation is done whenever an individual is admitted, transferred, or discharged. Medication reconciliation is done to prevent medication errors caused by omissions, duplications, errors in doses, or medication interactions (Joint Commission, 2010).

According to the Joint Commission (2010), medication reconciliation consists of five steps:

1. A list should be made of the medications an individual is currently taking.

2. A list should be made of the medications to be ordered by the individual's licensed HCP.

3. The licensed HCP should compare the medications on the two lists.

4. The licensed HCP should order medications for an individual based on the comparison of the two lists and the individual's clinical assessment.

5. The licensed HCP should communicate the new orders to the UAPs and to the individual.

Department of Public Health
Medication Administration Program
MEDICATION OCCURRENCE REPORT

Agency Name:_____ Name:_____
                                                (Consumer/Client)   Last   First
Site Address:_____ Date/Time of Occurrence:_____
            Street   Site Telephone Number(____)_____
                                                DPH Registration Number_____
            _____
            City/Town   Zip Code

TYPE of OCCURRENCE:
(As per regulation, contact consultant.)

(1)_____**Wrong Individual**   (4)_____**Wrong Dose**
(2)_____**Wrong Medication** (includes medication given without an order)   (5)_____**Wrong Route**
(3)_____**Wrong Time** (includes a "forgotten "dose)

MEDICATION(S) INVOLVED:

| | Name: | Dosage: | Frequency/Time: | Route: |

As Ordered:_____
As Given:_____
As Ordered:_____
As Given:_____
As Ordered:_____
As Given:_____

CONSULTANT CONTACTED
_____Registered Nurse   _____Registered Pharmacist   _____Licensed Practitioner

Name of Consultant:_____ Date Contacted:_____ Time Contacted:_____
                    Last   First
Recommended Action (Medical Intervention) _____Yes _____No
If Yes, check all those that apply:
(1)_____Lab Work or Other Tests (2)_____Physician Visit (3)_____Clinic Visit (4)_____Emergency Room Visit (5)_____Hospitalization
(6)_____Other (describe)_____

Did ☐ **medical intervention,** ☐ **illness,** ☐ **injury or** ☐ **death follow the Occurrence?** _____Yes _____No

If yes, notify DPH at (617) 983-6782 /FAX(617) 524-8062 within 24 hours. For ALL Occurrences,
forward written reports to your DMH/DMR MAP Coordinator within 7 days. (See reverse side for addresses.)

Supervisory Review/Follow-up
Contributing Factors: Check all that apply. If none apply, check none (g):

(a)___Failure to Accurately Record and/or Transcribe an Order   (d)___Medication Had Been Discontinued
(b)___Failure to Properly Document Administration   (e)___Improperly Labeled by Pharmacy
(c)___Medication Administered by Non-Certified Staff (Includes   (f)___Medication not Available (Explain below)
     instances where certification has expired or has been revoked) (g)___None

_____
_____
_____ **(If additional space is required, please use reverse side).**

Signature/Title:_____Print Name:_____Date:_____

0/30/96   **Occurrence Reporting is required by regulation at 105CMR 700.003(F)(1)(f).**
MAP9705.DOC   **Consultant Contact is required by regulation at 105CMR 700.003(F)(1)(g).**

DCP MAP Policy Manual May 2007

Figure 30-1 Massachusetts Department of Public Health, Medication Administration Program,
Medication Occurrence Report (reporting form used by UAPs to report medication errors in certain settings in the state of Massachusetts)

MEDICATION LOSSES

Whenever a medication is missing, a **medication loss** has occurred. Medication losses are serious. Medications that UAPs administer do have the potential to be abused by others. The medications, therefore, have value to the substance abuser as well as resale value on the street. When medications are missing, individuals no longer have the medications they need to keep themselves healthy and well. Depending on the type of insurance coverage an individual has, there may be difficulty in getting the medications replaced.

Most states have a process for reporting a medication loss. In the state of Massachusetts, as in some other states, the process requires that a form be completed and submitted. Figure 30-2 is a copy of a medication loss report form from the Massachusetts Department of Public Health (DPH), Division of Food and Drugs, Drug Control Program. The form, titled "Drug Incident Report," is used by DPH registrants to report drug losses.

Work settings also have policies and procedures for reporting medication losses. Most times, investigations will be performed to determine the cause of the loss. Laws permit the prosecution of individuals involved with or responsible for the loss of the medication.

UAPs need to know and follow the policies and procedures regarding the reporting of medication losses.

MEDICATION REFUSALS

Individuals refuse to take medications for many different reasons. Some of these reasons are:

1. The effects and side effects are unpleasant or unwanted.

2. The medications taste bad or leave an unpleasant taste in the individual's mouth.

3. The individual has difficulty swallowing the medication.

4. Religious beliefs.

5. Cultural beliefs.

6. Ethnic beliefs.

7. Moral beliefs.

8. Individual beliefs.

Each individual has different ideas and feelings about health, illness, and healing. At times, an individual may misunderstand the seriousness of a diagnosis and the medications prescribed for him. Other times, the individual may be in denial about the diagnosis and so will not take the medications or does not understand that the illness is chronic and will last a lifetime.

Whatever the issue may be, careful listening and attention to detail may help the UAP to better understand the individual. This understanding will provide the UAP with a foundation upon which he may be better able to explain to the individual the need for the medication and how the medication will work.

Department of Public Health
Division of Food and Drugs, Drug Control Program
DRUG INCIDENT REPORT

Pursuant to the Department's regulations at 105 CMR 700.005(D), registrants are required to report the loss of any controlled substances upon discovery. When a drug loss of discovered, kindly fill out this incident report and fax it to the Drug Control Program (617-524-8062) within twenty fours hours of discovery. Should you have questions or need to contact us, please see our website at www.mass.gov/dph/dcp or call 617-983-6700.

Date of Report	Report Prepared By	
Title	**Contact's Phone Number**	**Contact's e-mail**

Facility Information

Facility Name _____

Address _____

City _____ Zip Code _____

Facility Type

☐ Hospital ☐ Long Term Care ☐ Clinic ☐ Ambulance ☐ Manufacturer/Distributor

☐ MAP (DMR) ☐ MAP (DMH) ☐ Prison/House of Correction/Jail ☐ School

☐ Other (Please Specify) _____

Date of Loss	Specific location of loss (unit, floor, etc., if applicable)

Incident Type

☐ Diversion ☐ Loss ☐ Tampering ☐ Theft ☐ Documentation

☐ Other (Please Specify) _____

Drug (use additional sheets if needed)	Quantity	Strength	Dosage Form
_____	_____	_____	_____
_____	_____	_____	_____
_____	_____	_____	_____

Narrative (Please explain what happened, what factors may have contributed to loss, and any other relevant information. Please indicate if patient harm was involved. Please use additional sheets if necessary.)

_____
_____
_____
_____
_____
_____
_____
_____

For office use only

Received by Drug Unit	Staff initials	Intake number	Date facility contacted

Drug Incident Report   R20050817-01

Figure 30-2 Massachusetts Department of Public Health, Division of Food and Drugs, Drug Control Program, *Drug Incident Report* (reporting form used by the department's registrants to report missing medications)

These are some examples of individuals not wanting to take medication:

- An individual has high triglycerides and high cholesterol. He is at high risk for a stroke and/or heart attack. The licensed health care provider orders a medication to lower his cholesterol and places him on a special diet. However, the individual feels fine. He has no symptoms. He refuses to take the medication and refuses to follow the diet.

- An individual has schizophrenia. He is on medication to control the symptoms of his disease. He has been able to live alone and return to work. He feels that he has no symptoms at this time. He does not like taking medication when there is nothing wrong with him. He refuses to continue to take his medication.

- An individual has been diagnosed with depression. He is placed on an antidepressant. He is not permitted to drink alcohol while taking this medication. He does not like the fact that he cannot socialize with his friends on the weekends. The medication also affects his sexual drive. He does not like this effect. He refuses to take his medication.

- An individual is a diabetic. He has no symptoms of diabetes at this time. He feels well. He gets insulin on a daily basis by injection. Because he does not like getting an injection every day, he stops taking the insulin.

Active and Passive Refusals

active refusal
An individual directly refuses to take a medication.

passive refusal
The individual indirectly refuses to take the medication; for instance, the individual vomits his medication half an hour after taking it.

Individuals may actively or passively refuse to take a medication. **Active refusal** is when the individual directly refuses to take the medication. He may simply say "no" when the UAP goes to administer the medication. The individual may refuse to open his mouth when the UAP attempts to administer the medication.

Passive refusal requires closer observation and monitoring on the part of the UAP. Examples of passive refusal are:

- The individual takes the medication when offered by the UAP but then immediately spits the medication back out of his mouth.

- The individual takes the medication when offered by the UAP but at a later time spits the medication out; he may or may not try to hide the medication from the UAP.

- The individual takes the medication when offered by the UAP but then intentionally vomits within half an hour of taking the medications.

Ways to Deal with Refusals

To remain healthy, an individual does need to take his medications. This, of course, has to be balanced with an individual's right to refuse. To refuse care, however, an individual must be able to understand the consequences of his actions or inactions and must be informed of all possible outcomes of the refusal.

If an individual refuses his medications, here are a few questions the UAP should ask:

- Is the individual experiencing an unpleasant or unwanted side effect?

- Does the medication have an unpleasant taste, smell, or feel?

- Is the individual having difficulty swallowing the medication?

- Is the individual afraid of the medication for some reason? If so, why is he afraid of it?

- Is the individual refusing other medical care or just his medications?

Ways to deal with refusals include the following:

- If an individual refuses medication and does not give the UAP a specific reason for refusing, wait fifteen (15) minutes, then try to administer the medication again. If the individual refuses again, try again in another fifteen (15) minutes before considering this a final refusal.

- Notify one's supervisor immediately when an individual refuses to take medication.

- Notify the licensed health care provider of all medication refusals. It is very important that a licensed health care provider know when an individual is not taking his medication as prescribed. The licensed health care provider has the ability to make recommendations for administration of the medication, to change the way the medication is administered, or to change the medication to a new and different medication.

- Document all medication refusals on the medication sheet *and* in the progress notes.

- Observe and report any side effects of the medication, including the complaints the individual shares with the UAP about the medication.

- Consider changing the way the medication is given. Does the UAP always try to give the medication during the individual's favorite TV show? If the individual is currently getting the medication in solid form, would a liquid medication be better?

- Communicate with the licensed health care provider and the supervisor often. Both should know how the individual is doing.

- If refusal of medications becomes an ongoing problem, talk with the licensed health care team about the possibility of a consult with a social worker or behavior specialist.

- Be aware that some states have a law that may affect an individual's right to refuse antipsychotic medication.

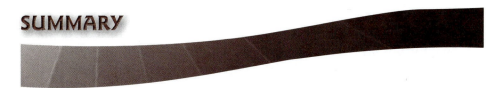

SUMMARY

Medication needs to be administered with careful planning and by following proper procedures. If medication is not given as ordered, there may be immediate and serious consequences on an individual's health. For example, a medication given incorrectly may result in an individual experiencing allergic reactions, side effects, medication interactions, and so on. The UAP needs to be observant. The UAP needs to know the emergency procedures for the setting in which he works. Emergency telephone numbers need to be posted near the telephones at his work site, including the telephone numbers for the Poison Control Center, police, ambulance, fire, and all designated numbers per the UAP's workplace policy.

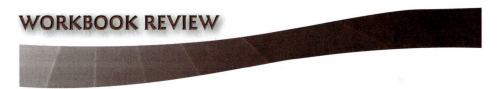

WORKBOOK REVIEW

Go to the workbook and complete the exercises for Chapter 30.

REVIEW QUESTIONS

1. In order to safely give an over-the-counter medication:
   a. obtain a licensed health care provider's order for each OTC medication to be given
   b. administer the medication according to the directions on the drug insert that accompanies the medication
   c. store OTC medications separate from prescription medications
   d. document OTC medication errors in the individual's progress notes
2. Synergism is:
   a. a medication reaction in which one medication prolongs or multiplies the effect of another medication
   b. a medication reaction in which one medication decreases or stops the effect of another medication
   c. a medication reaction in which one medication helps another for an effect that neither one could produce alone
   d. all of the above

3. Potentiation is:
   a. a medication reaction in which one medication prolongs or multiplies the effect of another medication
   b. a medication reaction in which one medication decreases or stops the effect of another medication
   c. a medication reaction in which one medication helps another for an effect that neither one could produce alone
   d. all of the above

4. Adverse effects:
   a. are minor reactions that need not be reported to the licensed HCP
   b. include physical or psychological dependence
   c. do not require documentation
   d. occur less as an individual ages

5. Anaphylaxis occurs most commonly:
   a. in the elderly
   b. with antibiotics, X-ray dyes containing iodide, and certain foods
   c. in children
   d. in the southeastern portion of the United States

6. A cumulative effect of a medication in an elderly individual is due to:
   a. adequate absorption
   b. the individual's ability to consume large amounts of fluid
   c. impaired excretion
   d. faster metabolism

7. A medication error occurs:
   a. any time a medication causes an adverse reaction
   b. when an individual refuses to take a medication
   c. if a medication is found on the floor
   d. any time a medication has not been given as prescribed by the licensed health care provider

8. To prevent medication errors:
   a. never use zeros
   b. never leave whole numbers standing alone
   c. use decimals whenever possible
   d. always question the order if you cannot interpret the medication name or dosage number or if the dose seems inappropriate

9. Reporting a medication error includes:
   a. blaming the individual because you have to do extra paperwork
   b. calling the individual's licensed health care provider to notify him of the error
   c. providing first aid even if one is not trained to do so
   d. completing a written report only if the individual has a reaction to the wrong medication administered

10. An individual's right to refuse a medication can be exercised when:
    a. he has a mental illness and does not want to take his medications
    b. he is able to understand the consequences of refusing his medication and all possible outcomes of the refusal
    c. he does not have any active symptoms
    d. he does not like the taste of his medication

CLINICAL SCENARIOS

1. During your shift you notice that you are missing 10 tablets of Ativan 1 mg. What is the first thing you should do? If the medication cannot be found, what must you do next?

2. Mr. Oliver has a prescription for a blood pressure medication. When you bring his medication to him, he tells you that he is not going to take it because he feels fine. As a UAP, what questions can you ask him? How could you deal with his refusal?

Chapter 31
Poison Control

Learning Objectives

After reading this chapter and completing the review exercises, you should be able to:

1. Spell and define terms.
2. List two groups of individuals at the greatest risk for accidental poisoning.
3. List four forms poisons are found in.
4. List ten of the most dangerous poisons.
5. Explain why prevention is the best form of treatment.
6. Describe the treatment for ingestion of a poison.
7. Describe the treatment for the inhalation of a poison.
8. Describe the treatment for poisoning of the skin and eyes.
9. List the steps for the emergency care of an individual with an accidental poisoning.
10. List the documentation guidelines for an accidental poisoning.
11. Describe a poison control center.

Key Terms

dermal exposure

ingestion

inhalation

ocular exposure

poison

vomitus

INTRODUCTION

Most poisonings are unintentional and accidental. According to the American Association of Poison Control Centers (AAPCC), there are nearly 2.5 million poison exposures reported every year in the United States. Of these exposures, adults over 19 years of age account for 91% of the deaths. Children and youth under 19 years of age account for 9% of the deaths. Children under the age of 6 are at the greatest risk. In fact, in the United States a child is poisoned every thirty (30) seconds (AAPCC, 2009).

A second group at risk for poisoning is the elderly. Medication overdoses may result in toxicity, leaving the elder confused, dizzy, weak, lethargic, and experiencing impaired coordination, tremors, and cardiac problems. An elder is at risk because:

- Medication may build up in the elder's body because of a slowdown in metabolism, impaired circulation, and changes in excretion.

- Incorrect dosing may occur because of poor vision or poor memory (the elder may have forgotten that she has taken her medication and take a double dose).

- Elders may self-administer many different prescription, herbal, and over-the-counter medications that may interact with each other.

- Elders may have medical conditions that affect the absorption of medication.

POISONS

ingestion
Taking a substance into the body by swallowing.

inhalation
Taking a substance into the body by breathing.

ocular exposure
Taking a substance into the body through the eyes.

dermal exposure
Taking a substance into the body through the skin.

A **poison** may be defined as any substance that can cause harmful effects in the body. A poison may be anything one eats (**ingestion**), breathes (**inhalation**), gets in the eyes (**ocular exposure**), or gets on the skin (**dermal exposure**) (AAPCC, 2009).

Poisons are found in four different forms:

- Solids

- Liquids: May cause damage quickly because a large amount of liquid may be swallowed in a short period of time and liquids are absorbed quickly

- Sprays

- Invisible: Gas or vapors, such as carbon monoxide and exhaust fumes from automobiles

Types of Poisons

According to the AAPCC, the most dangerous poisons may be:

- Medications:
    a. Pain medications, including OTC, prescriptions, and illegal medications
    b. Sedatives and hypnotics
    c. Antipsychotic medications

    d. Cardiovascular medications, including heart and blood pressure medications

    e. Antidepressants

    f. Iron supplements: According to the FDA, iron tablets are the leading cause of poisoning death in children under 6 years of age

    g. Alcohol

- Household products: Very caustic and leave scarring and other damage:
  a. Drain cleaners
  b. Oven cleaners
  c. Toilet bowl cleaners
  d. Furniture polish
  e. Pesticides
  f. Gasoline, kerosene
  g. Lamp oil
  h. Tiki-torch oil
  i. Antifreeze
  j. Windshield solution

- Personal care products:
  a. Mouthwash
  b. Nail polish remover
  c. Permanent wave solutions
  d. Hair removal products

- Plants:
  a. Wild mushrooms
  b. Philodendron
  c. Pokeweed
  d. Foxglove
  e. Holly berries
  f. Castor bean
  g. Dieffenbachia

- Environmental poisons:
  a. Carbon monoxide
  b. Lead paint
  c. Mercury

TREATMENT FOR POISONING

Prevention

The best treatment for poisoning is to prevent the poisoning in the first place. Figure 31-1 provides a list of tips from the American Medical Association to prevent poisoning.

    Many educational programs teach children, families, and elders about the prevention of poisonings and safe medication administration. One such educational program, "Mr. Yuk," is a warning sticker that may be applied to dangerous products (Figure 31-2). "Mr. Yuk" warns children

PATIENT EDUCATION CONCERNING POISONS

Public education is of greatest importance in preventing poisoning. The general public must be instructed in safety precautions with medications, and it is especially important to inform the parents and caretakers of young children and older adults. It is the responsibility of all health care workers to provide the necessary information to help prevent poisoning.

To prevent poisoning, the American Medical Association recommends the following precautions:

1. Keep all medicines, household chemicals, cleaning supplies, and pesticides in a locked cupboard. There is no place that is "out of reach of children."

2. Never transfer poisonous substances to unlabeled containers or to food containers such as milk or soda bottles or cereal boxes. Keep in original labeled container.

3. Never store poisonous substances in the same area with food. Confusion could be fatal.

4. Never reuse containers of chemical products.

5. When discarding medication, always flush down the toilet. Never discard it in a wastebasket.

6. Do not give or take medications in the dark.

7. Never leave medications on a bedside stand. Confusion while an individual is sleepy could result in a fatal overdose.

8. Always read the label before taking any medication or pouring any solution for ingestion.

9. Never tell children the medicine you are giving them is candy.

10. When preparing a baby's formula, taste the ingredients. Never store boric acid, salt, or talcum near the formula ingredients.

11. Never give or take any medication that is discolored, has a strange odor, or is outdated.

12. Don't take medicine in front of children.

13. Keep pocketbooks, purses, and pillboxes out of reach of children.

14. Rinse out containers thoroughly before disposing of them.

Figure 31–1 **Education concerning poisons** *(Source: Woodrow, R. (2007) Essentials of Pharmacology for health professions (5th ed). pages 144–145. Clifton Park, NY: Delmar, Cengage Learning.)*

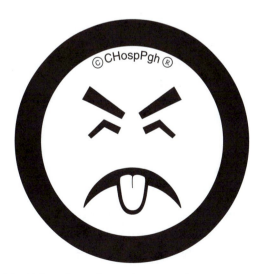

Figure 31–2 Mr. Yuk and similar stickers may be obtained from many poison control centers throughout the United States. The telephone number of the nearest poison control center is frequently printed on these stickers *(Permission to reproduce Mr. Yuk has been granted by Children's Hospital of Pittsburgh)*

who cannot read that a product is dangerous and may harm them. These stickers are available through poison control centers throughout the United States.

Treatment for Ingestion of a Poison

The most common type of poisoning is by ingestion. If an individual swallows the wrong medication or takes too much of a medication, immediately call the poison control center or the individual's licensed HCP. If an individual swallows a substance that is not food or medication, have the individual drink a small amount of milk or water and immediately call the poison control center or the individual's licensed HCP. *Do not administer ipecac syrup!* (AAPCC 2009).

Before 2004, ipecac syrup was used to cause vomiting in individuals who had ingested certain poisons. However, extensive research has found this practice to be ineffective and at times harmful. Therefore, in early 2004, the American Academy of Pediatrics (AAP) issued a policy statement against keeping ipecac syrup in the home and requesting that ipecac syrup presently in homes be discarded. Ipecac syrup is no longer the drug of choice for treating poison by ingestion.

Treatment for Inhalation of a Poison

When treating an individual for inhalation of a poison, the licensed health care provider treats the individual's symptoms. Fresh air, oxygen, and CPR are provided as needed. If the individual inhaled an insect spray, an antidote may need to be administered at the emergency medical care center.

Treatment for Poisoning of Skin and Eyes

If a poison enters the eyes or gets onto the skin, the eyes or skin should be immediately flushed with a constant flow of water for a minimum of fifteen (15) minutes. The individual must then be immediately transported to the nearest emergency medical care center for treatment. If the poison was absorbed through the skin into the body, an antidote may need to be administered at the emergency medical care center.

EMERGENCY CARE FOR AN ACCIDENTAL POISONING

Before an emergency ever occurs at the workplace, the UAP must know the emergency procedures at her workplace. The telephone numbers for the poison control center and the nearest emergency medical care center should be at each telephone in the workplace for easy access during an emergency. If possible, program the phone number for the poison control center into the phone at the workplace and the individual's home.

If a poisoning occurs, the UAP should follow these steps:

1. Remain calm.

2. Call 911 or the local emergency services telephone number if the individual:

   - Has collapsed

   - Is having a seizure

   - Is unconscious

   - Is not breathing or does not have a pulse.

Note: **If the UAP is certified in CPR and/or first aid, the UAP should provide care as she was trained.**

3. Remain with the individual at all times.

4. If an individual swallows the wrong medication or takes too much of a medication, immediately call the poison control center or the individual's licensed HCP. *Do not administer ipecac syrup!*

5. If an individual swallows a substance that is not food or medication, have the individual drink a small amount of milk or water. Immediately call the poison control center or the individual's licensed HCP. *Do not administer ipecac syrup!*

6. If the individual has inhaled a poison, get the individual to fresh air right away.

7. If the poison is on the skin, remove the individual's clothing and rinse the skin for at least fifteen (15) minutes.

8. If the poison is in the eye(s), flush the eyes for at least fifteen (15) minutes using large cups of lukewarm water held two (2) to four (4) inches away from the eye(s) and poured steadily across the eye(s).

9. Call the local poison control center or the individual's licensed health care provider.

10. Have the following information ready:

    - Name of the product and its ingredients

    - Amount of the product that was consumed

    - Time that the poisoning occurred

    - Location and phone number of the UAP's workplace

    - Age of the individual

    - Individual's condition; if possible, include the individual's vital signs

    - Weight and height of the individual

11. Follow the instructions of the poison control center and/or the licensed HCP.

12. Wash hands.

13. Transport the individual to the nearest emergency medical care enter. If the individual has vomited, take her **vomitus** to the center with her.

vomitus
The material vomited by an individual.

14. On return to the workplace, document per workplace policy.

Note: Many products have incorrect or outdated first aid instructions. The UAP needs to call either the individual's licensed health care provider for orders or the local poison control center.

Documentation Guidelines for Emergency Care of the Individual

When documenting emergency care of an individual for an episode of poisoning, the UAP needs to document the following information:

- Time and date of the accidental poisoning
- The individual's condition at the time of the poisoning
- The name of the harmful substance and the amount taken
- Circumstances of the accidental poisoning
- Names of the individuals who were with the individual at the time of the accident if the individual was not alone
- Care provided and individual's response to care provided

In addition to completing a progress note, the UAP needs to complete an incident report per workplace policy.

POISON CONTROL CENTERS

Poison control centers are located throughout the United States. Some centers are certified. Some centers are not certified. For quick reference, Figure 31-3 provides a map of poison control centers throughout the United States along with a list of detailed coverage information (AAPCC, 2009).

A poison control center is staffed with specially trained doctors, pharmacists, and registered nurses. The center is available twenty-four (24) hours a day, seven (7) days a week, 365 days a year. The centers provide emergency information and may refer the UAP or an individual to a licensed health care provider or to the local emergency medical care center. The poison control centers do not charge a fee for their service.

The specialists at the center are trained to provide information and treatment recommendations for a variety of concerns, including:

- Treatment for poisons
- Bites and stings
- Food poisoning
- Occupational poisoning

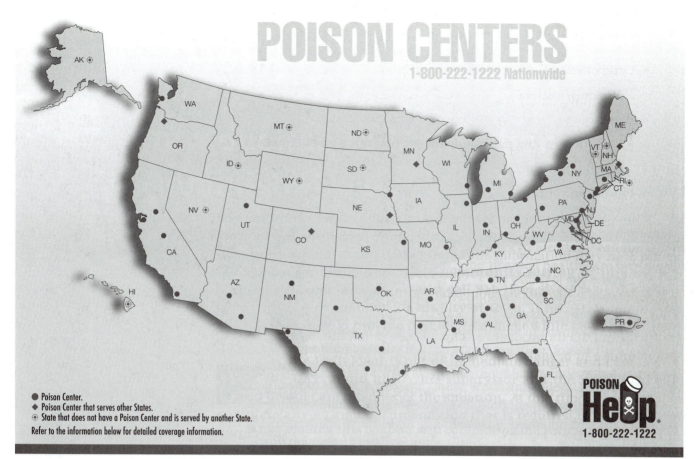

POISON CENTERS
1-800-222-1222 Nationwide

- ● Poison Center.
- ◆ Poison Center that serves other States.
- ✷ State that does not have a Poison Center and is served by another State.

Refer to the information below for detailed coverage information.

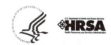

POISON Help ®
1-800-222-1222

Alabama
Regional Poison Control Center
Alabama Poison Center

Alaska ✷
Served by OR (Oregon Poison Center)

Arizona
Arizona Poison & Drug Information Center
Banner Poison Control Center

Arkansas
Arkansas Poison & Drug Information Center

California
California Poison Control System (locations in
Sacramento, San Francisco, Fresno and San Diego)

Colorado ◆
Rocky Mountain Poison & Drug Center
  serving CO, HI, ID, MT & NV

Connecticut
Connecticut Poison Control Center

Delaware ✷
Served by PA (Poison Control Center at
  the Children's Hospital of Philadelphia)

District of Columbia ◆
National Capital Poison Center
  serving DC, MD & VA

Florida
Florida Poison Information Center - Miami
Florida Poison Information Center - Jacksonville
Florida Poison Information Center - Tampa

Georgia
Georgia Poison Center

Hawaii ✷
Served by CO (Rocky Mountain Poison & Drug Center)

Idaho ✷
Served by CO (Rocky Mountain Poison & Drug Center)

Illinois
Illinois Poison Center

Indiana
Indiana Poison Center

Iowa
Iowa Statewide Poison Control Center

Kansas
Kansas Poison Control Center

Kentucky
Kentucky Regional Poison Center

Louisiana
Louisiana Drug & Poison Information Center

Maine ◆
Northern New England Poison Center
  serving ME, NH & VT

Maryland
Maryland Poison Center
Also served by DC (National Capital Poison Center)

Massachusetts ◆
Regional Center for Poison Control & Prevention
  serving MA & RI

Michigan
DeVos Children's Hospital Regional Poison Center
Children's Hospital of Michigan Regional
  Poison Control Center

Minnesota ◆
Hennepin Regional Poison Control Center
  serving MN, ND & SD

Mississippi
Mississippi Poison Control Center

Missouri
Missouri Regional Poison Center

Montana ✷
Served by CO (Rocky Mountain Poison & Drug Center)

Nebraska ◆
Nebraska Regional Poison Center
  serving NE & WY

Nevada ✷
Served by CO (Rocky Mountain Poison & Drug Center)

New Hampshire ✷
Served by ME (Northern New England Poison Center)

New Jersey
New Jersey Poison Information & Education System

New Mexico
New Mexico Poison & Drug Information Center

New York
Upstate New York Poison Center
Ruth A. Lawrence Poison and Drug Information Center
Long Island Regional Poison and Drug Information Center
New York City Poison Control Center
Western New York Poison Center

North Carolina
Carolinas Poison Center

North Dakota ✷
Served by MN (Hennepin Regional Poison Center)

Ohio
Greater Cleveland Poison Control Center
Cincinnati Drug & Poison Information Center
Central Ohio Poison Center

Oklahoma
Oklahoma Poison Control Center

Oregon ◆
Oregon Poison Center
  serving OR & AK

Pennsylvania ◆
Pittsburgh Poison Center
Poison Control Center at the Children's Hospital
  of Philadelphia serving PA & DE

Puerto Rico
Puerto Rico Poison Center

Rhode Island ✷
Served by MA (Regional Center for Poison Control
  & Prevention)

South Carolina
Palmetto Poison Center

South Dakota ✷
Served by MN (Hennepin Regional Poison Control Center)

Tennessee
Tennessee Poison Center

Texas
Texas Panhandle Poison Center
North Texas Poison Center
Central Texas Poison Center
Southeast Texas Poison Center
West Texas Regional Poison Center
South Texas Poison Center

Utah
Utah Poison Control Center

Vermont ✷
Served by ME (Northern New England Poison Center)

Virginia
Virginia Poison Center
Blue Ridge Poison Center
Also served by DC (National Capital Poison Center)

Washington
Washington Poison Center

West Virginia
West Virginia Poison Center

Wisconsin
Wisconsin Poison Center

Wyoming ✷
Served by NE (Nebraska Regional Poison Center)

HRSA
U.S. Department of Health and Human Services
Health Resources and Services Administration

PoisonHelp.hrsa.gov

Figure 31-3 A map of poison control centers throughout the United States along with a list of detailed coverage
information *(AAPCC, 2009)*

- Drug overdose

- Pill identification

- Plants

- Medication interactions and adverse reactions (side effects)

- Animal poisoning

- Poison prevention

The telephone number for the local poison control center may be found on the inside cover of the local telephone book or on the Internet at http://www.aapcc.org. Keep the telephone number near every telephone at the workplace and home for easy access during an emergency. If possible, program the phone number for the poison control center into the phone at the workplace and the individual's home.

SUMMARY

The UAP plays an important role at her workplace in preventing accidental poisonings. By following the recommendations from the AAPCC and the American Medical Association, the UAP can create a safe environment for the individuals she cares for. In addition, knowing the emergency procedures for her workplace before an emergency arises will allow the UAP to give care when needed in a timely fashion. Doing so can decrease the severity of any injuries should an accidental poisoning occur.

WORKBOOK REVIEW

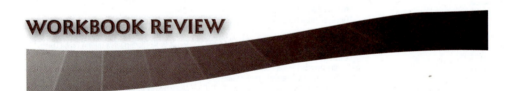

Go to the workbook and complete the exercises for Chapter 31.

REVIEW QUESTIONS

1. The group at the greatest risk for poisoning is:
   a. the elderly
   b. children under 6 years old
   c. children over 6 years old
   d. healthy adults

2. Elderly individuals are most at risk for poisoning from:
   a. household products
   b. personal care products
   c. environmental poisons
   d. medications
3. According to the FDA, the leading cause of poisoning death in children under 6 years of age is:
   a. ingestion of iron tablets
   b. ingestion of mouthwash
   c. ingestion of lead paint
   d. inhalation of insect spray
4. The best treatment for poisoning is:
   a. syrup of ipecac
   b. fresh air and oxygen
   c. prevention
   d. several 8- to 16-ounce glasses of water
5. The most common method of poisoning is by:
   a. inhalation
   b. ingestion
   c. absorption through the skin
   d. exposure of the eyes
6. If an individual takes too much medication, the first step the UAP should take is:
   a. immediately call the poison control center or the individual's licensed HCP
   b. have the individual drink a small amount of milk or water
   c. drive the individual to the nearest medical care center
   d. call 911 and begin CPR and/or first aid
7. If the individual has inhaled a poison:
   a. have the individual drink a small amount of milk or water
   b. immediately drive the individual to the nearest emergency medical care center
   c. call 911 and begin CPR and/or first aid
   d. get the individual to fresh air right away
8. If the individual gets a poison on her skin:
   a. observe the individual for twenty-four (24) hours
   b. arrange an appointment with her licensed HCP within three (3) days
   c. remove the individual's clothing and rinse the skin for at least fifteen (15) minutes
   d. get the individual to fresh air right away
9. If an individual gets a poison in her eyes:
   a. observe her for twenty-four (24) hours
   b. immediately drive her to the nearest emergency medical care center
   c. wash her eyes and the areas around her eyes with a mild soap and warm water solution then rinse well
   d. flush her eyes for at least fifteen (15) minutes using large cups of lukewarm water held two (2) to four (4) inches away from the eye(s) and poured steadily across the eye(s)

10. If an individual has vomited and is being taken to an emergency medical care center, the UAP needs to bring:

    a. the individual's vomitus

    b. the individual's medical record

    c. the address and phone number of the UAP's workplace

    d. the individual's photo identification

CLINICAL SCENARIOS

1. You are working at a group home. Part of your assignment today is to give care to Mary, a woman who has been showing signs of depression. You notice that she has not yet gotten up this morning, which is unusual for her. You enter her room. You find her lying on her bed with her eyes closed. As you approach her, you notice that she is unusually quiet and still. You kick something on the floor. You pick it up. It is a prescription pill bottle that is empty. You check the label. You see that it contained 30 tablets of Valium. When you get to Mary and try to wake her, you realize that she is not breathing.

    a. What do you do first?

    b. What do you do next?

    c. Describe the emergency care you should give to Mary.

    d. Write a note describing the event. Use today's date and the occurrence time of 7:30 a.m.

2. You are working at a day program. You are in the kitchen with John and Ted. John is preparing a bleach solution for sanitizing the sink. He accidentally pours full-concentration bleach on his arm. He is wearing a long-sleeved shirt.

    a. What do you do?

    b. Write a note documenting the event. Use today's date and the occurrence time of 1:30 p.m.

MODULE VII
Additional Knowledge and Skills

Chapter 32
Mathematics: Weights and Measures

Learning Objectives

After reading this chapter and completing the review questions, you should be able to:

1. Spell and define terms.
2. Express Arabic numerals as Roman numerals.
3. Express Roman numerals as Arabic numerals.
4. Define the apothecary system.
5. Define the household system.
6. Define the metric system.
7. Calculate oral forms of adult medication dosages.

Key Terms

apothecary system	household system	meter	Roman numerals
Arabic numerals	liter	numerals	volume
gram	metric system		

INTRODUCTION

Preparing and administering medications is a task the UAP will be asked to do in his work as a caregiver. Giving medications safely to another individual is a big responsibility. The UAP will need to be able to give the correct dose according to the licensed health care provider's order. Depending on the UAP's state regulations and workplace policies, this may mean that the UAP may need to measure or calculate the amount of medication to be given. The medication may be a liquid or a solid. If the medication is not measured correctly, the individual may have a bad reaction or become ill.

NUMERALS

Numerals are part of an organized system for counting. Both Arabic and Roman numerals belong to this system. "1," "2," and "3" are examples of **Arabic numerals**. "I," "II," and "III" are examples of **Roman numerals**. Medication orders are usually written in Arabic numerals. Roman numerals, however, may also be used at times for medication orders. Table 32-1 provides a list of Arabic and Roman numerals. Table 32-2 provides a list of

Table 32-1 Arabic and Roman Numerals

ARABIC NUMERALS	ROMAN NUMERALS
1	I
2	II
3	III
4	IV
5	V
6	VI
7	VII
8	VIII
9	IX
10	X
50	L
100	C
500	D
1000	M

Delmar/Cengage Learning

Table 32-2 Roman Numerals Commonly Used in Medication Orders and Their Arabic Equivalents

ROMAN NUMERALS	ARABIC EQUIVALENT
I	1
II	2
III	3
IV	4
V	5
VI	6
VII	7
VIII	8
IX	9
X	10

Delmar/Cengage Learning

Roman numerals commonly used in medication orders and their Arabic equivalents.

MEASUREMENT SYSTEMS

The health care industry uses three systems of measurement. These systems are as follows:

- Apothecary system
- Household system
- Metric system

Apothecary System

The **apothecary system** is the old pharmacy system. The apothecary system is rarely used today. However, because the apothecary system is used at times, it is important for the UAP to be familiar with the system. Table 32-3 provides a list of terms and abbreviations used for weight and **volume** in the apothecary system.

volume
The amount of space occupied by a liquid.

Household System

Although the **household system** is not widely used throughout the health care industry, the UAP may find that he uses household measures when he is working in a home care setting or when he is instructing an individual in self-administration. Household measures are estimates only. Most of the tools used are not the exact same size in every household and are not accurate enough to measure medication. For example, a household teaspoon may hold 4 mL of liquid or more than 5 mL of liquid. It all depends on the size of the teaspoon being used. The standard set by the American Standards Institute for an American teaspoon is 5 mL.

The difference is especially noted when administering medications by dropper. Drop sizes differ from dropper to dropper. Because of this fact, it is important to use the dropper that comes with the medication.

Table 32-3 A List of Terms and Abbreviations Used for Weight and Volume in the Apothecary System

APOTHECARY SYSTEM OF WEIGHT		APOTHECARY SYSTEM OF VOLUME	
TERM	ABBREVIATION	TERM	ABBREVIATION
dram	dr	fluidounce	floz
grain	gr	fluidram	fldr
ounce	oz	gallon	gal
pound	lb	minim	m
		pint	pt
		quart	qt

Delmar/Cengage Learning

Table 32-4 Household System Abbreviations with Equivalents

MEASUREMENT	ABBREVIATION	EQUIVALENT
drop	gtt	Depends on the size of the drop
ounce	oz	2T, 6 tsp
teaspoon	t or tsp	60 gtt
tablespoon	T or tbsp	3 tsp
teacup	tcp	6 oz
cup or glass	C	8 oz
pint	pt	16 oz, 2 cups
quart	qt	32 oz, 2 pt, 4 cups
gallon	gal	128 oz, 4 qt, 16 cups

Delmar/Cengage Learning

In addition, the size of a drop depends on the following factors:

• The size of the hole in the dropper

• The angle at which the dropper is held; for proper use of a dropper refer to Chapter 7, "Administration of Nonparenteral Medication"

• The pressure used to squeeze the dropper

• The thickness of the liquid

• The temperature of the liquid

Table 32-4 gives a list of household abbreviations with equivalents.

Figure 32-1 illustrates a comparison of drops, teaspoons, tablespoons, ounces, and cup.

Metric System

The **metric system** is widely used when ordering and measuring medications. The metric system is a decimal system based on 10 or multiples of 10. The basic units of the metric system are **gram** for weight, **liter** for volume, and **meter** for length.

Common Metric Prefixes

Below is a list of prefixes that can be used with any metric unit of measure—grams, liters, or meters.

• Milli: one-thousandth of a unit, written as 0.001

• Kilo: 1,000 units, written as 1,000

Table 32-5 gives a list of the basic metric units for weight and volume.

Table 32-6 gives a list of common metric equivalents.

Table 32-7 gives a list of common equivalents in metric, apothecary, and household for liquids.

Table 32-8 gives a list of common equivalents in metric and apothecary for solids.

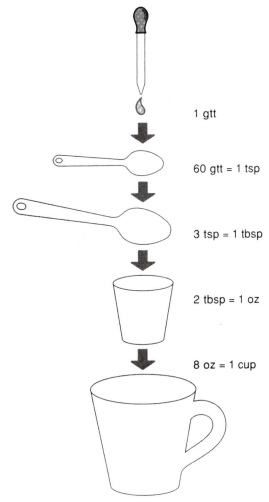

Figure 32-1 Comparing household measurements

Table 32-5 Basic Metric Units for Weight and Volume

WEIGHT		
TERM	**ABBREVIATION**	**EQUIVALENT**
milligram	mg	0.001 of a gram
gram	g	1000 milligrams
kilogram	kg	1000 grams
VOLUME		
TERM	**ABBREVIATION**	**EQUIVALENT**
milliliter	mL	0.001 of a liter
liter	L	1000 milliliters
kiloliter	kL	1000 liters

Delmar/Cengage Learning

Table 32-6 Common Metric Equivalents

Length
2.5 centimeters (cm) = 1 inch (in.)
Volume
1000 milliliters (ml) = 1 liter (L)
Weight
1 kilogram = 2.2 pounds (lb)
Delmar/Cengage Learning

Table 32-7 Common Equivalents in Metric, Apothecary and Household Systems for Liquids

METRIC	APOTHECARY	HOUSEHOLD
1 ml	15 m	
5 ml	1 dr	1 tsp
15 ml	4 dr	1 tbsp
30 ml	1 oz	2 tbsp
240 ml	8 oz	1 measuring cup (240 ml)
500 ml	1 pt (16 oz)	1 pt
1,000 ml	1 qt (32 oz)	1 qt

Based on Woodrow, R. (2007). *Essentials of pharmacology for health occupations* (5th ed.), Table 5-3. Clifton Park, NY: Delmar, Cengage Learning.

Table 32-8 Common Equivalents in Metric and Apothecary Systems for Solids

METRIC (GRAMS)	METRIC (MILLIGRAMS)	APOTHECARY
1 g	1,000 mg	15 gr
0.6 g	600 mg	10 gr
0.5 g	500 mg	7½ gr
0.3 g	300–325 mg	5 gr
0.2 g	200 mg	3 gr
0.1 g	100 mg	1½ gr
0.06 g	60–65 mg	1 gr
0.05 g	50 mg	3/4 gr
0.03 g	30 mg	1/2 gr
	0.4 mg	1/150 gr

Based on Woodrow, R. (2007). *Essentials of pharmacology for health occupations* (5th ed.), Table 5-4. Clifton Park, NY: Delmar, Cengage Learning.

CALCULATING ORAL FORMS OF ADULT DOSES

Oral medications are available in solid and liquid forms. There will be times when the amount of the solid or liquid oral medication that the UAP has on hand does not match the amount ordered by an individual's licensed HCP. When this happens, the UAP will need to determine how much medication to administer to the individual. There are several ways to determine the amount of medication to administer. Two ways to do this are as follows:

1. Use of the formula **"dose = strength × amount"** (see Example 1)

2. Use of the formula **"Desired/Have × Quantity"** (see Example 2)

Note: According to the National Counsel on State Boards of Nursing, Certified Medication Assistants (MA-C) do not calculate or convert medication dosages (National Council of State Boards of Nursing Delegate Assembly, 2007).

EXAMPLE 1:

The licensed health care provider orders 500 mg of Principen (ampicillin sodium) capsules. The dose on hand is 250-mg capsules.

"dose = strength × amount"

500 mg = 250 mg × 2

The *dose* is found in the licensed health care provider's order. Usually the dose is written right after the name of the medication. For example, in the order below,

Principen (ampicillin sodium) 500 mg by mouth q6h

the dose is *500 mg*.

The *strength* is found on the pharmacy label after the name of the medication. The strength is the measurement in which each unit of medication is available. For example, on a pharmacy label stating,

Principen (ampicillin sodium) 250 mg

the strength is *250 mg*. This means that each capsule in the bottle has 250 mg of Principen (ampicillin sodium) in it. Therefore, two capsules would be needed to satisfy the licensed health care provider's order calling for 500 mg of Principen (ampicillin sodium).

The licensed health care provider's order gives the UAP the written instructions for administering or giving a medication(s). The pharmacy label provides the UAP with a way to identify the medication he is giving. The *amount* to be given is found in the licensed health care provider's order as well as on the pharmacy label. The amount is the number of units of medication that are to be given. The amount may be the number of pills, tablets, capsules, and so on. For example, in the order below,

Principen (ampicillin sodium) two capsules by mouth every six (6) hours

the amount given each time the medication is given is *two capsules*.

EXAMPLE 2:

The licensed health care provider orders 100 mg of Topamax tablets. The dose on hand is 50-mg tablets.

"D/H × Q"

100 mg/50 mg = 2

First, figure out the amount of medication ordered and the amount of medication on hand. If the medications are not in the same unit of measure, contact the individual's licensed HCP, pharmacist, or other clinician for assistance in calculating the dose.

Next, place the information into the formula "D/H × Q" as above. The amount of medication *ordered* by the individual's licensed HCP is *100 mg*. The amount of medication *on hand* is *50 mg*.

Complete the calculation by *dividing* the amount on hand into the amount ordered by the individual's licensed HCP.

The result is the *quantity* to be administered: *two tablets of Topamax.*

Both of these formulas may be used to determine the amount of liquid medication to administer.

EXAMPLE 3:

The licensed health care provider orders Penicillin VK oral suspension 250 mg × ten (10) days. The dose on hand is 125 mg/5 mL.

"dose = strength × amount"

250 mg = 125 mg/5 mL × 2

The *dose* is found in the licensed health care provider's order. Usually the dose is written right after the name of the medication. For example, in the order below,

Penicillin VK oral suspension 250 mg q6h × ten (10) days

the dose is *250 mg.*

The *strength* is found on the pharmacy label, after the name of the medication. The strength is the measurement in which each unit of medication is available. For example, on a pharmacy label stating,

Penicillin VK oral suspension 125 mg/5 mL

the strength is *125 mg/5 mL*. This means that each 5 mL in the bottle has 125 mg of Penicillin VK oral suspension in it. Therefore, 10 mL would be needed to satisfy the licensed health care provider's order calling for 250 mg of Penicillin VK oral suspension.

The licensed health care provider's order gives the UAP the written instructions for administering or giving a medication(s). The pharmacy label provides the UAP with a way to identify the medication he is giving. The *amount* to be given is found in the licensed health care provider's order as well as on the pharmacy label. The amount is the number of units of medication that are to be given. The amount may be the number of pills, tablets, capsules, and so on. For example, in the order below,

Penicillin VK oral suspension 250 mg q6h for ten (10) days

the pharmacy label tells how many teaspoons, tablespoons, or mL to give,

Take 2 teaspoons (10 mL) by mouth every six (6) hours

the *amount* given each time the medication is given *2 teaspoons (10 mL).*

EXAMPLE 4:

The licensed health care provider orders 400 mg ibuprofen suspension q4h as needed for knee pain. The dose on hand is 100 mg/5 mL:

"D/H × Q"

400 mg/100 mg = 4

4 × 5 mL = 20 mL

First, figure out the amount medication ordered and the amount of medication on hand. If the medications are not in the same unit of measure, contact the individual's licensed HCP, pharmacist, or other clinician for assistance in calculating the dose.

Next, place the information into the formula "D/H × Q" as above. The amount of medication *ordered* by the individual's licensed HCP is *400 mg*. The amount of medication *on hand* is *100 mg/5 mL*.

Complete the calculation by *dividing* the amount of milligrams on hand into the amount of milligrams ordered by the individual's licensed HCP. Multiply the quantity by the number of milliliters (mL) per 100 mg to determine the dose of liquid medication to be administered.

The result is the *quantity* to be administered: 4 teaspoons *(20 mL) of ibuprofen suspension.*

When calculating the oral dose of medication to be administered to an individual, the UAP should have a second staff person check his calculations *before* administering the medication to the individual. Doing so helps to prevent medication errors and ensures the safety of the individual.

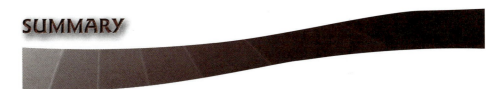

SUMMARY

Basic math skills are a necessity in the work of a UAP. The UAP needs to understand the three systems of measurement, including the basic equivalents between systems, to safely administer medications. The UAP needs to know how to safely calculate adult doses of oral medications if this is permitted by state regulations and workplace policy. Having these skills will allow the UAP to safely and effectively administer medications.

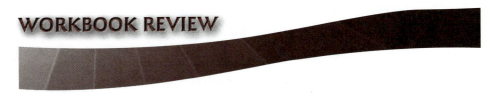

WORKBOOK REVIEW

Go to the workbook and complete the exercises for Chapter 32.

REVIEW QUESTIONS

1. Convert the following from Roman numerals to Arabic numerals:

    a. IV _____

    b. XII _____

    c. MCLIV _____

    d. V _____

    e. VIII _____

    f. XXXVI _____

    g. XIX _____

    h. CXC _____

    i. XX _____

2. Convert the following from Arabic numerals to Roman numerals:

    a. 2,003 _____

    b. 14 _____

    c. 98 _____

    d. 3,456 _____

    e. 231 _____

    f. 798 _____

    g. 465 _____

    h. 2 _____

    i. 72 _____

    j. 112 _____

Write your answers below in the space provided.

3. The basic units of the metric system are:

    a. _____ for weight

    b. _____ for volume

    c. _____ for length.

4. Write the name of the prefix for each of the following.

    a. _____ one-thousandth of a unit, written as 0.001

    b. _____ 1,000 units, written as 1000

5. Write in the correct equivalent for each of the following:

    a. 1,500 mL _____ liter

    b. 1 L _____ milliliters

    c. 1 g _____ mg

    d. 3,000 mg _____ gram

6. Write the correct abbreviation and unit of measurement for each of the following:

    a. one gram _____

    b. 2,000 milligrams _____

    c. three liters _____

    d. 500 milliliters _____

Household Measures and Apothecaries' Measures

7. Write the abbreviations for each of the following:

    a. _____ drops

    b. _____ teaspoon

    c. _____ tablespoon

    d. _____ ounce

    e. _____ cup

    f. _____ pint

    g. _____ quart

    h. _____ gallon

8. Write in the correct abbreviation for each of the following:

    a. 2 _____ = 1 oz

    b. 1 _____ = 6 tsp

    c. 16 _____ = 2 C

    d. 4 _____ = 2 pt

    e. 2 _____ = ½ gal

    f. 32 _____ = 1 qt

    g. 1 _____ = 16 oz

Calculating Oral Forms of Adult Dosage

9. Complete the problems below.

    a. The licensed health care provider ordered Apresoline (hydralazine hydrochloride) tablets, 25 mg. Available are Apresoline tabs, 10 mg. How many tablets will you give?

    b. The licensed health care provider ordered Prevacid (iansoprazole) capsules, 30 mg. On hand are Prevacid capsules, 15 mg. How many capsules will you give?

    c. The licensed health care provider ordered 200 mg of Monitan (acebutolol hydrochloride) tablets. Available are Monitan tablets, 400 mg. How many tablets will you give?

    d. The licensed health care provider ordered Hycodan (hydrocodone bitartrate) syrup 10 mg. On hand is 5 mg/5 mL. How many milliliters will you give?

e. The licensed health care provider ordered Mysoline (primidone) suspension, 125 mg. Available are Mysoline suspension, 250 mg/ 5 mL. How many milliliters will you give?

f. The licensed health care provider ordered 3 mg of Coumadin (warfarin sodium) orally. Available are Coumadin, 6-mg tablets. How many tablets will you give?

g. The licensed health care provider ordered 40 mg of Vasotec (enalapril maleate) tablets. On hand are Vasotec (enalapril maleate), 20-mg tablets. How many tablets will you give?

h. The licensed health care provider ordered 1000 mg of Carafate (sucralfate) orally. On hand are Carafate tablets, 1 g. How many tablets will you give?

Chapter 33
Vital Signs

Learning Objectives

1. Spell and define terms.
2. Identify the equipment needed to take an individual's vital signs.
3. Identify the range of normal values for each type of vital sign.
4. Demonstrate measuring temperature with an oral thermometer.
5. Demonstrate measuring temperature with a rectal thermometer.
6. Demonstrate measuring temperature with a tympanic thermometer.
7. Demonstrate counting a radial pulse.
8. Demonstrate counting an apical pulse.
9. Demonstrate counting respirations.
10. Demonstrate taking blood pressure using a standard blood pressure cuff and stethoscope.
11. Demonstrate taking blood pressure with an automatic blood pressure unit.

Key Terms

apical pulse

apnea

automatic blood pressure unit

blood pressure

body core

bpm

brachial artery

bradycardia

character

Cheyne-Stokes respirations

diastolic blood pressure

digital thermometer

electronic blood pressure unit

electronic thermometer

expiration

inspiration

pedal pulse

probe

pulse

pulse rate

radial pulse

rales	shallow	symmetry	tympanic thermometer
rate	sphygmomanometer	systolic blood pressure	vital signs
respiration	stertorous	tachypnea	volume
rhythm	stethoscope	temperature	

INTRODUCTION

Medication administration may require the UAP to take an individual's **vital signs**. Literally, these are life signs—measurements of body functions that keep an individual alive. There are four vital signs: temperature, pulse, respiration, and blood pressure. Each of these vital signs is reviewed briefly in this chapter. In addition, the equipment used to measure each vital sign is discussed. Some work settings may use separate equipment for each type of vital sign. Other settings may use one machine that can measure all four signs at once.

Note: When the UAP is taking an individual's vital signs, she is not to tell the individual the results of the measurements. Doing so is not the UAP's responsibility. The UAP is to document the results of the measurements in the individual's medical record and to report the results to the licensed health care provider. The UAP is to refer the individual to the licensed health care provider, who will discuss the results with her.

> **vital signs**
> Measurements of body functions that keep an individual alive.

TEMPERATURE

Temperature is a measure of body heat. It is:

- Fairly constant, and usually 1° to 3° higher in the afternoon and evening
- Much higher at the center of the body (the **body core**) than at the body surface
- Different in the same individual when taken at different areas, such as the ear, the mouth, or the rectum

An individual's body temperature may be affected by many different factors, including:

- Illness or infection
- Environmental temperature
- Medication
- Age
- Time of day
- Exercise
- Emotions

> **temperature**
> A measure of body heat; the balance between heat made and heat lost.

Table 33-1 Temperature Ranges and Averages

BODY AREA MEASURED	AVERAGE TEMPERATURE	NORMAL RANGE
Oral	98.6°F	97.6°F–99.6°F
Axillary (armpit)	97.6°F	96.6°F–98.6°F
Rectal	99.6°F	98.6°F–100.6°F

Delmar/Cengage Learning

- Pregnancy or menstrual cycle
- Hydration

Table 33-1 gives normal temperature averages and ranges for different areas of the body.

Measuring Body Temperature

Temperature is typically measured in one of four body areas:

- The mouth—oral temperature (the most common area)
- The ear—tympanic temperature (gives the quickest measurement)
- The rectum—rectal temperature (the most accurate)
- The armpit—axillary temperature (takes the longest to measure and is least accurate; this is usually used only if no other site can be measured safely or accurately)

Temperatures are routinely taken orally. If a different route is to be used, the UAP should be told by her supervisor or the individual's licensed health care provider of the alternate route to use.

GUIDELINES FOR USING AN ORAL AND RECTAL THERMOMETER

Oral Thermometer

Do not use if the individual is:

- Uncooperative or irrational
- Restless, confused, or disoriented
- Unconscious
- Very weak
- Chilled
- Coughing
- Recovering from oral surgery
- Receiving oxygen except by nasal cannula

- Unable to breathe through her nose
- On seizure precautions

Remember the following when taking an oral temperature:

- An oral reading could be false on an individual with dentures.

- If an individual has been smoking, eating, or drinking, the UAP must wait fifteen (15) minutes before taking the individual's temperature to get an accurate reading.

- Keep in mind that an individual who is restless or breathes through the mouth would not give an accurate oral temperature reading. It is the UAP's responsibility to notify a supervisor or licensed health care provider when an oral temperature may not be appropriate.

Rectal Thermometer

Do not use if the individual has:

- Combative behavior
- Diarrhea or fecal impaction
- Rectal bleeding or hemorrhoids
- A colostomy
- Had rectal surgery
- Rectal or colonic disease
- Recently had a heart attack or prostate surgery

Note: **In some work settings the UAP must have a licensed health care provider's order for a rectal temperature.**

Remember the following when taking a rectal temperature:

- Always hold a rectal thermometer in place the entire time to avoid possible injury to the individual.

THERMOMETERS

When asked to measure body temperature, the UAP will use one of four types of thermometers, depending on what is used at her workplace. The four types of thermometers are:

- The electronic thermometer
- The digital thermometer
- The tympanic thermometer
- A disposable oral thermometer

Refer to Figures 33-1, 33-2, 33-3, and 33-4 for pictures of the electronic, digital, tympanic, and disposable thermometers.

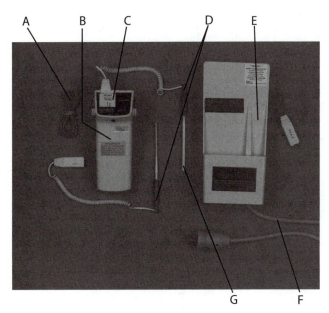

Figure 33-1 An electronic thermometer. The temperature is registered in large, easy-to-read numerals. The disposable protective sheath covering is placed over the probe tip. The probe is inserted into the individual's mouth. (A) The plastic cord goes around the UAP's neck when carrying the thermometer; (B) Thermometer; (C) Box of disposable probe covers; (D) Probe (blue = oral, red = rectal); (E) Charging unit; (F) Probe cord; (G) Disposable probe cover *(Source: Delmar/Cengage Learning)*

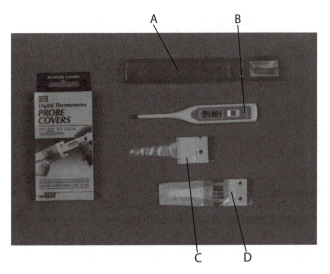

Figure 33-2 Digital thermometer. (A) Carrying case; (B) Digital thermometer; (C) Probe cover less backing; (D) Probe cover with backing *(Source: Delmar/Cengage Learning)*

probe
The portion of the thermometer that goes into the individual's body.

Electronic Thermometer

An **electronic thermometer** uses a **probe** that is placed into the individual. The probe sheath is covered in a disposable cover. A new disposable cover is used for each individual. After the UAP takes the temperature,

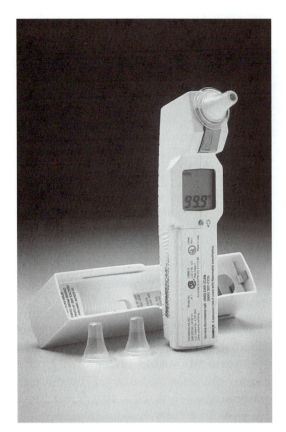

Figure 33-3 Cordless, handheld tympanic thermometer that measures the temperature of the tympanic membrane in the ear. The window on the handset shows the digital temperature reading. The thermometer can be set to provide an oral, rectal, Fahrenheit, or Celsius equivalent reading *(Source: Courtesy of Thermoscan® Inc., San Diego, CA)*

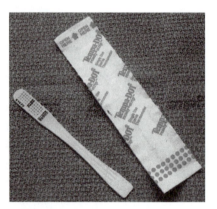

Figure 33-4 A disposable thermometer is used only for oral temperatures. It is used once, then discarded *(Source: Delmar/Cengage Learning)*

she throws the cover away. The thermometer reads the temperature in about thirty (30) seconds.

Digital Thermometer

The **digital thermometer** works in exactly the same way as the electronic thermometer. It is just a smaller handheld unit. A digital thermometer also uses a disposable sheath to cover the probe before use. A buzzer or beeper sounds when the temperature is reached. The measurement is displayed in the number window. A digital thermometer typically registers a temperature in anywhere from twenty (20) to sixty (60) seconds.

Using an Electronic or Digital Thermometer
The steps for using an electronic or digital thermometer are shown in Procedures 33-1, 33-2, and 33-3.

Procedure 33-1

Taking an Oral Temperature with an Electronic or Digital Thermometer

For an oral temperature reading:

1. Gather the equipment:
   - Electronic or digital thermometer
   - Disposable probe covers
   - Gloves (if glove use is the UAP's work setting policy)
2. Wash hands.
3. Tell the individual what will be done. Answer any questions.
4. Ask the individual if she has had anything to eat or drink or has smoked within the past fifteen (15) minutes. If she answers yes, the UAP must wait fifteen (15) minutes before taking her temperature to get an accurate reading.
5. Cover the probe with a disposable cover.
6. Insert the covered probe under the individual's tongue with the tip of the probe pointing toward the side of her mouth, not pointing directly toward the back of her mouth.
7. Hold the probe in position. Ask the individual to close her mouth and breathe through her nose.
8. When a buzzer signals that the temperature has been reached, remove the probe. Read the temperature.
9. Throw away the sheath. The UAP must not touch it with her hands. If wearing gloves, remove them. Throw the gloves in the trash.
10. Return the probe to its position in the thermometer case.
11. Wash hands.
12. Write the individual's temperature in the notes or on a notepad.
13. Return the thermometer to its charger.

Procedure 33-2

Taking a Rectal Temperature with an Electronic or Digital Thermometer

For a rectal temperature reading:

1. Follow steps 1 through 3 of Procedure 33-1. For equipment, also gather water-soluble lubricant and clean paper tissues with other supplies. Do not use petroleum jelly.
2. Lower the back of the bed so the individual is lying flat. Ask the individual to turn on her side. Help her as needed.

3. Cover the thermometer probe with a disposable sheath.

4. Put on gloves. Apply a small amount of water-soluble lubricant to the tip of the sheath. Remember, do not use petroleum jelly.

5. Fold back the bed linens to expose the buttocks.

6. Separate the buttocks with one hand. Insert the sheath-covered probe about one (1) inch into the rectum or as recommended by the thermometer company. Hold the probe in place, making sure to replace the linens over the individual as soon as the probe is in place.

7. Read the temperature when the buzzer goes off.

8. Remove the probe. Throw away the sheath. Use tissues to wipe lubricant from the individual's skin. Throw the tissues in the trash.

9. Remove gloves. Throw the gloves in the trash.

10. Return the probe to its position in the thermometer case.

11. Wash hands.

12. Write the individual's temperature in the notes or on a notepad.

13. Return the thermometer to its charger.

Procedure 33-3

Taking an Axillary Temperature with an Electronic or Digital Thermometer

1. Follow steps 1 through 3 of Procedure 33-1.

2. Wipe the axillary area dry.

3. Put the covered probe in place. Keep the individual's arm close to her body. Hold the probe in place until the buzzer signals that the temperature has been reached.

4. Remove the thermometer probe. Read the temperature. Throw away the cover in the trash.

5. Return the probe to its position in the thermometer case.

6. Wash hands.

7. Write the individual's temperature in the notes or on a notepad.

8. Return the thermometer to its charger.

Tympanic Thermometer

A **tympanic thermometer** measures the heat given off by the tympanic membrane, or eardrum. Like the electronic and digital thermometers, it is used with disposable probe covers. This is a good thermometer to use for many reasons:

- The temperature registers in just a few seconds, which makes it easier to take the temperature of an agitated individual.
- If the UAP cannot take a temperature orally, then she can use the tympanic method rather than taking a rectal or axillary temperature.
- The tympanic thermometer usually has a choice of core, oral, or rectal settings. This means that it can be used in the ear, and the reading will be the same as if the temperature was measured in the body center, mouth, or rectum.

Remember the following when taking a tympanic temperature reading:

- If an individual has been outside, the UAP must wait fifteen (15) minutes before taking the temperature.
- If the individual has been lying on the ear that the UAP will use to measure the temperature, the UAP must wait fifteen (15) minutes before taking the temperature or use the opposite ear.
- If an individual has a hearing aid, use the opposite ear to take the temperature or remove the hearing aid and wait fifteen (15) minutes.
- If an individual is directly in the path of cold air or is being fanned, the temperature reading may be low.
- Tympanic readings can be inaccurate if the user's technique is not correct. For correct technique, first insert the probe tip into the ear as far as it will go. Then rotate the handle until it is in line with the jaw, as if the individual is holding a telephone. Quickly press the button to get the measurement.

Using Tympanic Thermometer

The steps for using a tympanic thermometer are shown in Procedure 33-4.

Procedure 33-4
Taking a Temperature with a Tympanic Thermometer

The steps for using a tympanic thermometer are as follows:

1. Gather the equipment:
   - Tympanic thermometer
   - Disposable probe covers
   - Gloves (if glove use is the UAP's work setting policy)

2. Wash hands.

3. Tell the individual what will be done and answer any questions.

4. Place a clean probe cover on the probe.

5. Select the correct setting on the thermometer—core, oral, or rectal setting.

6. Put on gloves if there is a possibility of contact with blood or body fluids, open areas, or wet linens.

7. Position the individual so that the ear is easily reached.

8. Gently pull the top of the ear up and back to straighten the ear canal for an accurate measurement (Figure 33-5).

9. Gently place the probe into the ear canal as far as it can go. Do not apply pressure or force the probe in any way!

10. Rotate the handle until it is in line with the jaw, as if the individual is holding a telephone to the ear.

11. Quickly press the button to measure the temperature.

12. When the signal sounds, remove the probe from the individual's ear and throw the cover away. Read the temperature.

13. Wash hands.

14. Write down the temperature in the notes or on a notepad.

15. Return the thermometer to its charger.

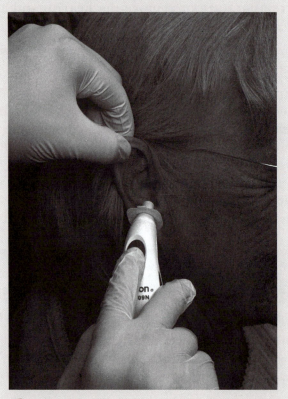

Figure 33-5 Gently pull the ear back and up
(Source: Delmar/Cengage Learning)

Disposable Oral Thermometers

A disposable oral thermometer is made of paper or plastic. It is used for taking an oral temperature. Once used, it is thrown away. A disposable thermometer has dots on it that change color from brown to blue, depending on an individual's temperature. The thermometer is used in the same manner as an electronic or digital thermometer for taking an oral temperature. After the temperature is reached on the thermometer, the UAP must remind the individual to open her mouth before the UAP removes the thermometer. If the individual's lips are closed when the UAP removes the thermometer, the thermometer may cause tears in the lips and inside the mouth.

PULSE AND RESPIRATIONS
Pulse

pulse
The pressure of the blood against the wall of an artery as the heart beats.

radial pulse
A pulse taken at the wrist.

pedal pulse
A pulse taken at the ankle/foot.

apical pulse
A pulse taken over the heart.

bpm
The abbreviation for "beats per minute."

The **pulse** is the pressure of the blood against the wall of an artery as the heart beats. The most commonly measured pulse is the **radial pulse**. It is measured at the radial artery at the wrist on the thumb side in line with the index, or pointer, finger. Other areas for taking a pulse include:

- The carotid artery on the side of the neck (a carotid pulse)
- The dorsalis pedis artery on the side of the ankle (a **pedal pulse**)
- Over the heart (an **apical pulse**)

Pulse measurement includes finding the:

- **Rate**, or speed, of an individual's pulse (**pulse rate**)
  - Bradycardia is an unusually slow pulse, a pulse less than 60 beats per minute (**bpm**)
  - Tachycardia is an unusually high pulse, a pulse above 100 bpm
- **Character**, the "feel," of an individual's pulse
  - **Rhythm**, or regularity of the pulse
  - **Volume** or fullness of a pulse beat; for example, pulse may be "hard," striking the fingers, or "thready," a soft pulse that feels like a thread under the fingers

Pulse rates may be affected by:

- Age
- Drugs or medications
- Exercise
- Elevated or lowered temperature
- Emotions
- Illness
- Position
- An individual's level of fitness
- Sexual activity

Table 33-2 Average Pulse Rates

GENDER	BEATS PER MINUTE
Adult men	60–70
Adult women	65–80
Delmar/Cengage Learning	

Average pulse rates for men and women are listed in Table 33-2.

When taking and recording an individual's pulse, the UAP must notify her supervisor right away if she notices tachycardia (100 bpm or more), **bradycardia** (less than 60 bpm), or irregularities in character (rhythm and volume).

Taking a Pulse

The steps for taking a pulse are shown in Procedure 33-5.

Procedure 33-5
Taking a Radial Pulse

When taking a radial pulse:

1. Gather equipment.
   - A watch with a second hand
   - Notepad or paper
   - A pen
2. Wash hands.
3. Tell the individual what will be done and answer any questions.
4. Have the individual sit or lie down comfortably. If she is sitting, rest her arm on a table or flat surface with her palm down. If she is lying down, rest her arm across her body.

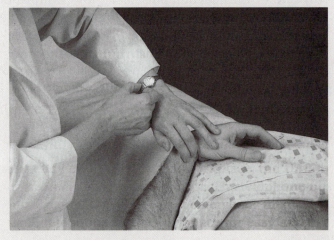

Figure 33-6 Locate the pulse on the thumb side of the wrist with the tips of your first three fingers *(Source: Delmar/Cengage Learning)*

5. Locate the pulse on the thumb side and palm side of her wrist, using the tips of the first three fingers (Figure 33-6).

Note: Do not use the thumb to take a pulse. It has its own pulse, which may be confused with the individual's pulse.

6. When the pulse is felt, push down slightly. Count the beats felt for sixty (60) seconds, or one (1) minute.

7. Remember the reading when counting respirations (described in the next section).

8. Write down the numbers for pulse and respirations after counting respirations.

9. Wash hands.

Respiration

respiration
A body function that brings in oxygen and takes away or removes carbon dioxide.

inspiration
Breathing in, or inhalation.

expiration
Breathing out, or exhalation.

The purpose of **respiration**, or breathing, is to bring oxygen to the cells of the body and to take carbon dioxide away from the cells of the body.

When respiration is affected by illness or disease, there is less oxygen in the blood as well as less carbon dioxide leaving the body. An individual who experiences this has a bluish or dusky color to her skin, known as cyanosis.

Respiration has two parts: **inspiration**, or breathing in, and **expiration**, or breathing out. When counting respirations, the UAP is to watch the individual's chest as it rises and falls. One respiration is equal to one full cycle of the chest rising and falling.

When counting respirations, as when counting pulse, there are certain traits to look for, including:

- **Character**—words used to describe the respiration, such as regular, irregular, shallow, deep, or labored
- **Rate**—the number of respirations per minute
- **Rhythm**—regularity of breathing
- **Symmetry**—whether the chest expands equally on both sides as air enters the lungs
- **Volume**—the depth of the respiration

Respirations may be affected by:

- Age
- Illness
- Elevated temperature
- Emotions
- Exercise
- Sexual activity

Different breathing patterns have different names, including:

- Normal—regular pattern, sixteen (16) to twenty (20) breaths per minute
- **Tachypnea**—fast, shallow breathing; similar to panting
- **Shallow**—a breath that only partially fills the lungs
- Dyspnea—difficult or labored breathing
- **Apnea**—a period of no respirations
- **Cheyne-Stokes respirations**—a repeating pattern of dyspnea and apnea
- **Stertorous**—respirations that are similar to snoring
- **Rales**—also called crackles; a moist respiration caused by fluid collecting in the air passages
- Wheezing—dyspnea with a sighing or whistling sound caused by a narrowing of the air passages in the lungs or by increased mucus in the air passages

When counting the respirations, remember that the average rate of respirations is sixteen (16) to twenty (20) per minute. The UAP must contact her supervisor if she notices a rate of *more than twenty-five (25) breaths per minute*, which is too fast, or a rate of *less than twelve (12) breaths per minute*, which is too slow.

Counting Respirations

The steps for counting respirations are shown in Procedure 33-6.

Procedure 33-6
Counting Respirations

When counting respirations:

1. Gather the equipment.
   - A watch with a second hand
   - Paper or a notepad
   - A pen
2. After counting the pulse rate, leave the fingers on the radial pulse and start counting the number of times the individual's chest rises and falls. Count for a total of one (1) minute. One respiration is equal to one full cycle of the chest rising and falling.
3. Notice the depth and regularity of the respirations.
4. Write down the time the respirations were counted, the rate, depth, and regularity of the respirations, along with the pulse rate, on the paper or notepad.
5. Wash hands.

Note: When taking an individual's pulse and respirations, the UAP needs to count the respirations without the individual being aware of the fact that the UAP is doing so. This allows the UAP to get an accurate count. This is because an individual's breathing pattern may change under certain conditions. For example, if an individual knows that her breaths are being watched and counted, her breathing pattern may change without her meaning to do so.

A more accurate way to count respirations is to count the respirations right after counting the pulse. The easiest way to do this is to just leave a hand on the spot where the pulse is being counted. Count the respirations. Then remove the hand. This way, it will be as though the pulse is being counted rather than the respirations.

BLOOD PRESSURE

blood pressure
The force of blood against the walls of the arteries during a heartbeat.

systolic blood pressure
The pressure when the heart is pumping.

diastolic blood pressure
The pressure when the heart is relaxed.

Blood pressure measures the force of the blood against the walls of the arteries during a heartbeat. There are two numbers in the measurement: **systolic blood pressure** is the first number, and **diastolic blood pressure** is the second number.

Table 33-3 shows average blood pressure readings.

Blood pressure may be higher because of:

* Age
* Conditions of blood vessels
* Diseases, including arteriosclerosis, high cholesterol, or diabetes mellitus
* Eating
* Emotional stress from anger or fear
* Exercise
* Heredity and gender—men have slightly higher blood pressure than women before menopause
* Obesity

Table 33-3 Average Blood Pressures

CATEGORY	SYSTOLIC BLOOD PRESSURE (mm Hg)	DIASTOLIC BLOOD PRESSURE (mm Hg)
Hypotension	100 or less	60 or less
Normal	<120	<80
Prehypertension (almost high blood pressure)	120–139	80–89
Stage I hypertension	140–159	90–99
Stage II hypertension	160 or higher	100 or higher

Note: mm Hg = millimeters or mercury, a measure of pressure.

Delmar/Cengage Learning

- Pain
- Some drugs or medications

Blood pressure may be lower because of:

- Abnormal conditions like hemorrhage (blood loss) or shock
- Dehydration
- Depressants, or medications that slow down body functions
- Diuretics, or medications that lower the volume or amount of body fluids
- Emotions such as grief
- Fasting, or not eating
- Rest
- Some medications such as antihypertensives, also called low blood pressure medications

An individual's typical blood pressure is affected by:

- Age
- Condition of blood vessels
- Emotion
- Gender
- Heredity
- The amount of sleep an individual has had
- Viscosity, or thickness, of the blood
- Weight

Blood pressure is typically measured in the upper arm, just above the elbow, at the **brachial artery**. It can be done in either arm *except*:

- *At the site of an IV infusion*
- *At the site of a dialysis access device*
- *On the same side as a recent surgical procedure in the arm or trunk*
- *On the same side as a pulse oximeter*
- *If the arm is paralyzed, injured, or swollen*

brachial artery
An artery in the arm used for taking blood pressure.

Guidelines for Measuring Blood Pressure

When getting ready to measure an individual's blood pressure, follow these steps first:

1. Before using the stethoscope, the UAP must clean the bell portion with an alcohol wipe and the earpieces with another wipe. The earpieces of the stethoscope should point forward when placed in the ears.

2. If the gauge is working slowly or not set at zero, the UAP must report this to her supervisor and use another sphygmomanometer.

3. The UAP should turn off the radio or television before taking an individual's blood pressure so that she can hear. She should also ask the individual not to talk while she is measuring blood pressure.

4. Remember these causes of inaccurate blood pressure readings:

- Use of a cuff that is too small or too large
- A cuff that is not wrapped correctly
- Incorrect positioning of the arm
- Not using the same arm for all readings
- Not having the gauge at eye level
- Deflating the cuff too slowly

Equipment for Measuring Blood Pressure

sphygmomanometer
Equipment used to measure blood pressure.

stethoscope
Equipment used to hear sounds produced by the body.

To measure blood pressure, a **sphygmomanometer** and **stethoscope** are used (Figures 33-7A, 33-7B, and 33-8). The sphygmomanometer contains the cuff and the gauge, while the stethoscope amplifies the sounds.

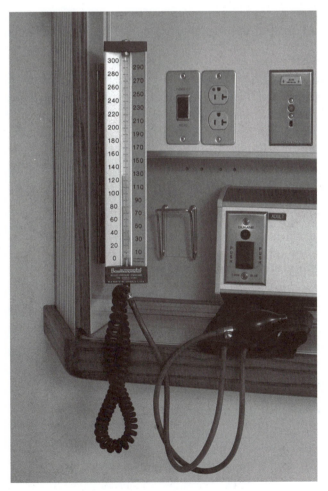

Figure 33-7a A mercury gravity sphygmomanometer *(Source: Delmar/Cengage Learning)*

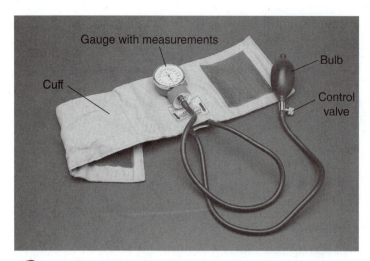

Figure 33-7b A dial (aneroid) sphygmomanometer
(*Source: Delmar/Cengage Learning*)

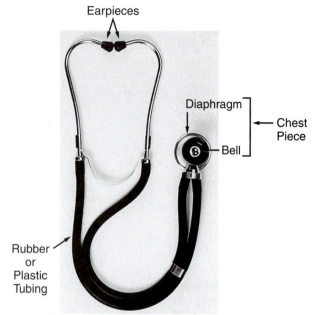

Figure 33-8 Stethoscope
(*Source: Delmar/Cengage Learning*)

The sphygmomanometer:

- Has a cuff that appropriately fits the individual's arm.

Note: **Cuffs that are too small or too large will give inaccurate readings. Check cuff size before taking blood pressure. The bladder of the blood pressure cuff should be at least 80% of the circumference of the individual's arm. If the UAP is unsure of the appropriate sizing, she should contact her supervisor.**

- Has two tubes; one connects the pressure bulb to the cuff, and the other connects the cuff to the gauge.

- Has a gauge which is either a column or a dial; both have numbers.

To read the gauge, follow these steps:

1. For a column or mercury gauge:

   - It should be at eye level.

   - It should not be tilted.

   - Take the reading at the top of the column of mercury inside the tube.

2. For a dial or aneroid gauge:

   - Observe it at eye level.

   - Do not read it at an angle.

The stethoscope:

- Has a diaphragm or a bell, or both, that is placed on the body.

- Has two tubes, one for each of the listener's ears.

- Has earpieces for each of the listener's ears.

Some work settings may have an electronic or automatic sphygmomanometer that does not require a stethoscope to be used. Instead, the electronic or automatic unit displays the blood pressure reading on a screen. The **electronic blood pressure unit** may be a large piece of equipment that is moved from room to room in a facility (Figure 33-9). The **automatic blood pressure unit** may be a small portable unit commonly used in a home setting (Figure 33-10).

When using both the electronic and the automatic units, it is very important to use the right size cuff. The width of the cuff should be equal to 40% of the size of the individual's upper arm. The UAP must also take at least one blood pressure reading using the standard method before using the electronic or automatic blood pressure unit. This reading then provides a baseline with which to compare the readings from the electronic unit.

The electronic blood pressure unit cannot be used for individuals with:

- Severe hypertension (high blood pressure) or hypotension (low blood pressure)

- Very fast heart rates (pulses)

- Irregular heart rhythms

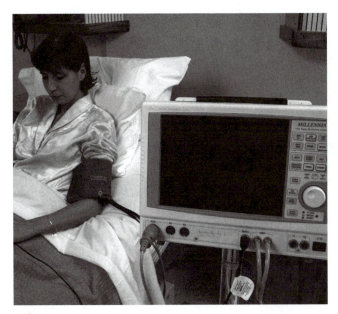

Figure 33-9 An electronic blood pressure unit. It is commonly used in a facility *(Source: Delmar/Cengage Learning)*

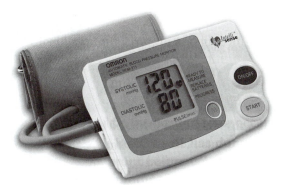

Figure 33-10 An automatic electronic blood pressure unit. It is commonly used in home settings *(Source: Courtesy of Omron Health Care, Inc. Bannockburn, IL)*

The individual's care plan, the work setting's communication logbook, or a similar document should clearly identify those individuals for whom an electronic or automatic blood pressure unit may not be used.

Measuring Blood Pressure

The steps for measuring blood pressure are shown in Procedures 33-7 and 33-8.

Procedure 33-7
Measuring Blood Pressure with a Sphygmomanometer and Stethoscope

To take an individual's blood pressure, follow these steps:

1. Gather the equipment.

   - Sphygmomanometer
   - Stethoscope
   - Alcohol wipes
   - Paper or notepad
   - A pen

2. Wash hands.

3. Tell the individual what will be done and answer any questions. During this time, have the individual rest for at least three (3) minutes. Activity may increase blood pressure.

4. Remove the individual's arm from her sleeve, or roll her sleeve five (5) inches above the elbow if it is not too tight.

5. Find the brachial artery with the fingertips (Figure 33-11).

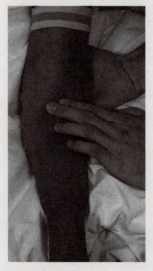

Figure 33-11 Locate the brachial artery with your fingertips
(Source: Delmar/Cengage Learning)

6. Rest the individual's arm on the table if she is sitting or on the bed next to her if she is lying down. Place her hand with her palm facing up.

7. Select the correct size blood pressure cuff.

8. Wrap the cuff around her arm, about one (1) inch above the elbow, and smooth it out so that there are no gaps.

9. Hold the pressure bulb in the dominant hand and find the brachial pulse with the fingertips of the other hand. Inflate the cuff until a pulse is no longer felt. Check the gauge number. Remember that number and add 30 to it to get the highest gauge number for inflation of the cuff for the blood pressure reading.

10. Quickly deflate the cuff and wait fifteen (15) to thirty (30) seconds before inflating it for the reading.

11. Place the stethoscope over the brachial artery.

12. Inflate the cuff quickly, up to the number figured from step 9.

13. Release the pressure slowly by turning the valve on the pressure gauge until a slow stream of air is being released.

14. Listen for at least two steady beats in a row from the stethoscope while watching the gauge. The number at which the first regular sound is heard is the first number of the blood pressure. This is the *systolic blood pressure.*

15. Keep deflating the cuff until the last sound is heard. The number at which the last sound is heard is the second blood pressure number. This is the *diastolic blood pressure.*

16. Keep letting the air out of the cuff, listening for any more sounds, until the cuff is empty.

17. Write down the numbers on the paper or notepad; for example, if the first sound heard was at 120 on the gauge and the last sound was at 80, write the blood pressure as 120/80.

18. Also write down which arm was used and whether the individual was sitting or lying down.

19. If the reading needs to be taken again, wait one (1) to two (2) minutes before doing so.

20. Clean the earpieces of the stethoscope with the alcohol wipes; also wipe the tubing if it has touched the individual or bed linens.

21. Put the equipment away.

22. Wash hands.

Procedure 33-8
Measuring Blood Pressure with an Electronic or Automatic Blood Pressure Unit

When measuring blood pressure with an electronic blood pressure unit, follow these steps:

1. Follow steps 1 through 6 of Procedure 33-7.

2. Locate the on/off switch and turn the electronic or automatic unit on. If need be, plug in the electronic blood pressure unit. The machine will signal when it is ready for use.

3. Select the correct size cuff for the individual.

4. Squeeze the excess air out of the cuff. Place the cuff on the individual's arm, following the directions in Procedure 33-7.

5. Make sure that the hose(s) between the cuff and the unit is not kinked.

6. If the unit has a frequency control switch, set it for automatic or manual.

7. If the unit has an inflation control switch, set it at 200 mm Hg.

8. Press the start button. The cuff will fill with air and then deflate.

9. When the measurement is complete, the blood pressure will be displayed on the screen. Some units may also display the pulse.

10. If the reading needs to be taken again, wait one (1) to two (2) minutes before doing so.

11. Record the results, including which arm was used and whether the individual was sitting or lying down.

12. Put the equipment away.

13. Wash hands.

Note: Each electronic and automatic blood pressure unit will work differently. Read the unit's instruction manual before using the unit. Refer to the instruction manual if any problems occur during the use of the unit.

Recording and Reporting Blood Pressure Readings

Once the UAP completes the blood pressure reading, she needs to record the reading in the assigned place(s) for her work setting. She then needs to report the following:

- If she was unable to hear a blood pressure reading

- If the blood pressure reading was higher than in previous readings

- If the blood pressure reading was lower than in previous readings

- If the site used to measure the blood pressure was a site other than the brachial artery

SUMMARY

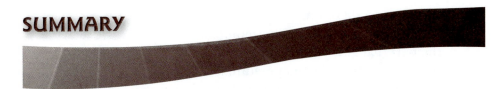

Taking vital signs is an important task because it allows the licensed health care provider to quickly identify any changes that may signal an illness. The UAP knows the individuals in her care and may help the licensed HCP by knowing how to take vital signs accurately, by recording them accurately, and by notifying the individual's licensed HCP of any unusual vital sign changes immediately.

WORKBOOK REVIEW

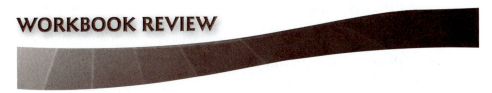

Go to the workbook and complete the exercises for Chapter 33.

REVIEW QUESTIONS

1. Temperature:
   a. is slightly higher in the afternoon and evening
   b. is much lower in the body core than at the body surface
   c. should be the same in an individual when measured at different areas
   d. all of the above
2. Oral temperature is:
   a. the quickest temperature measurement
   b. the longest and least accurate measurement
   c. the most common measurement
   d. the most accurate measurement
3. Tympanic temperature is:
   a. the quickest temperature measurement
   b. the longest and least accurate measurement
   c. the most common measurement
   d. the most accurate measurement
4. If an individual has been smoking, eating, or drinking before her oral temperature is taken:
   a. tell her not to do it again
   b. take a rectal temperature instead
   c. wait fifteen (15) minutes before taking her temperature
   d. contact your supervisor

5. The probe of a thermometer is:
   a. the disposable cover of a thermometer
   b. the part that goes into the body
   c. the screen where the temperature is displayed
   d. the charger for an electronic or digital thermometer

6. A rectal thermometer is held in place while taking a temperature:
   a. to avoid possible injury to the individual
   b. so the individual does not take it out
   c. to get a correct reading
   d. if there is no disposable sheath on it

7. When using a tympanic thermometer:
   a. one does not need to use probe covers
   b. use plenty of lubricant to avoid irritation
   c. insert the probe gently into the ear, then rotate the handle until it is in line with the jaw
   d. all of the above

8. Respirations are counted while taking the pulse because:
   a. they are the same thing
   b. it is the easiest way to avoid changes in an individual's breathing pattern
   c. if you tell the individual you are counting her breaths, she may refuse
   d. it is easier than taking blood pressure

9. Average blood pressure in adults is:
   a. around 120/80
   b. unusual in the elderly
   c. at least 33 points higher in women than in men
   d. all of the above

10. An individual's typical blood pressure can be affected by:
   a. sunlight
   b. driving
   c. the amount of water she drinks
   d. weight

CLINICAL SCENARIOS

1. You are asked to take Mrs. Pelletino's vital signs. When you enter her room to do so, you find that she is coughing and has a stuffy nose, causing her to breathe through her mouth. What is the best way to take her temperature? What is the correct technique for using this type of thermometer?

2. When you take her pulse and respirations, you get a pulse of 110 beats per minute with a thin, thready feel, and her respirations are twenty-six (26) per minute. What do you do?

Chapter 34
Care of Individuals with Epilepsy

Learning Objectives

After reading this chapter and completing the review exercises, you should be able to:

1. Spell and define terms.
2. Briefly describe the changes that occur in the body because of epilepsy.
3. List five possible causes of epilepsy.
4. Describe two major categories of seizures.
5. Describe emergency care of an individual having a seizure.
6. Explain why status epilepticus is a medical emergency.
7. Demonstrate the administration of Diastat gel.
8. Briefly describe four methods of treatment for an individual who has epilepsy.
9. List six anticonvulsants, their routes, side effects, and special considerations.
10. Explain the danger of discontinuing anticonvulsant medication for an individual who is in remission.
11. Describe a VNS implant and how it works.

Key Terms

absence seizures

anticonvulsant medications

antiepileptic drugs

atonic seizures

aura

epilepsy

generalized seizures

Lennox-Gastaut syndrome

medication interaction

myoclonic seizure	partial seizures	therapeutic range	Vagus nerve
neurons	seizures	tuberous sclerosis	stimulation
nonepileptic seizure	status epilepticus		(VNS therapy)

INTRODUCTION

According to the Epilepsy Foundation, more than three (3) million Americans of all ages have epilepsy. Approximately 200,000 additional new cases of seizure disorders and epilepsy are diagnosed each year. Over their lifetime, one (1) in ten (10) adults in the United States will have a seizure. Epilepsy:

- Is one of the most common disorders of the nervous system

- Affects people of all ages, races, and ethnic backgrounds

- May develop at any time of life, although it is more likely to develop in early childhood and in individuals over the age of sixty-five (65)

- Is more likely to affect males than females

Epilepsy is not a mental disorder. Epilepsy is a disorder of the nervous system. It is a seizure disorder caused by recurring and temporary periods of disrupted brain activity. Epilepsy may be caused by anything that affects the brain, including but not limited to a head injury, tumors, Alzheimer's disease, or stroke. Epilepsy may be inherited. About 70% of the time, the cause of epilepsy is not found.

There is no cure for epilepsy. Epilepsy is treatable, however, with medications, surgery, diet, and/or a device that stimulates the vagus nerve. Epilepsy is not contagious. Epilepsy, once under treatment, does not tend to get worse as one ages. In fact, most adults with epilepsy may expect to live a normal life span.

EPILEPSY

The nervous system is the "driver" of the human body. The nervous system controls and coordinates all body activities, from movement to breathing to hormone production. Some parts of this system control daily functions, while others become active only in dangerous situations.

Neurons are the cells of the nervous system. They conduct electrical charges through extensions called axons and dendrites. An axon carries the charge from the neuron and passes it on to the dendrites of the next neuron. Chemicals, called neurotransmitters, allow the charges to pass from one neuron to the next. Axons and dendrites are usually found in bundles, wrapped by connective tissue and resembling cables. These cables are the nerves of the body (Figures 34-1A and 34-1B).

During the normal functioning of the brain, millions of tiny electrical charges pass between the nerve cells (neurons) in the brain and to all parts of the body. **Epilepsy** is a disorder that results in a disruption of these tiny electrical charges. The disruption of the electrical charges

neurons
The cells of the nervous system; they conduct electrical charges.

epilepsy
A disorder of the nervous system that results in a disruption of the tiny electrical charges in the brain; causes seizures.

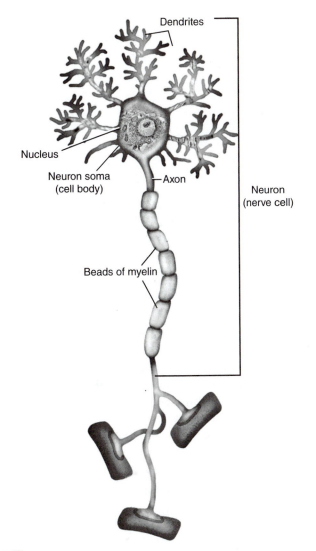

Figure 34-1a **The neuron** (*Source: Delmar/Cengage Learning*)

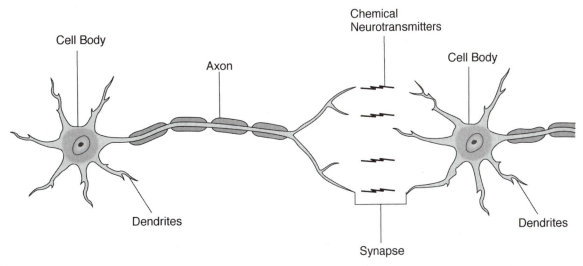

Figure 34-1b Chemicals called neurotransmitters help pass messages across the synapse from one neuron to another (*Source: Delmar/Cengage Learning*)

may cause physical changes in an individual for a short period of time. These physical changes may affect the individual's:

- Level of consciousness

- Body movements

- Sensations

These physical changes are known as **seizures** (convulsions).

Causes of Epilepsy

The factors that may cause an individual to have epilepsy may have been present in the brain since birth. For instance, the individual may have experienced a lack of oxygen during the birthing process, or the individual may have inherited the disorder. On the other hand, an individual may develop epilepsy later in life because of factors such as injury, infection, disease, exposure to chemicals, or other factors.

Having a single seizure does not mean that an individual has epilepsy. Many illnesses or severe injuries may affect the brain to produce a single seizure. It is only when the seizures continue or when the problem causing the seizures cannot be corrected that the disorder is known as epilepsy. A licensed health care provider needs to obtain a detailed history and perform diagnostic testing before making a diagnosis of epilepsy.

Some of the possible causes of epilepsy include the following:

- Lead poisoning

- Genetic causes such as **tuberous sclerosis**

- Infections like meningitis and encephalitis

- Problems in brain development before birth

- Lack of oxygen during birth

- Head injuries

- Stroke

- Alzheimer's disease

- Brain tumors

- Maternal drug use

SEIZURES

Seizures are physical changes in the body due to the disruption of the electrical charges in the brain. The type of seizure that occurs depends on the area(s) of the brain where the disruption occurs. A seizure may be just a momentary loss of consciousness, a disruption in the individual's senses, staring spells, or severe shaking and jerking of the body. Seizures are commonly called *convulsions*. Although each seizure has the same basic characteristics, seizures look different from one individual to another.

seizures
Convulsions; physical changes in the body due to the disruption of the electrical charges in the brain.

tuberous sclerosis
A rare, genetic disease that causes benign tumors to grow in the brain and on other organs, such as the kidneys, heart, eyes, lungs, and skin; commonly affects the central nervous system and results in a combination of symptoms, including seizures, developmental delay, behavioral problems, skin abnormalities, and kidney disease.

An individual may have only one type of seizure or he may have multiple types of seizures. The type or types of seizures an individual has will depend on (1) the area of his brain that is affected by the epilepsy and (2) how much of his brain is affected by the epilepsy. The more complicated an individual's seizure activity is, the more difficult it will be to control his seizures. The more difficult it is to control an individual's seizure activity, the greater the negative impact will be on his quality of life. The goal of treatment is always to stop an individual's seizures with the least amount of side effects possible.

Some individuals may experience an aura just before having a seizure. An **aura** is a warning of sorts. An aura involves an individual's senses. Right before having a seizure, an individual may smell, taste, or hear something different. For instance, an individual may taste a metallic taste or smell a certain odor right before having a seizure. This sensation will occur on a regular basis before each and every seizure.

An aura should serve as a warning sign to the individual. When the aura occurs, the individual should find a safe place. The UAP caring for an individual with epilepsy needs to be aware of the individual's aura. When the aura occurs, the UAP needs to help the individual get to a safe place. Once in a safe place, the UAP needs to remain with the individual during the seizure and needs to follow the individual's plan of care.

Some individuals may have a service dog. The service dog may warn them of an impending seizure. The service dog has been specially trained to smell a chemical change in the individual. The chemical change is believed to signal the beginning of a seizure. The UAP's facility most likely has a policy regarding service dogs. It is the UAP's responsibility to know and follow his workplace policy.

Seizures are classified into two major categories:

1. Partial seizures

2. Generalized seizures

Partial seizures are limited to a specific area of one side of the brain. Partial seizures are the most common type of seizure. Any movement, sensory, or emotional symptom may occur, including visual or auditory hallucinations. Partial seizures may spread into a generalized seizure. There are two types of partial seizures: (1) simple partial seizure and (2) complex partial seizure.

Generalized seizures affect both sides of the brain from the beginning of the seizure. The most common form of generalized seizure is grand mal seizure. Generalized seizures cause loss of consciousness. Loss of consciousness may be for brief periods of time or may last for much longer periods of time. There are four major types of generalized seizures: (1) generalized tonic-clonic, (2) myoclonic, (3) absence, and (4) atonic.

In addition, an individual may have a **nonepileptic seizure**. A nonepileptic seizure briefly changes an individual's behavior. This seizure may look like an epileptic seizure. A nonepileptic seizure, however, is *not* caused by electrical disruptions in the brain. A nonepileptic seizure may be caused by a lack of blood supply to the brain,

aura
A warning sign or sensation that an epileptic seizure is about to take place.

partial seizure
A type of seizure that is limited to a specific area of one side of the brain; may or may not cause loss of consciousness.

generalized seizures
Seizures that affect both sides of the brain from the beginning of the seizure; cause loss of consciousness.

nonepileptic seizure
A seizure caused by a physical condition, emotional trauma, or psychological stress; not related to epilepsy.

hypoglycemia (low blood glucose), sleep disorders, movement disorders, or other physical conditions. Nonepileptic seizures may also be caused by emotional trauma or stressful psychological experiences. Treatment of a nonepileptic seizure consists of treating the underlying cause of the disorder.

Partial Seizures

Important facts to remember about partial seizures are:

- Most partial seizures last only a minute or two, even though the recovery period after the seizure may last longer.

- Except in rare cases, the seizure will end naturally, on its own.

- Partial seizures cannot be stopped, although licensed health care providers may administer medications to end a seizure in an emergency, or a device known as a vagus nerve stimulator (VNS) may be used to help stop the seizure. For the most part, seizures stop on their own without any help.

- The movements caused by the seizures are not dangerous to other people. The UAP needs only to keep the individual safe by removing objects in the individual's path and by observing the individual until the seizure is over.

Simple Partial Seizures

Important facts to remember about simple partial seizures are:

- An individual remains conscious.

- An individual may be fully aware of what is happening. If so, the individual may or may not be able to talk or move during the seizure.

- An individual can usually remember what happened during the seizure.

- Movement, emotion, sensations, and feelings may be affected in unusual and even frightening ways:

  - An individual may experience uncontrolled movements in just about any part of the body; for instance, an individual's eyes may move from side to side, the face may twitch, a hand may shake, and then the shaking may spread to the entire arm.

  - The individual may have a sudden change in emotions, such as a sudden feeling of fear or a sense that something terrible is going to happen, or may become very angry and have a sudden outburst of anger that is totally unlike him.

  - Because all five senses are controlled by different areas of the brain, these seizures may produce strange sensations that are not really there, such as a feeling of a breeze on the skin when no breeze is present, an unusual hissing sound, strange smells, or distortions in vision.

- An individual's memory may be affected, causing disturbing memories of people and places from the past.

- Sudden nausea and/or stomach pain may be caused by simple partial seizures.

- Episodes of sweating, flushing, and/or becoming pale may occur.

- An individual may report an out-of-body experience with a distortion of time.

- An individual may report feeling uncomfortable with usual, familiar things and places.

- Well-known places may suddenly look unfamiliar, or new places may seem familiar; new events may seem as if they happened before, a feeling called déjà vu.

- An individual may experience a sudden outburst of uncontrolled laughter or crying.

Emergency Care for an Individual Having a Simple Partial Seizure. For an individual having a simple partial seizure, the UAP would provide the following emergency care:

1. Remain with the individual at all times.

2. Call for help.

3. Watch the individual closely.

4. Explain to others what is happening. Most people do not know or understand what is happening.

5. Do not restrain the individual.

6. Remove dangerous objects from the individual's path.

7. Speak quietly and calmly and direct the individual to sit down. Guide him away from dangerous situations. Use force only in an emergency to protect the individual from immediate harm, such as walking in front of an oncoming car.

8. Remain with the individual until he is fully alert.

Complex Partial Seizures

A larger part of the brain is affected by complex partial seizures, causing an individual's level of consciousness to be affected. Consciousness may be impaired or the individual may become unconscious. Important facts to remember about complex partial seizures are:

- During this seizure, the individual cannot interact normally with another person.

- The individual has no control over his movement, speech, or actions. He does not know what he is doing.

- The individual does not remember what happened during the seizure.

- The individual is in a dreamlike, trancelike state. His eyes are open. He can stand on his feet. He can move about.

- The individual may be able to speak, but his words do not make any sense.

- The individual does not respond appropriately to others.

Complex partial seizures may occur anywhere in the brain but usually take place in the temporal lobe of the brain. Complex partial seizures, therefore, are commonly called temporal lobe epilepsy or psychomotor epilepsy.

Complex partial seizures usually begin with a blank stare and a loss of contact with surroundings. The seizure then progresses to:

- Chewing movements with the mouth

- Picking at or fumbling with clothing

- Mumbling

- Performing simple, unorganized movements over and over again

- Agitation, screaming, running, or making flailing movements with his arms or bicycling movements with his legs

- Running in fear

- Crying out

- Repeating the same phrase over and over

- At times, the individual may wander, leaving a room, going downstairs, and even going out into the street, completely unaware of what he is doing

- The individual may also try to undress during the seizure

The individual's actions are usually unorganized, confused, and meaningless.

Emergency Care for an Individual Having a Complex Partial Seizure. For an individual having a complex partial seizure, the UAP would provide the following emergency care:

1. Remain with the individual at all times.

2. Call for help.

3. Do not restrain the individual.

4. Remove dangerous objects from the individual's path.

5. Calmly direct the individual to sit down. Guide him away from dangerous situations. Use force only in an emergency to protect the individual from immediate harm, such as walking in front of an oncoming car.

6. Observe but do not approach an individual who is aggressive or angry.

7. Remain with the individual until he is fully alert.

Generalized Seizures

Generalized Tonic-Clonic Seizures

This type of seizure happens in two phases:

1. Tonic phase—stiffening of the arms and legs
2. Clonic phase—jerking of the arms, legs, and face

During the tonic phase of a generalized tonic-clonic seizure, breathing may slow or stop. When this happens, the UAP may note a grayish-blue color (cyanosis) of the lips, nail beds, and face. An individual usually begins breathing again during the clonic phase when the arms, legs, and face are jerking. Breathing, however, may be irregular during the clonic phase. The clonic phase usually lasts less than one (1) minute (Figure 34-2).

It is possible for individuals to experience different patterns in a generalized tonic-clonic seizure. These various patterns include:

- Only a tonic phase
- Only a clonic phase
- A tonic-clonic-tonic pattern

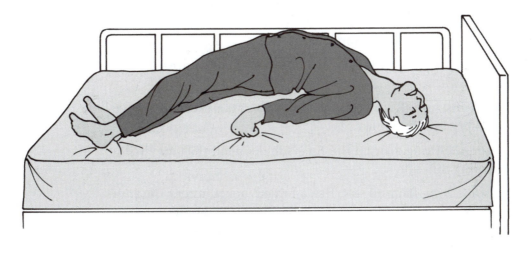

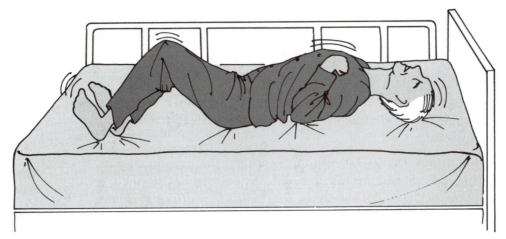

Figure 34-2 Generalized tonic-clonic seizures involve the entire body
(Source: Delmar/Cengage Learning)

Important facts to remember about generalized tonic-clonic seizures are:

- Incontinence may or may not occur during the seizure.

- The individual may bite his tongue or the inside of his mouth during the seizure.

- The individual's breathing after the seizure may be noisy or appear to be labored.

- Following the seizure, the individual may be confused, lethargic, and want to sleep.

- After a seizure, the individual may have a headache.

- Depending on the individual, it may take several minutes to several hours after the seizure is over for the individual to fully recover.

Emergency Care for an Individual Having a Generalized Tonic-Clonic Seizure. For an individual having a generalized tonic-clonic seizure, the UAP would provide the following emergency care:

1. Remain with the individual at all times.

2. Call for help.

3. Keep calm. Reassure others who may be nearby.

4. Time the seizure with a watch.

5. To protect the individual, move objects from the area around the individual.

6. Do not restrain the individual's movements unless the movements put him in danger.

7. Loosen anything around the individual's neck that may make breathing difficult.

8. Put something flat and soft, like a folded jacket, under the individual's head. If nothing is available, the UAP should kneel on the floor and place the individual's head in his lap.

9. *DO NOT* try to force the individual's mouth open. *DO NOT* try to put anything in his mouth. It is *not* true that an individual having a seizure may swallow his tongue. Trying to hold the tongue may injure the individual's teeth or jaw.

10. Once the seizure ends, gently turn the individual onto his side to keep his airway open and drain secretions (saliva).

11. Do not give the individual liquids, food, or medications until he is fully awake.

12. Do not attempt artificial respiration unless the individual does not begin breathing on his own *after* the seizure has stopped. *If the individual does not start breathing on his own after the seizure stops, the UAP should call 911 or the telephone number for the local emergency medical services. If the UAP is trained in CPR, he should begin CPR.*

13. Let the individual rest until he is fully awake.

14. Be friendly and courteous as the individual returns to consciousness.

15. Offer assistance if the individual is confused.

Note: A generalized tonic-clonic seizure is not an emergency unless:

- *It lasts longer than five (5) minutes*
- *A second seizure occurs soon after the first seizure finishes*
- *The individual does not begin to regain consciousness shortly after the shaking from the seizure stops*
- *It is the first time the individual experiences a seizure*
- *The individual is pregnant*
- *The individual is injured*
- *The individual has diabetes*
- *The individual is having difficulty breathing*
- *The seizure occurs in the water (e.g., the individual is swimming)*

If any of these conditions exist, the UAP should call 911 and/or the telephone number for his local emergency medical services. The individual should be transported immediately by ambulance to the nearest emergency medical care center.

Myoclonic Seizure

myoclonic seizure
A seizure consisting of rapid, brief contractions of muscles that occur at the same time on both sides of the body.

A **myoclonic seizure** consists of rapid, brief contractions of muscles that occur at the same time on both sides of the body. Myoclonic seizures may at times involve only one hand or one foot. An individual might think he is just being clumsy or is having a jerking reaction of his hand and foot. The sensation resembles that of an individual having a jerking sensation of a foot while sleeping.

First aid is usually not needed. However, the individual does need to be evaluated by his licensed health care provider when this type of seizure occurs for the first time.

Atonic Seizures

atonic seizures
Seizures during which there is a sudden loss of muscle tone; also called a drop attack.

Atonic seizures are also known as drop attacks, astatic seizures, or akinetic seizures. In an atonic seizure, there is a sudden loss of muscle tone. The head drops, posture may go limp, or an individual may suddenly collapse. Because atonic seizures happen without any warning (aura) and because an individual falls with significant force, atonic seizures may cause injuries to the head, face, or other parts of the body.

Atonic seizures tend to be resistive to medications. To prevent injuries, an individual may be required to wear headgear such as a helmet. No first aid is needed unless the individual is injured from a fall. The individual does, however, need to be evaluated by his licensed health care provider when this type of seizure occurs for the first time or if the number of atonic seizures increases.

Absence Seizures

Absence seizures are more commonly known as petit mal seizures. During a petit mal seizure, an individual may experience a lapse in awareness. The individual may appear to be daydreaming or staring for only a few seconds. Absence or petit mal seizures have no warning (aura) and no aftereffect. At times, absence seizures may be accompanied by myoclonic jerking movements of the eyelids or facial muscles or by a loss of muscle tone.

Absence seizures are more common in children. These seizures tend to be so short in length that the seizures tend to be missed. Absence seizures may happen for several months before a child is medically evaluated and treated.

No first aid is needed for an absence seizure. However, the individual does need to be evaluated by his licensed health care provider when this type of seizure occurs for the first time.

absence seizures
Seizures during which an individual experiences a lapse in awareness; also called a petit mal seizure.

Status Epilepticus

Status epilepticus is a condition of nonstop seizure activity. Instead of stopping after a short period of time, an individual's seizure develops into a series of seizures. Status epilepticus is a medical emergency. Death may occur if the individual does not receive emergency care. The seizures should be immediately brought under control. The individual should be transported by ambulance to the nearest emergency medical center for care. The UAP should call 911 or the telephone number for his local medical emergency services. *The UAP is NEVER to transport the individual in any form of personal or work vehicle!*

When caring for an individual with epilepsy, particularly for an individual with a history of status epileticus, the UAP should:

- Ask the individual's licensed health care provider if there are any emergency medications that may be administered to the individual if he experiences status epilepticus.

- Know the emergency protocol for the individual in his care.

- Ask the individual's licensed health care provider to establish standing orders and an emergency protocol with the local emergency medical center for care of the individual. Place a copy of the standing orders and emergency plan in the individual's record. When transporting the individual to the emergency medical center for care, the UAP should take a copy of the standing orders and/or emergency plan of care with him. The UAP is to share this information with the health care professionals at the emergency medical center on arrival.

Treatment of Status Epilepticus

For an individual in status epilepticus, the treatment of choice is the administration of diazepam (Valium) intravenously. However, it may be difficult to start an intravenous line while an individual is experiencing a seizure. In addition, if the individual has an episode of status epilepticus while he is out in the community or at home, starting an intravenous line may not be an option. During these times, diazepam (Valium) may be administered rectally. See Procedure 34-1 for the rectal administration of Valium (diazepam).

Note: The brand name for the rectal form of Valium (diazepam) is Diastat.

Procedure 34-1
Administration of Diastat (Diazepam)

When administering Diastat gel rectally, follow these guidelines:

1. When arriving at work and before an emergency arises:

   A. Compare the medication sheet, pharmacy label, and licensed health care provider order.

   B. Check the expiration date on the Diastat package.

2. When an emergency arises, identify the right individual.

3. Move objects from the area around the individual. Protect his head.

4. Obtain the Diastat, gloves, and water-soluble gel.

5. Provide privacy.

6. Remove the syringe from the box.

7. To remove the protective cover from the syringe, push the cover with the thumb and pull.

8. Put on gloves.

9. Remove the individual's clothing (slacks and/or underclothing).

10. Lubricate the rectal tip of the syringe with a water-soluble gel. Do not use petroleum-based gel.

11. Turn the individual onto his side facing away from the UAP. Make sure he will not fall.

12. Bend the individual's upper leg forward toward his abdomen.

13. Separate the buttocks. Gently insert the tip of the syringe into the rectum past the sphincter muscle, about one (1) inch for adults.

14. Slowly count to three (3) while gently pushing the plunger of the syringe. Push the plunger until the plunger stops and all of the medication has entered the rectum.

15. Slowly count to three (3) before removing the syringe from the rectum.

16. Slowly remove the empty syringe.

17. Slowly count to three (3) while holding the buttocks together to prevent the medication from leaking out.

18. Redress the individual.

19. Leave the individual on his side. Provide for the individual's safety.

20. Care for the equipment. Discard the empty syringe as per work place policy.

21. Remove gloves.

22. Wash hands.

23. Document per workplace policy.

24. Observe the individual.

Note: Call 911 or the telephone number for the local emergency medical services if any of the following occur:

- Seizure(s) occurs for fifteen (15) minutes after the Diastat has been administered or as ordered by the licensed health care provider.
- An individual's seizure(s) is different than in the past.
- The UAP is concerned by the frequency or severity of the individual's seizure(s).
- The UAP is concerned by the color or breathing of the individual.
- The individual is having an unusual or serious problem(s).

TREATMENT OF EPILEPSY

According to the Epilepsy Foundation, it is estimated that at least 50% of individuals with epilepsy may gain complete control of their seizure activity for long periods of time. An additional 20% of individuals may have a significant decrease in the number of seizures that they have. The remainder of individuals will struggle with frequent seizures, memory and cognitive effects, and other impairments that greatly affect their quality of life.

The goal of treatment is to stop seizures without side effects or with minimal side effects. The first choice of treatment for epilepsy is medication. If medications fail, surgery and a device known as a vagal nerve stimulator (VNS therapy) may be alternatives. For children, parents and licensed health care providers may choose treatment with a ketogenic diet, which is discussed later in this chapter.

Anticonvulsant Medications

Anticonvulsant medications, also known as **antiepileptic drugs**, are the most common treatment for an individual with epilepsy. Anticonvulsant medications are thought to work by preventing the disruption of the electrical charges in the brain. Anticonvulsant medications do not cure epilepsy. These medications control an individual's seizures. An individual with more than one type of seizure may need to take more than one type of anticonvulsant medication.

anticonvulsant medications Medications used to treat epilepsy, to prevent or control seizures (convulsions).

The individual's licensed health care provider prescribes an individual's medication based on several factors. These factors include the following:

- Seizure type/epilepsy syndrome
- Therapeutic blood level
- Medication side effects
- Age of the individual
- Lifestyle of the individual
- Childbearing potential of the individual
- Other medications and treatments the individual is receiving

An anticonvulsant medication will not begin to work until the medication reaches a certain level in the bloodstream. This blood level may or may not be within a **therapeutic range**. For the medication to reach a therapeutic level, the individual must receive the medication as prescribed by his licensed health care provider. The desired blood level for each individual varies depending on the individual's needs and reaction to medication. The licensed health care provider may decide to maintain an individual's blood level below, within, or above the therapeutic range.

Several classes of medications are used in the treatment of epilepsy, including the following:

- Barbiturates: When used properly, this is one of the safest forms of long-term anticonvulsant therapy.
- Hydantoins: Used mainly to prevent and treat generalized tonic-clonic seizures and psychomotor seizures.
- Succinimides: Used in the treatment of absence seizures.
- Oxazolidinediones: Also used in the treatment of absence seizures but usually used when other medications have failed to control the seizures.
- Benzodiazepines: Have been effective with absence seizures as well as other disorders. Diazepam administered intravenously is usually the medication of choice for status epilepticus. Diazepam may also be administered rectally during status epilepticus if unable to start an IV.
- Valproic acid and divalproex sodium: Effective for the treatment of absence seizures and used with other anticonvulsants to treat other seizure disorders.
- Tegretol: Used for treatment of partial seizures and generalized tonic-clonic seizures that have not responded well to other anticonvulsants.
- Felbamate: Effective for treatment of partial seizures and in combination with other anticonvulsant medications for treatment of **Lennox-Gastaut syndrome**.
- Neurontin: Effective in combination with other anticonvulsants in the treatment of partial seizures.

therapeutic range
A guide to the licensed health care provider as to the amount of medication that should be in an individual's bloodstream.

Lennox-Gastaut syndrome
A seizure disorder seen especially in young children; often accompanied by a type of petit mal seizure.

- Lamotrigine: Used in combination with other anticonvulsant medications for treatment of partial seizures, generalized tonic-clonic seizures, myoclonic seizures in adults, and Lennox-Gastaut syndrome in children.

- Other medications: Diamox, Phenurone, and paraldehyde may also be used.

Table 34-1 lists anticonvulsant medications currently in use, along with their brand names, generic names, route of administration, common side effects, and special considerations.

Table 34-1 Anticonvulsant Medications with Dosage Information and Adverse Reactions

GENERIC NAME	BRAND NAME	DOSAGE INFORMATION	ADVERSE REACTIONS	COMMENTS
Acetazolamide	Diamox Novo-Zolamide	Oral, 8–30 mg/kg daily in divided doses	Numbness, tingling, feeling of "pins and needles," loss of appetite, frequent urination	Treatment for absence seizures in children.
Carbamazepine	Tegretol	Oral, 200 mg twice a day on first day, gradually increase by 200 mg weekly in divided doses administered every 6–8 hours, do not give more than 1,200 mg/day	Dizziness, vertigo, drowsiness, edema, arrhythmias, skin rashes, nausea, vomiting, abdominal pain, aplastic anemia, blurred vision, weight gain	Instruct the individual to report complaints of fever, sore throat, mouth ulcers, or easy bruising. Do not suddenly stop the medication. Instruct the individual to avoid performing dangerous tasks or driving because the medication may cause dizziness and drowsiness. Give with food. Medication may interact with multiple other medications.
Clonazepam	Klonopin	Oral, initial dose do not administer more than 1.5 mg/day divided into 3 doses, dose may be increased in amounts of 0.5–1 mg every 3 days until seizures are controlled or side effects occur, do not give more than 20 mg/day	Depression, behavioral changes, confusion, drowsiness, impaired coordination, unsteady gait, muscle weakness, increase production of saliva, loss of appetite, bradycardia	Do not suddenly stop the medication. Should not be used in individuals with chronic respiratory disorders. Drowsiness, impaired coordination, and unsteady gait caused by this medication often improve with continued use of the medication. Instruct the individual to avoid performing dangerous tasks or driving because the medication may cause dizziness and drowsiness. Should not be used in individuals with history of allergy to benzodiazepines.

Table 34-1 Anticonvulsant Medications with Dosage Information and Adverse Reactions—*continued*

GENERIC NAME	BRAND NAME	DOSAGE INFORMATION	ADVERSE REACTIONS	COMMENTS
Diazepam	Valium Diastat	Oral, 15–30 mg daily Rectal, gel IV by licensed HCP only for status epilepticus	Drowsiness, slurred speech, muscle weakness, vertigo, low blood pressure, tachycardia, urinary retention, nausea, blurred vision, hiccups, coughing, liver dysfunction, jaundice	Observe elderly and very ill individuals closely when administering this medication. Medication may cause apnea and/or cardiac arrest.
Ethosuximide	Zarontin	Oral, 500 mg/day, increase dose by 250 mg every 4–7 days until seizures are controlled or side effects develop	Blood dyscrasias, kidney damage, impaired coordination, drowsiness, dizziness, epigastric distress, nausea, vomiting	Take with food if GI upset occurs. Do not suddenly stop the medication. Instruct the individual to avoid driving and other tasks that require alertness. Individual's licensed HCP should monitor the individual's blood status regularly.
Felbamate	Felbatol	Oral, initial 1,200 mg/day in 3–4 divided doses, increase dose in 600 mg amounts every 2 weeks, do not administer more than a total of 3,600 mg/day	Photosensitivity, loss of appetite, nausea, vomiting, constipation, insomnia, headache, fatigue, fever, weight loss, anxiety	Shake suspension well before using. Instruct the individual to avoid unprotected exposure to sunlight. Individual should use sunscreen and wear appropriate clothing when outdoors.
Gabapentin	Neurontin	Oral, 300 mg on first day, 300 mg twice daily on day 2, then 300 mg three times a day, dose may be increased to a total of 3,600 mg/day if needed	Dizziness, drowsiness unsteady gait, abnormal involuntary movements of the eyes, tremors	Instruct the individual to avoid performing dangerous tasks or driving because the medication may cause dizziness and drowsiness. Do not administer with antacids.
Lamotrigine	Lamictal	Oral, 25–150 mg daily in 1 or 2 doses	Dizziness, visual disturbances, skin rash, sedation, nausea, vomiting	Instruct the individual to avoid driving and other tasks that require alertness. Medication may increase sensitivity to ultraviolet light and sunlight. Instruct the individual to avoid unprotected exposure to sunlight and ultraviolet light.

(continues)

Table 34-1 Anticonvulsant Medications with Dosage Information and Adverse Reactions—*continued*

GENERIC NAME	BRAND NAME	DOSAGE INFORMATION	ADVERSE REACTIONS	COMMENTS
Levetiracetam	Keppra	Oral, initial 500 mg twice a day, may increase by 1,000 mg/day every 2 weeks to a total of 3,000 mg/day	Somnolence, dizziness, unsteady gait, impaired coordination, depression, nervousness, dizziness, amnesia, mental status changes, personality changes, numbness, tingling, feeling of "pins and needles," psychotic symptoms, constipation, diarrhea, nausea, vomiting, headache, loss of appetite, double vision, withdrawal seizures	Administer medication with a full glass of water. May give the medication with or without food. Do not suddenly stop the medication. Instruct the individual to avoid driving and other tasks that require alertness. Instruct individual to rise slowly from a sitting or lying position. Instruct individual to use a reliable birth control method.
Oxcarbazepine	Trileptal	Oral, 300–600 mg twice a day	Slowing of psychomotor skills, somnolence, unsteady gait, vertigo, dizziness, anxiety, dry mouth, insomnia, emotional issues, nervousness, agitation, mental status changes	Instruct the individual to avoid driving and other tasks that require alertness. Instruct individual to rise slowly from a sitting or lying position. Instruct individual to use a reliable birth control method.
Phenobarbital	Luminal	Oral, 100–320 mg daily at bedtime	Respiratory depression, skin rash, nausea, vomiting, nightmares, insomnia, hangover, dizziness, bradycardia, nausea, liver damage	Instruct the individual to avoid performing dangerous tasks or driving while on this medication. Prolonged use may cause physical or psychological dependence. Do not suddenly stop the medication. Do not use in individuals with obstructive pulmonary disease.
Phenytoin, phenytoin sodium	Dilantin	Oral, initial 100–125 mg three times a day, gradually increase dose to 600 mg/day	Gingival hyperplasia, abnormal movements of the eyes, changes in vision, drowsiness, impaired coordination, slurred speech, low blood pressure, nausea	Individual receiving continuous tube feedings administered by G-tube, J-tube, or NG tube must have the feedings turned off for at least one (1) hour before and one (1) hour after the administration of the liquid preparation of the medication through the tube because many tube feeding formulas interfere with the absorption of this medication. Observe the individual for signs of gingival hyperplasia. Individuals should be encouraged to practice good mouth care.

Table 34-1 Anticonvulsant Medications with Dosage Information and Adverse Reactions—*continued*

GENERIC NAME	BRAND NAME	DOSAGE INFORMATION	ADVERSE REACTIONS	COMMENTS
				Observe the individual for signs of folate deficiency and anemia. If the individual is receiving a folate supplement, do not stop the supplement without first getting the written approval of the individual's licensed HCP.
Primidone	Mysoline	Oral, 100–125 mg at bedtime on days 1–3, 100–125 mg twice a day on days 4–6, 100–125 mg 3 times a day on days 7–9, on day 10 administer 250 mg 3–4 times a day, do not administer more than a total of 2,000 mg/day	Respiratory depression, drowsiness, sedation, vertigo, nausea, loss of appetite, skin rash, nausea, vomiting, liver damage, hair loss, swelling of the eyelids	Instruct the individual to avoid performing dangerous tasks or driving while on this medication. Prolonged use may cause physical or psychological dependence. Do not suddenly stop the medication. Do not use in individuals with obstructive pulmonary disease.
Topiramate	Topamax	Oral, initial 25–50 mg daily, increase dose 25–50 mg weekly up to 200 mg twice a day	Dizziness, drowsiness, fatigue, malaise, poor memory and concentration, nervousness, psychomotor slowing, speech and language problems, agitation, anxiety, confusion, depression, impaired coordination, tremor, generalized weakness, abnormal vision, nausea, constipation, loss of appetite	Instruct the individual to swallow the medication without chewing. May give the medication with or without food. Do not suddenly stop the medication. Instruct the individual to avoid performing dangerous tasks or driving while on this medication.
Trimethadone	Tridione	Oral, 300 mg twice a day	Blood dyscrasias, liver damage, kidney damage, nausea, vomiting, skin rash, photophobia	Do not suddenly stop the medication. Instruct the individual to report complaints of fever, sore throat, mouth ulcers, or easy bruising.
Valproic acid	Depakene Depakote	Oral, initial 15 mg/kg/day, increase by 5–10 mg/kg/day weekly, do not administer more than a total of 60 mg/kg/day	Nausea, vomiting, weakness, drowsiness, dizziness, impaired coordination, liver damage, depression, skin rash	Instruct the individual to avoid performing dangerous tasks or driving while on this medication. Observe the individual for signs of liver damage.

(continues)

Table 34-1 Anticonvulsant Medications with Dosage Information and Adverse Reactions—*continued*

GENERIC NAME	BRAND NAME	DOSAGE INFORMATION	ADVERSE REACTIONS	COMMENTS
Valproic acid *(continued)*				To decrease GI upset, administer with food. Instruct the individual to swallow the capsule form of the medication without chewing to avoid irritation of the mouth or teeth. Do not suddenly stop the medication. Medication may interact with multiple other medications. Do not suddenly stop the medication. Use with caution in individuals with respiratory disorders. Instruct the individual to avoid performing dangerous tasks or driving because the medication may cause dizziness and drowsiness.
Zonisamide	Zonegran	Oral, 100–120 mg daily	Slowing of psychomotor skills, somnolence, unsteady gait, vertigo, difficulty concentrating, insomnia, decrease sex drive, depression, agitation, mental status changes	Offer plenty of fluids. Instruct the individual to avoid performing dangerous tasks or driving. Instruct individual to rise slowly from a sitting or lying position. Instruct individual to use a reliable birth control method.

Based on Schull, P. D. (2007). *Premier 2008 edition nursing spectrum drug handbook*. USA: Nursing Spectrum.

Side Effects of Anticonvulsant Medications

The most common side effects of anticonvulsant medications are:

- Rash
- Clumsiness
- Drowsiness
- Irritability
- Nausea

In addition, some anticonvulsant medications cause changes in emotions, memory, and behavior and affect learning. At times, anticonvulsant medications may increase the number of seizures an individual has.

Warning signs of possible serious side effects of anticonvulsant medications include the following:

- Prolonged fever
- Rash
- Severe sore throat
- Mouth ulcers
- Easy bruising
- Pinpoint bleeding or bruising
- Weakness
- Severe fatigue
- Swollen glands
- Lack of appetite
- Increased seizure activity

Note: If the UAP observes any of these warning signs, the UAP should immediately contact his supervisor and the individual's licensed health care provider.

Medication Interactions

Whenever more than one medication is taken by an individual, it is possible that the combination of those medications will change the effect of each of the individual medications. One medication may increase, decrease, or cancel out the effects of the other. This is known as a **medication interaction**.

A medication interaction is of great concern in an individual with epilepsy. Increasing the level of medication in the individual's bloodstream may cause the individual to have side effects from his anticonvulsant medications. A decrease in the amount of anticonvulsant medication in an individual's bloodstream may cause breakthrough seizures or status epilepticus. An individual with epilepsy needs to make sure that his blood level(s) of anticonvulsant medication(s) stays within his therapeutic range at all times.

It is, therefore, very important that the licensed health care provider know *all* of the medications that the individual is taking to prevent unwanted medication interactions. This includes all prescription, over-the-counter medications, and herbal medications. The UAP and the individual need to make sure that the individual takes only those medications that are ordered by his licensed HCP.

As a point of reference, Table 34-2 lists some of the common medication interactions that may occur with anticonvulsant medications.

Special Considerations for Anticonvulsant Medications

A serious concern with anticonvulsant medications is the difference between brand-name medications and generic medications. Although this difference does not play a significant role with other medications, the difference may be serious in regard to anticonvulsant medications.

Table 34-2 Possible Medication Interactions with Common Anticonvulsants

MEDICATION	INTERACTION	MEDICATION	INTERACTION
carbamazepine	acetaminophen	phenytoin	acetaminophen
	bupropion		alcohol, ethyl
	charcoal		allopurinol
	cimetidine		amiodarone
	contraceptives, oral		antacids
	cyclosporine		anticoagulants, oral
	danazol		antidepressants, tricyclic
	diltiazem		barbiturates
	doxycycline		benzodiazepines
	erythromycin		carbamazepine
	felbamate		charcoal
	felodipine		chloramphenicol
	fluoxetine		chlorpheniramine
	fluvoxamine		cimetidine
	grapefruit juice		clonazepam
	haloperidol		contraceptives, oral
	isoniazid		corticosteroids
	lamotrigine		cyclosporine
	lithium		diazoxide
	macrolide antibiotics (e.g., Clarithromycin, Troleandomycin)		dicumarol
			digitalis glycosides
	methylphenidate		disopyramide
	muscle relaxants, nondepolarizing		disulfiram
			dopamine
	phenobarbital		doxycycline
	phenytoin		estrogens
	primidone		fluconazole
	propoxyphene		folic acid
	ticlopidine		furosemide
	tricyclic antidepressants (TCAs)		haloperidol
			ibuprofen
	valproic acid		isoniazid
	vasopressin		levodopa
	verapamil		levonorgestrel
	warfarin sodium		lithium
			loxapine

Table 34-2 Possible Medication Interactions with Common Anticonvulsants—*continued*

MEDICATION	INTERACTION	MEDICATION	INTERACTION
phenytoin (continued)	mebendazole	valproic acid	alcohol
	meperidine		carbamazepine
	methadone		charcoal
	metronidazole		chlorpromazine
	metyrapone		cimetidine
	mexiletine		clonazepam
	miconazole		CNS depressants
	milk thistle (herb)		diazepam
	nitrofurantoin		erythromycin
	omeprazole		ethosuximide
	phenothiazines		felbamate
	primidone		lamotrigine
	pyridoxine		phenobarbital
	quinidine		phenytoin
	rifampin		salicylates (aspirin)
	salicylates		warfarin sodium
	sucralfate		zidovudine
	sulfonamides		
	sulfonylureas		
	theophylline		
	trimethoprim		
	valproic acid		

Delmar/Cengage Learning

Generic medications are approved with a 10% to 15% difference in their composition as compared to the equivalent brand-name medications. This difference may cause breakthrough seizures in an individual with epilepsy. It is extremely important for the UAP to make certain that an individual's medication is *not* changed from a brand-name form of anticonvulsant to a generic form of medication or vice versa without the written order of the individual's licensed health care provider. Changing the individual's medication may result in an increase in his seizure activity and even in a bout of status epileticus.

Discontinuing Anticonvulsant Medications

Under certain circumstances, an individual may not need to take anticonvulsant medication for his entire life. If his seizures have been well controlled for several years, the individual may have entered remission. The individual's licensed health care provider may decide to slowly withdraw the individual's anticonvulsant medication over a set period of time. The individual will require close observation by the UAP and his licensed health care provider as he goes through this change. In addition, during this time seizure precautions will need to be followed.

When discontinuing an individual's medication, the medication is withdrawn slowly over a one (1)- to three (3)-month period. Medication is never stopped suddenly. Doing so may cause not only a seizure but also status epilepticus as well as other potential complications.

Making the decision to discontinue an individual's anticonvulsant medication is always a difficult one, especially for an adult. An adult with stable epilepsy tends to be leading a productive life, driving and working daily. Having a seizure during the discontinuation of his medication may disrupt an individual's daily life. If the individual has a seizure while his medication is being discontinued, the individual may not be able to drive and might not be able to fulfill his work duties. The decision to discontinue anticonvulsant medication is, therefore, a difficult one made by the individual and his licensed health care provider.

An individual meeting the following criteria has the greatest chance of successfully discontinuing his medication:

- Has only one type of primary generalized seizures
- Is younger than thirty (30) years of age
- Has seizures that are well controlled with medication
- Has a series of normal EEGs on medication
- Has been seizure-free for two (2) to five (5) years

Surgery

When medication alone has not been successful in controlling an individual's seizures, brain surgery may be an alternative treatment for the individual. Brain surgery is not for every individual, however. Brain surgery is most likely to be considered for an individual with epilepsy when:

- Diagnostic work-up has documented that the individual's seizures are due to epilepsy and not due to other causes.
- Anticonvulsant medications have not been successful in controlling the individual's seizure activity.
- The individual has had adverse reactions to anticonvulsant medications.
- The seizures always begin in one localized, specific area of the brain that may be removed without damaging other areas of the brain, specifically the more important areas that control speech, memory, or eyesight.

Brain surgery is a very delicate operation. The operation is performed by highly trained and skilled specialists at a medical center. Local hospitals do not usually have the equipment or the trained health care professionals to perform this type of surgery.

Even with surgery, the individual may need to take anticonvulsant medications for several years, usually for one (1) to two (2) years until healing is complete. Anticonvulsant medications are then slowly discontinued, as discussed previously. Once healing is complete, many individuals have a good chance to live a seizure-free life, free of medication. Some individuals do not benefit from the surgery.

Ketogenic Diet

The ketogenic diet is used mainly to treat children with epilepsy. The diet is very high in fats and low in carbohydrates and proteins, getting almost 80% of its calories from fat. The body burns the fats it consumes for energy. In doing so, the body enters a state of starvation. In some way, not fully understood by licensed health care providers, it prevents seizures in some children.

This is a strict diet. The child's family must be committed to following the diet if there is to be a chance of success. When the diet is followed as it should be, the diet helps two (2) out of three (3) children control their seizures and may prevent seizures completely in one (1) out of three (3) children. As with all forms of treatment, a ketogenic diet may have side effects depending on the individual child.

Children stay on this diet for two (2) years. At the end of the two (2)-year period, children slowly resume their original diet.

Vagus Nerve Stimulation (VNS Therapy)

vagus nerve stimulation (VNS therapy)
A nondrug therapy used to treat epilepsy.

Vagus nerve stimulation (VNS therapy) is a nondrug therapy. It is the first to be approved by the FDA in more than 100 years. VNS therapy uses a small device, similar to a pacemaker, which is implanted into the chest to control seizures.

The device, called a VNS implant, stimulates the vagus nerve. The vagus nerve is located on the left side of the neck. When the nerve is stimulated, the vagus nerve carries electrical impulses to the brain. The number of seizures and/or the intensity of seizures may be decreased by VNS therapy.

VNS therapy is another form of therapy that is tried when medication alone fails to control an individual's seizures. Currently the therapy is approved for individuals

- Twelve (12) years of age and older

- Who have partial seizures

- When other methods fail to control their seizure activity

The device is about the size of a silver dollar. It is surgically implanted in the chest. Surgery is usually done on an outpatient basis. Surgery takes about an hour to perform.

Thin wires called electrodes are passed under the skin from the device up to the vagus nerve on the left side of the neck. The wires are then wound around the vagus nerve. A battery in the device generates the energy that passes from the device through the wires to the vagus nerve and stimulates the nerve. The battery is programmed by the health care team to send a few seconds of electrical energy to the vagus nerve.

When an individual feels a seizure coming on, he can activate the discharge of energy by passing a small magnet over the battery. In some individuals, this will stop the seizure. The individual may also choose to shut the VNS device off by holding a magnet over the battery for a period of time.

Complete seizure control with VNS therapy is not usually achieved. However, most individuals do have fewer seizures. In addition, the effectiveness of VNS therapy tends to improve over time. As with surgery and the ketogenic diet, it is almost always necessary for an individual to continue to take his anticonvulsant medication along with the VNS therapy.

According to the Epilepsy Foundation, approximately 32,000 individuals have received the VNS therapy. Individuals using VNS therapy report an improved quality of life. Studies show that about one-third of individuals have a major improvement in seizure control. Another one-third of individuals have some improvement in seizure control. However, one-third of the individuals studied continue to have seizures as they did before receiving VNS therapy. As with all forms of treatment for epilepsy, seizure control and improved quality of life are the main goals.

Side Effects of VNS Therapy

Side effects of VNS therapy are minor. Most common side effects include:

- Hoarseness

- Tickling in the throat

- A change in voice quality during the actual passing of the magnet over the battery to prevent a seizure

- Increased coughing

- Infection after surgery

Rejection of the device is not a problem. If the device has to be removed, the most common reason is that the device is not effective. One percent of the time, the device is removed because of infection after surgery or malfunction of the device.

Special Considerations with VNS Therapy

- According to the manufacturer, properly operating microwave ovens, toasters, hair dryers, or other electrical appliances should not affect a VNS implant.

- According to the manufacturer, cell phones should not affect a VNS implant.

- According to the manufacturer, metal detectors at airports and other locations should not affect a VNS implant.

- An individual with a VNS implant should not have any kind of diathermy (deep heat treatments).

- An individual with a VNS implant *may* have X-rays but does need to tell health care providers, *before* he has a procedure, that he has a VNS implant.

- Health care providers need to take special precautions for an individual with a VNS implant when performing an MRI scan. Only certain MRI scanners should be used. The VNS implant should be turned off temporarily for the MRI scan.

- An individual needs to show his manufacturer-supplied identification (ID) card to all licensed health care providers (physicians, nurses, dentists, rehabilitation providers, and so on) *before* treatment and care are provided.

- An individual with a VNS implant may experience sleep apnea or other sleep interruptions when the VNS implant turns on during sleep. If so, the UAP needs to contact the individual's licensed health care provider.

- If the magnet no longer prevents seizures when passed over the individual's device, the UAP needs to immediately contact the individual's licensed health care provider and the supervisor.

- According to the manufacturer, the battery in the VNS implant may last up to twelve (12) years, depending on several factors. The battery, however, may have to be replaced after six (6) years. The individual and the UAP need to check periodically with the individual's licensed health care provider on the functioning of the VNS implant.

Additional information on VNS therapy is available at http://www.vnstherapy.com/epilepsy/patient.

Complementary Treatment

Because of the nature of epilepsy, the social stigmas and myths that surround it, its incurable nature, and the impact the disease has on an individual's quality of life, an individual may choose to seek out an alternate form of treatment. Complementary treatment in particular will be of interest to an individual when his seizures are not well controlled or when he is experiencing side effects from his medication. An individual, his family, and his caregivers need to keep in mind the fact that not all complementary treatments may have undergone the scrutiny and evaluation that approved treatments have. This does not mean that alternative treatments are not effective or should not be considered. It does mean that an individual needs to consult with his licensed health care provider before discontinuing one treatment and beginning another.

Alternative or complementary treatments may include folk medicines, herbal medications, special diets, megavitamin therapy, and other options. If the individual's licensed health care provider has no objections and the treatments do not contain any harmful substances or include any harmful practices or effects, the individual may choose to try them. The individual should consider, however, the cost of the treatment, including not just the financial cost but also the cost to his health.

CARE OF THE INDIVIDUAL WITH EPILEPSY

The UAP's responsibilities when caring for an individual with epilepsy include:

- Assist the individual in dealing with the stigma and myths surrounding epilepsy. Society as a whole has believed over the years that epilepsy is a sign of mental retardation or a form of mental illness. The individual may need help in dealing with the stigmas and stereotypes these beliefs have created as well as the discrimination he may face in school, work, and other areas of his life.

- Ensure that the individual takes his medication as ordered. Many factors may cause an individual to refuse to take his anticonvulsant medication. The UAP needs to observe the individual when administering medication to ensure that the medication is taken as ordered. If the individual refuses to take his medication as ordered, the UAP needs to immediately contact the individual's licensed health care provider. Medication refusals are discussed further in Chapter 30.

- Provide frequent mouth care, gum massage, and dental care for an individual taking Dilantin. Inspect the mouth daily. In addition, assist the individual in scheduling visits to his dentist at least twice a year for cleaning, more often if treatment is needed. A side effect of long-term Dilantin therapy is gingival hyperplasia (Figure 34-3).

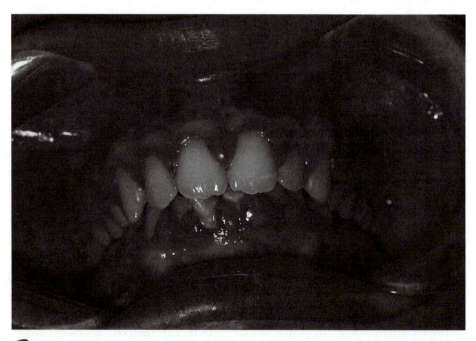

Figure 34-3 Gingival hyperplasia. The gum tissue has grown over the teeth in this individual, who is on long-term Dilantin (phenytoin) therapy *(Source: Courtesy of Joseph L. Konzelman, Jr., DDS)*

- Do not discontinue or start a new medication without a written order from the individual's licensed health care provider. This includes herbal medications, OTC medications including vitamins, and other forms of alternative treatments.

- If using medication in suspension form, shake the medication well before administering the medication.

- Observe an individual closely whenever medication is added, discontinued, or changed. This includes anticonvulsant medication, over-the-counter medications, herbal medications, and other prescription medications.

- Immediately report observations of fever, sore throat, mouth ulcers, and easy bruising to the individual's licensed HCP.

SUMMARY

The UAP plays an important role in the care of the individual with epilepsy. Because anticonvulsant medications are the first choice of treatment, proper administration of these medications has a significant effect on the treatment an individual will receive for the remainder of his life. Anticonvulsant medications administered as ordered will control seizures for the majority of individuals with epilepsy. However, medications administered at improper times or in incorrect amounts or with the wrong foods or liquids may increase an individual's number of seizures. When this occurs, an individual's quality of life is affected. Doses of medications may be increased or decreased, increasing the risk of side effects or placing the individual at risk for breakthrough seizures or status epilepticus. The individual may be considered for surgery or VNS therapy when in reality anticonvulsant medication would have controlled his seizures. The UAP is the frontline caregiver and as such has a significant effect on an individual's life.

WORKBOOK REVIEW

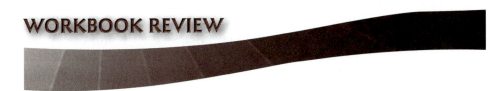

Go to the workbook and complete the exercises for Chapter 34.

REVIEW QUESTIONS

1. Epilepsy is a disorder of the:
   a. musculoskeletal system
   b. nervous system
   c. endocrine system
   d. cardiovascular system

2. Seizures are also known as:
   a. convulsions
   b. contortions
   c. epilepsy
   d. tuberous sclerosis

3. When treating epilepsy, the goal is to:
   a. eliminate the aura an individual experiences right before a seizure
   b. change the type of seizures an individual has
   c. cure the individual so he no longer has epilepsy
   d. stop the seizures with the least amount of side effects

4. An aura is:
   a. the trigger in the brain that causes a seizure
   b. a sensory warning sign that an individual is about to have a seizure
   c. a type of seizure in an individual with epilepsy
   d. a type of convulsion in an individual with epilepsy

5. When an individual with epilepsy experiences an aura, the UAP should:
   a. help the individual to a safe place
   b. leave the individual and go get help
   c. tell other staff members that the individual is having an aura
   d. immediately call the workplace supervisor and the individual's licensed HCP

6. When providing emergency care to an individual having a seizure, it is important for the UAP to:
   a. restrain the individual so he does not hurt himself
   b. go and get help immediately
   c. stay with the individual at all times during the seizure
   d. immediately contact the individual's licensed HCP and the workplace supervisor

7. When giving emergency care to an individual who is having a tonic-clonic seizure, the UAP should:
   a. restrain the individual's movements so he does not hurt himself
   b. put a small, flat object in the individual's mouth
   c. begin CPR as soon as the seizure is over
   d. time the seizure with a watch

8. A tonic-clonic seizure is an emergency if:
   a. the individual has trouble breathing
   b. the seizure lasts for three (3) minutes or less
   c. the individual is restrained
   d. the individual loses consciousness

9. Status epilepticus is:
   a. another name for a generalized tonic-clonic seizure
   b. another name for epilepsy
   c. a condition of nonstop seizure activity that may cause death
   d. an evaluation of an individual with epilepsy by his licensed HCP

10. The medication of choice for treatment of status epilepticus is:
    a. diphenhydramine
    b. diazepam
    c. Dilantin
    d. didanosine

11. Anticonvulsant medications are used to:
    a. cure epilepsy
    b. reduce an aura
    c. control seizures
    d. reduce the severity of a seizure

12. The therapeutic range of a medication is:
    a. the level in the bloodstream at which the medication works
    b. the level in the bloodstream reached when the individual's licensed HCP discontinues the medication
    c. the level in the bloodstream when an individual first takes the medication
    d. the level in the bloodstream when the individual's licensed HCP changes the medication

13. Warning signs of possible serious side effects of anticonvulsant medications include:
    a. increased appetite and agitation
    b. weakness and bruising
    c. high blood pressure and increased heart rate
    d. low blood pressure and decreased heart rate

14. A ketogenic diet is used to treat:
    a. adults with epilepsy
    b. men with epilepsy
    c. women with epilepsy
    d. children with epilepsy

15. A VNS implant may help to:
    a. decrease the number and intensity of seizures
    b. eliminate the need for anticonvulsant medications
    c. reduce the occurrence of auras before a seizure
    d. adapt a child to a ketogenic diet

CLINICAL SCENARIOS

1. Part of your assignment today is to give care to Jennifer, a woman who has epilepsy. As you are assisting her with self-care, Jennifer says, "Do you smell oranges? I smell oranges." She suddenly turns to you and yells, "Get away from me, don't touch me, I hate you!" Her face begins to twitch on the right side. You notice that she is sweating and her skin is pale. Then Jennifer bursts into tears.

   a. What is happening to Jennifer?

   b. What might her report of smelling oranges be? What should you do?

   c. What type of seizure is Jennifer having?

   d. Describe how you would help Jennifer during this event.

   e. Write a note for Jennifer's record, describing this event. Use today's date and the time of 7:45 a.m.

2. You are on an outing with a group from a day program. Part of your assignment today is to monitor Frank, who has epilepsy. You are sitting with Frank on a bench when his legs suddenly stiffen. Frank falls off the bench. His arms and legs begin jerking and then stiffen again. Frank stops breathing for a moment. His arms and legs begin to jerk again. After that, Frank's body relaxes. He begins to breathe again. You notice that Frank's breathing is irregular and that he is gasping.

   a. What type of seizure is Frank having?

   b. What should you do to give emergency care to Frank during this event?

   c. What should you do when the seizure is over?

   d. Write a note describing this event. Use today's date. Presume that the seizure started at 1:30 p.m. and lasted for three (3) minutes.

Chapter 35
Substance Abuse

Learning Objectives

After reading this chapter and completing the review questions, you should be able to:

1. Spell and define key terms.
2. Describe four commonly abused substances in the United States today.
3. List three routes of administration for abused substances.
4. List the street names for six commonly abused substances in the United States.
5. Describe five adverse reactions due to the use of abused substances.
6. Discuss the role of the UAP in recognizing and reporting suspected substance abuse.

Key Terms

addiction

anabolic steroids

anterograde amnesia

cannabinoids

club drugs

cocaine

depressants

flashbacks

hallucinogens

huffing

inhalants

injecting

LSD

marijuana

nicotine

PCP (phencyclidine)

peripheral neuropathies

physical addiction

psychological addiction

psychotropic

smoking

snorting

stimulants

substance abuse

tolerance

withdrawal

INTRODUCTION

Drug abuse and addiction are common problems in the United States today. Approximately 9.4% of individuals in the United States currently have a problem with addiction (Woodrow, 2007). This chapter discusses substances that are most commonly abused, including prescription medications, illegal substances, and alcohol. Street names for these substances are identified along with routes of administration, DEA schedules, and adverse events that may occur with abuse of the substance.

BASIC DEFINITIONS

These are some of the basic definitions used when talking about substance abuse:

- **Substance abuse** is the misuse of a substance that causes the individual mental, physical, social, or emotional harm.

- Abuse can lead to dependency or **addiction**. Addiction can be physical or psychological in nature.

- **Injecting** is the when the individual uses a syringe and needle to directly insert the substance into her body.

- **Physical addiction** occurs when one or more of the body's functions become dependent on the presence of a drug. Without the drug, the body experiences withdrawal symptoms.

- **Psychological addiction** occurs when a mental or emotional craving exists for the effects produced by a substance. Without the drug, there are no physical withdrawal symptoms.

- **Smoking** is when an individual inhales the substance into the lungs.

- **Snorting** is when the individual inhales the substance into the nose, where the substance is then directly absorbed into the bloodstream through the nasal tissues.

- **Tolerance** occurs when the individual's body adjusts to the dose of the substance being abused and a larger amount of substance is needed to achieve the desired or wanted effect.

- **Withdrawal** is an illness that happens when an individual with a **physical addiction** to a substance is no longer given that substance. Symptoms include nausea, shakes, sweats, tremors, and acute cravings for the substance.

substance abuse
The misuse of a legal or illegal substance enough to cause an individual mental, physical, social, or emotional harm.

physical addiction
One or more of the body's functions becomes dependent on the presence of a drug; without it, the body experiences withdrawal symptoms.

psychological addiction
A mental or emotional craving for the effects produced by a substance; without it, there are no physical withdrawal symptoms.

COMMONLY ABUSED SUBSTANCES

There are numerous substances that are abused in the United States today. This chapter discusses only the most common. These are divided into the following six categories:

- Cannabinoids

- Depressants

- Hallucinogens
- Opioids and morphine derivatives
- Stimulants
- Miscellaneous substances

Cannabinoids

Cannabinoids include **marijuana** and hashish. According to the National Institute on Drug Abuse (2009a), twenty-five (25) million individuals age twelve (12) and older have abused marijuana at least once in 2006 in the year prior to being surveyed.

Table 35-1 provides additional information on marijuana and hashish, including street names, routes of administration, DEA schedules, and adverse effects.

Depressants

Depressants include both prescription medications and illegal drugs. The prescription medications are used as sedatives to treat insomnia, anticonvulsants to control seizures, and antianxiety medications to relieve anxiety.

GHB (Xyrem) and Rohypnol (flunitrazepam) are two commonly used **club drugs**. Club drugs tend to be abused by teens and young adults at nightclubs, bars, raves, and trance scenes.

Rohypnol (flunitrazepam) is known as the "date rape" drug. Rohypnol (flunitrazepam) causes **anterograde amnesia**. It is often secretly given to an individual before a sexual assault.

Table 35-1 provides additional information on depressants, including street names, routes of administration, DEA schedules, and adverse effects.

anterograde amnesia The lack of recall of events that happen while an individual is under the influence of a substance.

Hallucinogens

Hallucinogens include **LSD** (d-lysergic acid diethylamide) and **PCP** (phencyclidine). The effects of hallucinogens are inconsistent, making these drugs dangerous. Hallucinogens affect every individual differently. In addition, the effect on an individual will be different each time the individual abuses the drug.

Individuals who abuse LSD often experience **flashbacks**. Flashbacks occur suddenly and without warning. These may occur a few days or even a year after the individual uses a dose of LSD. In some individuals the flashbacks may continue for long periods of time.

flashbacks Recurrences of certain aspects of their drug experience (their trip).

Table 35-1 provides additional information on hallucinogens, including street names, routes of administration, DEA schedules, and adverse effects.

Opioids and Morphine Derivatives

Opioids and morphine derivatives include both prescription medications and illegal drugs. The prescription medications are used to relieve pain.

Table 35-1 Commonly Abused Substances with Street Names, Brief Descriptions, and Adverse Effects

SUBSTANCE	STREET NAMES	ROUTES OF ADMINISTRATION	DEA SCHEDULE	BRIEF DESCRIPTION	ADVERSE EFFECTS
Cannabinoids					
Hashish	Boom, chronic, gangster, hash, hash oil, hemp	Smoked, swallowed	I	A more concentrated form of THC, a black sticky liquid.	Same as marijuana.
Marijuana	Blunt, dope, ganja, grass, herb, joints, Mary Jane, pot, reefer, sinsemilla, skunk, weed	Usually smoked as a cigarette commonly called a joint or in a pipe, can also be mixed with food or brewed as tea and swallowed	I	Most commonly used illegal drug in the United States. Main active chemical is THC.	Memory and learning problems, distorted perception, difficulty thinking and problem solving, impaired coordination, increased heart rate and pulse, decreased capacity to carry oxygen to the body. Effects can last for days or weeks. Long-term use may lead to addiction.
Depressants					
Barbiturates Amytal Nembutal Phenobarbital Seconal	Barbs, reds, red birds, phennies, tooies, yellows, yellow jackets	Injected, swallowed	II, III, V	Prescription medications used as sedatives and to treat seizures.	Physically addictive and causes withdrawal if stopped suddenly, confusion, fatigue, impaired coordination, poor memory and judgment, poor concentration, and respiratory depression and arrest.
Benzodiazepines					
Ativan Halcion Librium Valium Xanax	Candy, downers, sleeping pills, tranks	Injected, swallowed	IV	Prescription medications used as sedatives and to relieve anxiety.	Physically addictive and causes withdrawal if stopped suddenly, sedation, drowsiness, depression, unusual excitement, fever, irritability, poor judgment, slurred speech, and dizziness.
Club Drugs					
GHB	G, Georgia, home boy, grievous bodily harm, liquid ecstasy	Swallowed	I	A central nervous system depressant that was approved by the FDA in 2002 for the treatment of narcolepsy, a sleep disorder. Approval came with severe restrictions and close patient monitoring.	Coma, seizures, amnesia, and withdrawal effects, including insomnia, anxiety, tremors, and sweating.

Methaqualone	Quaalude, Sopor, Parest, ludes, mandrex, quad, quay	Injected, swallowed	I	Illegal drug that produces euphoria	Depression, poor reflexes, slurred speech, and coma.
Rohypnol	Forget-me pill, Mexican Valium, R2, Roche, roofies, roofinol, rope, rophies	Snorted, swallowed	IV	Not approved for use in the United States.	May lead to tolerance and dependence. May be lethal (deadly) when mixed with alcohol and/or other central nervous system depressants.
Hallucinogens					
LSD	Acid, blotter, boomers, cubes, microdot, yellow sunshines	Swallowed, absorbed through tissues of the mouth—available as tablets, capsules, liquid, or on absorbent paper	I	One of the strongest mood-altering drugs available.	Unpredictable psychological effects; visual hallucinations; delusions; increased body temperature, heart rate, and blood pressure; sleeplessness; and loss of appetite. Produces rapid, intense emotional swings. Tolerance develops.
PCP	Angel dust, boat, hog, love boat, peace pill	Injected, swallowed, smoked—sold as tablets, capsules, or colored powder	I, II	Illegally made in labs. Never approved for human use because of problems during clinical trials.	Physically addictive and causes withdrawal if stopped suddenly. Often causes overdose and unpleasant psychological effects. Produces rapid, intense emotional swings. Increased heart rate and blood pressure, shallow respirations, flushing, heavy sweating, numbness of extremities, loss of coordination, nausea, vomiting, blurred vision, drooling, and loss of balance.
Opioids and morphine derivatives					
Codeine	Captain Cody, schoolboy, doors and fours, loads, pancakes and syrup	Injected, swallowed.	II, III, IV, V	A prescription medication used to relieve pain.	Tolerance and addiction develops, causes withdrawal if stopped suddenly. Drowsiness, nausea, constipation, confusion, sedation, respiratory depression and arrest, unconsciousness, coma, and death.

(continues)

Table 35-1 Commonly Abused Substances with Street Names, Brief Descriptions, and Adverse Effects—*continued*

SUBSTANCE	STREET NAMES	ROUTES OF ADMINISTRATION	DEA SCHEDULE	BRIEF DESCRIPTION	ADVERSE EFFECTS
Fentanyl	Apache, China girl, China white, dance fever, friend, goodfella, jackpot, murder 8, TNT, Tango and Cash	Injected, swallowed, snorted	I, II	A prescription medication used to relieve pain.	Tolerance and addiction develops, causes withdrawal if stopped suddenly. Drowsiness, nausea, constipation, confusion, sedation, respiratory depression and arrest, unconsciousness, coma, and death.
Heroin	Brown sugar, dope, H, horse, junk, skag, skunk, smack, white horse	Injected, swallowed, snorted	I	Addictive drug processed from morphine.	Tolerance and physical dependence develops, causes withdrawal if stopped suddenly. Fatal overdose, respiratory depression. spontaneous abortion, infection of heart lining and valves, liver and kidney disease, and infectious diseases such as hepatitis and HIV/AIDS.
Morphine	M, Miss Emma. monkey, white stuff	Injected. swallowed, smoked	II, III	A prescription medication used to relieve pain.	Tolerance and addiction develops, causes withdrawal if stopped suddenly. Drowsiness, nausea, constipation, confusion, sedation, respiratory depression and arrest, unconsciousness, coma, and death.
Opium	Big O. black stuff, block, gum, hop	Swallowed, smoked	II, III	A prescription medication used to relieve pain.	Tolerance and addiction develops, causes withdrawal if stopped suddenly. Drowsiness, nausea, constipation, confusion, sedation, respiratory depression and arrest, unconsciousness, coma, and death.
Oxycodone HCL	Oxy, O.C., killer	Injected, swallowed, snorted	II	A prescription medication used to relieve pain.	Tolerance and addiction develops, causes withdrawal if stopped suddenly. Drowsiness, nausea, constipation, confusion, sedation, respiratory depression and arrest, unconsciousness, coma, and death.

Drug	Common/Street Names	How Taken	Schedule	Effects
Hydrocodone bitartrate	Vike, Watson-387	Swallowed	II	A prescription. medication used to relieve pain.	Tolerance and addiction develops, causes withdrawal if stopped suddenly. Drowsiness, nausea, constipation, confusion, sedation, respiratory depression and arrest, unconsciousness, coma, and death.

Stimulants

Drug	Common/Street Names	How Taken	Schedule	Description	Effects
Amphetamines	Bennies, black beauties, crosses, hearts, LA turnaround, speed, truck drivers, uppers	Injected, swallowed, smoked, snorted	II	A prescription medication used to treat ADHD and narcolepsy. Increases energy and mental alertness.	Physically addictive and causes withdrawal if stopped suddenly. Increased heart rate and blood pressure, rapid or irregular heart rate, decrease appetite, weight loss, heart failure, nervousness, and insomnia.
Cocaine	Blow, bump, C, candy, Charlie, coke, crack, flake, rock, now, toot	Injected, smoked, snorted	II	A very addictive drug, provides a feeling of euphoria and energy.	Physically addictive and causes withdrawal if stopped suddenly. Heart attacks, respiratory failure, strokes, seizures, bizarre and violent behavior, and death. Increases body temperature, heart rate, and blood pressure. Causes headaches, GI complications, abdominal pain, and nausea. If snorted, causes nosebleeds, loss of sense of smell, swallowing difficulties, hoarseness, and a chronic runny nose.
MDMA	Adam, clarity, ecstasy, Eve, lover's speed, peace, STP, X, XTC	Swallowed, a tablet or capsule	I	A man-made stimulant with psychedelic effects, produces feelings of mental stimulation, emotional warmth, increased sensory stimulation, and increased physical energy.	Confusion, depression, sleep problems, craving for the drug, severe anxiety, nausea, chills, sweating, teeth clenching, muscle cramping, blurred vision, increased heart rate and blood pressure, and hyperthermia. May cause brain damage. Adverse effects may occur days or even weeks after taking the drug.

(continues)

Table 35-1 Commonly Abused Substances with Street Names, Brief Descriptions, and Adverse Effects—continued

SUBSTANCE	STREET NAMES	ROUTES OF ADMINISTRATION	DEA SCHEDULE	BRIEF DESCRIPTION	ADVERSE EFFECTS
Methamphetamine	Chalk, crank, crystal, fire, glass, go fast, ice, meth, speed	Injected, swallowed, smoked, snorted	II	A prescription medication that is very addictive, increases alertness and physical activity, decreases appetite, and increases respirations, heart rate, blood pressure, and body temperature.	Physically addictive and causes withdrawal if stopped suddenly. Psychotic behavior, hallucinations, stroke, hyperthermia (severe increase in body temperature), severe dental problems, anxiety, confusion, insomnia, mood disturbances, and violent behavior.
Methylphenidate	JIF, MPH, R-ball, Skippy, the smart drug, vitamin R	Injected, swallowed, snorted	II	A prescription medication used to treat ADHD.	Tolerance and addiction develop, causes withdrawal if stopped suddenly. Aggression, violence, psychotic behavior, memory loss, cardiac and neurological damage, and impaired memory and learning.
Nicotine	Cigarettes, cigars, smokeless	Smoked, snorted, snuff, spit tobacco, bidis, chew	Not scheduled	One of the most heavily used addictive drugs in the United States.	Highly addictive, causes withdrawal if stopped suddenly. Increases individual's risk for lung cancer, emphysema, bronchial lung disorders, and cardiovascular diseases.
Miscellaneous substances					
Anabolic steroids	Roids, juice	Injected, swallowed, topical (applied to the skin) Usually taken in cycles of weeks or months interrupted by shorter rest periods. This is known as "cycling."	III	Most are synthetic (man-made) substances similar to male hormones. Abused, especially by athletes, to improve performance and appearance.	In males, shrinking of the testicles, reduced sperm count, infertility, baldness, and breast development. In females, growth of facial hair, changes in menstrual cycle, baldness, and deepening of voice. Other effects include severe acne, high blood pressure, jaundice, aggression, extreme mood swings, paranoia, delusions, impaired judgment, liver and kidney tumors, and cancer.

Dextromethorphan (DXM)	Robotripping, Robo, Triple C	Swallowed	Not scheduled	OTC cough and cold medication.	Distorted visual perception, memory loss, numbness, delirium, depression, and respiratory depression and arrest.
Inhalants	Laughing gas, poppers, snappers, whippets	Inhaled through the nose and mouth. Known as "huffing."	Swallowed	Breathable chemical vapors intentionally inhaled for their mind-altering effects. Substances inhaled include but are not limited to spray paints, glues, cleaning fluids, degreasers, dry-cleaning fluids, gasoline, lighter fluid, correction fluids, felt-tip marker fluid, electronic contact cleaners, hair or deodorant sprays, vegetable oil sprays, whipped cream aerosols, refrigerant gases, chloroform, and nitrous oxide.	Produce a rapid high similar to alcohol, slurred speech, lack of coordination, dizziness, euphoria, lightheadedness, hallucinations, delusions, confusion, nausea, vomiting, and hypoxia. Most cause a loss of sensation and even unconsciousness. May cause irreversible effects, such as hearing loss, peripheral neuropathies, brain damage, liver and kidney damage, and "sudden sniffing death" from suffocation.

Note: Club drugs used by teens and young adults at nightclubs, bars, raves, and/or trance scenes include but are not limited to GHB, Rohypnol, MDMA (ecstasy), methamphetamine, and LSD (acid).

Based on Information obtained from National Institute of Drug Abuse, http://www.drugabuse.gov/drugpages.

Table 35-1 provides additional information on opioids and morphine derivatives, including street names, routes of administration, DEA schedules, and adverse effects.

Stimulants

Stimulants include prescription medications, illegal drugs, and legal substances such as **nicotine**. **Cocaine** is a powerful, addictive, illegal drug. A form of cocaine, known as crack cocaine, is easily accessible. When smoked, it produces an almost immediate sense of euphoria followed by a significant depression. This depression brings on a strong urge to smoke more, leading to a cycle of dependency.

Long-term methamphetamine use causes severe structural and functional changes in the areas of the brain that deal with emotion and memory, causing emotional and cognitive problems.

Nicotine is highly addictive. According to the National Institute on Drug Abuse (2009b), nearly seventy-three (73) million individuals age twelve (12) and older had used a tobacco product at least once in 2006 in the month prior to being surveyed.

Cigarette smoking accounts for 90% of all cancers. Cigarette smoking is a leading cause of cardiovascular disease. In addition, cigarette smoking is linked to cataracts, leukemia, and pneumonia. An adult who smokes dies, on average, fourteen (14) years earlier than an individual who does not smoke.

Table 35-1 provides additional information on stimulants, including street names, routes of administration, DEA schedules, and adverse effects.

Miscellaneous Substances

Anabolic Steroids

Anabolic steroids are man-made substances. Anabolic steroids mimic male hormones. Abuse of anabolic steroids can lead to serious, irreversible health problems.

Table 35-1 provides additional information on anabolic steroids, including street names, routes of administration, DEA schedules, and adverse effects.

Dextromethorphan (DXM)

Dextromethorphan (DXM) is a substance found in OTC cough and cold medications.

Table 35-1 provides additional information on dextromethorphan (DXM), including street names, routes of administration, DEA schedules, and adverse effects.

Inhalants

Inhalants are substances that are breathed in from a plastic bag or by stuffing a rag soaked with the chemical into the mouth, called **huffing**. Use of inhalants can be fatal. Serious and irreversible effects include

peripheral neuropathies
Permanent damage to the nerves, particularly in the hands, feet, and lower legs.

brain damage, hearing loss, **peripheral neuropathies**, and cardiovascular damage. They can also cause death.

Table 35-1 provides additional information on inhalants, including street names, routes of administration, DEA schedules, and adverse effects.

ALCOHOL

Although alcohol is a legal substance, it is the number one drug problem in the United States (Woodrow, 2007). According to the National Institute on Alcohol Abuse and Alcoholism (2009), there are approximately 10.8 million underage drinkers in the United States.

Adolescents in the United States choose alcohol as their drug of choice. Three-fourths (3/4) of 12th graders, more than two-thirds (2/3) of 10th graders, and approximately two-fifths (2/5) of 8th graders have consumed more than a few sips of alcohol in their lifetime. In fact, teens use alcohol more than cigarettes and marijuana combined. Forty percent of teens get alcohol from adults twenty-one (21) years or older at no cost. A smaller percentage gets alcohol from their parents, guardian, or other family members (National Institute on Alcohol Abuse and Alcoholism, 2009).

In addition, underage drinking is common in the military with 62.3% of underage military members drinking at least once a year. Twenty-one percent of active military personnel age twenty (20) or younger report heavy alcohol use. A similar percentage of college age students report binge drinking (National Institute on Alcohol Abuse and Alcoholism, 2009).

Alcohol is responsible for 100,000 deaths per year and for more than half of all traffic accidents. These traffic accidents account for 30% of all U.S. traffic fatalities (Woodrow, 2007).

Alcohol is a fast-acting depressant on the central nervous system. In addition, alcohol also has a **psychotropic** effect on the body, producing a feeling of excitement, sedation, and finally anesthesia. Large amounts of alcohol can cause a stupor, cerebral edema, depressed respiration, and death.

psychotropic
Affecting the mind, behavior, and emotions.

Prolonged alcohol use affects all organs of the body and can cause permanent damage. Damage may include the following:

- Liver damage
- Pancreatitis
- Cancer of the liver and pancreas
- Esophageal varices
- GI ulcers
- GI hemorrhage
- Disorders in the absorption of nutrients
- Malnutrition
- Cardiac myopathy

- Cardiac arrhythmias due to potassium deficiency
- Seizure disorders
- Mental deterioration
- Memory loss
- Ataxia (impaired coordination)

SUBSTANCE ABUSE IN THE WORKPLACE

The UAP may come into contact with individuals who have a history of substance abuse or who are active abusers. Because of their history of substance abuse, these individuals may sustain accidental injuries or infections more often than usual. They may try to trick the UAP into thinking they have a disease that could be treated by addictive prescription drugs. The individuals may be the individuals to whom the UAP gives care, or they may be coworkers.

Whenever the UAP meets an individual who she thinks might be abusing substances, she needs to report it to her supervisor immediately. If it is an individual the UAP is caring for, the individual's licensed health care provider needs to know as well. If it is a coworker, the UAP needs to—and in some states must—report it just as she would report any other type of abuse. An individual under the influence of drugs or alcohol should not be given the responsibility of taking care of others. It can pose a danger to everyone.

Substance abuse of legal or illegal substances can also cost the UAP her certification(s) and her job. Substance abusers may find help and support from many organizations and help groups. Here is a list of phone numbers, e-mail addresses, and Web sites of support groups and organizations:

- Al-Anon/Alateen:
  http://www.al-anon.org

- Alcoholics Anonymous:
  http://www.alcoholics-anonymous.org
  212-870-3400

- American Council for Drug Education:
  http://www.acde.org
  E-mail: acde@phoenixhouse.org
  718-222-6641

- Cocaine Anonymous:
  http://www.ca.org
  E-mail: cawso@ca.org
  310-559-5833

- Marijuana Anonymous:
  http://www.marijuana-anonymous.org
  office@marijuana-anonymous.org
  800-766-6779

- Mothers Against Drunk Driving: 800-438-6233

- Narcotics Anonymous: 818-773-9999

- National Clearinghouse for Alcohol and Drug Information:
  http://www.health.org
  800-729-6686

- National Council on Alcoholism and Drug Dependency:
  http://www.ncadd.org
  E-mail: national@ncadd.org
  800-611-1155

- National Institute on Drug Abuse:
  http://www.nida.nih.gov
  E-mail: information@nida.nih.gov
  301-443-1124

- National Institute on Alcohol Abuse and Alcoholism:
  http://www.niaaa.nih.gov
  301-443-3860

- National Clearinghouse for Drug Abuse Information

- Nicotine Anonymous:
  http://www.nicotine-anonymous.org
  877-879-6422

SUMMARY

Substance abuse is a serious issue. It affects not only the individual who is abusing the medication or drug but also everyone with whom that individual comes in contact. The UAP has a legal, moral, and ethical responsibility to report substance abuse. It is the UAP's responsibility to know her state regulations and workplace policies. She is responsible to report knowledge of substance abuse to her supervisor and to the appropriate authorities.

WORKBOOK REVIEW

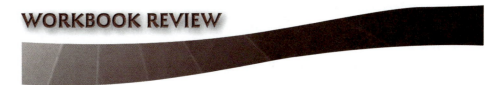

Go to the workbook and complete the exercises for Chapter 35.

REVIEW QUESTIONS

1. Physical addiction to a substance:
   a. occurs when an individual has a mental or emotional craving for a substance
   b. occurs when one or more body functions become dependent upon a substance
   c. is a legal or illegal substance misused by an individual
   d. is an illness that causes flulike symptoms

2. Psychological addiction to a substance:
   a. occurs when an individual has a mental or emotional craving for a substance
   b. occurs when one or more body functions become dependent upon a substance
   c. is a legal or illegal substance misused by an individual
   d. is an illness that causes flulike symptoms

3. Stimulants:
   a. depress the nervous system
   b. cause symptoms such as drowsiness and slurred speech in an individual who abuses them
   c. are physically addictive substances that may cause withdrawal symptoms if abruptly stopped
   d. are psychologically addictive substances that do not cause physical withdrawal symptoms

4. Depressants:
   a. are a central nervous system stimulant
   b. increase anxiety
   c. are a central nervous system depressant
   d. are also called club drugs

5. Adverse effects from inhalants may include:
   a. brain damage
   b. blindness
   c. sterility
   d. hunger

6. An individual who snorts cocaine may have symptoms including:
   a. nosebleeds and a constant runny nose
   b. weakness and increase appetite
   c. relaxation and drowsiness
   d. involuntary kicking movements

7. Opiates are used medically to:
   a. provide local anesthesia
   b. treat diarrhea and abdominal cramps
   c. relieve pain
   d. reduce symptoms of the flu

8. Tobacco smoke contains substances that may:
   a. increase an individual's risk for lung cancer, emphysema, bronchial disorders, and cardiovascular disease
   b. cause increased anger and aggression in an individual who smokes
   c. relieve symptoms of a bronchial illness
   d. cause chills, fever, and nausea

9. PCP is dangerous because:
   a. it may cause tachycardia
   b. it may significantly increase the appetite
   c. it is illegally made in labs
   d. it is easy to overdose on PCP

10. If a UAP suspects a coworker of abusing substances, she should:
   a. ask the individual if she is abusing substances
   b. report it just as she would report any other type of abuse
   c. not say anything so she does not get in trouble
   d. tell other coworkers of her suspicions

CLINICAL SCENARIOS

1. When you are at work one day, you see a coworker who is extremely talkative—more so than usual. Her pupils are dilated and her skin is pale. You notice that she becomes dizzy after assisting an individual to stand up. You know she has been working two jobs over the past six (6) months and used to complain of being tired a lot. Now she has not mentioned her fatigue in the past few weeks. What do you think might be happening? What do you do about it?

2. You work in a place where individuals are allowed to self-administer medications if they are able to do so. You know that Mr. Luango can self-administer his medications. He has recently had tendon surgery and was given a prescription for Demerol. In the past few days, he has been vomiting frequently and complaining of itching on his arms and legs. Now he seems to be much happier than usual and is napping frequently during the day. What do you think might be happening? What can you do about it as a UAP?

References

American Association of Poison Control Centers. (2009). *Poison control in action.* Retrieved June 22, 2009, from http://www.aapcc.org/dnn/PoisonPrevention/FAQ/tabid/117/Default.aspx

American Cancer Society. (2009a). *Chemotherapy: What it is, how it works.* Retrieved May 22, 2009, from http://www.cancer.org/docroot/ETO/content/ETO_1_2X_Chemotherapy_What_It_Is_How_It_Helps.asp?sitearea = ETO&viewmode = print&

American Cancer Society. (2009b). *Detailed guide: Cancer (general information).* Retrieved June 11, 2009, from http://www.cancer.org/docroot/CRI/CRI_2_3x.asp?dt = 72

American Society for Pharmacology and Experimental Therapeutics. (2008). Retrieved December 8, 2008, from http://www.aspet.org

Asacol. (2009). *What is inflammatory bowel disease?* Retrieved June 8, 2009, from http://www.asacol.com/ulcerative-colitis/inflammatory-bowel-disease.jsp?utm_source = google&utm_medium

Broyles, B. E., Reiss, B. S., & Evans, M. E. (2007). *Pharmacological aspects of nursing care* (7th ed.). Clifton Park, NY: Delmar, Cengage Learning.

Centers for Disease Control and Prevention. (2009). *Introduction.* Retrieved May 10, 2009, from http://www.cdc.gov/obesity/index.html

Cerner Corporation. (2008). *Medication administration record (eMAR).* Retrieved August 27, 2008, from http://www.cerner.com/public/Cerner_3.asp?id = 27047

Deter, L. L., & Polesky, W. (1999). *MAP trainer's manual: The five rights of medication administration.* Boston: Center for Community Health.

Dey, L. P. (2009). *Epipen [epinephrine] auto-injector.* Retrieved May 5, 2009, from http://www.epipen.com

Doylestown Hospital. (2008). *Electronic medication administration record (eMAR).* Retrieved August 27, 2008, from http://doylestownhospital.org/body.cfm?id = 434

Epilepsy Foundation. *First aid.* Retrieved June 23, 2009, from http://www.epilepsyfoundation.org/about/firstaid/index.cfm

Epilepsy Foundation. *Seizures and syndromes.* Retrieved June 23, 2009, from http://www.epilepsyfoundation.org/about/types/types/statusepilepticus.cfm

Epilepsy Foundation. *Complementary treatment: Complementary therapies.* Retrieved June 23, 2009, from http://www.epilepsyfoundation.org/about/treatment/complementary/incex.cfm

Epilepsy Foundation. *Treatment options: Ketogenic diet.* Retrieved June 23, 2009, from http://www.epilepsyfoundation.org/about/treatment/ketogenicdiet/index.cfm

Epilepsy Foundation. *Treatment options: Medications.* Retrieved June 23, 2009, from http://www.epilepsyfoundation.org/about/treatment/medications/medsside.cfm

Epilepsy Foundation. *Treatment options: Surgery.* Retrieved June 23, 2009, from http://www.epilepsyfoundation.org/about/treatment/surgery/index.cfm

Epilepsy Foundation. *Treatment options: Vagus nerves stimulation.* Retrieved June 23, 2009, from http://www.epilepsyfoundation.org/about/treatment/vns/vnssurgery.cfm

Epilepsy Foundation. *What is epilepsy?* Retrieved June 23, 2009, from http://www.epilepsyfoundation.org/about

Frechette & Massachusetts Department of Public Health. (1982). *Request for authorization to proceed to public hearing on regulations which would allow for medication administration in community programs for mentally ill or mentally retarded persons by employees who have completed an approved training program.* Jamaica Plain, MA: Frechette & Massachusetts Department of Public Health.

Garner, B. (Ed.). (2000). *Black's law dictionary* (7th ed.). St. Paul, MN: West Group.

Hebrew Senior Life. (2008a). *Computerized physician online entry (CPOE).* Boston: Hebrew Senior Life.

Hebrew Senior Life. (2008b). *Electronic medication administration record (eMAR).* Boston: Hebrew Senior Life.

Hegner, B. R., Acello, B., & Caldwell, E. (2008). *Nursing assistant: A nursing process approach* (10th ed.). Clifton Park, NY: Delmar, Cengage Learning.

The Joint Commission. (2009). *"Do not use" list.* Retrieved February 9, 2009, from http://www.jointcommission.org/PatientSafety/DoNotUseList/default.htm?print=yes

Joint Commission. (2010). *Using medication reconciliation to prevent errors.* Retrieved January 23, 2010, from http://www.jointcommission.org/SentinelEvents/SentinelEventAlert/sea_35.htm

Medline Plus. (2009a). *Smoking.* Retrieved June 11, 2009, from http://www.nlm.nih.gov/medlineplus/smoking.html

Medline Plus. (2009b). *Erectile dysfunction.* Retrieved June 13, 2009, from http://www.nlm.nih.gov/medlineplus/erectiledysfunction.html

Medquest Communications. (2008). *Electronic medication administration record (eMAR).* Retrieved August 27, 2008, from http://findarticles.com

Myers, T. (Ed.). (2006). *Mosby's pocket dictionary of medicine, nursing, and health professions* (5th ed.). St. Louis, MO: Mosby Elsevier.

National Council of State Boards of Nursing Delegate Assembly. (2007). *Medication assistant (MA-C) model curriculum.* Chicago: National Council of State Boards of Nursing.

National Health and Blood Institute. (2009). *Facts about menopausal hormonal therapy.* Retrieved June 13, 2009, from http://www.nhlbi.nih.gov/health/women/pht_facts.pdf

National Institutes on Alcohol Abuse and Alcoholism. (2009). *Statistical snapshot.* Retrieved June 24, 2009, from http://www.niaaa.nih.gov

National Institute of Allergy and Infectious Diseases. (2008). *Antimicrobial (drug) resistance.* Retrieved October 5, 2008, from http://www3.niaid.nih.gov/topics/antimicrobialResistance/Understanding/causes.htm

National Institute of Drug Abuse. Retrieved June 23, 2009, from http://www.drugabuse.gov/DrugPages.

National Institute of Drug Abuse. (2009a). *Marajuana.* Retrieved June 23, 2009, from http://www.drugabuse.gov/DrugPages/Marajuana.html

National Institute of Drug Abuse. (2009b). *Tobacco/nicotine*. Retrieved June 23, 2009, from http://www.drugabuse.gov/DrugPages/Nicotine.html

National Kidney and Urological Disease Information Clearinghouse. (2009). *Erectile dysfunction*. Retrieved June 13, 2009, from http://kidney.niddk.nih.gov/kudiseases/pubs/impotence/index.htm#cause

Office of National Drug Control Policy. (2007). *Proper disposal of prescription drugs*. Retrieved November 8, 2008, from http://whitehousedrugpolicy.gov/drugfact/factsht/proper_disposal.html

Schull, P. D. (2007). *Premier 2008 edition nursing spectrum drug handbook*. New York: Nursing Spectrum.

Smith, S., & Gove, J. E. (2005). *Physical changes of aging* (2nd ed.). Gainesville: University of Florida, Florida Cooperative Extension Service.

Sorrentino, S. (2008). *Mosby's textbook for nursing assistants* (7th ed.). St. Louis, MO: Mosby.

THELEAPFROGGROUP. (2010). *Fact sheet computerized physician order entry*. Retrieved January 4, 2010, from http://www.leapfroggroup.org/media/file/Leapfrog-Computer_Physician_Order_Entry_Fact_Sheet.pdf

U.S. Food and Drug Administration. (2008). *How to dispose of unused medications*. Retrieved June 24, 2008, from http://www.fda.gov/consumer/updates/drug_disposal062308.html

U.S. Food and Drug Administration. (2009). *The new over-the-counter medicine label: Take a look*. Retrieved February 9, 2009, from http://www.fda.gov/Drugs/EmergencyPreparedness/BioterrorismandDrugPreparedness/ucm133411.htm

Williams, S. J., & Torrens, P. R. (1993). *Introduction to health services* (4th ed.). Clifton Park, NY: Delmar, Cengage Learning.

Woodrow, R. (2007). *Essentials of pharmacology for health occupations* (5th ed.). Clifton Park, NY: Delmar, Cengage Learning.

Yoder, M., & Collins, S. (1999). *Controlled substance count book*. Sturbridge, MA: SCRRI.

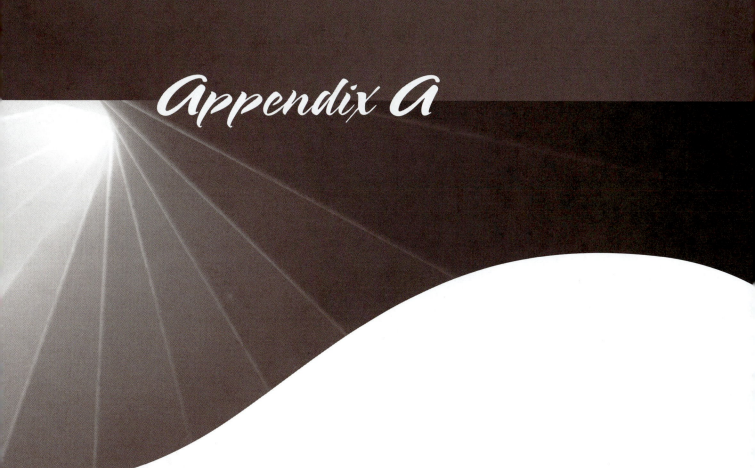

Appendix A

Table of Authorities

Addington v. Texas, 441 U.S. 418 (1979)

Lessard v. Schmidt, 379 F. Supp. 1376 (1974)

Matter of Stokes, 546 A.2d 356 (D.C. App. 1988)

O'Connor v. Donaldson, 422 U.S. 563 (1975)

Humphrey v. Cady, 405 U.S. 504 (1972)

Foucha v. Louisiana, 504 U.S. 71 (1992)

Doe by Doe v. Austin, 848 F.2d 1386, 1395–96 (6th Cir. 1988)

Clark v. Cohen, 794 F.2d 79, 86 (3rd Cir. 1986)

Best v. St. Vincents Hospital, Docket No. 03-Cv. 0365 (S.D.N.Y. 2003)

In Re Qawi, 32 Cal. 4th 1, 81 P.3d 224 (2004)

Appendix B

Source: Reprinted with permission from the Center for the Advancement of Patient Safety.

A Publication of the USP Center for the Advancement of Patient Safety   April 2004   No. 79

USP Quality Review

USE CAUTION—AVOID CONFUSION

This updated resource now includes reports submitted to both USP medication error reporting programs—MEDMARX℠ and the USP Medication Errors Reporting (MER) Program—from their inception through December 31, 2002. Similarity of drug names involves confusion between look-alike and/or sound-alike brand names, generic names, and brand to generic names. This confusion is compounded by illegible handwriting, lack of knowledge of drug names, newly available products, similar packaging or labeling, and incorrect selection of a similar name from a computerized product list.

Below is a list of similar drug names reported to MEDMARX and MER. It is important to remember that these names may not sound alike as you read them or look alike in print, but when handwritten or communicated verbally, these names have caused or could cause confusion. (Brand names are *italicized* and new entries are highlighted in brown).

Accolate . . . . *Accupril*	*Actonel* . . . . *Actos*	*Allegra* . . . . *Viagra*
Accolate . . . . *Accutane*	*Actos* . . . . *Actonel*	*Allegra-D* . . . . *Allegra*
Accupril . . . . *Aciphex*	*Acular* . . . . Ocular Lubricants	*Allegra-D* . . . . *Allerx-D*
Accupril . . . . *Accolate*	Acyclovir . . . . Acetazolamide	*Allerx-D* . . . . *Allegra-D*
Accupril . . . . *Accutane*	Acyclovir . . . . Famciclovir	Allopurinol . . . . *Apresoline*
Accupril . . . . *Altace*	*Adalat CC* . . . . *Aldomet*	*Alora* . . . . *Aldara*
Accupril . . . . *Aricept*	*Adalat CC* . . . . *Allegra*	Alprazolam . . . . Clonazepam
Accupril . . . . *Monopril*	*Adderall* . . . . *Inderal*	Alprazolam . . . . Diazepam
Accutane . . . . *Accolate*	Adenosine . . . . Adenosine Phosphate	Alprazolam . . . . Lorazepam
Accutane . . . . *Accupril*	Adenosine Phosphate . . . . Adenosine	*Altace* . . . . *Accupril*
Acebutolol . . . . Albuterol	*Apidex-P* . . . . *Aciphex*	*Altace* . . . . . *Amaryl* . . . . . *Amerge*
Acetaminophen . . . . Acetaminophen and Codeine and Hydrocodone	*Adriamycin* . . . . *Aredia*	*Altace* . . . . *Artane*
Acetaminophen . . . . Acetaminophen and Codeine and Oxycodone	*Adriamycin* . . . . *Idamycin*	*Altace* . . . . *Norvasc*
Acetaminophen . . . . Acetaminophen and Hydrocodone and Codeine	*Advair* . . . . *Advicor*	*Alupent* . . . . *Atrovent*
Acetaminophen . . . . Acetaminophen and Oxycodone and Codeine	*Advicor* . . . . *Advair*	Amantadine . . . . Amiodarone
Acetazolamide . . . . Acetohexamide	*Aggrastat* . . . . *Aggrenox*	Amantadine . . Ranitidine . . Rimantadine
Acetazolamide . . . . Acetylcysteine	*Aggrastat* . . . . Argatroban	*Amaryl* . . . . . *Altace* . . . . . *Amerge*
Acetazolamide . . . . Acyclovir	*Aggrenox* . . . . *Aggrastat*	*Amaryl* . . . . *Avandia*
Acetohexamide . . . . Acetazolamide	*Akarpine* . . . . Atropine	*Amaryl* . . . . *Reminyl*
Acetylcysteine . . . . Acetazolamide	Albuterol . . . . Acebutolol	*Amaryl* . . . . *Symmetrel*
Aciphex . . . . *Accupril*	*Aldara* . . . . *Alora*	*Ambien* . . . . *Amen*
Aciphex . . . . *Adipex-P*	Aldesleukin . . . . Oprelvekin	*Ambien* . . . . *Ativan*
Aciphex . . . . *Aricept*	*Aldomet* . . . . *Adalat CC*	*Ambien* . . . . *Coumadin*
Aciphex . . . . *Vioxx*	*Alkeran* . . . . *Leukeran*	*Amen* . . . . *Ambien*
Activase . . . . *Retavase*	*Allegra* . . . . *Adalat CC*	*Amerge* . . . . . *Altace* . . . . . *Amaryl*
	Allegra . . . . *Allegra-D*	*Amicar* . . . . *Amikin*
	Allegra . . . . *Asacol*	Amikacin . . . . Anakinra
		Amikin . . . . *Amicar*

Amiloride . . . . Amlodipine	Asacol . . . . Os-Cal	Benadryl . . . . Benylin	
Aminophylline . . . . Amitriptyline	Asparaginase. . . . . Pegaspargase	Benazepril . . . . Benadryl	
Amiodarone . . . . Trazodone	Atacand . . . . Antacid	Benazepril . . . . Benzonatate	
Amiodarone . . . . Amantadine	Atacand . . . . Avandia	Benazepril . . . . Donepezil	
Amiodarone . . . . Amlodipine	Atarax . . . . Amoxicillin	Benazepril . . . . Lisinopril	
Amiodarone . . . . Amrinone (Former nomenclature for Inamrinone)	Atarax . . . . Ativan	Bentyl . . . . Benadryl	
	Atenolol . . . . Metoprolol	Bentyl . . . . Bumex	
	Atgam . . . . Ratgam (Synonym for Thymoglobulin)	Bentyl . . . . Proventil	
Amitriptyline. . . . . Aminophylline		Benylin . . . . Benadryl	
Amitriptyline. . . . . Imipramine		Benylin . . . . Ventolin	
Amitriptyline. . . . . Nortriptyline	Ativan . . . . Ambien	Benzonatate . . . . Benazepril	
Amlodipine. . . . . Amiloride	Ativan . . . . Atarax	Benzonatate . . . . Benztropine	
Amlodipine. . . . . Amiodarone	Atorvastatin . . . . Pravastatin	Benztropine . . . . Benzonatate	
Amlodipine. . . . . Felodipine	Atropine . . . . Akarpine	Bepridil . . . . Prepidil	
Amoxicillin. . . . . Amoxil	Atrovent . . . . Alupent	Betagan . . . . Betoptic	
Amoxicillin . . . . Ampicillin	Atrovent . . . . Azmacort	Betapace . . . . Betapace AF	
Amoxicillin. . . . . Atarax	Atrovent . . . . Flovent	Betapace AF . . . . Betapace	
Amoxicillin. . . . . Augmentin	Atrovent . . . . Natru-Vent	Betoptic . . . . Betagan	
Amoxil . . . . Amoxicillin	Atrovent . . . . Serevent	Betoptic . . . . Betoptic S	
Amphotericin B, ... Amphotericin B, Lipid Complex Liposomal	Attenuvax . . . . Meruvax	Betoptic S . . . . Betoptic	
	Augmentin . . . . Amoxicillin	Biaxin. . . . . Bactrim	
Amphotericin B, ... Amphotericin B, Liposomal . . . . Lipid Complex	Augmentin . . . . Ampicillin	Bisacodyl . . . . Bisoprolol	
	Avandia . . . . Amaryl	Bisacodyl . . . . Visicol	
Ampicillin . . . . Amoxicillin	Avandia . . . . Atacand	Bisoprolol . . . . Bisacodyl	
Ampicillin. . . . . Augmentin	Avandia . . . . Avelox	Bisoprolol . . . . Fosinopril	
Ampicillin . . . . Oxacillin	Avandia . . . . Coumadin	Boost bar . . . . Buspar	
Amrinone . . . . Amiodarone (Former nomenclature for Inamrinone)	Avandia . . . . Prandin	Brevibloc . . . . Brevital	
	Avapro. . . . . Anaprox	Brevital. . . . . Brevibloc	
	Avapro . . . . Avelox	Bumex . . . . Bentyl	
Anaflex . . . . Zanaflex	Avelox . . . . Avandia	Bumex . . . . Buprenex	
Anakinra . . . . Amikacin	Avelox . . . . Avapro	Bumex . . . . Nimbex	
Anaprox . . . . Avapro	Avelox . . . . Cerebyx	Bumex . . . . Permax	
Anaspaz. . . . . Antispas	Avinza . . . . Invanz	Bupivacaine . . . . Ropivacaine	
Anbesol . . . . Anusol	Avonex . . . . Lovenox	Buprenex . . . . Bumex	
Ansaid . . . . Asacol	Azithromycin . . . . Erythromycin	Bupropion. . . . . Buspirone	
Antacid . . . . Atacand	Azithromycin . . . . Vancomycin	Buspar . . . . Boost bar	
Antispas. . . . . Anaspaz	Azithromycin . . . . Aztreonam	Buspirone . . . . Bupropion	
Anusol . . . . Anbesol	Azmacort . . . . Atrovent	Butalbital, ... Butalbital, Acetaminophen, Aspirin, and and Caffeine Caffeine	
Anusol . . . . Anusol-HC	Azmacort . . . . Nasacort		
Anusol-HC . . . . Anusol	Aztreonam . . . . Azithromycin	Butalbital, ... Butalbital, Aspirin, and Acetaminophen, Caffeine and Caffeine	
Anzemet. . . . . Aricept	Bactrim. . . . . Biaxin		
Apresoline . . . . Allopurinol	Bactrim DS . . . . Bancap HC	Cafergot . . . . Carafate	
Apresoline . . . . Priscoline	Bancap HC. . . . . Bactrim DS	Calan. . . . . Calan SR	
Aredia . . . . Adriamycin	Baycol . . . . Bellergal	Calan. . . . . Colace	
Argatroban. . . . . Aggrastat	Beclovent . . . . Beconase	Calan SR . . . . Calan	
Argatroban. . . . . Orgaran	Beconase . . . . Beclovent	Calan SR . . . . Cardizem CD	
Aricept . . . . Accupril	Beconase . . . . Beconase AQ	Calan SR . . . . Cardizem SR	
Aricept . . . . Aciphex	Beconase AQ . . . . Beconase	Calciferol . . . . Calcitriol	
Aricept . . . . Anzemet	Bellergal . . . . Baycol	Calcitriol. . . . . Calciferol	
Artane . . . . Altace	Benadryl . . . . Benazepril	Calcium Acetate . . . . Calcium Carbonate	
Asacol . . . . Allegra	Benadryl . . . . Bentyl		
Asacol . . . . Ansaid			

804

Calcium Carbonate . . . . . . Calcium Acetate
Calcium Carbonate . . . . . . Calcium Gluconate
Calcium Chloride. . . . . . . Calcium Gluconate
Calcium Gluconate . . . . . Calcium Carbonate
Calcium Gluconate . . . . . . Calcium Chloride
Capoten . . . . *Catapres*
Captopril. . . . . Carvedilol
Carafate . . . . *Cafergot*
Carbatrol . . . . *Carbrital*
(Carbamezapine   (Pentobarbitone
in U.S.)   Sodium in
                     Australia)
Carbidopa . . . . Levodopa and
                     Carbidopa
Carboplatin . . . . Cisplatin
Carbrital. . . . . *Carbatrol*
(Pentobarbitone   (Carbamezapine
Sodium in Australia) in U.S.)
Cardene . . . . *Cardizem*
Cardene . . . . *Cardura*
Cardene . . . . Codeine
Cardene SR. . . . . *Cardizem SR*
Cardiem . . . . *Cardizem*
Cardizem . . . . *Cardene*
Cardizem . . . . *Cardiem*
Cardizem . . . . *Cardizem SR*
Cardizem . . . . Clonidine
Cardizem CD . . . . *Calan SR*
Cardizem CD . . . . *Cardizem SR*
Cardizem SR. . . . . *Calan SR*
Cardizem SR. . . . . *Cardene SR*
Cardizem SR. . . . . *Cardizem*
Cardizem SR. . . . . *Cardizem CD*
Cardura . . . . *Cardene*
Cardura . . . . *Cordarone*
Cardura . . . . *Coumadin*
Cardura . . . . *K-Dur*
Cardura . . . . *Ridaura*
Carteolol. . . . . Carvedilol
Cartia. . . . . *Cartia XT*
(Aspirin in   (Diltiazem in U.S.)
New Zealand)
Cartia XT. . . . . *Diltia XT*
Cartia XT. . . . . *Procardia XL*
Cartia XT. . . . . *Cartia*
(Diltiazem in U.S.) (Aspirin in
                     New Zealand)
Carvedilol . . . . Captopril
Carvedilol . . . . Carteolol
Cataflam . . . . *Catapres*
Catapres. . . . . *Capoten*
Catapres. . . . . *Cataflam*

Ceclor. . . . . *Ceclor CD*
Ceclor CD. . . . . *Ceclor*
Cefaclor . . . . Cephalexin
Cefazolin . . . . Cefepime
Cefazolin . . . . Cafotaxime
Cefazolin . . . . Cefotetan
Cefazolin . . . . Cefoxitin
Cefazolin . . . . Cefprozil
Cefazolin . . . . Ceftazidime
Cefazolin . . . . Ceftizoxime
Cefazolin . . . . Ceftriaxone
Cefazolin . . . . Cefuroxime
Cefazolin . . . . Cephalexin
Cefepime. . . . . Cefazolin
Cefepime. . . . . Cefotetan
Cefepime. . . . . *Cefotan*
Cefixime . . . . Cefpodoxime
Cefobid. . . . . Celecoxib
Cefobid. . . . . *Levbid*
Cefol. . . . . *Cefzil*
Cefotan. . . . . *Ceftin*
Cefotan. . . . . *Claforan*
Cefotan. . . . . Cefepime
Cefotan. . . . . Ceftriaxone
Cefotaxime . . . . Cefazolin
Cefotaxime . . . . Cefotetan
Cefotaxime . . . . Cefoxitin
Cefotaxime . . . . Ceftazidime
Cefotaxime . . . . Ceftizoxime
Cefotaxime . . . . Ceftriaxone
Cefotaxime . . . . Cefuroxime
Cefotetan . . . . Cefazolin
Cefotetan . . . . Cefepime
Cefotetan . . . . Cefotaxime
Cefotetan . . . . Cefoxitin
Cefotetan . . . . Ceftazidime
Cefotetan . . . . Ceftizoxime
Cefotetan . . . . Ceftriaxone
Cefoxitin. . . . . Cefazolin
Cefoxitin. . . . . Cefotaxime
Cefoxitin. . . . . Cefotetan
Cefoxitin. . . . . Ceftriaxone
Cefoxitin. . . . . Cefuroxime
Cefpodoxime. . . . . Cefixime
Cefprozil. . . . . Cefazolin
Cefprozil. . . . . Cefuroxime
Ceftazidime . . . . Cefazolin
Ceftazidime . . . . Cafotaxime
Ceftazidime . . . . Cefotetan
Ceftazidime . . . . Ceftizoxime
Ceftazidime . . . . Ceftriaxone

Ceftazidime . . . . Cefuroxime
Ceftin. . . . . *Cefotan*
Ceftin. . . . . *Cefzil*
Ceftin. . . . . *Cipro*
Ceftin. . . . . *Rocephin*
Ceftizoxime . . . . Cefazolin
Ceftizoxime . . . . Cefotaxime
Ceftizoxime . . . . Cefotetan
Ceftizoxime . . . . Ceftazidime
Ceftizoxime . . . . Cefuroxime
Ceftriaxone . . . . Cefazolin
Ceftriaxone . . . . Cefotaxime
Ceftriaxone . . . . Cefotetan
Ceftriaxone . . . . Cefoxitin
Ceftriaxone . . . . Ceftazidime
Ceftriaxone . . . . Cefuroxime
Ceftriaxone. . . . . *Cefotan*
Cefuroxime . . . . Cefazolin
Cefuroxime . . . . Cefotaxime
Cefuroxime . . . . Cefprozil
Cefuroxime . . . . Ceftazidime
Cefuroxime . . . . Ceftizoxime
Cefuroxime . . . . Ceftriaxone
Cefuroxime . . . . Cephalexin
Cefuroxime . . . . Deferoxamine
Cefuroxime . . . . Cefoxitin
Cefzil . . . . *Cefol*
Cefzil . . . . *Ceftin*
Cefzil . . . . *Kefzol*
Celebrex . . . . . *Celexa* . . . . . *Cerebyx*
Celebrex . . . . . *Celexa* . . . . . *Cerebra*
Celecoxib . . . . *Cefobid*
Celexa . . . . *Zyprexa*
Celexa . . . . *Celebrex*.. . . . . *Cerebra*
Celexa . . . . *Cerebyx* .. . . . . *Celebrex*
Cephalexin . . . . Cefaclor
Cephalexin . . . . Cefazolin
Cephalexin . . . . Cefuroxime
Cephalexin . . . . Ciprofloxacin
Cerebra . . . *Celebrex*. . . . . *Celexa*
Cerebyx . . . . *Avelox*
Cerebyx . . . *Celebrex*. . . . . *Celexa*
Cetirizine . . . . Cyclobenzaprine
Chlordiazepoxide . . . . Chlorpromazine
Chlorhexidine . . . . Chlorpromazine
Chlorpromazine . . . . Chlordiazepoxide
Chlorpromazine . . . . Chlorhexidine
Chlorpromazine . . . . Chlorpropamide
Chlorpromazine . . . . Chlorthalidone
Chlorpromazine . . . . Prochlorperazine
Chlorpromazine . . . . Thioridazine

Chlorpropamide . . . . Chlorpromazine

Chlorthalidone . . . . Chlorpromazine

Cipro . . . . Ceftin

Ciprofloxacin. . . . . Cephalexin

Ciprofloxacin. . . . . Levofloxacin

Ciprofloxacin. . . . . Olloxacin

Cisplatin . . . . Carboplatin

Citracal . . . . Citrucel

Citrucel . . . . Hydrocil

Citrucel . . . . Citracal

Claforan. . . . . Cefotan

Claritin. . . . . Claritin-D

Claritin-D. . . . . Claritin

Clinoril. . . . . Clozaril

Clinoril. . . . . Oruvail

Clomiphene . . . . Clomipramine

Clomipramine . . . . Clomiphene

Clomipramine . . . . Desipramine

Clonapam . . . . Corlopam
(Clonazepam   (Fenoldopam
in Canada)   in U.S.)

Clonazepam . . . . Alprazolam

Clonazepam . . Clonidine . . Klonopin

Clonazepam . . . . Clorazepate

Clonazepam . . . . Diazepam

Clonazepam . . . . Lorazepam

Clonidine . . . . Colchicine

Clonidine . . . . Cardizem

Clonidine . . . Klonopin . . . Clonazepam

Clorazepate. . . . . Clonazepam

Clozaril . . . . Clinoril

Clozaril . . . . Colazal

Codeine . . . . Cardene

Codeine . . . . Iodine

Codeine . . . . Lodine

Codiclear DH . . . . Codimal DH

Codimal DH . . . . Codiclear DH

Cognex. . . . . Corgard

Colace . . . . Calan

Colace . . . . Peri-Colace

Colace . . . . Colace
(Docusate Sodium)   (Glycerin
                     suppository)

Colace . . . . Colace
(Glycerin suppository) (Docusate Sodium)

Colazal . . . . Clozaril

Colchicine. . . . . Clonidine

Combivir . . . . Epivir

Cordarone . . . . Cardura

Cordarone . . . . Coumadin

Corgard . . . . Cognex

Corgard . . . . Cozaar

Corlopam . . . . Clonapam
(Fenoldopam in U.S.) (Clonazepam in
                      Canada)

Cortane . . . . Cortane-B

Cortane-B. . . . . Cortane

Cortef. . . . . Lortab

Cortisone . . . . Hydrocortisone

Cortisporin . . . . Cortisporin
(Ophthalmic)   (Otic)

Cortisporin . . . . Cortisporin
(Otic)   (Ophthalmic)

Cosopt . . . . Trusopt

Coumadin . . . . Avandia

Coumadh . . . . Cardura

Coumadin . . . . Cordarone

Coumadin . . . . Ambien

Covera . . . . Provera

Cozaar. . . . . Corgard

Cozaar. . . . . Hyzaar

Cozaar. . . . . Zocor

Cyclobenzaprine . . . . Cetirizine

Cyclobenzaprine . . . . Cyproheptadine

Cyclophosphamide . . . . . . Cyclosporine

Cycloserine . . . . Cyclosporine

Cyclosporine. . . . . Cyclophosphamide

Cyclosporine. . . . . Cycloserine

Cyproheptadine. . . . . Cyclobenzaprine

Cytarabine . . . Cytosar. . . . Cytoxan

CytoGam . . . . Gamimune N

Cytosar. . . . . Cytovene

Cytosar. . . . Cytoxan. . . . . Cytarabine

Cytosar-U . . . . Neosar

Cytotec. . . . . Cytoxan

Cytovene . . . . Cytosar

Cytoxan . . . . Cytosar . . . . Cytarabine

Cytoxan . . . . Cytotec

Danazol . . . . Dantrium

Danocrine. . . . . Dantrium

Dantrium . . . . Danazol

Dantrium . . . . Danocrine

Darvocet. . . . . Percocet

Darvocet-N. . . . . Darvon

Darvocet-N. . . . . Darvon-N

Darvon. . . . . Darvocet-N

Darvon . . . . Diovan

Darvon-N . . . . Darvocet-N

Datril . . . . Detrol

Daunorubicin . . . . Doxorubicin

Deferoxamine . . . . Cefuroxime

Demadex . . . . Demerol

Demeclocycline. . . . . Dicyclomine

Demerol . . . . Demadex

Demerol . . . . Desyrel

Demerol . . . . Dilaudid

Denavir . . . . Indinavir

Depakene . . . . Depakote

Depakote . . . . Depakene

Depakote . . . . Senokot

Depakote . . . . Depakote ER
(Delayed Release)   (Extended Release)

Depakote ER . . . . Depakote
(Extended Release)   (Delayed Release)

Depo-Estradiol . . . . Depo-Testadiol

Depo-Medrol. . . . . Depo-Provera

Depo-Provera . . . . Depo-Medrol

Depo-Testadiol . . . . Depo-Estradiol

Deseril . . . . Desyrel
(Methysergide   (Trazodone
Maleate in Australia) in U.S.)

Desferal . . . . DexFerrum

Desipramine . . . . Imipramine

Desipramine . . . . Clomipramine

Desipramine . . . . Nortriptyline

Desyrel . . . . Demerol

Desyrel . . . . Deseril
(Trazodone in U.S.) (Methysergide
                     Maleate in Australia)

Detrol. . . . . Datril

Detrol. . . . . Dextrostat

DexFerrum . . . . Desferal

Dextroamphetamine . . . . . . Dextroamphetamine
                     and Amphetamine

Dextroamphetamine . . . . . . Dextroamphetamine
and Amphetamine

Dextrostat. . . . . Detrol

DiaBeta . . . . Zebeta

Diamox . . . . Dobutrex

Diastix . . . . Keto-Diastix

Diatex . . . . Diatx
(Diazepam   (Multivitamin
in Mexico)   in U.S.)

Diatx . . . . Diatex
(Multivitamin   (Diazepam
in U.S.)   in Mexico)

Diazepam . . . . Alprazolam

Diazepam . . . . Clonazepam

Diazepam . . . . Ditropan

Diazepam. . . . . Ditropan XL

Diazepam . . . . Lorazepam

Diazepam . . . . Midazolam

Dicloxacillin . . . . Doxycycline

Dicyclomine . . . . Demeclocycline

Dicyclomine . . . . Diphenhydramine

Dicyclomine . . . . Doxycycline

Diflucan. . . . . Dilantin

Diflucan . . . . *Diprivan*
Digoxin . . . . Doxepin
Dilantin . . . . *Diflucan*
Dilaudid . . . . Demerol
Diltia XT . . . . *Cartia XT*
Dimetapp . . . . *Donnatal*
Diovan . . . . Darvon
Diovan . . . . Zyban
Diphenhydramine . . . . Dicyclomine
Diphenhydramine . . . . Dipyridamole
Diphtheria and . . . . Tetanus Toxoid
Tetanus Toxoid
Diprivan . . . . *Diflucan*
Diprivan . . . . *Ditropan*
Dipyridamole . . . . Diphenhydramine
Ditropan . . . . Diazepam
Ditropan . . . . *Diprivan*
Ditropan XL . . . . Diazepam
Dobutamine . . . . Dopamine
Dobutrex . . . . *Dlamox*
Dobutrex . . . . Dopamine
Docetaxel . . . . Paclitaxel
Docusate Calcium . . . . Docusate Sodium
Docusate Sodium . . . . Docusate Calcium
Dolobid . . . . *Slo-bid*
Donepezil . . . . Benazepril
Donepezil . . . . Doxazosin
Donnatal . . . . *Dimetapp*
Donnatal . . . . *Donnatal Extentabs*
Donnatal Extentabs . . . . . . *Donnatal*
Dopamine . . . . *Dobutrex*
Dopamine . . . . Dobutamine
Doxazosin . . . . Terazosin
Doxazosin . . . . Donepezil
Doxepin . . . . Digoxin
Doxepin . . . . Doxycycline
Doxorubicin . . . . Daunorubicin
Doxorubicin . . . . Doxorubicin
                            Liposomal
Doxorubicin . . . . Idarubicin
Doxorubicin . . . . Doxorubicin
Liposomal
Doxycycline . . . . Dicloxacillin
Doxycycline . . . . Dicyclomine
Doxycycline . . . . Doxepin
Duratuss . . . . *Duratuss-G*
Duratuss-G . . . . *Duratuss*
Dynabac . . . . *DynaCirc*
Dynacin . . . . *DynaCirc*
DynaCirc . . . . *Dynabac*
DynaCirc . . . . *Dynacin*
Edecrin . . . . *Eulexin*

Efavirenz . . . . Nelfinavir
Effexor . . . . *Effexor XR*
Effexor XR . . . . *Effexor*
Efudex . . . . *Eurax*
Elavil . . . . *Enbrel*
Elavil . . . . *Oruvail*
Elavil . . . . *Plavix*
Eldepryl . . . . Enalapril
Eldopaque Forte . . . . *Eldoquin Forte*
Eldoquin Forte . . . . *Eldopaque Forte*
Elidel . . . . *Eligard*
Eligard . . . . *Elidel*
Elmiron . . . . *Imuran*
Enalapril . . . . *Eldepryl*
Enalapril . . . . Lisinopril
Enbrel . . . . *Elavil*
Enoxacin . . . . Enoxaparin
Enoxaparin . . . . Enoxacin
Entex LA . . . . *Eulexin*
Entuss . . . . *Entuss-D*
Entuss-D . . . . *Entuss*
Ephedrine . . . . Epinephrine
Epinephrine . . . . Ephedrine
Epinephrine . . . . *Neo-Synephrine*
Epinephrine . . . . Norepinephrine
Epivir . . . . *Combivir*
Epogen . . . . *Neupogen*
Equagesic . . . . *EquiGesic*
EquiGesic . . . . *Equagesic*
Erex . . . . *Urex*
Erythrocin . . . . *Ethmozine*
Erythromycin . . . . Azithromycin
Eskalith . . . . *Estratest*
Esmolol . . . . *Osmitrol*
Esomeprazole . . . . Omeprazole
Estrace . . . . *Evista*
Estraderm . . . . *Testoderm*
Estradiol . . . . Ethinyl Estradiol
Estradiol . . . . *Risperdal*
Estramustine . . . . Exemestane
Estratab . . . . *Estratest*
Estratest . . . . *Eskalith*
Estratest . . . . *Estratab*
Estratest . . . . *Estratest HS*
Estratest HS . . . . *Estratest*
Ethinyl Eatradiol . . . . Estradiol
Ethinyl Estradiol . . . . Ethinyl Estradiol
and Levonorgestrel   and Norgestrel
Ethinyl Estradiol . . . . Ethinyl Estradiol
and Norgestrel   and Levonorgestrel
Ethmozine . . . . *Erythrocin*
Etidronate . . . . Etomidate

Etomidate . . . . Etidronate
Eulexin . . . . *Edecrin*
Eulexin . . . . *Entex LA*
Eurax . . . . *Efudex*
Evista . . . . *Estrace*
Evista . . . . *E-Vista*
                            (Monograph in
                            Nursing Drug
                            References)
E-Vista . . . . *Evista*
(Monograph in
Nursing Drug
References)
Exemestane . . . . Estramustine
Famciclovir . . . . Acyclovir
Famotidine . . . . Fluoxetine
Famotidine . . . . Furosemide
Felodipine . . . . Amlodipine
Felodipine . . . . Nifedipine
Felodipine . . . . Ranitidine
Fentanyl Citrate . . . . Sufentanil Citrate
Fer-in-Sol . . . . *Poly-Vi-Sol*
Fioricet . . . . *Fiorinal*
Fioricet . . . . *Florinef*
Fiorinal . . . . *Fioricet*
Fleet Enema . . . . *Fleet Phospho-Soda*
Fleet Phospho-Soda . . . . . . *Fleet Enema*
Flomax . . . . *Flonase*
Flomax . . . . *Flovent*
Flomax . . . . *Fosamax*
Flomax . . . . *Volmax*
Flonase . . . . *Flomax*
Flonase . . . . *Flovent*
Florinef . . . . *Floricet*
Florinef . . . . Fluoride
Flovent . . . . *Atrovent*
Flovent . . . . *Flomax*
Flovent . . . . *Flonase*
Flucytosine . . . . Fluorouracil
Fludara . . . . *FUDR*
Fludarabine . . . . *Flumadine*
Flumadine . . . . Fludarabine
Fluocinolone . . . . Fluocinonide
Fluocinonide . . . . Fluocinolone
Fluocinonide . . . . Fluorouracil
Fluoride . . . . *Florinef*
Fluorouracil . . . . Flucytosine
Fluorouracil . . . . Fluocinonide
Fluoxetine . . . . Fluphenazine
Fluoxetine . . . . Fluvoxamine
Fluoxetine . . . . Famotidine
Fluoxetine . . . . Fluvastatin

Fluoxetine . . . . Furosemide	
Fluoxetine . . . . Paroxetine	
Fluphenazine . . . . Fluoxetine	
Fluphenazine . . . . Perphenazine	
Fluphenazine . . . . Trifluoperazine	
Flurazepam . . . . Temazepam	
Fluvastatin . . . . Fluoxetine	
Fluvoxamine . . . . Fluoxetine	
FML Forte . . . . FML S.O.P	
FML S.O.P. . . . . FML Forte	
Folic Acid . . . . Folinic Acid	
Folinic Acid. . . . . Folic Acid	
Foltex PFS . . . . FOLTX	
FOLTX. . . . . Foltex PFS	
Foradil . . . . Toradol	
Fortovase . . . . Invirase	
Fosamax. . . . . Flomax	
Fosinopril . . . . Bisoprolol	
Fosinopril . . . . Furosemide	
Fosinopril . . . . Lisinopril	
Fosinopril . . . . Minoxidil	
Fosphenytoin . . . . Phenytoin	
FUDR . . . . Fludara	
Furosemide . . . . Famotidine	
Furosemide . . . . Fluoxetine	
Furosemide . . . . Fosinopril	
Furosemide . . . . Torsemide	
Gamimune N . . . . CytoGam	
Gemzar . . . . Zinecard	
Gengraf . . . . Prograf	
Gentamicin . . . . Tobramycin	
Gentamicin . . . . Vancomycin	
Glipizide . . . . Glyburide	
Glucophage . . . . Glucophage XR	
Glucophage . . . . Glucotrol	
Glucophage . . . . Glutofac	
Glucophage . .Glucophage XR . .Glucotrol	
Glucophage XR. . . . . Glucotrol XL	
Glucophage XR. . . . . Glucophage	
Glucophage XR. . Glucotrol . . . .Glucophage	
Glucotrol . . Glucophage . . Glucophage XR	
Glucotrol . . . . Glucophage	
Glucotrol . . . . Glucotrol XL	
Glucotrol . . . . Glyburide	
Glucotrol XL. . . . . Glucophage XR	
Glucotrol XL . . . . Glucotrol	
Glutofac . . . . Glucophage	
Glyburide . . . . Glipizide	
Glyburide . . . . Glucotrol	
Glycerin . . . . Nitroglycerin	
Granulex . . . . Regranex	

Guaifenesin . . . . Guanfacine	
Guanfacine . . . . Guaifenesin	
Halcion. . . . . Haldol	
Haldol . . . . Halcion	
Haldol . . . . Haldol Decanoate	
Haldol . . . . Inderal	
Haldol . . . . Stadol	
Haldol Decanoate. . . . . . . Haldol	
Haloperidol. . . . . Halotestin	
Halotestin . . . . Haloperidol	
Hemoccult . . . . Seracult	
Heparin . . . . Levaquin	
Heparin . . . . Hespan	
Herceptin . . . . Perceptin	
Hespan . . . . Heparin	
Humalog. . . . . Humalog Mix	
Humalog Mix . . . . Humalog	
Humalog, Insulin . . . . Humulin, Insulin	
Human	Human
Humulin 70/30 . . . . Humulin N	
Humulin 70/30 . . . . Humulin R	
Humulin L. . . . . Humulin N	
Humulin L. . . . . Humulin U	
(Lente)	(Ultralente)
Humulin N . . . . Humulin 70/30	
Humulin N . . . . Humulin R	
Humulin N . . . . Humulin U	
Humulin N . . . . Novolin N	
Humulin N . . . . Humulin L	
Humulin R . . . . Humulin 70/30	
Humulin R . . . . Humulin N	
Humulin R . . . . Humulin U	
Humulin R . . . . Novolin R	
Humulin U . . . . Humulin N	
Humulin U . . . . Humulin R	
Humulin U . . . . Humulin L	
(Ultralente)	(Lente)
Humulin, Insulin. . . . . Humalog, Insulin	
Human	Human
Hydralazine . . . . Hydrochlorothiazide	
Hydralazine. . . . . Hydrocortisone	
Hydralazine. . . . . Hydroxyzine	
Hydrochlorothiazide . . . . . Hydralazine	
Hydrochlorothiazide . . . . . Hydroxychloroquine	
Hydrocil . . . . Citrucel	
Hydrocodone . . . . Hydrocortisone	
Hydrocodone and . . . . . . Oxycodone and	
Acetaminophen	Acetaminophen
Hydrocodone and . . . . . . Hydromorphone	
Acetaminophen	
Hydrocortisone . . . . Cortisone	
Hydrocortisone . . . . Hydralazine	

Hydrocortisone . . . . Hydrocodone	
Hydromorphone . . . . Hydrocodone and	
	Acetaminophen
Hydromorphone . . . . Morphine	
Hydroxychloroquine. . . . . Hydrochlorothiazide	
Hydroxyurea . . . . Hydroxyzine	
Hydroxyzine . . . . Hydralazine	
Hydroxyzine . . . . Hydroxyurea	
Hypergel . . . . MPM GelPad	
	Hydrogel Saturated
	Dressing
Hyzaar . . . . Cozaar	
Idamycin . . . . Adriamycin	
Idarubicin . . . . Doxorubicin	
IMDUR. . . . . Imuran	
IMDUR. . . . . Inderal LA	
IMDUR. . . . . K-Dur	
Imipenem . . . . Meropenem	
Imipenem. . . . . Omnipen	
Imipramine . . . . Amitriptyline	
Imipramine . . . . Desipramine	
Imodium. . . . . Indocin	
Imovax. . . . . Imovax I.D.	
Imovax I.D.. . . . . Imovax	
Imuran . . . . Elmiron	
Imuran . . . . IMDUR	
Imuran . . . . Tenormin	
Inapsine . . . . Lanoxin	
Inderal . . . . Adderall	
Inderal . . . . Haldol	
Inderal . . . . Isordil	
Inderal . . . . Toradol	
Inderal LA . . . . IMDUR	
Indinavir. . . . . Denavir	
Indocin. . . . . Imodium	
Infliximab . . . . Rituximab	
Insulin . . . . Integrilin	
Insulin Human . . . . Lispro, Insulin	
	Human
Insulin Human . . . . Isophane, Insulin	
	Human
Integrilin . . . . Insulin	
Invanz . . . . Avinza	
Invirase. . . . . Fortovase	
Iodine . . . . Codeine	
Iodine. . . . . Lodine	
Ismo . . . . Isordil	
Isophane, Insulin. . . . . . . Insulin Human	
Human	
Isopto Carpine . . . . Propine	
Isordil. . . . . Inderal	
Isordil . . . . Ismo	

Isosorbide . . . . Isosorbide
Dinitrate   Mononitrate
Isosorbide . . . . Isosorbide
Mononitrate   Dinitrate
Kaletra . . . . Keppra
Kaopectate . . . . Kayexalate
Kayexalate . . . . Kaopectate
Kayexalate . . . . Potassium Acetate
K-Dur . . . . Cardura
K-Dur . . . . IMDUR
K-Dur . . . . K-Lor
Keflex . . . . Kefzol
Keflex . . . . Norflex
Kefurox . . . . Kefzol
Kefzol . . . . Cefzil
Kefzol . . . . Keflex
Kefzol . . . . Kefurox
Kenalog . . . . Ketalar
Keppra . . . . Kaletra
Ketalar . . . . Kenalog
Keto-Diastix . . . . Diastix
Ketorolac . . . . Ketotifen
Ketotifen . . . . Ketorolac
Klonopin . . . Clonidine . . . Clonazepam
K-Lor . . . . K-Dur
K-Lor . . . . K-Lyte
K-Lyte . . . . K-Lor
K-Lyte . . . . K-Lyte Cl
K-Lyte Cl . . . . K-Lyte
Kogenate Kogenate-2
Kogenate-2 . . . . Kogenate
K-Phos Neutral . . . . Neutra-Phos-K
Labetolol . . . . Lamictal
Lacrilube . . . . Surgilube
Lamicel . . . . Lamisil
Lamictal . . . . Labetolol
Lamictal . . . . Lamisil
Lamictal . . . . Lomotil
Lamictal . . . . Ludiomil
Lamisil . . . . Lamicel
Lamisil . . . . Lamictal
Lamisil . . . . Lomotil
Lamivudine . . . . Lamotrigine
Lamivudine . . . . Zidovudine
Lamotrigine . . . . Lamivudine
Lanoxin . . . . Levothyroxine
Lanoxin . . . . Inapsine
Lanoxin . . . . . Lasix . . . . . . Lomotil
Lanoxin . . . . Levoxyl
Lanoxin . . . . Levsin
Lanoxin . . . . Lonox
Lanoxin . . . . Lovenox

Lanoxin . . . . Xanax
Lantus, Insulin . . . . Lente, Insulin
Human   Human
Lasix . . . . . . Lomotil . . . . . Lanoxin
Lasix . . . . Luvox
L-Dopa . . . . Levodopa . . . . Methyldopa
Lente, Insulin . . . . Lispro, Insulin
Human   Human
Lente, Insulin . . . . Lantus, Insulin
Human   Human
Leucovorin . . . Leukine . . . Leukeran
Leucovorin . . . . Levothyroxine
Leukeran . . . . Alkeran
Leukeran . . Leucovorin . . . . Leukine
Leukine . . . . Leukeran . . . . . Leucovorin
Levaquin . . . . Heparin
Levaquin . . . . Lovenox
Levaquin . . . . Tequin
Levbid . . . . Cefobid
Levbid . . . . Lithobid
Levbid . . . . Lopid
Levbid . . . . Lorabid
Levlen . . . . Tri-Levlen
Levobunolol . . . . Levocabastine
Levocabastine . . . . Levobunolol
Levocarnitine . . . . Levofloxacin
Levodopa . . L-Dopa . . . . . Methyldopa
Levodopa and . . . . Carbidopa
Carbidopa
Levofloxacin . . . . Ciprofloxacin
Levofloxacin . . . . Levocarnitine
Levothyroxine . . . . Lanoxin
Levothyroxine . . . . Leucovorin
Levothyroxine . . . . Liothyronine
Levoxyl . . . . Lanoxin
Levoxyl . . . . Luvox
Levsin . . . . Lanoxin
Lexapro . . . . Loxapine
Librax . . . . Librium
Librium . . . . Librax
Lioresal . . . . Lotensin
Liothyronine . . . . Levothyroxine
Lipitor . . . . Zocor
Lisinopril . . . . Benazepril
Lisinopril . . . . Enalapril
Lisinopril . . . . Fosinopril
Lisinopril . . . . Quinapril
Lisinopril . . . . Risperdal
Lispro, ... Insulin Human
Insulin Human
Lispro, ... Lente,
Insulin Human   Insulin Human

Lithobid . . . . Levbid
Lithobid . . . . Lithostat
Lithostat . . . . Lithobid
Lodine . . . . Codeine
Lodine . . . . Iodine
Lomotil . . . . Lamictal
Lomotil . . . . Lamisil
Lomotil . . . . Lanoxin . . . . . Lasix
Loniten . . . . Lotensin
Lonox . . . . Lanoxin
Loperamide . . . . Lorazepam
Lopid . . . . Levbid
Lopid . . . . . . Lorabid . . . . . Slo-bid
Lorabid . . . . Levbid
Lorabid . . . . Lortab
Lorabid . . . . . Slo-bid . . . . . Lopid
Loratadine . . . . Losartan
Lorazepam . . . . Alprazolam
Lorazepam . . . . Clonazepam
Lorazepam . . . . Diazepam
Lorazepam . . . . Loperamide
Lorazepam . . . . Midazolam
Lorazepam . . . . Temazepam
Lorcet . . . . Lortab
Lortab . . . . Cortef
Lortab . . . . Lorabid
Lortab . . . . Lorcet
Lortab . . . . Luride
Losartan . . . . Loratadine
Losartan . . . . Valsartan
Lotensin . . . . Lioresal
Lotensin . . . . Loniten
Lotensin . . . . Lovastatin
Lotrimin . . . . Lotrisone
Lotrisone . . . . Lotrimin
Lotronex . . . . Lovenox
Lotronex . . . . Protonix
Lovastatin . . . . Lotensin
Lovenox . . . . Avonex
Lovenox . . . . Lanoxin
Lovenox . . . . Levaquin
Lovenox . . . . Lotronex
Lovenox . . . . Luvox
Loxapine . . . . Lexapro
Loxitane . . . . Soriatane
Ludiomil . . . . Lamictal
Luride . . . . Lortab
Luvox . . . . Lasix
Luvox . . . . Levoxyl
Luvox . . . . Lovenox
Magnesium Citrate . . . . . . Magnesium Sulfate

Magnesium Sulfate . . . . . . Magnesium Citrate

Maxipime . . . . *Moxapen*
(Cefepime   (Amoxicillin
Hydrochloride   Trihydrate
in U.S.)   in Thailand)

Meclofenamate . . . . Mycophenolate

Medigesic . . . . *Medi-Gesic*

Medi-Gesic . . . . *Medigesic*

Medroxyprogesterone . . . . Methylprednisolone

Medroxyprogesterone . . . . Metolazone

Mefloquine . . . . Meloxicam

Megace . . . . *Raglan*

Mellaril . . . . Melphalan

Meloxicam . . . . Mefloquine

Melphalan . . . . *Mellaril*

Melphalan . . . . *Myleran*

Meperidine . . . . Methadone

Meperidine . . . . Morphine

Mepron . . . . *Mepron*
(Atovaquone   (Meprobamate
in U.S.)   in Australia)

Meropenem . . . . Imipenem

Meruvax . . . . *Attenuvax*

Mesalamine . . . . Sulfasalazine

Metadate CD . . . . *Metadate ER*

Metadate ER . . . . *Metadate CD*

Metaxalone . . . . Metolazone

Metformin . . . . Metronidazole

Methadone . . . . Meperidine

Methadone . . . . Methylphenidate

Methazolamide . . . . Methimazole

Methazolamide . . . . Metronidazole

Methimazole . . . . Methazolamide

Methohexital . . . . Methotrexate

Methotrexate . . . . Methohexital

Methotrexate . . . . Metolazone

Methyldopa . . . L-Dopa . . . Levodopa

Methylphenidate . . . . Methadone

Methylprednisolone . . . . . .
Medroxyprogesterone

Methylprednisolone . . . . . . Prednisone

Metoclopramide . . . . Metolazone

Metoclopramide . . . . Metoprolol

Metoclopramide . . . . Metronidazole

Metolazone . . . .
Medroxyprogesterone

Metolazone . . . . Metaxalone

Metolazone . . . . Methotrexate

Metolazone . . . . Metoclopramide

Metolazone . . . . Metoprolol

Metoprolol . . . . Atenolol

Metoprolol . . . . Metoclopramide

Metoprolol . . . . Metolazone

Metoprolol . . . . Metronidazole

Metoprolol . . . . Misoprostol

Meteprolol Succinate . . . . . Metoprolol Tartrate

Metoprolol   Metoprolol
Tartrate   Succinate

MetroGel . . . . *MetroGel-Vaginal*

MetroGel-Vaginal . . . . *MetroGel*

Metronidazole . . . . Metformin

Metronidazole . . . . Methazolamide

Metronidazole . . . . Metoclopramide

Metronidazole . . . . Metoprolol

Metronidazole . . . . Miconazole

Miacalcin . . . . *Micatin*

Micatin . . . . *Miacalcin*

Miconazole . . . . Metronidazole

Micro-K . . . . *Micronase*

Micronase . . . . *Micro-K*

Micronase . . . . *Microzide*

Microzide . . . . *Micronase*

Midazolam . . . . Diazepam

Midazolam . . . . Lorazepam

Midodrin . . . . *Midrin*

Midodrine . . . . Molindone

Midrin . . . . Midodrin

Mifepristone . . . . Misoprostol

Minoxidil . . . . Fosinopril

Minoxidil . . . . *Monopril*

MiraLax . . . . *Mirapex*

Mirapex . . . . *MiraLax*

Misoprostol . . . . Metoprolol

Misoprostol . . . . Mifepristone

Mitomycin . . . . Mitoxantrone

Mitoxantrone . . . . Mitomycin

Moban . . . . *Mobic*

Mobic . . . . *Moban*

Molindone . . . . Midodrine

Monoket . . . . *Monopril*

Monopril . . . . *Accupril*

Monopril . . . . Minoxidil

Monopril . . . . *Monoket*

Morphine . . . . Hydromorphone

Morphine . . . . Meperidine

Moxapen . . . . *Maxipime*
(Amoxicillin   (Cefepime
Trihydrate in   Hydrochloride
Thailand)   in U.S.)

MPM GelPad . . . . *Hypergel*
Hydrogel Saturated
Dressing

MS Contin . . . . *OxyContin*

Murocel *Murocoll-2*

Murocoll-2 . . . . *Murocel*

Mycelex . . . . *Mycolog*

Mycolog . . . . *Mycelex*

Mycophenolate . . . . Meclofenamate

Mylanta . . . . *Mylicon*

Myleran . . . . Melphalan

Mylicon . . . . *Mylanta*

Naprelan . . . . *Naprosyn*

Naprosyn . . . . *Naprelan*

Naprosyn . . . . *Niaspan*

Narcan . . . . *Norcuron*

Narcan . . . . *Nubain*

Nasacort . . . . *Azmacort*

Nasalcrom . . . . *Nasalide*

Nasalide . . . . *Nasalcrom*

Nasarel . . . . *Nizoral*

Natru-Vent . . . . *Atrovent*

Navane . . . . *Norvasc*

Nebcin . . . . *Nubain*

Nefazodone . . . . Nelfinavir

Nelfinavir . . . . Efavirenz

Nelfinavir . . . . Nefazodone

Nelfinavir . . . . Nevirapine

Neoral . . . . *Neurontin*

Neoral . . . . *Nizoral*

Neosar . . . . *Cytosar-U*

Neo-Synephrine . . . . Epinephrine

Neo-Synephrine . . . . *Neo-Synephrine*
12-Hour

Neo-Synephrine . . . . Norepinephrine

Neo-Synephrine . . . . *Neo-Synephrine*
12-Hour

Nephrox . . . . *Niferex*

Neumega . . . . *Neupogen*

Neupogen . . . . *Epogen*

Neupogen . . . . *Neumega*

Neurontin . . . . *Neoral*

Neurontin . . . . *Noroxin*

Neutra-Phos . . . . *Neutra-Phos-K*

Neutra-Phos-K . . . . *K-Phos Neutral*

Neutra-Phos-K . . . . *Neutra-Phos*

Nevirapine . . . . Nelfinavir

Niacin . . . . Niaspan

Niaspan . . . . *Naprosyn*

Niaspan . . . . Niacin

Nicardipine . . . Nifedipine . . . Nimodipine

Nicoderm . . . . *Nitroderm*

NicoDerm CQ . . . . *Nitro-Dur*

Nifedipine . . . . Felodipine

Nifedipine . . . . Nicardipine . . . Nimodipine

Niferex . . . . *Nephrox*

Nimbex . . . . *Bumex*

Nimbex	Revex
Nimodipine. . . Nicardipine . . . Nifedipine	
Nitro-Bid.	Nitro-Dur
Nitroderm.	Nicoderm
Nitro-Dur	NicoDerm CQ
Nitro-Dur	Nitro-Bid
Nitro-Dur	NitroQuick
Nitroglycerin.	Glycerin
NitroQuick	Nitro-Dur
Nizatidine.	Tizanidine
Nizoral	Nasarel
Nizoral	Neoral
Nolvadex	Norvasc
Norcuron	Narcan
Norepinephrine.	Epinephrine
Norepinephrine.	Neo-Synephrine
Norepinephrine.	Phenylephrine
Norflex.	Keflex
Norflex . . . . Noroxin.	Norfloxacin
Norflex.	Norvasc
Norfloxacin. . . Norflex . . . Noroxin	
Noroxin	Neurontin
Noroxin . . . . Norflex	Norfloxacin
Norpramin	Nortriptyline
Nortriptyline.	Amitriptyline
Nortriptyline.	Desipramine
Nortriptyline	Norpramin
Norvasc	Altace
Norvasc	Navane
Norvasc	Nolvadex
Norvasc	Norflex
Norvasc	Vasotec
Norvir.	Retrovir
Novolin 70/30	Novolin N
Novolin L	Novolin N
Novolin N.	Humulin N
Novolin N.	Novolin 70/30
Novolin N.	Novolin L
Novolin N.	Novolin R
Novolin R.	Humulin R
Novolin R.	Novolin N
Nubain.	Narcan
Nubain.	Nebcin
Nutropin.	Nutropin AQ
Nutropin AQ.	Nutropin
Ocufen	Ocuflox
Ocufen	Ocupress
Ocuflox.	Ocufen
Ocular Lubricants.	Acular
Ocumycin.	Ocu-Mycin
Ocu-Mycin	Ocumycin

Ocupress.	Ocufen
Ofloxacin	Ciprofloxacin
Olanzapine	Oxcarbazepine
Omeprazole	Esomeprazole
Omnipen.	Imipenem
Opium Tincture, ... Deodorized	Opium, Camphorated
Opium, ... Camphorated	Opium Tincture, Deodorized
Oprelvekin	Aldesleukin
Orgaran	Argatroban
Ortho Tri-Cyclen	Ortho-Cyclen
Ortho Tri-Cyclen	Tri-Levlen
Ortho-Cept	Ortho-Cyclen
Ortho-Cept	Ortho-Est
Ortho-Cyclen	Ortho-Cept
Ortho-Cyclen	Ortho Tri-Cyclen
Ortho-Est.	Ortho-Cept
Oruvail.	Clinoril
Oruvail.	Elavil
Os-Cal	Asacol
Osmitrol	Esmolol
Oxacillin.	Ampicillin
Oxazepam	Oxycodone
Oxazepam	Temazepam
Oxcarbazepine	Olanzapine
Oxybutynin	OxyContin
Oxycodone.	Oxazepam
Oxycodone	OxyContin
Oxycodone and. . . . . Acetaminophen	Hydrocodone and Acetaminophen
Oxycodone and. . . . . Acetaminophen	Oxycodone and Aspirin
Oxycodone. . . . . and Aspirin	Oxycodone and Acetaminophen
OxyContin	MS Contin
OxyContin	Oxybutynin
OxyContin	Oxycodone
Paclitaxel	Docetaxel
Paclitaxel	Paroxetine
Paclitaxel	Paxil
Pamelor	Panlor SS
Panlor SS	Pamelor
Papaverine	Propafenone
Parafon Forte DSC.	Profen Forte
Paraplatin	Platinol
Parlodel	Pindolol
Parlodel	Provera
Paroxetine.	Fluoxetine
Paroxetine.	Paclitaxel
Paroxetine.	Pyridoxine
Paxil.	Paclitaxel

Paxil.	Plavix
Paxil.	Taxol
Pediapred.	Pediazole
Pediapred.	Risperdal
Pediazole	Pediapred
Pegaspargase.	Asparaginase
Penicillamine.	Penicillin
Penicillin	Penicillamine
Penicillin G . . . . Potassium	Penicillin G Procaine
Penicillin G . . . . Procaine	Penicillin G Potassium
Pentobarbital.	Phenobarbital
Pepcid	Prevacid
Perative	Periactin
Perceptin	Herceptin
Percocet	Darvocet
Percocet	Percodan
Percocet	Procet
Percodan	Percocet
Percodan	Peri-Colace
Percodan	Vicodin
Periactin.	Perative
Peri-Colace	Colace
Peri-Colace	Percodan
Peri-Colace	Procardia
Permax.	Bumex
Permethrin	Pyrethrins, Piperonyl Butoxide
Perphenazine	Fluphenazine
Phenazopyridine	Promethazine
Phenobarbital	Pentobarbital
Phenylephrine	Norepinephrine
Phenylephrine.	Phenytoin
Phenytoin	Fosphenytoin
Phenytoin	Phenylephrine
Physostigmine.	Pyridostigmine
Pilocar	Polocaine
Pilocarpine	Proparacaine
Pindolol	Parlodel
Pindolol	Plendil
Pioglitazone	Rosiglitazone
Pitocin	Pitressin
Pitressin	Pitocin
Platinol.	Paraplatin
Plavix.	Elavil
Plavix.	Paxil
Plendil	Pindolol
Plendil	Pletal
Plendil	Prilosec
Plendil	Prinivil
Pletal	Plendil

Pneumococcal . . . . Pneumococcal
Vaccine, 23-Valent   Vaccine, 7-Valent
(Polyvalent)

Pneumococcal . . . . Pneumococcal
Vaccine, 7-Valent   Vaccine, 23-Valent
                        (Polyvalent)

Polocaine . . . . Pilocar
Poly-Vi-Sol . . . . Fer-In-Sol
Potassium . . . . Prednisone
Potassium Acetate . . . . Kayexalate
Potassium Acetate . . . . Potassium Chloride
Potassium . . . . Potassium
Bicarbonate and   Bicarbonate and
Potassium Chloride   Potassium Citrate
Potassium . . . . Potassium
Bicarbonate and   Bicarbonate and
Potassium Citrate   Potassium Chloride
Potassium Chloride . . . . . . Potassium Acetate
Potassium Chloride . . . . . Potassium Citrate
Potassium Chloride . . . . . . Sodium Chloride
Potassium Citrate . . . . Potassium Chloride
Potassium Phosphates . . . . Sodium Phosphates
Prandin . . . . Avandia
Pravachol . . . . Prevacid
Pravachol . . . . Prinivil
Pravachol . . . . Propranolol
Pravastatin . . . . Atorvastatin
Prazosin . . . . Terazosin
Precare . . . . Precose
Precose . . . . Precare
Prednisolone . . . . Prednisone
Prednisone . . . . Methylprednisolone
Prednisone . . . . Potassium
Prednisone . . . . Prednisolone
Prednisone . . . . Prilosec
Prednisone . . . . Primidone
Prednisone . . . . Pseudoephedrine
Premarin . . . . Prempro
Premarin . . . . Prevacid
Premarin . . . . Primaxin
Premarin . . . . Provera
Premphase . . . . Prempro
Premphase . . . . Vancenase
Prempro . . . . Premarin
Prempro . . . . Premphase
Prepidil . . . . Bepridil
Prevacid . . . . Prinivil
Prevacid . . . . Pepcid
Prevacid . . . . Pravachol
Prevacid . . . . Premarin
Prevacid . . . . Prilosec
Preven . . . . Preveon

Preveon . . . . Preven
Prilosec . . . . Plendil
Prilosec . . . . Prednisone
Prilosec . . . . Prevacid
Prilosec . . . . Prinivil
Prilosec . . . . Prozac
Primacor . . . . Primaxin
Primatene . . . . ProAmantine
Primaxin . . . . Premarin
Primaxin . . . . Primacor
Primidone . . . . Prednisone
Prinivil . . . . Plendil
Prinivil . . . . Pravachol
Prinivil . . . . Prevacid
Prinivil . . . . Prilosec
Prinivil . . . . Prinzide
Prinivil . . . . Proventil
Prinzide . . . . Prinivil
Priscoline . . . . Apresoline
ProAmantine . . . . Primatene
Probenecid . . . . Procanbid
Procainamide . . . . Prochlorperazine
Procan SR . . . . Proscar
Procanbid . . . . Probenecid
Procardia . . . . Peri-Colace
Procardia . . . . Provera
Procardia XL . . . . Cartia XT
Procet . . . . Percocet
Prochlorperazine . . . . Chlorpromazine
Prochlorperazine . . . . . . Procainamide
Prochlorperazine . . . . . . Promethazine
Proctocort . . . . Proctocream HC
Proctocream HC . . . . Proctocort
Profen . . . . Profen II . . . . . Profen LA
Profen Forte . . . . Parafon Forte DSC
Profen II . . . . Profen . . . . . Profen LA
Profen LA . . . Profen . . . . . Profen II
Prograf . . . . Gengraf
Promethazine . . . . Phenazopyridine
Promethazine . . . . Prochlorperazine
Promethazine VC . . . . . . Promethazine
                        w/ Codeine
Promethazine VC . . . . . . Promethazine
w/ Codeine   w/ Codeine
Promethazine . . . . Promethazine VC
w/ Codeine   w/ Codeine
Promethazine . . . . Promethazine VC
w/ Codeine
Propafenone . . . . Papaverine
Proparacaine . . . . Pilocarpine
Propine . . . . Isopto Carpine
Propranolol . . . . Pravachol

Propranolol . . . . Propulsid
Propulsid . . . . Propranolol
Propylthiouracil . . . . Purinethol
Proscar . . . . Procan SR
Proscar . . . . ProSom
Proscar . . . . ProSom . . . . . Prozac
Proscar . . . . Provera
ProSom . . . . Proscar
ProSom . . . . Prozac . . . . . Proscar
Protonix . . . . Lotronex
Proventil . . . . Bentyl
Proventil . . . . Prinivil
Provera . . . . Covera
Provera . . . . Parlodel
Provera . . . . Premarin
Provera . . . . Procardia
Provera . . . . Proscar
Prozac . . . . Prilosec
Prozac . . . . . Proscar . . . . . ProSom
Pseudoephedrine . . . . Prednisone
Pulmicort . . . . Pulmozyme
Pulmozyme . . . . Pulmicort
Purinethol . . . . Propyithiouracil
Pyrazinamide . . . . Pyridostigmine
Pyrethrins, ... Permethrin
Piperonyl Butoxide

Pyridium . . . . Pyridoxine
Pyridostigmine . . . . Physostigmine
Pyridostigmine . . . . Pyrazinamide
Pyridostigmine . . . . Pyridoxine
Pyridoxine . . . . Paroxetine
Pyridoxine . . . . Pyridium
Pyridoxine . . . . Pyridostigmine
Pyridoxine . . . . Pyrimethamine
Pyrimethamine . . . . Pyridoxine
Quibron . . . Quibron-T . . . . Quibron-T/SR
Quibron-T . . . . Quibron . . . Quibron-T/SR
Quibron-T/SR . . Quibron . . Quibron-T
Quinacrine . . . . Quinidine
Quinapril . . . . Lisinopril
Quinidine . . . . Quinacrine
Quinidine . . . . Quinine
Quinine . . . . Quinidine
Raloxifene . . . . Ropinirole
Ramipril . . . . Rifampin
Ranitidine . . Amantadine . . Rimantadine
Ranitidine . . . . Felodipine
Ratgam . . . . Atgam
(Synonym for
Thymoglobulin)
ReFresh . . . . Refresh (lubricant
(breath drops)   eye drops)

Refresh . . . . ReFresh
(lubricant eye drops)   (breath drops)
Reglan . . . . Megace
Reglan . . . . Renagel
Reglan . . . . Robitussin
Reglan . . . . Zofran
Regranex . . . . Granulex
Relafen . . . . Rezulin
Remegel . . . . Renagel
Remeron . . . . Restoril
Remeron . . . . Zemuron
Reminyl . . . . Amaryl
Reminyl . . . . Robinul
Renagel . . . . Reglan
Renagel . . . . Remegel
Reno-60 . . . . Renografin-60
Renografin-60 . . . . Reno-60
Reopro . . . . Rheomacrodex
Repaglinide . . . . Rosiglitazone
Requip . . . . Risperdal
Reserpine . . Risperdal . . . Risperidone
Restoril . . . . Remeron
Restoril . . . . Risperdal
Restoril . . . . Vistaril
Retavase . . . . Activase
Retrovir . . . . Norvir
Retrovir . . . . Ritonavir
Revex . . . . Nimbex
Revex . . . . ReVia
ReVia . . . . Revex
Rezulin . . . . Relafen
Rheomacrodex . . . . Reopro
Ridaura . . . . Cardura
Rifabutin . . . . Rifampin
Rifadin . . . . Rifater
Rifampin . . . . Ramipril
Rifampin . . . . Rifabutin
Rifater . . . . Rifadin
Rimantadine . . Amantadine . . Ranitidine
Risedronate . . . . Risperidone
Risperdal . . . . Estradiol
Risperdal . . . . Lisinopril
Risperdal . . . . Pediapred
Risperdal . . . . Requip
Risperdal . . . . Reserpine . . . . . Risperidone
Risperdal . . . . Restoril
Risperidone . . . Reserpine . . . . . Risperdal
Risperidone . . . . Risedronate
Risperidone . . . . Ropinirole
Ritalin . . . . Ritalin SR
Ritalin SR . . . . Ritalin
Ritonavir . . . . Retrovir

Rituximab . . . . Infliximab
Robinul . . . . Reminyl
Robitussin . . . . Reglan
Robitussin . . . . Robitussin DM
Robitussin AC . . . . Robitussin DAC
Robitussin AC . . . . Robitussin DM
Robitussin DAC . . . . Robitussin AC
Robitussin DM . . . . Robitussin
Robitussin DM . . . . Robitussin AC
Robitussin DM . . . . Rondec DM
Rocephin . . . . Ceftin
Rondec DM . . . . Robitussin DM
Ropinirole . . . . Raloxifene
Ropinirole . . . . Risperidone
Ropivacaine . . . . Bupivacaine
Rosiglitazone . . . . Pioglitazone
Rosiglitazone . . . . Repaglinide
Roxanol . . . . Roxicet
Roxanol . . . . Roxicodone
Roxanol . . . . Roxicodone Intensol
Roxicet . . . . Roxanol
Roxicet . . . . Roxicodone
Roxicodone . . . . Roxanol
Roxicodone . . . . Roxicet
Roxicodone . . . . Roxicodone
Intensol
Roxicodone Intensol . . . . . Roxanol
Roxicodone Intensol . . . . . Roxicodone
Rynatan . . . . Rynatuss
Rynatuss . . . . Rynatan
Salagen . . . . Seleginine
Salbutamol . . . . Salmeterol
(Albuterol in
other countries)
Salmeterol . . . . Salbutamol
(Albuterol in other
countries)
Salsalate . . . . Sulfasalazine
Sarafem . . . . Serophene
Seleginine . . . . Salagen
Seleginine . . . Serentil . . . Sertraline . . . Serzone
Seleginine . . . . Sertraline
Senna . . . . Soma
Senokot . . . . Depakote
Senokot . . . . Sinemet
Seracult . . . . Hemoccult
Serentil . . . Seleginine . . . Sertraline . . . Serzone
Serentil . . . . Seroquel
Serentil . . . . Serzone
Serentil . . . . Sinequan
Serevent . . . . Atrovent
Serevent . . . . Serevent Diskus

Serevent Diskus . . . . Serevent
Serophene . . . . Sarafem
Seroquel . . . . Serentil
Seroquel . . . Serzone . . . . . Sinequan
Seroquel . . . . Symmetrel
Seroquel . . . . Sertraline
Sertraline . . . Seleginine . . . Serentil . . . Serzone
Sertraline . . . . Seroquel
Serzone . . . Seroquel . . . . Sinequan
Serzone . . . . Sertraline . . . Seleginine . . . Serentil
Sinemet . . . . Senokot
Sinemet . . . . Sinemet CR
Sinemet CR . . . . Sinemet
Sinequan . . . . Serentil
Sinequan . . . Seroquel . . . Serzone
Sinequan . . . . Singulair
Singulair . . . . Sinequan
Slo-bid . . . . Dolobid
Slo-bid . . . . Lopid . . . . . Lorabid
Slow Fe . . . . Slow-K
Slow-K . . . . Slow Fe
Sodium . . . . Sodium Chloride
Bicarbonate
Sodium Chloride . . . . Potassium Chloride
Sodium Chloride . . . . Sodium
Bicarbonate
Sodium . . . . Potassium
Phosphates   Phosphates
Solu-Cortef . . . . Solu-Medrol
Solu-Medrol . . . . Depo-Medrol
Solu-Medrol . . . . Solu-Cortef
Soma . . . . Senna
Soma . . . . Soma Compound
Soma Compound . . . . Soma
Soriatane . . . . Loxitane
Sotalol . . . . Subdue
Stadol . . . . Haldol
Stadol . . . . Toradol
Subdue . . . . Sotalol
Sufentanil Citrate . . . . Fentanyl Citrate
Sulfadiazine . . . . Sulfasalazine
Sulfasalazine . . . . Mesalamine
Sulfasalazine . . . . Salsalate
Sulfasalazine . . . . Sulfadiazine
Sulfasalazine . . . . Sulfisoxazole
Sulfisoxazole . . . . Sulfasalazine
Sumatriptan . . . . Zolmitriptan
Suprax . . . . Surfak
Surfak . . . . Suprax
Surgilube . . . . Lacrilube
Symmetrel . . . . Amaryl
Symmetrel . . . . Seroquel

813

Symmetrel.	Synthroid
Synagis.	Synvisc
Synthroid	Symmetrel
Synvisc.	Synagis
Tambocor.	Temodar
Tamiflu.	Tamoxifen
Tamiflu.	Theraflu
Tamoxifen.	Tamiflu
Tamoxifen.	Tamsulosin
Tamsulosin	Tamoxifen
Taxol	Paxil
Taxol	Taxotere
Taxotere	Taxol
Tegretol	Toradol
Tegretol	Trental
Tegretol	Trileptal
Tegretol-XR	Toprol-XL
Temazepam.	Flurazepam
Temazepam.	Lorazepam
Temazepam.	Oxazepam
Temodar	Tambocor
Tenormin	Imuran
Tenormin	Thiamine
Tenormin	Trovan
Tequin	Levaquin
Tequin	Ticlid
Terazosin	Prazosin
Terazosin	Doxazosin
Testoderm.	Estraderm
Tetanus Toxoid	Diphtheria and Tetanus Toxoid
Tetracycline.	Tetradecyl Sulfate
Tetradecyl Sulfate	Tetracycline
Thalitone	Thalomid
Thalomid	Thalitone
Theraflu	Tamiflu
Thiamine	Tenormin
Thioridazine	Chlorpromazine
Thorazine	Thioridazine
Thioridazine	Thorazine
Tiagabine	Tizanidine
Tiazac	Tigan
Tiazac	Ziac
Ticlid	Tequin
Tigan	Tiazac
Timoptic.	Timoptic-XE
Timoptic-XE	Timoptic
Tizanidine.	Nizatidine
Tizanidine.	Tiagabine

TNKase.	t-PA (Synonym for Alteplase, recombinant)
Tobradex	Tobrex
Tobramycin.	Gentamicin
Tobrex	Tobradex
Tolazamide	Tolbutamide
Tolbutamide	Tolazamide
Tolcapone	Tolterodine
Tolterodine	Tolcapone
Topamax	Toprol-XL
Topiramate.	Torsemide
Toprol-XL	Tegretol-XR
Toprol-XL	Topamax
Toradol.	Foradil
Toradol.	Inderal
Toradol.	Stadol
Toradol.	Tegretol
Toradol.	Torecan
Toradol.	Tramadol
Torecan	Toradol
Torsemide	Furosemide
Torsemide	Topiramate
t-PA	TNKase (Synonym for Alteplase, recombinant)
Tramadol.	Toradol
Tramadol	Trandolapril
Tramadol	Trazodone
Tramadol	Voltaren
Trandate.	Trental
Trandate	Tridrate
Trandolapril.	Tramadol
Trazodone	Amiodarone
Trazodone	Tramadol
Trental	Tegretol
Trental	Trandate
Triad . . . . (Butalbital/ Acetaminophen/ Caffeine)	Triad (topical)
Triad . . . . (topical)	Triad (Butalbital/ Acetaminophen/ Caffeine)
Triamterene.	Trimethoprim
Tridrate	Trandate
Trifluoperazine	Fluphenazine
Trifluoperazine	Trihexyphenidyl
Trihexyphenidyl	Trifluoperazine

Trileptal	Tegretol
Tri-Levlen	Levlen
Tri-Levlen	Ortho Tri-Cyclen
Trimethoprim	Triamterene
Tri-Nasal	Triphasil
Tri-Norinyl	Triphasil
Triphasil	Tri-Nasal
Triphasil	Tri-Norinyl
Trovan	Tenormin
Trusopt.	Cosopt
Tylenol	Tylenol w/ Codeine
Tylenol Children's.	Tylenol w/ Codeine
Tylenol w/ Codeine.	Tylenol
Tylenol w/ Codeine.	Tylenol Children's
Ultane	Ultram
Ultracef . . . . (Cefadroxil in other countries)	Ultracet (Acetaminophen/ Tramadol Hydrochloride in U.S.)
Ultracet . . . . (Acetaminophen/ Tramadol Hydrochloride in U.S.)	Ultracef (Cefadroxil in other countries)
Ultram	Ultane
Ultram	Voltaren
Unasyn.	Zosyn
Uniretic	Univasc
Univasc	Uniretic
Univasc	Urispas
Urex	Erex
Uridon	Vicodin
Urised.	Urocit-K
Urispas.	Univasc
Urispas.	Uro-Mag
Urocit-K	Urised
Uro-Mag.	Urispas
Valacyclovir	Valgancyclovir
Valcyte.	Valtrex
Valgancyclovir	Valacyclovir
Valium	Versed
Valium	Vicodin
Valsartan	Losartan
Valtrex	Valcyte
Vancenase	Premphase
Vancenase	Vanceril
Vancenase AQ	Vanceril DS
Vanceril	Vancenase
Vanceril DS	Vancenase AQ
Vancomycin	Azithromycin
Vancomycin	Gentamicin

814

Vancomycin . . . . Vecuronium
Vancomycin . . . . *Vibramycin*
Vantin . . . . Ventolin
Vasocon . . . . *Vasocon A*
Vasocon A . . . . *Vasocon*
Vasotec . . . . *Norvasc*
Vecuronium . . . . Vancomycin
Ventolin . . . . *Benylin*
Ventolin . . . . *Vantin*
Vepesid . . . . *Versed*
Verapamil . . . . *Verelan*
Verelan . . . . Veraparmil
Verelan . . . . *Virilon*
Versed . . . . *Valium*
Versed . . . . *Vepesid*
Versed . . . . *Vistaril*
Vexol . . . . *VoSol*
Viagra . . . . *Allegra*
Vibramycin . . . . Vancomycin
Vicodin . . . . *Percodan*
Vicodin . . . . *Uridon*
Vicodin . . . . *Valium*
Vicodin . . . . *Vicodin ES*
Vicodin . . . . *Vioxx*
Vicodin ES . . . . *Vicodin*
Vinblastine . . . . Vincristine
Vincristine . . . . Vinblastine
Vioxx . . . . *Aciphex*
Vioxx . . . . *Vicodin*
Vioxx . . . . *Zyvox*
Viracept . . . . Viramune
Viramune . . . . Viracept
Virilon . . . . Verelan
Visicol . . . . Bisacodyl
Vistaril . . . . *Restoril*
Vistaril . . . . Versed
Vistaril . . . . Zestril
Vitamin C . . . . Vitamin E
Vitamin D . . . . Vitamin E
Vitamin E . . . . Vitamin C
Vitamin E . . . . Vitamin D

Volmax . . . . *Flomax*
Voltaren . . . . Tramadol
Voltaren . . . . *Ultram*
VoSol . . . . Vexol
Wellbutrin . . . . *Wellbutrin SR*
Wellbutrin SR . . . . *Wellbutrin*
Xalatan . . . . *Xalcom*
(Latanoprost/
Timolol in other
countries)
Xalcom . . . . *Xalatan*
(Latanoprost/
Timolol in other
countries)
Xanax . . . . *Lanoxin*
Xanax . . . . *Zanaflex*
Xanax . . . . *Zantac*
Xanax . . . . . *Zantac* . . . . . *Zyrtec*
Xigris . . . . *Zydis*
(Dosage Form
Trademark)
Yocon . . . . *Zocor*
Zagam . . . . *Zyban*
Zaleplon . . . . Zolpidem
Zanaflex . . . . *Anaflex*
Zanaflex . . . . *Xanax*
Zantac . . . . *Xanax*
Zantac . . . . . *Xanax* . . . . . *Zyrtec*
Zantac . . . . *Zofran*
Zaroxolyn . . . . *Zyprexa*
Zebeta . . . . *DiaBeta*
Zemuron . . . . Remeron
Zerit . . . . Zestril
Zestril . . . . Vistaril
Zestril . . . . Zerit
Zestril . . . . Zocor
Zestril . . . . Zyrtec
Ziac . . . . Tiazac
Ziac . . . . Zocor
Zidovudine . . . . Lamivudine
Zidovudine . . . . Zidovudine and
Lamivudine

Zidovudine . . . . Ziprasidone
Zidovudine . . . . Zidovudine
and Lamivudine
Zinacef . . . . Zithromax
Zinecard . . . . Gemzar
Ziprasidone . . . . Zidovudine
Zithromax . . . . Zinacef
Zocor . . . . Cozaar
Zocor . . . . Lipitor
Zocor . . . . Yocon
Zocor . . . . Zestril
Zocor . . . . Ziac
Zocor . . . . Zoloft
Zofran . . . . Reglan
Zofran . . . . Zantac
Zofran . . . . Zosyn
Zolmitriptan . . . . Sumatriptan
Zoloft . . . . Zocor
Zoloft . . . . *Zyloprim*
Zolpidem . . . . Zaleplon
Zonalon . . . . *Zone A Forte*
Zone A Forte . . . . *Zonalon*
Zosyn . . . . Unasyn
Zosyn . . . . Zofran
Zovirax . . . . *Zyvox*
Zyban . . . . *Zagam*
Zydis . . . . *Xigris*
(Dosage Form
Trademark)
Zyloprim . . . . Zoloft
Zyprexa . . . . *Celexa*
Zyprexa . . . . *Zaroxolyn*
Zyprexa . . . . *Zyprexa Zydis*
Zyprexa . . . . *Zyrtec*
Zyprexa Zydis . . . . *Zyprexa*
Zyrtec . . . . . . *Xanax* . . . . . *Zantac*
Zyrtec . . . . *Zestril*
Zyrtec . . . . *Zyprexa*
Zyvox . . . . *Vioxx*
Zyvox . . . . *Zovirax*

Appendix C
Drugs That Should Not Be Crushed

As a rule of thumb, any sustained-release or extended-release formulation should never be crushed. Instead, attempt to get a liquid formulation of the product so that it can be administered in that form. Coated products should also not be crushed. They were coated for a specific purpose, e.g., to prevent stomach irritation by the product, to prevent destruction of the product by stomach acid, to prevent an unwanted reaction, or to produce a prolonged or extended effect.

These are some of the drugs that should not be crushed:

Accutane	Arthrotec	Ceclor CD	Crixivan
Aciphex	ASA E.C.	Ceftin	Cymbalta
Actiq	ASA Enseal	Cefuroxime	Cytovene
Actonel	Augmentin XR	CellCept	Depakote ER
Adalat cc SR	Avinza	Chlortrimeton SR	Detrol LA
Adderall XR	Avodart	Choledyl SR	Dilacor XR
Advicor ER	Azulfadine Entab	Cipro XR	Ditropan XL
Afrinol Repetab	Betaphen-VK	Claritin-D	Divalproex XR
Aggrenox	Biaxin XL	Colace	Drixoral tablet
Allegra D	Biscodyl EC	Colestid	Ducolax EC
Allerest capsule	Boniva	Commit	DynaCirc CR
Alprazolam ER	Budeprion SR	Compazine Spansule	Ecotrin tablet
Altoprev	Calan SR	Concerta	Effexor XR
Ambien CR	Cardene SR	Concerta SR	E-Mycin tablet
Aminodur Duratab	Cardizem LA, SR	Covera-HS	Erythromycin EC
Aptivus	Cardura XL	Creon EC	Evista

Feldene

Fentora

Feosol Spansule

Ferro Grad-500
    tablet/sequels

Flagyl ER

Flomax

Fosamax

Geocillin

Gleevec

Glipizide

Glucatrol XL

Glucophage XR

Imdur SR, LA

Inderal LA

Indocin SR

Innopran XL

Intelence

Isoptin SR

Isordil Tembids,
    Dinitrate

Isordil sublingual

Kadian

Kaon tablet

Kapidex

K-Dur, K-tab

Keppra XR

Ketek

Klor-Con

Lamictal XR

Lescol XL

Levbid SR

Lithobid SR

Luvox CR

Macrobid SR

Mestinon
    Timespans

Metadate CD, SR

Metoprolol ER

Motrin

MS Contin

Mucinex

Nexium

Niaspan

Nicotinic acid

Nifediac CC

Nifedipine ER

Nitroglycerin tablet

Nitrospan capsule

Norpace CR

OxyContin

Pancrease EC, MT

Paxil CR

Plendil SR

Prevacid

Prilosec SR

Procardia XL

Propecia

Proscar

Protonix

Prozac weekly

Ranexa

Razadyne ER

Renagel

Requip XL

Revlimid

Risperdal M-tab

Ritalin LA/SR

Rythmol SR

Seroquel XR

Sinemet CR

Slo-Niacin

Slow K tablet; Slow
    Mag, Slow Fe

Strattera

Sudafed SA capsule

Sular

Tasigna

Tegretol XR

Temodar

Tessalon Perles

Theobid Duracaps

Tiazac SR

Topamax

Toprol XL

Tracleer

Trental SR

Treximet

Tylenol ER

Ultram ER

Uniphyl SR

Uroxatral

Valcyte

Verapamil SR

Verelan PM

Videx EC

Voltaren EC

Wellbutrin SR

Xanax SR

ZORprin

Zerit XR

Zolinza

Zomig ZMT

Zyban

Zyflo CR

Zyrtec-D

Reprinted from Spratto, G. and Woods, A. (2011) *Delmar Nurse's Drug Handbook: Special 20 Year Anniversary*, 1st ed. Clifton Park, NY: Delmar, Cengage Learning.

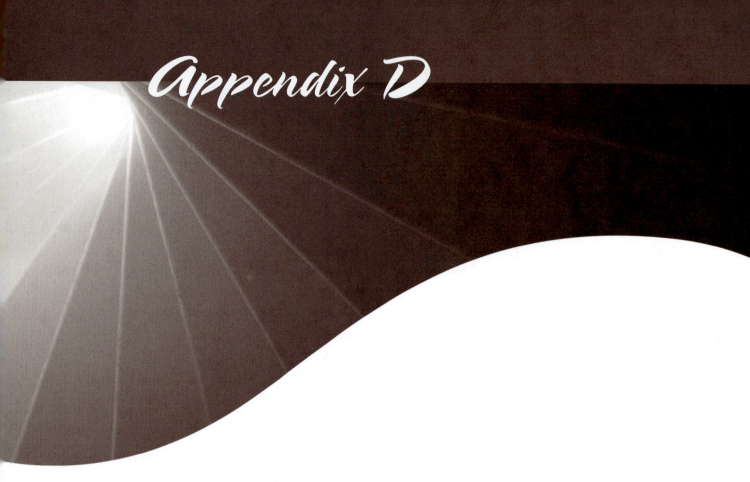

Appendix D

Suggested Readings and Resources

Agnes, M., & Laird, C. (Eds.). (2002). *Webster's new world dictionary and thesaurus* (2d ed.). Cleveland, OH: John Wiley & Sons.

Curran, A. M. (2009). *Math for meds: Dosages and solutions* (10th ed.). Clifton Park, NY: Delmar, Cengage Learning.

Cyberonics, Inc. *A comprehensive resource for patients living with seizure disorders for their families and friends.* Retrieved June 24, 2009, from http://www.vnstherapy.com/epilepsy/patient/index.asp.

Delaune, S. C., & Ladner, P. K. (2006). *Fundamentals of nursing* (3rd ed.). Clifton Park, NY: Delmar, Cengage Learning.

Deter, L. (2006). *Basic medication administration skills.* Clifton Park, NY: Delmar, Cengage Learning.

Deter, L. (2007). *Advanced medication administration skills.* Clifton Park, NY: Delmar, Cengage Learning.

Ebersole, P. & Hess, P. (2001). *Geriatric nursing and healthy aging.* St. Louis, MO: Mosby.

Gaylene, Bouska, & Altman. (2004). *Delmar's fundamental and advanced nursing skills* (2nd ed.). Clifton Park, NY: Delmar, Cengage Learning.

Institute for Safe Medication Practices. *ISMP's list of error-prone abbreviations, symbols, and dose designations.* Retrieved February 9, 2009, from http://www.ismp.org/tools/errorproneabbreviations.pdf.

Kennamer, M. (2005). *Math for health care professionals.* Clifton Park, NY: Delmar, Cengage Learning.

Moini, J. (2009). *Fundamental pharmacology for pharmacy technicians.* Clifton Park, NY: Delmar, Cengage Learning.

Mulvihill, M. L. (1995). *Human diseases: A systemic approach* (4th ed.). Norwalk, CT: Appleton & Lange.

National Institute of Drug Abuse. *Club Drugs.* Retrieved June 23, 2009, from http://www.drugabuse.gov/DrugPages/Clubdrugs.html.

National Institute of Drug Abuse. *Cocaine*. Retrieved June 23, 2009, from http://www.drugabuse.gov/DrugPages/Cocaine.html.

National Institute of Drug Abuse. *Commonly abused drugs*. Retrieved June 23, 2009, from http://www.drugabuse.gov/DrugPages/Drugs of abuse.html.

National Institute of Drug Abuse. *Heroin*. Retrieved June 23, 2009, from http://www.drugabuse.gov/DrugPages/Heroin.html.

National Institute of Drug Abuse. *Inhalants*. Retrieved June 23, 2009, from http://www.drugabuse.gov/DrugPages/Inhalants.html.

National Institute of Drug Abuse. *MDMA (ecstasy)*. Retrieved June 23, 2009, from http://www.drugabuse.gov/DrugPages/MDMA.html

National Institute of Drug Abuse. *Methamphetamine*. Retrieved June 23, 2009, from http://www.drugabuse.gov/DrugPages/Methamphetamine.html.

National Institute of Drug Abuse. *PCP/Phencyclidine*. Retrieved June 23, 2009, from http://www.drugabuse.gov/DrugPages/PCP.html.

National Institute of Drug Abuse. *Prescription drug abuse chart*. Retrieved June 23, 2009, from http://www.drugabuse.gov/DrugPages/PrescripDrugsChart.html.

National Institute of Drug Abuse. *Prescription medications*. Retrieved June 23, 2009, from http://www.drugabuse.gov/DrugPages/prescription.html.

National Institute of Drug Abuse. (2009). *Steroids (anabolic)*. Retrieved June 23, 2009, from http://www.drugabuse.gov/DrugPages/Steroids.html.

Nicol, M., Bavin, C., Cronin, P., & Rawlings-Anderson, K. (2008). *Essential nursing skills* (3rd ed.). New York: Mosby/Elsevier.

Potter, P. A., & Perry, A. G. (2009). *Fundamentals of nursing* (7th ed.). St. Louis, MO: Mosby.

Semela, T. P., Beizer, J. L., & Higbee, M. D. (2005). *Lexi-Comp's geriatric dosage handbook* (10th ed.). Hudson, OH: Lexi-Comp.

Silverman, H. M. (Ed.). (2008). *The pill book* (13th ed.). New York: Bantam Dell.

St. Mary Medical Center. *Handwashing Facts and Tips*. Retrieved March 14, 2009, from http://www.stmaryhealthcare.org/body.

University of Massachusetts Medical School. (2000). *Massachusetts Department of Mental Retardation curriculum on gastrostomy and jejunostomy tubes*. Boston: Massachusetts Department of Mental Retardation.

Glossary

abbreviations A shortened way to write health care orders.

abrasion A scrape on the skin.

absence seizure A seizure during which an individual experiences a lapse in awareness; also called a petit mal seizure.

absorption The passage of substances across and into tissues.

abuse Intentional mistreatment or misuse.

acne A condition of the skin most common in adolescence and early adulthood that is usually on the face, neck, chest, back, and shoulders.

acquired immune deficiency syndrome (AIDS) A set of symptoms and infections resulting from damage to the immune system caused by the human immunodeficiency virus (HIV).

active immunization Immunization occurs when a vaccine is given, causing the body to form antibodies.

active refusal An individual directly refuses to take a medication.

acute pain Occurs suddenly and without warning. Usually is the result of injury or surgery. Decreases over time as healing takes place.

addiction The compulsive, uncontrollable use of a substance.

administer To dispense or to give, for example, to give medication.

Adult Foster Care A state-funded program that offers disabled and/or elderly individuals the opportunity to live in private homes in the community.

advance directive A document stating an individual's wishes for treatment (or no treatment)—completed before it is needed for use when the individual is unable or incapable to communicate.

adverse reaction An unwanted action or effect of a medication that is harmful to the body.

aerosol A type of liquid medication packaged in a pressurized container.

agonist action An action in which a medication mixes with special sites on specific cells, causing a response to the medication.

agoraphobia An irrational fear of leaving the house and of open spaces.

aiding and abetting To assist or help another individual in the committing of an illegal act, crime, or other inappropriate act, including the failure to report unethical and/or illegal acts that one witnesses.

AIDS Acquired immune deficiency syndrome is a set of symptoms and infections resulting from damage to the immune system caused by the human immunodeficiency virus (HIV).

akathisia An inability to sit down, with symptoms including agitation, fidgeting, and pacing.

allergen An allergy-causing substance.

allergic reaction Hypersensitivity, many times noted by a rash or hives.

allergy An individual's hypersensitivity to a substance that causes a physical reaction.

almshouses Privately financed homes for the poor.

Alzheimer's disease A progressive disorder recognized by a devastating mental decline.

amenorrhea Without a menstrual cycle.

amount The number of units of medication to be given.

amputation The surgical removal of a limb, for example, an arm or a leg.

amyotropic lateral sclerosis (ALS) Lou Gehrig's disease; a progressive disease that causes muscle weakness and paralysis and is almost always fatal.

anabolic steroids Man-made substances that mimic male hormones

analgesic-antipyretics Medications that relieve pain and reduce fever.

analgesics Medications used to relieve pain caused by many different conditions.

anaphylactic reaction A severe allergic reaction that *may cause death* if not treated immediately; anaphylaxis.

anaphylaxis A rapid, severe allergic reaction; an anaphylactic reaction.

asthenia Absence or loss of strength; weakness.

anesthetics Medications used to (1) prevent pain, (2) relax muscles, and (3) induce lack of sensation during surgery and other procedures.

angina pectoris Chest pain caused by a lack of blood supply to the heart.

angioedema Swelling of the face, neck, lips, larynx, hands, feet, genitalia, or internal organs.

anorexia Loss of appetite.

antacids Medications that neutralize hydrochloric acid in the stomach; used to treat indigestion, heartburn, and pain; to promote healing of ulcers; to manage esophageal reflux.

antagonism The opposing action of two medications in which one medication decreases or cancels out the effect of the other medication.

antagonist action An action in which one medication blocks the effect of a second medication through different actions in the body.

anterograde amnesia The lack of recall of events that happen while an individual is under the influence of a substance.

antiangiogenesis A cancer treatment that uses medications or substances to stop tumors from making new blood vessels.

antianxiety medications Medications that counteract or relieve anxiety.

antiarrhythmic Medications that are used to treat an arrhythmia (irregular heartbeat).

antibacterials Medications used to treat bacterial infections.

antibiotics Medications used to treat infectious diseases.

anticoagulants Medications that prevent or delay clotting of the blood.

anticonvulsants Medications used to treat seizures in individuals with epilepsy.

antidepressants Medications that elevate mood.

antidiabetics Oral medications that are used to manage and treat non–insulin-dependent diabetes mellitus (NIDDM), or Type 2 diabetes.

antidiarrhea medications Medications that decrease the number of loose, watery stools an individual is having.

antiemetics Medications that prevent or stop vomiting.

antiepileptic drugs Medications used to treat seizures in individuals with epilepsy.

antiflatulents Medications used to treat (1) the symptoms of gastric bloating and (2) pain from flatus after surgery.

antifungals Medications that control conditions caused by fungi.

antiglaucoma medications Medications used to treat glaucoma.

antihelmintics Medications used to treat helminthiasis, an infestation of the intestine with parasitic worms.

antihistamines Medications that relieve allergy symptoms.

antihypertensives Medications used to treat hypertension (high blood pressure).

anti-infectives Medications that prevent and treat infections.

anti-inflammatory medications Medications used to relieve inflammation.

antilipidemic medications Medications used to lower high levels of lipids in the blood.

antimanic medications Medications that treat the manic phase of bipolar disorder.

antimicrobials Medications that kill or prevent the growth of microorganisms.

antimigraine medications Medications used to treat migraine headaches.

antineoplastic medications Medications used to destroy the abnormal, damaged, "cancer" cells (malignant cells).

antioxidants Chemical substances that neutralize free radicals.

antiparkinsonian medications Medications used to give relief of the symptoms of Parkinson's disease.

antiprotozoals Medications used to treat diseases caused by parasites, for example, malaria.

antipruritics Medications that relieve itching.

antipsychotic medications Medications that modify psychotic behavior; also called neuroleptics.

antiseptics Substances that are used to prevent or slow the growth of microorganisms.

antithyroid medications Medications used for treatment of hyperthyroidism, preparation for removal of the thyroid, and radioactive iodine therapy.

antitubercular Medications used to treat tuberculosis.

antitussives Medications that prevent coughing in an individual who does not need to have a productive cough; allow an individual to sleep better, decreasing fatigue.

antivirals Medications used to treat viral infections.

anxiety A general feeling of worry or dread.

aphasia Difficulty expressing oneself or understanding communication or language.

apical pulse A pulse that is taken over the heart.

apnea A period of no breathing.

apothecary system An old pharmacy system used when ordering and measuring medications.

aqueous humor A clear, watery fluid that fills the eye.

Arabic numerals Examples are "1," "2," and "3."

arrhythmia An irregular heartbeat caused by a disruption of the sinoatrial node, which sets the rhythm of the heartbeat.

arteriosclerosis Thickening, hardening, and loss of elasticity of the artery walls.

arthritis Inflammation of the joints.

ascites An abnormal collection of fluid in the abdomen.

aspiration The entrance of stomach contents, liquids, or other substances into the respiratory tract; may cause pneumonia.

assessment An evaluation.

assisted living facilities Facilities that provide daily supervision and/or assistance with daily activities as needed to individuals who are able to live on their own. Medical care and nursing care are not provided.

asthma A chronic disorder of the bronchial airways that results in narrowed, inflamed, and sensitive bronchial tubes.

atelectasis A collapse of a lung.

ataxia Impaired coordination.

atonic seizure A seizure during which there is a sudden loss of muscle tone; also called a drop attack.

atrial fibrillation An irregular heart rate occurring in the atria of the heart.

atrial flutter A type of atrial fibrillation with a heart rate of 230 to 380 beats per minute.

aura A warning sign or sensation that an epileptic seizure is about to take place.

autoimmune response A condition in which the body's defense system malfunctions and begins to attack itself.

automatic blood pressure unit A small portable unit to measure blood pressure, commonly used in a home setting.

average dose The amount of medication proven most effective with the least amount of side effects.

avitaminosis An illness caused by a lack of vitamins in the diet.

benign prostatic hypertrophy A non-cancerous, noninflammatory enlargement of the prostate, most common in men over fifty (50) years of age.

bisphosphonates Medications that directly act to (1) increase bone thickness at the hip and spine and (2) decrease first fractures and future fractures; used to treat osteoporosis.

bipolar disorder Manic depression or manic-depressive psychosis.

blood dyscrasia An abnormal condition of the elements (parts) of the blood or of parts needed for clotting of the blood.

blood pressure The force of blood against the walls of the arteries during a heartbeat.

body core The center of the body.

body language Using one's body to communicate a message.

bolus A large amount of liquid instilled into the stomach or small intestine.

bpm The abbreviation for "beats per minute."

brachial artery An artery in the arm used for taking blood pressure.

bradycardia A pulse of less than 60 beats per minute (bpm).

bradykinesia A decrease in spontaneous movement.

brachytherapy Also called internal radiation: a radioactive source in the form of a seed, wire, or pellet is implanted in (placed into) the body or near the tumor.

breach A break or violation of a particular duty or standard of care.

bronchitis Chronic inflammation of the lining of the air passages in the lungs.

bronchodilator A medication that opens the airway, allowing an individual to breathe.

buccal medications Medications that are dissolved in the mouth in a pouch between the cheek and gum at the back of the mouth.

buccal tablets Tablets that are dissolved in the mouth in a pouch between the cheek and gum at the back of the mouth.

bursitis An inflammation of the bursa sacs around a joint.

cannabinoids Illegal substances including marijuana and hashish.

caplet A type of solid medication that has the same size and shape as a capsule but has the consistency of a tablet.

capsule A small two-part container usually made of gelatin that contains medication.

carcinogenic A substance that can produce cancer.

cardiac glycosides Medications that (1) strengthen the heartbeat, (2) slow the heart rate (pulse), and (3) improve the contractions of the heart muscle as it pumps blood throughout the body.

cardiomyopathy Any disease that affects the structure and function of the heart.

cardiovascular disease (CVD) Diseases of the heart and blood vessels.

cardiovascular system Circulatory system; brings oxygen and nourishment to the cells and removes waste products.

carpopedal spasm Spasms and rigidity in the hands and feet.

cataract The lens of the eye becomes cloudy and no light can pass through.

causation A connection between a breach of duty and the harm to the individual resulting from that breach.

cavities Spaces in the body that contain the organs.

cell The basic unit of the body.

central nervous system stimulant Medications that improve the function of the central nervous system.

cerebrovascular accident (CVA) A stroke caused by complete or partial loss of blood flow to the brain.

character The rhythm and volume, or "feel," of an individual's pulse; also words to describe respiration.

chemical name The molecular (chemical) formula for a medication.

chemotherapy Treatment of disease by using anticancer medications that destroy cancer cells.

chewable tablets Tablets that are made to be chewed and then swallowed.

Cheyne-Stokes respirations A repeating pattern of dyspnea (labored breathing) and apnea (no breathing).

cholecystitis Inflammation of the gallbladder.

cholelithiasis Gallstones.

cholinesterase inhibitors Medications that prevent the breakdown of acetylcholine in the brain; used to treat Alzheimer's disease.

chronic bronchitis Prolonged inflammation in the bronchi.

chronic pain Lasts longer than six (6) months. May be caused from multiple medical conditions.

civil liability Being held legally responsible for inappropriate conduct; usually results in the payment of damages to an injured individual, her family, or her representative.

Client's Bill of Rights A document that states the rights of individuals receiving home health care.

club drugs Illegal substances that are usually abused by teens and young adults at nightclubs, bars, raves, and trance scenes.

colon Part of the large intestine (bowel).

colony-stimulating factors (CSFS) Medications that stimulate an individual's bone marrow to make more red blood cells.

cognitive disorders Affect intellect, memory, and/or attention.

communication A two-way process in which individuals share information.

communication book A written form of communication used by staff to report on the condition of the individuals for whom they are caring.

comparative negligence A legal rule under which a determination is made as to who is more negligent than another when multiple individuals are involved in a situation.

Computerized Physician Online Entry (CPOE) A computerized, organized method by which licensed healthcare providers are able to enter (write) orders for the treatment of individuals.

congestive heart failure A heart condition that is the result of the heart failing to pump the blood adequately throughout the body.

conjunctivitis The inflammation of the mucous membrane that lines the eyelids and covers the eye.

constipation The infrequent and difficult movement of the bowel.

continuous positive airway pressure (CPAP) A device that delivers pressure to the individual's airway while the individual sleeps.

contraindications Conditions making medication dangerous to use.

Controlled Substance Count Book A book used for the documentation of the administration of controlled substances.

controlled substances Prescription medications that, because of their danger for addiction and abuse, have additional federal regulations.

COPD Chronic obstructive pulmonary disease; a condition that interferes with normal breathing over a long period of time, such as emphysema or bronchitis.

corticosteroids Medications used topically to treat conditions of the skin; used orally to treat asthma and COPD.

Cox 2 Inhibitors Medications that relieve inflammation; pose less risk for GI bleed and fewer gastric problems than NSAIDs.

criminal liability Being held legally responsible for illegal conduct; usually results in being sent to jail or prison and/or the payment of a fine issued by the court.

culture A laboratory test done to determine the type of invading organism causing an infection.

cumulative effect Increasing in effect.

curative use The use of medications to kill or remove the cause of a disease.

Cushing's syndrome A condition that is the result of an excess amount of adrenal cortex hormones.

cyanosis A blue or purplish discoloration of the skin caused by a lack of oxygen.

cystitis Inflammation of the urinary bladder.

cystocele A hernia at the wall between the bladder and the vagina.

cystoscopy The direct visualization of the urinary tract and bladder with use of a scope inserted into the urethra.

decongestants Medications that shrink the swollen linings of the respiratory tract and open nasal passages; used to relieve symptoms of nasal congestion.

decubitus ulcers Pressure ulcers.

deinstitutionalization The process of moving or shifting individuals from living in large facilities, hospitals, state schools, and other large settings to living in homes, apartments, and other community settings.

delegation The legal act of assigning tasks or duties.

demulcents Medications that soothe irritation.

dependence An acquired need for a medication that may produce psychological and/or physical symptoms of withdrawal when the medication is discontinued.

depressants Medications that decrease actions in the body.

dermal exposure Taking a substance into the body through the skin.

diabetes mellitus A metabolic disorder that causes an inability to use insulin; an imbalance of carbohydrates in the body; diabetes.

digital thermometer A small handheld unit with a probe used to measure temperature.

diagnostic use The use of medications in radiology (X-ray).

diaphoresis Sweating, perspiration.

diastolic blood pressure The pressure when the heart is relaxed.

diffuse peritonitis The widespread inflammation of the lining of the abdominal cavity.

discontinuing To stop a medication, done only with a licensed health care provider's order.

discrimination Treating any individual differently because of her race, color, sex, national origin, sexual orientation, age, religious beliefs, or defined protected category.

disease-modifying antirheumatic medications (DMARDS) Medications used to treat rheumatoid arthritis.

disinfectants Substances that can quickly kill microorganisms on any surface.

disposal form A form used for the documentation of the disposal of medication(s); also called a disposal record.

disposal record A form used for the documentation of the disposal of medication(s); also called a disposal form.

distribution The location of medications in various organs and tissues after administration.

diuresis An excessive production of urine in the body.

diuretics Medications that increase urine output and relieve or prevent edema.

diversion Theft of controlled substances (C-II through C-V). In some states, this includes substances in C-VI.

divided dose Portions of the dose administered over a period of time.

dosage The amount of medication that is prescribed (ordered) for administration.

dose The amount of medication ordered by the licensed health care provider.

douche An irrigation of the vaginal canal with medicated or normal saline solution.

drug A substance used in medicine that may affect how the body works.

drug-resistant organism A microorganism that is not killed by medication and which can potentially cause death.

drug standards Rules made so that we, the people, get what we pay for when we fill our prescription medications.

drug substitution laws Laws that allow generic medications to be substituted for trade-name medications.

duty An obligation to provide an established standard of care for an individual receiving care.

dyspepsia Upset stomach.

dyspnea Difficult or labored breathing.

dystonia Literally, difficult or bad tone; symptoms include spasms and rigidity in various muscle groups.

dysuria Difficulty or pain during urination.

ecchymosis A bruise.

edema A local or general collection of fluid in the body tissues.

effervescent tablets Tablets that, when placed in water, release active ingredients, making a solution.

electrolytes Acid, base, and salt particles formed by the breakdown of mineral compounds in body fluids.

electrolyte imbalance An imbalance of the basic minerals and salts important to our body functions. These are sodium, potassium, calcium, chloride, bicarbonate, and sulfate.

electronic blood pressure unit A large piece of equipment used to measure blood pressure that is moved from room to room in a facility.

electronic Medication Administration Record (eMAR) A computerized record that eliminates all paper records and creates an organized system for medication administration.

electronic thermometer An electronic unit with a probe used to measure temperature.

elixir A type of liquid medication; medications dissolved in a solution of alcohol and water that has been sweetened and flavored.

embolus A blood clot that has disconnected from the point where it was formed.

emetics Medications used to induce vomiting.

emollients Medications that soothe irritation.

emphysema A chronic respiratory disease with damage to the air sacs in the lungs, causing loss of elasticity and decrease in the exchange of oxygen and carbon dioxide.

emulsion A type of liquid medication; fine droplets of oil in water or water in oil.

endocrine system Made up of glands or distinct clusters of cells that release hormones.

endoscopy Visual inspection of the inside of a body cavity using special instruments.

enema A way to administer a liquid solution or liquid medication into the rectum and colon (part of the bowel); may also be used to clean the bowel.

enteric-coated tablets Tablets that are dissolved in the small intestine.

enterocutaneous fistulae Abnormal passages or pathways from the intestines to the skin.

epigastric distress Heartburn.

epilepsy A seizure disorder caused by recurring and temporary episodes of disrupted brain function.

EpiPen Auto-Injector A syringe-needle unit prefilled with the medication epinephrine.

erectile dysfunction The inability for a male to achieve or maintain an erection; also called impotence.

erosive esophagitis A condition in which stomach acids travel back up through the bottom of the esophagus causing irritation and tissue damage.

***Escherichia coli* (*E. coli*)** The most common cause of a urinary tract infection.

esophagitis Inflammation of the lining of the esophagitis.

ethical standards Guides to moral behavior.

ethics committee An advisory group of individuals from multiple professions who are consulted in an attempt to resolve a conflict or issue.

euphoria Excitement.

exacerbation The time when a disease process and its symptoms are most severe and debilitating.

excoriation A part of the skin has been scratched or scraped away.

excretion The process of removing substances from the body.

expectorants Medications that help loosen mucus, liquify bronchial secretions, and remove phlegm (sputum).

expiration Breathing out, or exhalation.

external medications Medications that are applied or put onto the outside of the body.

external radiation therapy A machine delivers high-energy waves of radiation from outside the body to the tumor and some nearby tissue.

extrapyramidal symptoms (EPS) Abnormalities of movement that mimic movements that would be brought on after an injury to the brain.

fat-soluble vitamins Vitamins that are stored in fat tissue and in the liver.

faxed orders Written orders that are faxed to the UAP by the licensed health care provider.

feces Stool; semisolid waste passed out of the body through the rectum; bowel movement, or BM.

fibromyalgia A chronic pain syndrome.

financial abuse Use of money to control an individual.

Five Rights of Delegation Guidelines followed by a nurse when he or she delegates a task(s) to a UAP.

flashbacks Recurrences of certain aspects of one's drug experience (one's trip).

flatus Gas or air in the stomach or intestines; commonly passed out of the body by belching or through the rectum.

fracture Any break in any bone.

friction Skin rubbing against another surface, even another area of skin.

free radicals Unstable and highly reactive molecules that can cause significant cell damage.

function One's ability to do daily tasks such as eating, dressing, bathing, and toileting.

fungus A plantlike organism that may be parasitic or may grow in dead and decaying organic matter.

gastroesophageal reflux disease (GERD) A condition in which stomach acids travel back up into the esophagus, causing inflammation and discomfort.

gastrointestinal system The digestive tract; helps the body to break down, transport, and absorb nutrients (food) as well as to remove waste.

gastrostomy tube (G-tube) A tube that is placed directly into the stomach through a surgical incision(cut) in the skin; feedings, liquids, and medications are provided through the tube.

generalized seizure A seizure that affects both sides of the brain from the beginning of the seizure; causes loss of consciousness.

generic equivalents Generic medications that cost less than trade- or brand-name medications but that are "equivalent" or equal in effectiveness.

generic name The common or general name used for a medication.

gene therapy A type of cancer treatment still under research.

geriatric clients or patients Individuals age sixty-five (65) years and older; the elderly.

gigantism A condition that causes excessive growth of the body or a body part.

GI ischemia Decreased blood supply to the gastrointestinal system.

GI protectants Medications that protect the lining of the stomach.

glaucoma A condition of the eye in which there is increased intraocular pressure due to the blockage of the outflow of the fluid in the eye.

glycosuria Sugar in the urine.

gout A metabolic disease that causes painful swelling of certain joints. The most common site is the great toe.

gram Measurement for weight in the metric system.

Graves' disease A condition in which there is too much thyroid hormone in the blood.

grievance A situation in which an individual feels she wishes to file a complaint.

habilitation model Allows an individual to participate as fully as possible in all aspects of his life, including his family, community, and social life. Staff provide a wide range of support, from providing personal care (activities of daily living), health care, transportation, and advocacy to social and recreational assistance and employment support, depending on the setting in which one works. As a coach and partner, one may actually help the individual to direct his own life.

hallucinogens Illegal substances including LSD (d-lysergic acid diethylamide) and PCP (phencyclidine); their effects are inconsistent, affecting every individual differently each time the individual abuses the drug.

handheld inhaler A type of inhaler that is held in an individual's hand.

harm Physical or emotional injury.

Helicobacter pylori An infection in the lining of the stomach that is related to stomach and peptic ulcers as well as stomach cancer.

helminthiasis A condition in which there is an intestinal infestation with parasitic worms.

hemoglobin A part of the blood that carries oxygen from the lungs to the cells.

hernia Occurs when a structure pushes through a weakened area in a body wall that usually holds it in place.

herpes An acute viral disorder of which there are many different types.

herpes simplex Cold sores or genital herpes.

herpes zoster Shingles.

HIPAA The Health Insurance Portability and Accountability Act of 1996; a federal law that guarantees that an individual's health information is protected.

hirsutism Abnormal hair growth.

histamine H$_2$ blockers Medications used for short term relief of indigestion, heartburn, gastroesophageal reflux disease (GERD), upper GI bleeding, and esophagitis.

hives Red, raised bumps on the skin.

homeostasis A state of normal balance of electrolytes in body fluids.

hormone A substance made by the body that controls growth and regulates body activities.

hormone replacement therapy (HRT) Medications used to replace or maintain a level of estrogen and/or progesterone.

hospice A facility or program that provides care to individuals who are dying and to their families.

household system A system used when ordering and measuring medications, especially in home care and when teaching self-administration.

huffing Breathing illegal substance into the body from a plastic bag or by stuffing a rag soaked with the chemical into the mouth.

human immunodeficiency virus (HIV) A retrovirus that causes acquired immuno-deficiency syndrome, or AIDS.

humidifier A bottle of water that is attached to the oxygen administration equipment.

hydronephrosis A buildup of fluid in the kidney because of a blocked ureter or distended bladder, which causes damage to kidney cells.

hypercalcemia A high level of calcium in the blood.

hyperglycemia A condition in which there is too much sugar in the blood.

hyperglycosuria Too much sugar in the urine.

hyperkalemia A high level of potassium in the blood.

hypersensitivity An allergic response to a medication.

hypertension High blood pressure; a systolic blood pressure equal to or greater than 140, or a diastolic blood pressure equal to or greater than 90.

hypertensive crisis A life-threatening situation requiring immediate emergency care. Symptoms include severe headache, palpitations, sweating, chest pain, possible intracranial hemorrhage, and death.

hyperthermia A treatment for cancer that uses heat to kill cancer cells.

hypervitaminosis A condition caused by an excessive amount of a vitamin in the body, which can lead to an illness; particularly due to taking too many vitamin pills.

hypesthesia Decreased sensitivity.

hypnotic A medication that causes sleep.

hypochloremia A low level of chloride in the blood.

hypoglycemia A condition in which there is too little sugar in the blood.

hypokalemia A low level of potassium in the blood.

hypotension Low blood pressure.

hypovitaminosis A condition caused by a lack of vitamins in the body, often due to poor nutrition; may lead to avitaminosis.

hypoxemia Insufficient oxygen in the blood.

hysteroid dysphoria A general dissatisfaction, restlessness, depression, and anxiety that can escalate to hysteria.

idiosyncrasy A unique, unusual response to medication.

idiosyncrasies Special characteristics of an individual.

immunity The state of being protected from or resistant to a specific disease due to the development of antibodies.

immunization The process of inducing or providing immunity artificially by administering an immunobiologic.

immunotherapy A treatment for cancer in which the individual's immune system is used to fight cancer.

implications for administration The medical conditions that are treated by the medication; the reason why the medication is being used.

incentive spirometer A device used to help an individual breathe deeply.

incision A cut or wound in the body.

infection Microorganisms enter the body or a body part, multiply, and produce injury or illness.

inflammation A normal response to infection, injury, or irritation of living tissue.

informed consent Permission given for care or treatment after knowing all information.

ingestion Taking a substance into the body by swallowing.

inhalation The act of breathing.

inhalants Illegal substances breathed into the body that cause serious and irreversible effects including brain damage, hearing loss, peripheral neuropathies, and cardiovascular damage; they may also cause death.

inhalant medications Medications used to treat diseases of the respiratory tract; also called pulmonary medications.

inhaler A sealed container of medication that is under pressure.

initial dose The first dose of medication administered.

injecting When the individual uses a syringe and needle to directly insert an illegal substance into the body.

inspiration Breathing in or inhalation.

integumentary system Includes the skin; protects the other systems from infection; helps to regulate temperature and eliminate some waste.

intermittent positive-pressure breathing (IPPB) machine A machine that combines an aerosol that administers a fine mist of liquid medication deep into the lungs with a mechanical breather to assist patients who are unable to take a deep breathe on their own.

internal medications Medications that are taken into the body.

internal radiation therapy, also called brachytherapy; a radioactive source in the form of a seed, wire, or pellet is implanted (placed into) in the body or near the tumor.

intraocular pressure The pressure within the eyeball.

involuntary seclusion The separation from others against the wishes of the individual.

jejunostomy tube (J-tube) A tube that is placed directly into the individual's jejunum (small bowel) through a surgical incision (cut) in the skin; feedings, liquids, and medications are provided through the tube.

jejunum A part of the small bowel (colon).

keratolytics Medications that control conditions of abnormal scaling or peeling of the skin.

kyphoscoliosis Severe curvature of the spine.

laceration A cut, a break in the skin.

lactic acidosis A buildup of an end product of metabolism in the bloodstream.

larynx Voice box.

layered tablets Tablets that have two or more layers of medication.

laxatives Medications that aid the body in the elimination of waste.

least restrictive setting Caring for an individual in a setting that permits him to have as much freedom as possible while at the same time providing care that meets all of his needs.

legal standards Guides to legal behavior.

Lennox-Gastaut syndrome A seizure disorder seen especially in young children; often accompanied by a type of petit mal seizure.

lesions Changes in the skin caused by injury or disease or as part of the aging process.

lethal dose The amount of medication that could kill an individual.

lethargic Overly drowsy or tired.

liable Being held responsible.

licensed health care providers Individuals licensed within each state to provide medical care, for example, LPN, RN, nurse practitioner, nurse-midwife, pharmacist, physician assistant, dentist, podiatrist, physician, and doctor.

liniment A type of liquid medication used externally, with massage, to produce a feeling of heat to an area of the body.

lipids Fatty substances in the blood.

liquid oxygen canister A type of oxygen administration equipment that makes liquid oxygen by cooling oxygen gas.

liter Measurement for volume in the metric system.

local action A term used to describe an external medication that is made to act on an area of the body to which it is applied.

local anesthesia Loss of sensation at the site of application of a topical medication or anesthetic.

local hyperthermia, also called thermal ablation; a small area of cancer cells are destroyed by very high temperatures.

long-term care facilities Nursing homes and other facilities that provide care to individuals who are chronically ill, disabled, or severely injured.

lotion A type of liquid medication used externally, without massage, to treat skin conditions.

Lou Gehrig's disease A progressive disorder that destroys the motor nerves that control voluntary movement.

lozenge A hard, circular or oblong piece of medication with a candylike base.

LSD An illegal substance, a type of hallucinogen that may produce flashbacks without warning.

maintenance dose The amount of medication that will keep medication at a therapeutic level in an individual's bloodstream.

malaise A feeling of illness.

malignant cells Cells or groups of cells that invade local tissue and destroy normal cells.

malpractice Improper, negligent, or unethical behavior that results in harm, injury, or loss to an individual.

marijuana An illegal substance, a type of cannabinoid.

masks Devices that deliver oxygen to an individual. Masks come in many different varieties.

maximum dose The largest amount of a medication that can be safely administered to an individual.

Medicaid A government reimbursement system through which the federal government issues money to the states. The states use the monies to pay for the care of individuals who have no money of their own.

Medicare A government program that partially pays for health care for individuals over the age of sixty-five (65) or who are permanently disabled.

Medication Administration Process The steps for administering medication to an individual: (1) observation, (2) reporting, and (3) recording.

medication administration system A system used in some hospitals, long-term care facilities, and individual care facilities to document medication administration.

medication cart A cart that is used to administer medications in some work settings.

medication error A medication is *not* given as prescribed by the licensed health care provider.

medication interaction The interaction between two or more medications that results in the increase, decrease, or cancellation of the effects of one or more of the medications.

medication loss Whenever a medication is missing.

medication orders Written instructions from the licensed health care provider to the UAP.

medication progress note A written note used to document events occurring during medication administration.

medication reconciliation A method used to compare the medications an individual is taking to the medications ordered by the individual's licensed HCP.

medication record sheet A form used to document medication administration; a medication sheet.

medication refusal An individual refuses to take medication.

medication sheet A form used to document medication administration; a medication record sheet.

membranes Sheets of tissue that line the body cavities.

menopausal symptoms The symptoms that occur as a normal result of aging when a woman's ovaries stop functioning and her menstrual cycle stops.

menopause The time when a woman's ovaries stop working and menstruation stops.

menstruation The fourth phase of the menstrual cycle. A period of uterine bleeding that usually lasts three (3) to five (5) days.

mental health The overall health or well-being of the mind.

mental retardation Not a disease or a medical disorder or mental disorder. It is the manner in which an individual functions. Begins in childhood and limits an individual's level of intelligence and adaptive behavior skills (communication skills, activity of daily living skills, social skills, leisure, health and safety, self-direction, basic literacy skills [reading, writing, and math], community use, and work). An individual is considered to have mental retardation if the following three factors are present: the individual's IQ is approximately 70 or below, the individual is severely limited in two or more adaptive behavior skill areas, and the condition was present before the age of eighteen (18) years. (Based on the American Association on Mental Retardation).

mental status One's awareness of his surroundings, knowing who he is, where he is, and the date and time.

metabolism The chemical and physical changes continuously occurring in the body.

metastasis The spread of malignant cells to other areas of the body through lymph or blood vessels or by passing through the body cavities.

meter Measurement for length in the metric system.

metric system A system used when ordering and measuring medications.

microorganism A living thing, whether plant or animal, too small to be seen with the naked eye.

migraine The most common type of vascular headache.

minerals Inorganic substances that are essential to the function of all body cells.

minimum dose The smallest amount of medication that can be administered to an individual that will be effective.

minimum oxygen saturation level The minimum level of oxygen to be maintained in an individual's blood.

miotics Medications that work by contracting the pupil.

misappropriation of funds Unauthorized use of an individual's money or funds for individual use.

mistreatment Treating an individual wrongly or badly.

mixture A type of liquid medication; medications that have been mixed with a liquid but are not dissolved in it.

monthly quality review A monthly review of all medication orders.

mucous membranes The lining of the body cavities that open to the outside of the body.

multidisciplinary team A team of professionals and paraprofessionals who work together to provide care to an individual and his family.

multiple sclerosis A nervous disorder caused by a loss of myelin around central nervous system fibers.

muscle relaxants Medications that relax the muscles of the body; used to treat pain, muscle spasms, and other conditions affecting the muscles of the body.

muscle stimulants Medications used to treat the symptoms of progressive musculoskeletal disorders such as myasthenia gravis.

muscle spasms Involuntary contractions of one or more muscles, usually accompanied by pain and limited movement.

musculoskeletal system Made up of the skeleton, or the bony frame of the body, and of the muscles, or fibers and cells that produce movement.

mute The inability to speak because of a physical defect or emotional problem.

myalgia Muscle pain usually accompanied by a feeling of weakness, distress, or discomfort.

myasthenia gravis A progressive musculoskeletal disorder with symptoms of chronic fatigue and muscle weakness, especially in the face and throat. The onset is gradual with eventual extension to other muscles, including the respiratory system.

mydriasis Dilation of the pupils.

mydriatics Medication used to dilate the pupil.

myocardial infarction (MI) Heart attack.

myoclonic seizure A seizure consisting of rapid, brief contractions of muscles that occur at the same time on both sides of the body.

myopathy An abnormal condition of skeletal muscle with muscle weakness, wasting, and changes in the muscle tissue.

myopia Nearsightedness.

narcolepsy Uncontrolled attacks of drowsiness or sleep during the daytime.

nasal cannula A device used to deliver oxygen to an individual.

nasal medications Medications for the nose.

nasogastric (NG) tube A tube that is placed through the nose into the stomach; feedings, liquids, and medications are provided through the tube.

National Drug Code (NDC) numbers Numbers used to identify the manufacturer, the medication, and the size of the medication container.

national origin Country where an individual comes from.

navel Belly button.

nebulizer A machine that is used to administer a fine mist of liquid medication deep into the lungs.

neglect Failure to do what can be done or should be done.

negligence Failing to provide appropriate care or providing improper or inappropriate care that results in injury or harm, whether physical or emotional, to the individual being cared for; carelessness.

nephritis An inflammation of the kidney.

nervous system Controls and coordinates all body activities.

neuroleptics Antipsychotic medications.

neurons The cells of the nervous system; they conduct electrical charges.

nicotine A legal substance that is highly addictive, an ingredient in cigarettes and chewing tobacco.

NMDA receptor antagonist Medications used to treat Alzheimer's disease.

nocturia A condition of more frequent urination, especially at night.

nonepileptic seizure A seizure caused by a physical condition, emotional trauma, or psychological stress; not related to epilepsy.

nonparenteral medications Medications that enter the body through any route other than injection.

nonsteroidal anti-inflammatory medications (NSAIDs) Medications used to treat inflammation.

normalization A principle or concept that helps us to create an environment for individuals with developmental disabilities that is as close to normal as possible. It allows us to offer the individuals the same types of treatment and care as others of their own age. Focus is on the positive qualities and strengths of the individual rather than the negative qualities or weaknesses.

nostrils Openings of the nose.

numerals A part of an organized system for counting.

nutrients Food.

nystagmus Involuntary jerking movement of the eyes.

obesity An excess of fat in relation to lean body mass, with a body weight of 20% or more over ideal weight for height.

objective observation An observation made through the use of one's senses.

observation A fact that becomes known to an individual either through the use of her senses or by a report from the individual experiencing the problem.

ocular exposure Taking a substance into the body through the eyes.

oculogyric crisis Severe and repeated upward rolling of the eyeballs.

official name The name of the medication as it appears in the official reference, usually the same as the generic name.

ointment A type of topical medication.

Omnibus Budget Reconciliation Act of 1987 (OBRA) The law that regulates the education and certification of nursing assistants in long-term care facilities.

ophthalmic medications Medications for the eye.

opiates Medications used in the relief of moderate to severe pain; also called opiods.

opioids Medications used in the relief of moderate to severe pain; also called opiates.

opportunistic An organism that can only cause disease in a host whose resistance is already lowered by other diseases or medications.

oral By mouth.

oral suspension A thick liquid medication that has to be shaken well before it is poured and administered.

organ Performs specific activities that help the body to work as a whole.

orthostatic hypotension A drop in blood pressure after an individual sits up from lying down or stands up from a sitting position too quickly.

osteoarthritis A type of arthritis that affects the cartilage in between the bones that form the joint.

osteoporosis A disease involving the loss of bone thickness and deterioration of bone tissue. The result is an increase in fractures, especially of the hip, spine, and wrist.

otic medications Medications administered into the ear.

otitis media An infection of the middle ear.

otosclerosis A progressive form of deafness.

ototoxicity Damage to the eight cranial nerve and the organs of hearing and balance.

over-the-counter (OTC) medications Nonprescription medications bought and used without medical supervision.

oxygen An odorless, colorless, tasteless gas.

oxygen concentrator A type of oxygen administration equipment that provides low liter flows of oxygen.

pain An abnormal sensation that causes suffering or distress.

palliative use Medications used to promote the quality of life by relieving or soothing the symptoms of a disease or disorder without curing it.

pancreatitis An inflammation of the pancreas with symptoms including sudden severe abdominal pain, nausea, and fever.

pancytopenia A decrease in the number of white blood cells, platelets, and mature red blood cells in the bloodstream.

papules A solid, raised, red area on the skin.

paralysis The loss of the ability to move or feel.

paralytic ileus Bowel obstruction due to paralysis of the bowel wall.

parasympatholytics Medications that cause local bronchodilation.

parenteral medications Medications that are injected into the body.

paresthesias An abnormal sensation of crawling or burning of the skin.

Parkinson's disease A nervous disorder that causes tremors, muscle rigidity, and difficulty with voluntary movement.

partial seizure A type of seizure that is limited to a specific area of one side of the brain; may or may not cause loss of consciousness.

passive immunization Immunization occurs when a preformed antibody or antitoxin is given.

passive refusal The individual indirectly refuses to take the medication; for instance, the individual vomits his medication half an hour after taking it.

Patient Care Partnership: Understanding Expectations, Rights and Responsibilities A document developed by the American Hospital Association that describes the basic rights that a patient is entitled to while in the hospital or outpatient clinic.

PCP (phencyclidine) An illegal substance, a type of hallucinogen.

pedal pulse A pulse taken at the ankle/foot.

pediatric clients or patients Infants, children, and teenagers.

pediculicides Medications that treat scabies or lice.

pediculosis Head lice or nits.

perforated eardrum A hole in the eardrum.

peripheral neuropathies Permanent damage to the nerves, particularly in the hands, feet, and lower legs.

perioral dermatitis Inflammation of the skin in and/or around the mouth.

peristalsis The rhythmic, involuntary movement in the GI tract that moves food from the esophagus to the rectum.

peritonitis Inflammation of the lining of the abdominal wall.

petechiae Tiny purple or red spots appearing on the skin due to tiny hemorrhages under the skin.

pharmaceutical company A company that makes and sells medications.

pharmacist A licensed individual who prepares and dispenses medication according to the written instructions of a licensed health care provider.

pharmacodynamics The study of how drugs act on living things.

pharmacokinetics Deals with the study of the action of drugs within the body.

pharmacology The science dealing with the effects of drugs on living things.

pharmacy patient profile A system used in the pharmacy to document and track an individual's medications.

pharynx Throat.

phantom pain Is the result of an amputation. Pain is real, not imaginery.

photodynamic therapy (PDT) A treatment that uses medications, known as photosensitizing medications, along with light to kill cancer cells.

photophobia Sensitivity to light.

photosensitivity Sensitivity to the sun.

physical abuse Causing physical harm through hitting, pinching, slapping, biting, or by other inappropriate or improper physical contact.

physical addiction One or more of the body's functions becomes dependent on the presence of a drug; without it, the body experiences withdrawal symptoms.

physical dependence The body's cells actually have a need for a medication; symptoms of physical withdrawal occur when the medication is stopped.

phytochemical Any one of a hundred natural chemical substances found in plants.

platelet inhibitors Medications that stop platelets from sticking together to form clots.

pneumonia An infection of the lungs.

poison Any substance that can cause harmful effects in the body.

polyuria Frequent urination.

posting The first step in a two-step process in transcribing medication orders onto a medication sheet.

potentiation The action of two medications in which one medication prolongs or multiplies the effect of the other medication.

prescription A written order from the licensed health care provider to the pharmacist.

pressure ulcers Decubitus ulcers, bedsores.

preventive use The use of medications to prevent or lessen the severity of a disease.

prevocational programs Programs that prepare individuals to enter work programs.

probe The portion of the thermometer that goes into the individual's body.

proctoscopy Visual inspection of the rectum using an instrument called a proctoscope.

progress note A brief note written by the UAP that provides an explanation of an individual's condition.

prophylactic use The use of medications to prevent or lessen the severity of a disease.

proton pump inhibitors Medications that decrease secretion of gastric acid; used for short-term relief of GERD, confirmed gastric and duodenal ulcer, erosive esophagitis, and heartburn.

prn order An order for a medication to be given "as necessary" or "when needed."

protrusion Sticking out of the tongue.

pruritus Itching.

pseudoparkinsonism A collection of symptoms that mimics those of parkinsonism.

psychological abuse Causing mental harm by threatening, belittling, or by other means; also known as emotional abuse.

psychological addiction A mental or emotional craving for the effects produced by a substance; without it, there are no physical withdrawal symptoms.

psychological dependence An acquired psychological need for a medication.

psychotic behavior A significant distortion of reality that affects an individual's ability to function in daily life.

psychotropic Affecting the mind, behavior, and emotions.

psychotropic medications Medications that affect the function, behavior, or experience of the mind.

pulmonary medications Medications used to treat diseases of the respiratory tract; also called inhalant medications.

pulse The pressure of the blood against the wall of an artery as the heart beats.

pulse oximeter A device used to measure the amount of oxygen in the blood.

pulse oximetry A reliable method used to determine the amount of oxygen in the blood.

pulse rate The speed of an individual's pulse.

purpura Hemorrhage into the skin.

pyrosis Another name for heartburn.

radial pulse A pulse taken at the wrist.

radiating pain Pain that moves from place of origin to other places, for instance, chest pain moving to the arm or jaw.

radiation therapy A treatment that uses high-energy particles or waves to destroy or damage cancer cells.

rales Also called crackles; a moist respiration caused by fluid collecting in the air passages.

rate The number of respirations or heartbeats per minute.

rebound bronchospasm A spasm in the airways due to a response to overuse of an inhalant medication.

rebound hyperacidity A reaction in which the body produces even more stomach acid.

rebound nasal congestion A reaction to the overuse of a nasal spray or decongestant in which the nose becomes more congested.

rectal medications Medications administered directly into the rectum.

rectocele A hernia at the wall between the vagina and the rectum.

rectum The opening of the body that leads into the bowel.

regional hyperthermia Also called whole body hyperthermia; used along with other cancer treatments such as radiation therapy, chemotherapy, or immunotherapy. The temperature of the entire body or a part of the body is raised to higher-than-normal level.

regulations A set of guidelines and procedures that have the effect of laws.

remission The time when the symptoms of a disease are stable or absent.

remote action A term used to describe a medication affecting a part of the body that is away from the area where it is administered.

renal calculi Kidney stones.

replacement use The use of medications to replace substances that are normally found in the body.

reproductive system Produces reproductive cells and hormones that control sex characteristics.

Resident's Bill of Rights A document that states the rights of residents living in long-term care facilities.

respiration A body function that brings in oxygen and takes away or removes carbon dioxide.

respiratory system Brings in oxygen for the blood and removes a waste product, carbon dioxide, from it.

Respondeat Superior A legal doctrine that holds the employer or superior responsible for actions of its employees that are performed in the scope of employment.

retinal or macular degeneration A break-down of the retina inside the eye that causes loss of central vision.

rheumatoid arthritis A type of arthritis that affects the joint tissue and lining.

rhythm Regularity of pulse and breathing.

Roman numerals Examples are "I," "II," and III."

rosacea A chronic form of acne seen in adults of all ages, usually on the nose, forehead, and cheeks.

route The way the medication enters the body.

routine order A detailed medication order that must be followed regularly.

sanatorium A facility for the care of the chronically ill.

scabicides Medications that treat scabies.

scabies Body lice.

schedules The groups or levels of certain prescription medications that have the danger for addiction and abuse.

scope of function The legal limits within which the UAP may work.

scope of practice The legal limits within which one may work.

scored tablets Tablets whose surface has a groove or slit cut into them, making it easy for the tablet to be cut or broken into halves or quarters.

sedative A medication that calms, soothes, or quiets without causing sleep.

seizures Convulsions; physical changes in the body due to the disruption of the electrical charges in the brain.

selective action An action by a medication upon certain body tissues or on a specific body part.

senses Seeing, hearing, smell, taste, and feeling.

sexual abuse Use of physical, psychological, or verbal means to force an individual to perform sexual acts.

sexual orientation The preference of an individual to live a heterosexual (straight), homosexual (gay or lesbian), or bisexual lifestyle.

shallow A breath that only partially fills the lungs.

shearing An action in which the skin moves in one direction and the structures underneath move in the opposite direction.

shock A state in which the circulation of the body is disrupted and the blood pressure is dangerously low.

side effect An unwanted action or effect of a medication.

single order A medication order given for one-time use only.

sigmoidoscopy Visual inspection of the sigmoid colon using special instruments.

sleep apnea A period of time during sleep when respirations stop for ten (10) seconds or more.

smoking The act of smoking tobacco, accounts for 90% of all cancers, a leading cause of cardiovascular disease linked to cataracts, leukemia, and pneumonia. An adult who smokes dies, on average, fourteen (14) years earlier than an individual who does not smoke.

snorting The act of inhaling a substance into the nose where the substance is then directly absorbed into the blood stream through the nasal tissues.

solution A type of liquid medication; one or more medications dissolved in an appropriate liquid.

somnolence Drowsiness.

spansules Capsules made to release medication at a steady rate over a period of hours.

specific action A term used to describe a medication that has a particular effect on certain bacteria or other pathogens.

sphygmomanometer Equipment used to measure blood pressure.

spondylitis Inflammation of the vertebra.

spray A type of liquid medication used mainly to treat nose and throat conditions.

standing order A medication order or set of medication orders that are prewritten by the licensed health care provider (or group of licensed health care providers).

stat order An order for a medication that is to be given immediately.

status epilepticus A condition of nonstop seizure activity.

statute of limitations A set time period to bring a legal claim in court.

sterile Being free from bacteria.

sternum Breastbone.

stertorous Respirations that are similar to snoring.

stethoscope Equipment used to hear sounds produced by the body, for example, heart and lung sounds.

Stevens-Johnson syndrome A serious, sometimes fatal, inflammatory disease. Signs and symptoms include the sudden onset of fever, blisters on the skin, and ulcers on the mucous membranes of the lips, eyes, mouth, nose, and genitals.

stimulants Medications that increase actions in the body.

stomatitis Inflammation inside the mouth.

strength The measurement in which each unit of medication is available.

subjective observation An observation made through information reported by the individual experiencing the problem.

sublingual medications Medications administered under the tongue, where they dissolve and are absorbed into the body.

sublingual tablets Tablets that are dissolved under the tongue.

substance abuse The misuse of a legal or illegal substance enough to cause an individual mental, physical, social, or emotional harm.

supportive housing Offers disabled individuals ongoing levels of support so that they may live in their own apartments in the community.

suppository A form of semisolid medication that when placed into the rectum, vagina, or urethra dissolves and has an effect on the surrounding area.

suspension A type of liquid medication; medications that have been mixed with a liquid but are not dissolved in it.

sympathomimetics Medications that relieve spasms in the air passages of the lungs and increase the aeration of the lungs; strong bronchodilators with serious side effects.

symmetry Whether the chest expands equally on both sides as air enters the lungs.

syncope Fainting.

synergism The action of two medications working together in which one medication helps the other for an effect that neither one could produce alone.

syrup A type of liquid medication; medications mixed in a concentrated solution of sugar and water, then flavored with a substance.

system A group of organs organized to work together, for example, the respiratory system.

systemic action A term used to describe a medication that, once absorbed or injected into the bloodstream, is carried throughout the entire body, affecting all the cells.

systemic lupus erythematosis A chronic inflammatory disease affecting many systems of the body.

systemic radiation therapy Radioactive medications called radiopharmaceuticals are administered by mouth or by injection. The medication travels throughout the body to the cancer cells.

systolic blood pressure The pressure when the heart is pumping.

tablet A small, solid, compressed form of medication that is found in many sizes, shapes, and colors.

tachycardia A pulse of more than 100 beats per minute (bpm).

tachypnea Fast, shallow breathing; similar to panting.

tardive dyskinesia Involuntary movements of the face, trunk, and extremities that develop as a side effect of long-term use of neuroleptics.

targeted therapy A treatment that uses medications or other substances to recognize and attack only cancer cells.

telephone orders (TO) Orders that are told to the UAP over the telephone by the licensed health care provider.

temperature A measure of body heat; the balance between heat made and heat lost.

teratogenic effect Administration of certain medications to pregnant women that cause birth defects in newborns.

theft Stealing.

therapeutic dose The amount of medication needed to be effective or to produce the desired effect.

therapeutic range A guide to the licensed health care provider as to the amount of medication that should be in an individual's bloodstream.

therapeutic use The use of medications in the treatment of diseases.

thermal ablation Also called local hyperthermia; a small area of cancer cells are destroyed by very high temperatures.

thrombolytic medications Medications that work with an individual's body to dissolve clots.

thrombophlebitis Inflammation of the vein along with the formation of a clot.

thrombus A blood clot that has formed inside a blood vessel.

thyroid medications Medications used for replacement therapy and treatment after the thyroid gland has been surgically removed or the gland has undergone radiological treatment to destroy its cells.

timed-release medication A type of medication that contains particles of medication that have various coatings that differ in the amount of time needed before the coatings dissolve; this medication is made to deliver a dose of medication over an extended period of time. This medication cannot be crushed or chewed.

tincture A type of liquid medication; medications dissolved in alcohol or alcohol and water.

tinnitus Ringing in the ears.

tissue A collection of specialized cells that perform a particular activity in the body.

tolerance A condition in which the individual's body adjusts to the dose of a medication and a larger amount of the medication is needed to achieve the desired or wanted effect.

topical An external medication made for use on the skin.

topical medications Medications applied to and having effects on a local area of the body.

torticollis A muscle spasm of the neck in which the head is pulled to one side and turned so the chin is pointing to the other side of the body.

total joint replacement A joint is surgically removed and an artificial one is inserted.

toxic dose The amount of medication that causes signs and symptoms of poisoning.

toxicity A condition that results from exposure to a poison or to poisonous amounts of a substance.

trachea Windpipe.

tracheostomy A surgical opening in the trachea.

trade name The brand name of a medication.

transcribe To write down or to copy.

transdermal system A small adhesive patch or disk filled with medication that is applied directly to the body near the area to be treated.

transient ischemic attack (TIA) A temporary decrease in blood flow to the brain causing symptoms similar to a stroke; however, symptoms are temporary and reversible.

trismus Spasms in the jaw muscles.

troche A hard, circular or oblong piece of medication with a candylike base.

tuberous sclerosis A rare, genetic disease that causes benign tumors to grow in the brain and on other organs, such as the kidneys, heart, eyes, lungs, and skin; commonly affects the central nervous system and results in a combination of symptoms, including seizures, developmental delay, behavioral problems, skin abnormalities, and kidney disease.

tuberculosis (TB) A chronic infectious disease, mainly of the lungs; may be contagious.

tympanic thermometer Measures the heat given off by the tympanic membrane, or eardrum.

ulcer A lesion caused by loss of tissue, usually combined with inflammation; sores.

unit dose A premeasured amount of a medication, individually packaged on a single dose basis.

unit dose container A container that holds a single dose of medication.

Unlicensed Assistive Personnel (UAP) Unlicensed direct care staff working in health care or in the human service field.

urinary incontinence The involuntary release of urine.

urinary system Excretes liquid wastes, manages blood chemistry, and manages fluid balance in the body.

urinary tract infection An infection of one or more parts of the urinary system, most commonly caused by *Escherichia coli* (*E. coli*).

uticaria Hives.

vagina The opening of the body that leads to the cervix and uterus.

vaginal medications Medications administered directly into the vagina.

vaginal tablets Tablets that are placed into the vagina with an applicator.

vagus nerve stimulation (VNS therapy) A nondrug therapy used to treat epilepsy.

varicella zoster Chickenpox.

vasoconstrictors Medications that (1) constrict blood vessels and (2) increase blood pressure.

vasodilators Medications that (1) dilate (enlarge) blood vessels and (2) increase their ability to carry blood.

verbal abuse Use of communication to cause physical or mental harm.

verbal orders (VO) Orders that are given verbally to the staff by the licensed health care provider.

verifying The second step in a two-step process in transcribing medication orders onto a medication sheet.

vertigo A condition in which an individual feels like he is moving in space or feels that objects around him are moving.

vesicles Blisters.

virus A parasitic organism that may cause disease by invading normal cells.

vital signs Measurements of body functions that keep an individual alive; blood pressure, temperature, pulse, respirations.

vitamins Substances found in a variety of foods that are basic to good health.

volume Fullness of a pulse beat; for example, pulse may be "hard," striking the fingers, or "thready," "soft," like a thread under the fingers; also the depth of the respiration.

volume The amount of space occupied by a liquid.

vomitus The material vomited by an individual.

vulvovaginitis A type of vaginal infection caused by a fungus.

water-soluble vitamins Vitamins that are not stored in the body and that need to be replenished daily.

wax emulsifier Medication used to remove a buildup of wax from an individual's ear(s).

wheals Hives.

wheezing Dyspnea (labored breathing) with a sighing or whistling sound caused by a narrowing of the bronchioles in the lungs or by increased mucus in the bronchi.

whole body hyperthermia Also called regional hyperthermia; used along with other cancer treatments such as radiation therapy, chemotherapy, or immunotherpay. The temperature of the entire body or a part of the body is raised to a higher-than-normal level.

withdrawal An illness that causes flulike symptoms in an individual who is not given a substance to which he has a physical addiction.

written orders Orders that are written by the licensed health care provider.

xanthines Medications that cause bronchodilation; used for acute asthma attacks.

Index

Page numbers followed by *t* or *f* indicate tables or figures, respectively. Those followed by *n* indicate margin notes. Medications are in **boldface.**

Brainstem, 293*f*
Breach, 37*n*, 38
Brimonidine (Alphagan-P), 344*t*, 346
Bromocriptine (Parlodel), 409, 410*t*
Bronchi, 299
Bronchitis, 569*n*
Bronchodilators
    definition of, 261*n*
    description of, 60*t*, 577
    parasympatholytics, 62*t*, 579–581, 581*t*
    sympathomimetics, 577–579, 579*t*
"Bubble" packaging, 21, 119
Buccal medications
    description of, 145, 145*n*
    tablets, 55
Budesonide (Pulmicort, Rhinocort), 581*t*
Bulk-forming laxatives, 540, 540*t*
Bumetanide (Bumex), 596*t*
Bupivacaine hydrochloride (Marcaine hydrochloride), 397*t*
Bupropion (Wellbutrin, Wellbutrin-SR), 366*t*, 372–373, 588, 589*t*
Burn medications, 60*t*, 327*t*, 332
Bursa, 286
Buspirone (Buspar), 361*t*, 361–362
Butalbital/caffeine/ acetaminophen (Esgic, Fioricet), 389*t*
Butorphanol (Stadol), 387*t*

Calcitonin-salmon (Miacalcin), 563–565, 564*t*
Calcium, 310*t*
Calcium carbonate (Tums), 529*t*
Calcium channel blockers, 481–482, 490, 491*t*
Cancer
    antiangiogenesis for, 471
    chemotherapy for. *See* Chemotherapy
    description of, 461–462

    gene therapy for, 471
    hyperthermia for, 470
    immunotherapy for, 470, 470*n*
    photodynamic therapy for, 471
    radiation therapy for, 469, 469*n*
    surgery for, 469–470
    targeted therapy for, 471
Cannabinoids, 783, 784*t*
Capillaries, 279
Caplet, 55
Capsaicin, 313*t*
Capsule, 55, 56*f*
Captopril (Capoten), 490, 491*t*
Carbamazepine (Tegretol, Tegretol XR), 366*t*, 392*t*, 406*t*, 763, 764*t*
Carbamide peroxide (Debrox, Murine Ear Wax Removal System, Bausch & Lomb Wax Removal System), 350*t*
Carbenicillin (Geocillin), 432*t*
Carbidopa/levodopa (Sinemet), 408, 410*t*, 411
Carbonic anhydrase inhibitor diuretics, 599
Carbonic anhydrase inhibitors, 342–343, 344*t*
Cardiac arrest, 599
Cardiac glycosides, 60*t*, 476–479, 479*t*
Cardiac muscle, 277, 287, 289*f*
Cardiomyopathy, 475, 475*n*
Cardiovascular disease, 475, 475*n*
Cardiovascular medications
    antiarrhythmics. *See* **Antiarrhythmics**
    anticoagulants, 500–503, 503*t*
    antihypertensives. *See* **Antihypertensives**
    antilipidemics. *See* **Antilipidemics**
    cardiac glycosides, 476–479, 479*t*
    colony-stimulating factors, 504–505
    indications for, 476
    platelet inhibitors, 503*t*, 503–504, 686*t*
    thrombolytic medications, 504

    vasoconstrictors, 488
    vasodilators, 486–487, 488*t*
Cardiovascular system, 279*n*, 279*t*, 279–281
Carisoprodol (Soma), 552*t*
Carpopedal spasm, 377
Carvedilol (Coreg), 491*t*
Cascara sagrada, 540*t*
Case management, 8
Cataract, 294
Causation, 38*n*
Cavities, 277*n*, 277–278, 278*f*
Cefaclor (Ceclor), 428*t*
Cefadroxil (Duricef), 428*t*
Cefdinir (Omnicef), 428*t*
Cefixime (Suprax), 428*t*
Cefpodoxime (Vantin), 428*t*
Cefuroxime (Ceftin), 428*t*
Celecoxib (Celebrex), 556*t*, 557–558
Cells, 276, 276*n*
Central nervous system, 290
Cephalexin (Keflex), 428*t*
Cephalosporins, 426–427, 428*t*
Cerebellum, 293*f*
Cerebrovascular disease, 293
Cetirizine (Zyrtec), 571*t*
Chamomile, 313*t*
Charting
    description of, 644–645
    guidelines for, 645, 647, 649*t*
Checks, 114
Chemical name, 53, 53*n*
Chemotherapy
    antineoplastic medications used in, 462–465, 464*t*
    care of individuals receiving, 465–468
    definition of, 462, 462*n*
    infection risks during, 465–467
    nutritional needs during, 468
    self-care needs during, 467
    special considerations for, 468
Chewable tablets, 55
Cheyne-Stokes respirations, 738
Chickenpox, 441
Chlamydia, 298
Chloral hydrate (Aquachloral), 399, 400*t*
Chloramphenicol (AK-Chlor), 438*t*

Curative surgery, 470
Cushing's syndrome, 322n
Cyanosis, 424n
Cyclobenzaprine (Flexeril), 552t, 687t
Cyclopentolate (Cyclogyl), 348t
Cycloserine (Seromycin), 449t
Cystitis, 300, 593n
Cystocele, 298
Cystoscopy, 607n

Danazol (Danocrine), 617t
Dantrolene (Dantrium), 552t
Darbepoetin alfa (Aranesp), 504
ddC (Hivid), 446t
ddI (Videx), 446t
Debulking surgery, 470
Decongestants, 61t, 569–570, 571t, 687t
Decubitus ulcers, 285
Deinstitutionalization
    definition of, 5n
    history of, 5–6
    legal cases, 5
Delavirdine (Rescriptor), 446t
Delegation
    definition of, 10n
    of duties, 7–8, 10
    of medication
        administration, 11–12
    refusal of, 12–13
    rights of, 11–12
Demeclocycline hydrochloride (Declomycin), 435t
Dementia, 415
Demulcents, 61t, 320, 322t, 323
Dendrites, 290, 291f, 750, 751f
Dependence, 682
Depressants, 64, 783, 784t
Depression
    antidepressants for. *See*
        Antidepressants
    description of, 362–363
Dermal exposure, 701, 701n
Dermis, 285
Desipramine (Norpramin), 365t
Desloratadine (Clarinex), 571t
Dexamethasone, 342t
Dexamethasone (Decadron), 513t

Dextromethorphan (Benylin, Robitussin DM), 575t, 789t, 790
Diabetes mellitus
    antidiabetic medications for.
        See **Antidiabetics**
    definition of, 282, 282n, 513
    insulin-dependent, 513
    non–insulin-dependent, 513
    signs and symptoms of, 514t
Diagnostic surgery, 469
Dialose, 540t
Diaphoresis, 368
Diarrhea, 537
Diastolic blood pressure, 739, 739n
Diazepam (Valium, Diastat), 361t, 550, 552t, 685t, 760–762, 765t, 784t
Dibucaine (Nupercainal), 322t
Diclofenac (Voltaren, Voltaren XR), 556t
Didanosine (Videx), 446t
Dietary supplements, 312–315
Diffuse peritonitis, 236n
Digital thermometer, 730–732
Digitalis, 477–478, 478t
Dilantin, 250, 254
Diltiazem (Cardizem), 490, 491t
Dimenhydrinate (Dramamine), 541t
Diphenhydramine (Benadryl, Caladryl), 322t, 571t, 575t, 686t
Diphenoxylate/atropine (Lomotil), 530t, 538–539
Dipivefrin (Propine), 344t
Dipyridamole (Persantine), 503t, 686t
Dipyridamole/aspirin (Aggrenox), 503t
Discontinuing of medication, 666–667, 771–772
Discrimination, 36, 36n
Disease-modifying antirheumatic medications, 61t, 558–560, 560t
Disinfectants, 329n, 329–330, 331t
Disopyramide (Norpace), 482–483, 686t

Disposal of medications
    documentation of, 124, 128f
    federal guidelines for, 124, 125f–127f
    reasons for, 122, 124
    rules of, 124, 125f–127f
Disposal record, 76, 76n, 86–87, 87f
Distribution, 684, 684n
Diuresis, 593n
Diuretics
    carbonic anhydrase inhibitor, 599
    definition of, 593n
    description of, 61t
    loop, 595–597, 596t
    osmotic, 596t, 599
    physiologic effects of, 593
    potassium-sparing, 596t, 597–599
    thiazide, 593–595, 596t
Divalproex sodium, 763
Diversion, 41, 41n
Divided dose, 66
Documentation
    computerized medical records, 649t
    continuous positive airway pressure, 201
    disposal of medications, 124, 128f
    enema administration, 216–217
    EpiPen Auto-Injector, 268
    gastrostomy tube
        care, 240
        flushing, 243
    incentive spirometer, 199
    incorrect completion of, 689
    jejunostomy tube
        care, 240
        flushing, 243
    medication administration, 113–114
    on medication sheet, 663–665
    overview of, 644–645
    principles of, 655
    pulse oximetry, 184
    residual feeding, 245–246
    tube feedings, 237
Dolasetron (Anzemet), 541t
Donepezil (Aricept), 417, 418t

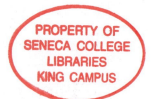